Textbook of

Traumatic Brain Injury

Textbook of
Traumatic Brain Injury

Editors

AK Mahapatra MS MCh DNB MAMS FNASc
Professor and Head
Department of Neurosurgery
All India Institute of Medical Sciences
New Delhi, India

Ex-Director
Sanjay Gandhi Postgraduate Institute of Medical Sciences
Lucknow, Uttar Pradesh, India

Raj Kumar MS MCh FASET FRCS MRCS MAMS MNASc
Professor and Head
Department of Neurosurgery
Chief
Trauma Center
Sanjay Gandhi Postgraduate Institute of Medical Sciences
Lucknow, Uttar Pradesh, India

Raj Kamal MS MCh
Former Assistant Professor
Department of Neurosurgery
All India Institute of Medical Sciences
New Delhi, India

Foreword

DK Gupta

JAYPEE BROTHERS MEDICAL PUBLISHERS (P) LTD

New Delhi • Panama City • London

Jaypee Brothers Medical Publishers (P) Ltd.

Headquarter

Jaypee Brothers Medical Publishers (P) Ltd
4838/24, Ansari Road, Daryaganj
New Delhi 110 002, India
Phone: +91-11-43574357
Fax: +91-11-43574314
Email: jaypee@jaypeebrothers.com

Overseas Offices

J.P. Medical Ltd.
83 Victoria Street London
SW1H 0HW (UK)
Phone: +44-2031708910
Fax: +02-03-0086180
Email: info@jpmedpub.com

Jaypee-Highlights Medical Publishers Inc.
City of Knowledge, Bld. 237, Clayton
Panama City, Panama
Phone: +507-301-0496
Fax: +507-301-0499
Email: cservice@jphmedical.com

Website: www.jaypeebrothers.com
Website: www.jaypeedigital.com

Inquiries for bulk sales may be solicited at: jaypee@jaypeebrothers.com

Textbook of Traumatic Brain Injury

First Edition: 2012

ISBN 978-93-80704-76-0

Printed at: Ajanta Offset & Packagings Ltd., New Delhi

Dedicated to

Our Respected Parents

and

Teachers

Head injury does not mean clot in brain, nor clot in brain means an operation, nor operation means cure.

— AK Mahapatra

- Raj Kumar

— Raj Kamal

Contributors

A Jindal MCh
Former Assistant Professor
Department of Neurosurgery
All India Institute of Medical Sciences
New Delhi, India

Abrar Ahad Wani MS, MCh
Associate Professor
Soch Kral Memorial College of
Education, Kashmir
Jammu and Kashmir, India

Aditya Gupta MBBS MCh
Associate Professor
Department of Neurosurgery
All India Institute of Medical Sciences
New Delhi, India

AK Mahapatra MS MCh DNB
MAMS FNASc
Professor and Head
Department of Neurosurgery
All India Institute of Medical Sciences
New Delhi, India

Ex-Director
Sanjay Gandhi Postgraduate Institute of
Medical Sciences, Lucknow
Uttar Pradesh, India

Arun Kumar Singh MS MCh
Professor and Head
Department of Plastic Surgery
Chhatrapati Sahuji Maharaj Medical
University, Lucknow
Uttar Pradesh, India

Arun Kumar Srivastava MS MCh
Assistant Professor
Department of Neurosurgery
Sanjay Gandhi Postgraduate Institute of
Medical Sciences, Lucknow
Uttar Pradesh, India

Chitra Sarkar MD
Professor
Department of Pathology
All India Institute of Medical Sciences
New Delhi, India

Deepak Agarwal MS MCh
Assistant Professor
Department of Neurosurgery
All India Institute of Medical Sciences
New Delhi, India

Devi Prasad Mohapatra MCh
Specialist of Plastic Surgery
Department of Plastic Surgery
Chhatrapati Sahuji Maharaj Medical
University, Lucknow
Uttar Pradesh, India

MC Sharma MD
Associate Professor
Department of Pathology
All India Institute of Medical Sciences
New Delhi, India

P Sarat Chandra MBBS MCh
Additional Professor
Assistant Professor
Department of Neurosurgery
All India Institute of Medical Sciences
New Delhi, India

PK Gupta MS MCh FRCS
Consultant
Department of Neurosurgery
Bahrain

Priyanka Kawal PhD Scholar
Senior Research Fellow
Department of Neurosurgery
Sanjay Gandhi Postgraduate Institute of
Medical Sciences, Lucknow
Uttar Pradesh, India

Raj Kamal MS MCh
Former Assistant Professor
Department of Neurosurgery
All India Institute of Medical Sciences
New Delhi, India

Raj Kumar MS MCh FASET FRCS MRCS
MAMS MNASc
Professor and Head
Department of Neurosurgery
Sanjay Gandhi Postgraduate Institute of
Medical Sciences, Lucknow
Uttar Pradesh, India

RR Sharma MS MCh
Consultant
Department of Neurosurgery
Khoula Hospital
Muscat
Sultanate of Oman

RV Devadas MCh
Specialist
Department of Neurosurgery
Khoula Hospital
Muscat
Sultanate of Oman

Sanjay Pawar MS MCh
Junior Specialist
Department of Neurosurgery
Khoula Hospital
Muscat
Sultanate of Oman

SD Lal MS MCh
Consultant
Department of Neurosurgery
Khoula Hospital
Muscat
Sultanate of Oman
All India Institute of Medical Sciences
New Delhi, India

Foreword

Textbook of Traumatic Brain Injury published by Professors AK Mahapatra, Raj Kumar and Raj Kamal is not just another book in the field of Neurosurgery. The book deals with various chapters, dealing with the practical management of the patients presenting with various types of head injuries. The book is a ready-reference not only for the specialists but also to the general surgeons, the postgraduate students and all others engaged in treating children and adults with head trauma.

Trauma is a major problem not only in the developed world but also in developing countries and head injury tops it all; contributing for about 10% of the five million deaths occurring each year globally due to various kinds of injuries. In India, over 270 individuals are killed in various road-traffic accidents each day and over, 5,000 individuals suffer from long-term disabilities.

Presently, there are very few specialized trauma centers in the country; however, due to a recent awakening; many trauma centers even with postgraduate teaching and training programs are being established throughout the length and breadth of this country. Once established, there would be large need for the intensivists, researchers, general surgeons, neurosurgeons and paramedical staff tuned to handle the emergency services with promptness, compassion and care.

The contributors are very eminent and highly competent neurosurgeons of national and international fame. They have many decades of experience to back them. This is reflected very well in the book. The chapters have been written in a simple language with a clear flow of thought. The book clearly emphasizes the importance of preventive strategies at the regional and national levels including the three-tier-system of trauma management promoted by the Government of India. The book also carries the much-needed recent information in improving the outcome of the roadside accident victims.

This textbook will certainly contribute to the better understanding and management of patients with head injuries. I am sure that the book would prove very handy to the undergraduate and postgraduate students as well as to the specialists equally. The book is a welcome addition to all departmental and institutional libraries as well as being a personal asset to all the neuroscientists.

DK Gupta MS MCh FAMS FRCS (Edins Glas) DSc (HC)
Vice Chancellor
Chhatrapati Sahuji Maharaj Medical University
(Formerly KG Medical University)
Lucknow, Uttar Pradesh, India

Preface

Injuries claim approximately 5 million lives every year worldwide. India with its 1.25 billion population has a large share of this. Two hundred and seventy people are killed every day in India following road-traffic accidents and about 1000 people sustain permanent injuries every day. Surprisingly, there is a limited exposure to medical students during undergraduate teaching. This is by and large due to lack of neurosurgery departments and teachers. Similarly, the situation is not much different in the postgraduate courses in general surgery. Even today, many neurosurgical centers do not treat head and spinal injury patients, as a policy and send their MCh and DNB students to another neurosurgical centers for a few months training. This has raised a big question about the quality of head injury care.

Currently, there are more than 1,200 neurosurgeons in India and with over 75% working in the large cities; hence there is very little scope of having neurosurgery department in many peripheral medical colleges. In years to come, we expect head injuries to be managed by general surgeons. Realizing India's vast population and area, it is impossible to think of a neurosurgeon in each district hospital. Hence, our aim should be to provide MBBS and MS (General Surgery) students adequate exposure and skills to manage neurological injuries, though we do not expect them to operate. At this stage, it is important to realize that 90% head injuries are minor and where patient may not require either neurosurgical intervention or ICU care. What they really need is primary care, skilled observation and assurance for confidence building. Doctors and paramedics should also be trained to prehospital care including transport of severely injured patients.

With these considerations in mind, 56 chapters in the book include all important academic and clinical aspects involved in management of head injury. Some important aspects like fluid and electrolytes management which are usually overlooked. This is especially important as a large number of severely head injury patients develop metabolic and electrolyte disturbances requiring meticulous management. Endocrine problems not only occur in severely injured patients, minor head-injured patients with short- and long-term effects, adversely affect the outcome. Infective complications, like meningitis and brain abscess, are not uncommon and require special mention. Coagulopathies also in head injury patients play an important role in the management of head injuries. Rare aspects, like post-traumatic basal ganglia hematoma, traumatic cerebellar hematoma, dural sinus thrombosis, CSF otorrhea and skull base fractures, facial injuries and atlantoaxial injuries, are also included to complete the list of complications of neurosurgical trauma.

The book has been written in such a manner that it will benefit young trainee neurosurgeons, trauma experts, medical students, teachers and also academicians practicing in the area of head injury and its management. It will give some important insight to researchers in the area of genetic and molecular aspects of head injury.

AK Mahapatra
Raj Kumar
Raj Kamal

Contents

Abbreviations

A

AAMVAs – American Association of Motor Vehicle Administrators
AANS – American Association of Neurological Surgeons
ABGs – Arterial Blood Gases
ACA – Anterior Central Artery
ADH – Antidiuretic Hormone
AMPA – (2-amino-3-(5-methyl-3-oxo-1, 2-oxazol-4-yl) propanoic acid)
ANP – Atrial Natriuretic Peptide
APV – Anterior Posterior View
APP – Amyloid Precursor Protein
APTT – Activated Partial Thromboplastin Time
ARDS – Adult Respiratory Distress Syndrome
ATLS – Acute Trauma Life Support
$AVDO_2$ – Arteriovenous Desaturation of Oxygen
AVM – Arteriovenous Malformation

B

BAEP – Brainstem Auditory Evoked Potential
BBB – Blood-brain Barrier
BISIG – Brain Injury Interdisciplinary Special Interest Group
BNP – Brain Natriuretic Peptide
BSH – Brainstem Hematoma

C

CNG – Compressed Natural Gas
CBF – Cerebral Blood Flow
CCF – Caroticocavernous Fistula
CCT – Central Conduction Time
CG – Ciliary Ganglion
$CMRO_2$ – Cerebral Metabolism Rate of Oxygen
COAD – Chronic Obstructive Airway Disease
CPP – Cerebral Perfusion Pressure
CS – Cavernous Sinus
CSF – Cerebrospinal Fluid
CSWS – Cerebral Salt Wasting Syndrome
CT – Computed Tomography
CVP – Central Venous Pressure
CVR – Cerebral Vascular Resistance

D

DAI – Diffuse Axonal Injury
DCS – Dorsal Column Stimulation
DI – Diabetes Insipidus
DIC – Disseminated Intravascular Coagulation
DNA – Deoxyribonucleic Acid
DSA – Digital Subtraction Angiography
DSI – Day Since Injury
DTPA – Diethylene Triamine Pentaacetic Acid

E

EM – Excitatory Amino Acid
EACA – Epsilon Aminocaproic Acid
ECA – External Carotid Artery Special Interest Group
ECD – Ethylene Cytosine Dimer
ECF – Extracellular Fluid
EDH – Extradural Hematoma
EEG – Electroencephalography
EO – Evidence of
EP – Evoked Potential
EVD – External Ventricular Drainage

F

FDP – Fibrin Degradation Product
FFA – Free Fatty Acid
FFP – Fresh Frozen Plasma
FIB – Fibrinogen Assay
FSH – Follicular Stimulating Hormone
FV – Flow Velocity

G

GH – Growth Hormone
GABA – Gamma Aminobutyric Acid
GCS – Glasgow Coma Scale
GOS – Glasgow Outcome Scale

GR – Good Recovery
GnRH – Gonadotropin Releasing Hormone

I

ICF – Intracellular Fluid
ICH – Intracerebral Hematoma
ICP – Intracranial Pressure
ICU – Intensive Care Unit
IIT – Insulin Tolerance Test
IVH – Intraventricular Hemorrhage

L

LED – Light Emitting Diode
LGB – Lateral Geniculate Body
LP – Lumbar Puncture

M

MAP – Mean Arterial Pressure
MCA – Middle Cerebral Artery
MCTC – Metrizamide Computed Tomograpy Cisternography
MD – Mild Disability
MLF – Medial Longitudinal Fasciculus
MOFS – Multiple Organ Failure Syndrome
MP – Methylprednisolone
MRC – Medical Research Council
MRI – Magnetic Resonance Imaging

N

NHDS – National Hospital Discharged Survey
NIH – National Institute of Health
NMDA – N-Methyl-D-Aspartate
NOS – Nitric Oxide Synthetase
NSI – Neurological Society of India

P

PCA – Posterior Cerebral Artery
PCS – Post-concussion Syndrome
PDS – Paroxysmal Depolarization Shift
PEEP – Positive End-expiratory Pressure
PET – Positron Emission Tomography
PFEH – Posterior Fossa Extradural Hematoma
PGD – Prostaglandin
PI – Pulsatility Index
PT – Prothrombin Time
PTA – Post-traumatic Amnesia
PTE – Post-traumatic Epilepsy
PTH – Post-traumatic Hydrocephalus
PTN – Pretectal Nucleus
PTT – Partial Thromboplastin Time
PVS – Persistent Vegetative State

R

RBC – Red Blood Corpuscle
REM – Resting Metabolic Expenditure
RIA – Radioimmune Assay
RN – Red Nucleus

S

SAH – Subarachnoid Hemorrhage
SD – Severe Disability
SDH – Subdural Hematoma
SEPs – Sensory Evoked Potentials
SIADH – Syndrome of Inappropriate ADH Secretion
SO – Suggestive of
SOV – Superior Ophthalmic Vein
SPECT – Single Photon Emission Computed Tomography
SSS – Superior Sagittal Sinus

T

TBGH – Traumatic Basal Ganglia Hematoma
TBI – Traumatic Brain Injury
TCD – Transcranial Doppler
TPN – Total Parenteral Nutrition
TCDB – Traumatic Coma Data Bank
TCT – Thrombin Clotting Time
TDAI – Traumatic Diffuse Axonal Injury
THAM – Tris-hydroxymethyl aminomethane
TIA – Transient Ischemic Attack
TPFL – Traumatic Posterior Fossa Lesion
TSH – Thyroid Stimulating Hormone

V

VOC – Voltage Operated Channel
VOR – Vestibulo-ocular Reflex
VP – Ventriculoperitoneal

W

WHO – World Health Organization

1 Introduction

AK Mahapatra

Head injury continues to be a nightmare, not only for the public but also for the neurosurgeon, because of high morbidity and mortality. Study published in Journal of Neurotrauma June 2001, which was a leading article from International Neurotrauma Conference, concluded that no change in last 30 years in mortality or morbidity of severe head injury. Unfortunately, incidence of head injury is rapidly increasing in the world, especially in developing countries including India. While in US, Australia or in Japan head injury incidence has fallen significantly. Loss of young people at their productive age, is a great financial loss for family as well as for the country. In India, problem has become more acute over last two decades, basically due to increased vehicular traffic and poor maintenance of the road. The number of head injuries are expected to increase further, due to urbanization, industrialization and increase in vehicular population.

Head injury defines an injury to the head and brain. Hence, injury to head which does not involve the brain, is not considered as head injury. It is not unusual for a neurosurgeons to get a call for treating a head injured patient from casualty, which turn out to be a simple case of scalp laceration or scalp hematoma. It means the people who send a calls to neurosurgeons do not even know, what is head injury. This occurs at small as well as large hospitals like AIIMS. It indicates, how casual is our approach towards diagnosis of head injury, a condition, which not only all doctors should know, but even general public must know. Hence, when a doctor is confronted with a situation, he must know, if the patient he is dealing with has or has not suffered from head injury.

Head injury is a neurosurgical problem, and operation if required, should be performed by a neurosurgeon. However, the question then remains, is it practically possible that every head injury can be seen, diagnosed and treated by neurosurgeon? This has been possible in US, Japan and many other countries where the trained personnels are available. In 3rd world countries it is not possible due to lack of facilities. For example, India with more than 1250 million people have over 1200 neurosurgeons.[1,2] Mostly, the neurosurgeons are available in metropolis or Govt. Medical College-based cities. Even today large number of our medical colleges do not have neurosurgical facilities. Hence, where is the question of district or subdivisional hospitals having the facility. Similarly in Nepal, for 30 million people there are only 6 to 8 neurosurgeons as compared to Japan, where for 130 million people there are over 6000 neurosurgeons. While in Oman there are 10 neurosurgeons for 2 million population. This means, in India and other developing countries, head injury has to be primarily managed by general surgeons, with a adequate (6 months to 1 year) training in head injury management.[5]

I remember my undergraduate days, when no one taught us anything about head injury. When a severe head injury patient got admitted in the general surgical wards in coma, we used to inform patient's relatives poor prognosis and 0 percent chance of survival.[1] The scenario is changed in large cities with improved educational standard and medical facilities. Whereas conditions are more or less same in small towns. It is not out of place to mention that 35 years have passed since I completed my MBBS. The medical college still does not have a neurosurgeon. The entire city, with a population of one million lacks a neurosurgeon. This is the ground reality in many medical colleges in India.

In Delhi, over 2200 people died due to road accidents in 1997[1] also in 2000 and over 15000 had nonfatal head injury and the number is increasing. Recently, over 2 to 3 years the incidence of head injury has fallen in Delhi 10 percent every year. This is basically because, strict implementation of helmet, seat belt, and banning of old vehicle to operate in Delhi road. Introduction of CNG uses has also helped in reduction of accidents. What is surprising, however, in many large cities like Bangalore, Chennai, Ahmedabad, Lucknow, Kanpur, Pune and Trivandrum, etc. helmet is not still compulsory for two wheeler driver.

Large number of young people die, which does not evoke much reaction except occasional photos and write up in newspapers. School bus accidents have rocked India in last few years and there were several incidents in Delhi. People react, discuss for few days then forget, till another school bus disaster takes place. Our authorities and public have become immune to elicit any response. Unfortunately, a death occurring outside India gets much more attention and publicity, like Raman Lamba's case, who died in Dhaka due to cricket ball injury or Indian people dieing in Australia. There was a great deal of reaction by the press people. While similar incidences occurring in India does not gets any attention. I must tell, I have seen and managed many cricket ball injuries to head, including major and minor. I have operated patients with clot following cricket ball injury. Unfortunately,

I have also seen many children, who became blind following the head injury by a cricket ball.

A Study to see the trends in head injury mortality among 0 to 14 years in Scotland revealed that the children residing in less affluent areas seems to be at relatively greater risk of sustaining fatal head injury than their affluent counterpart.[10] It means that the affluency and availability of health services at a reasonable distance also have bearing in the outcome of head injury.

All above emphasize the concern and need for proper management of head injury. Hence, it is important for all medical graduates and even public to have some knowledge of head injuries. Most important among that is, how to define head injury? As I have mentioned a head injury is synonymus with brain injury and the telltale evidence of head injury is loss of consciousness. Even if patient does not loose consciousness, he or she must have altered consciousness, it means patient is not fully conscious and oriented. Sometimes, it may be difficult to know whether a patient had really lost consciousness or not. If a patient developed memory loss for the events following the injury it is 100 percent certain that the patient had lost consciousness. The period following injury when a patient fails to register the events, despite of being conscious and alert, is called post-traumatic amnesia (PTA). Thus, PTA is a sure shot evidence of head injury. After having defined head injury it is worth at this stage to classify head injury. Head injury by and large is classified as: (a) minor, (b) moderate, and (c) severe. In a simple way one can say, head injury is minor, **when loss of consciousness is for less than 30 minutes, it is moderate, if the duration of unconsciousness is between 30 minutes and 6 hours**. If the duration of unconsciousness is longer than 6 hours, head injury is categorized as severe (Tables 1.1A and B). Fortunately 80 percent head injuries are minor.[6] However, I must state here is that "No head injury is minor enough to be neglected nor severe enough to be given up", Each head injury must be treated according to its own merit. I have personally seen large number of patients, whom the neurosurgeons had written off, they not only survived but also become alright. Sadly enough, this situation is rare, nevertheless, few examples only remind us to do our best, even if a patient is bad and carries a small chance of survival.[11,12]

Large number of factors determine the outcome in a head injury patients. Age, sex, severity of injury, intracranial pathology (Figs 1.1A to D), intracranial pressure and associated injuries are few significant prognostic factors (Fig. 1.2). Recently, genetic basis of head injury outcome is reported. Presence of Apolipoprotein E4 alleles is recognized as a poor prognostic factor. Patients who are homozygous or heterozygous for APO E4 allele have 14 times greater likelyhood of having poor outcome.[7-10]

All above facts emphasis a sound theoretical and practical knowledge on head injury management. There is a tremendous degree of nonuniformity in management of head injury, not only between general surgeons and neurosurgeons, but also the difference is apparent between neurosurgeons, depending on experience, availability of facilities and even between nonpracticing and practicing neurosurgeons.

Table 1.1A: Classification of head injury

	Duration of unconsciousness	*GCS (Glasgow coma scale)*
1. Minor or mild head injury	Less than 30 minutes	
2. Moderate head injury	More than 30 minutes and less than 6 hours	
3. Severe head injury	More than 6 hours	8 or less

Table 1.1B: Head injury classification

1. **Simple:** When there is no communication to outside. Hence, no CSF leak or brain matter coming out from scalp wound. No CSF rhinorrhea or otorrhea
2. **Compound:** (a) Open compound, (b) Closed compound
   a. *Open compound:* This head injury means, brain is exposed to outside through scalp wound and skull fracture
   b. *Closed compound:* When there is CSF rhinorrhea, CSF otorrhea and X-ray skull or CT scan head shows intracranial air

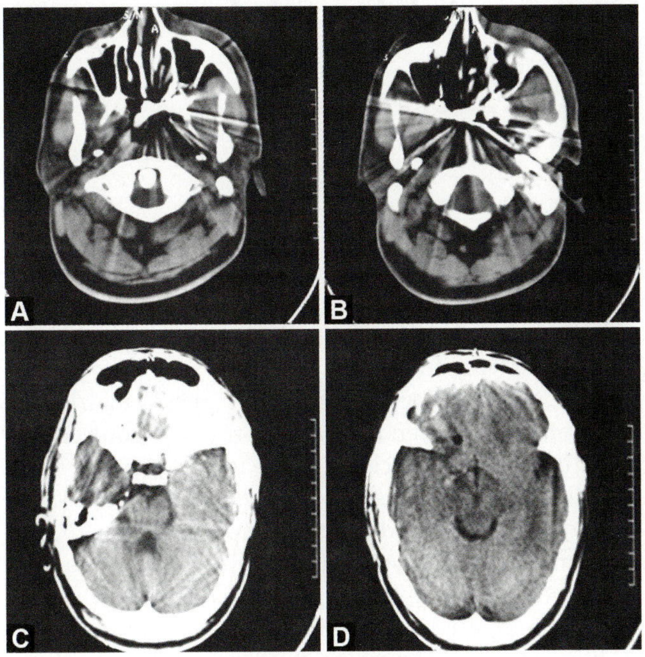

Figs 1.1A to D: CT skull base cut showing a bullet in the region of left optic canal and maxilla

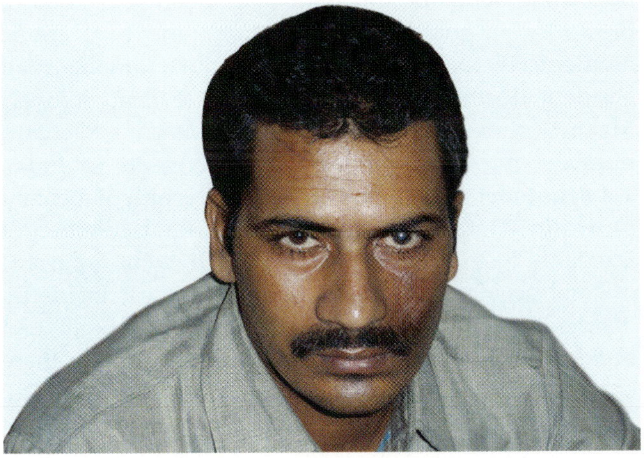

Fig. 1.2: Clinical photograph of patient with bullet injury showing opacity of left lense and dilated pupil

Considering all above points, the American Association of Neurological Surgeons (AANS) and Neurotrauma Subcommittee of Neurological Society of India (NSI), decided to develop guidelines for management of head injuries, with an aim to evolve uniform policy in management of head injury,[3,4] which is important both from medical, legal and ethical point of view. In India, so far head injury is a neglected fields, and has not attracted the attention of public or authority.

Overall, with tremendous increase in number of head injury, the management of head injury has gained an important place today. There are only a few books written on head injury by Indian authors. Hence, we visualized the need for a comprehensive books on head injury, which would provide overall knowledge on head injury, However, I must confess that, head injury is a vast subject and there is growing literature on various aspects of head injury. From this point of view no book can provide everything on the subject, however, having said that and knowing fully our limitations, we have made a venture to bring out this book only to provide our students and trainee an adequate knowledge on head injury management.

REFERENCES

1. Mahapatra AK. Management of Head Injury. Neurosciences Today 1997;2:197-204.
2. Bagchi AK. An Introduction to Head Injury. Calcutta, Oxford University Press 1980.
3. Guidelines for the management of "Severe Head Injury" a joint initiative, the Brain Trauma Foundation. The AANS and the joint section of Neurotrauma and Critical Care 1996.
4. Ramani PS, Mahapatra AK. Basic Manual for the Management of Head and Spinal injury, Published by Neurotraumatology Committee (NSI) Nirman Associate Mumbai 1996.
5. Head injuries—a neglected field in India. Editorial National Medical Journal of India (NMJI) 1991;4:53-64.
6. Kunter KC, Evlanger Dun, Tsai J, et al. Lower Cognitive performance of older football players positive for apolipoprotein E Epsilon 4 Neurosurg 2001;47:651-7.
7. Jordan BD, Relkin NR, Ravdin LD, et al. Apolipoprotein E Epsilon 4 associated with chronic traumatic brain injury in Boxing. JAMA 1997;278:136-40.
8. Friedman G, Froom P, Suzbon L, et al. Apolipoprotein E Epsilon 4 genotype predict poor outcome in Survivors & Traumatic brain injury. Neurology 1999;15:244-8.
9. MaC Farlane DP, Nicoll JA, Smith C, et al. APOE epsilony allele and amyloid beta protein deposition in long-term survivors of head injury. Neuroreport 1999;10:3945-8.
10. Williamson LM, Morrison A, Stone DH. Trends in head injury mortality among 0-14 year's olds in Scotland. J. of Epedemiol and comm. Health 2002;56:285-8.
11. Mahapatra AK, Tandon PN, Bhatia R, Banerji AK. Bilateral decerebration in head injury patients—an analysis of 62 cases. Surg Neurol 1985;25:536-40.
12. Sausa J, Sharma RR, Mahapatra AK, Lad SD. Bilateral dilated pupils in pediatric patients following severe head injury. Long-term outcome. Pan Arab J Neurosurg 2002;6:39-46.

2 Epidemiology of Head Injury

AK Mahapatra

INTRODUCTION

Head injury is an important public health problem today. In terms of the number of cases and the number of deaths, head injury is one of the front runner. Moreover, severe head injury is a great challenge to neurosurgeons and basic neuroscientists, as the mortality and morbidity is depressingly high and there is a great deal of efforts required to get marginally improved results. There are only few epidemiological studies[1-7] (Table 2.1). From India, the incidences are basically from metropolis, and based on medicolegal reports which may not be absolutely correct.[8-11]

Boys and children residing in relatively less affluent areas have highest head injury mortality rates. Pedestrian accidents are the leading cause of mortality.[31]

The incidence of head injury per 100,000 population per year ranges from 56 to 430.[2-7] The incidence varies in urban and rural population. The overall incidence in US is around 200 per 100,000 per year.[1] Fife et al 1986[7] reported the lowest incidence 152/100,000 population, on the contrary, Field 1976[2] reported an incidence as high as 430/100,000 population. Detailed epidemiological studies are done from small county like San Diego and Wales.[2,5,7] Some of the epidemiological studies are hospital based.[6] In India, the studies are either from traffic police records or from the hospitals.[10,12,13] Nearly 1.6 million people per year suffered from head injury in US.[24,28,29] In Spain incidence of head injury 91/100,000 as reported in 1988. However, report from China recorded a lowest incidence of 56 per 100,000 person per year in 1986.[27]

Table 2.1: Incidence of brain injury, selected reports

Authors	*Years*	*Study from*	*Rate per 100,000*
1. Jennett and MacMillan	1981	UK	270
2. Klauber et al	1981	San Diego, USA	294
3. Selecki et al	1981	New South Wales and Australia	377
4. Kraus et al	1984	San Diego, USA	180
5. Edna and Cappelen	1984	Norway	200
6. Fife et al	1986	Rhode Island	152
7. Wang et al	1996	China	56

An epidemiological study of head injuries in the population attending an emergency showed the head injury attendance accounts for 3.4 percent of all attendances per year. An overall rate of 453 per 100,000 was found for all head injuries, of which 40 per 100,000 were moderate to severe (10.9%). Urban residents have greater risk of presenting with moderate to severe injuries compared with residents of mixed/rural areas. A high attendance rate of moderate to severe head injuries (MSHIs) was found in the $<$ 5-year-old age group in urban areas of both sexes.[30]

In India, the incidence of head injury is steadily increasing with urbanization and increasing number of vehicular population.[10,13] Among the road traffic accidents 70 percent have head injury, among road accident deaths 70 percent are due to head injury.[12] Majority of deaths occur during first 72 hours. Recently, number of fatal accidents have increased in India. Total number of vehicles in India are only 1 percent of world's total vehicles, however, total number of accidents in India as reported in 1991 were 6 percent of total accidents,[9] thus, making it highest incidence of accident rate in the world. Currently annual road accidents in India is over 600,000. Every minute there is an accident and every eighth minute there is a death. In 1987[14] New York Times reported that fatality rate in India for 10,000 vehicles is 55, which was that time reported to be highest in the world. Today, I suppose the things have gone worse than what it was 10 years back. The incidence in Delhi has steadily increased (Table 2.2), however, over last 3 to 4 years incidence of head injury has shown a decline approximately 10 percent each year. Indian statistic as reported over a 12 years from 1980 to 1992, showed unacceptably high accidents and deaths.[10] Baker et al 1986 reported over 8 percent of total deaths in US were due to injury.[15] Approximately in US each year, 50,000 die from head injuries.[25,26] However, from the hospital statistic there is a 50 percent fall of head injury admission in 2002 compared to 1980.

Table 2.2: Road accidents and fatal accidents in Delhi

Year	No. of non-fatal accidents	No. of deaths
1991	6414	1651
1992	6878	1626
1993	6815	1686
1994	7260	1790
1995	7216	2003
1996	11315	2286
1997	15584	2176
2000	8439	1919
2001	8113	1778
2002	6800	1660
2009	15000	2250
2010 Till 30 June	7000	960

The number of accidents are directly proportional to number of vehicles on the road. At the time of independence the total vehicles in India were 300,000 and in 1995 the number increased by 270,00,000. In Delhi alone the vehicle has increased tremendously. The motor vehicle registration in Delhi, shows 500 registrations per day and number of vehicles has reached almost 6 million in 2009, as compared to 5 lakhs in 1980 (The Times of India, Feb. 2010). The statistics, as reported has shown a tremendous growth (Table 2.3), which shows increased number of vehicles, increased accidents and deaths. However, it is interesting to note number of accidents per 1000 vehicles in 1970 was 80 as compared to 14.7 in 1990. This shows the incidence of injury is decreased per 10,000 vehicles. However, the figure 14.7/1000 vehicle is very high as compared to other countries.[12] Table 2.4 shows the number of accidents per 1000 vehicles in India was 2.5 times more compared to US, however, the number of deaths were 10 times more. Thus, showing much higher mortality in India.

Table 2.3: Some Indian statistics

Parameters	Years 1970	1980	1990
	(Numbers in thousands)		
1. Number of accidents	114	153	282
2. Number of injured	70	109	224
3. Number of dead	14	24	54
4. Number of accidents per 1000 vehicles	80.3	33.8	14.7
5. Total number of vehicles	1401	4514	19177

Table 2.4: Number of accidents and deaths per 1000 vehicles in various countries

Country	Accidents per 1000 vehicles	Deaths per 1000 vehicles
Australia	3.1	0.39
Brazil	1.3	0.34
France	8.7	0.40
Japan	9.8	0.20
UK	14.0	0.52
USA	12.2	0.25
India	31.8	2.5

TYPES OF INJURY

Roughly 5 to 10 percent of injuries are fatal (Tables 2.3 and 2.4). Kraus et al 1984[7] reported 30 deaths per 100,000 population from San Diego. In India, over 60,000 people died due to road accidents every year. Fortunately, 75 to 80 percent[1,6,8] head injuries are minor or moderate. The proportion of severe head injury increases with age. The incidence of severe head injury is much lower in children. Besse in 1980[16] reported that 90 percent of head injuries in children were minor. National Hospital Discharged Survey (NHDS) of USA in 1985 showed 50 percent of all head injury discharged from the hospital were patients with concussion. The data from US reported an overall mortality 20 to 30 per 100,000 population. Several studies from USA (San Diego, Minnesota, Chicago) reported 63 to 86 percent head injury in San Diego to be mild. Kraus et al 1984[7] reported 91 percent of all head injury in San Diego were mild or moderate head injuries, while the figure from Central Virginia was 75 percent.[1] The variation can be due to the admission practice for head injury person. Hence, hospital-based data can be falacious.

Kalyanaraman 1971[17] reported head injury death to be the common cause of death in Madras General Hospital. Over 120,000 people die in India every year due to road accidents. Thus, head injury has acquired a major health hazard in most cities of India today.[10-14] In Delhi alone over 2200 deadhs occuted in 2009. Report from most cities and states of India show a rising trend (Table 2.5).[32,33]

ETIOLOGY OF HEAD INJURY AND AGE INCIDENCES

Head injury is most frequent in young people between 20 to 40 years. Around 60 to 70 percent head injury occurs in human beings in thirties and forties of their life. In India 40 percent population belongs to pediatric

Table 2.5: Death in five cities in India—2005

	City	% of all head injury
1.	Delhi	1717
2.	Chennai	1055
3.	Bangalore	835
4.	Mumbai	787
5.	Kanpur	598

Table 2.6: Incidence of head injury in different age groups in India

Age group	% of all head injury
Children below 20 years	30
Young/adults 20-40 years	60
Elderly above 60 years	10

age group and around 25 to 27 percent of all head injury victims are children under 16 years of age.[18,19] Studies from different county of USA showed peak incidence of head injury in 3rd decades and head injury rate ranged from 300 to 600/100,000 populationl. Not surprisingly, the incidence of head injury is lowest in extremes of age, below five years and above 60 years, and the rate is around 125 to 150/100,000 population (Table 2.6).[1,22,23]

The most common cause of head injury is the road accidents.[1,5,7,10,12,13] However, in the children fall is the most frequent cause.[20] Overall, 60 percent of injuries are due to road accidents and 25 to 30 percent of all injuries are due to fall.[1] In neonates, birth trauma is the most frequent cause.[1] However, etiology of head injury in pediatric age group vary considerably.[19,20] The pediatric population divided into: (a) below 3 years, (b) 3 to 9 years, and (c) 10 to 16 years. Among the children, more frequently involved group is the children between 3 and 10 years.[20] Older children are susceptible to bicycle injury, which contributed to around 10 percent of all head injury in children.[20,22,23]

GENDER AND HEAD INJURY

Overall head injury is less common in females.[1,20] The rate of accidents are related to driving and activities outside the house. Six of the eight US studies reported male to female ratio of incidence of head injury 3:2. Males had higher incidence of head injury as compared to females in all age group except infants and elderly patients above 65 years of age. Study from US showed peak incidence for male reaching 600 to 700/100,000 population around 15 to 25 years of age,[1] while in female the peak incidence of injury was in 15 to 25 years of age group, however, the rate of injury was even less than 50 percent than that of corresponding age group in males (500-700 in males vs 150 to 250 in females/100,000 population). In the children, boys outnumber girls in incidence in head injury and incidence is 1:1. 6 to 1.9 in different age groups.[20]

Table 2.7: Reasons for increasing number of accidents in India

A. Problems in Roads
- a. Poor design of roads
- b. Lack of safety measures
- c. Poor lighting
- d. Poor maintenance
- e. Lack of bilane system

B. Problems in Vehicles
- a. Poor standards of vehicles
- b. Lack of proper break system
- c. Lack of seat belt
- d. Running of other non-motorised vehicles like bicycle, cycle-rickshaw, bullock cart, camel cart, etc.

C. Problems in Driving and Drivers
- a. Inadequate training
- b. Easy availability of driving licence
- c. Not following traffic rules
- d. Poor visual acuity
- e. Consumption of drug and alcohol

REASONS FOR ROAD ACCIDENTS IN INDIA

There are large number of causes which lead to road accidents in India (Table 2.7). It is encouraging to know that the number of road accidents are reducing in developed countries. This is due to improved highway engineering leading to well-designed roads, improvisation and innovations by the automobile engineering leading to manufacturing of good vehicles with large number of safety measures. Most importantly, public awareness of prevention of accidents play an important role. Few obvious among them are use of helmets, seat belt, knowledge of traffic rules, and the long-term implications of severe accidents. Sadly, in India, above factors are not operating due to various reasons, most important among them is apathy by people and authorities.[9,10,14]

Among 43000 km long national highway, only 1 percent road in India is according to international standard. In US, highways are considered the safest in the world and there is 1 death per each 160 million kilometer driven. In India, there are 6 deaths per everyone million kilometers driven. Thus, number of deaths in India are (160 × 6) 960 times more frequent than US. Poor design of roads, inadequate maintenance, poorly maintained vehicle with no safety facilities, apathy by authorities and above all poorly trained drivers are by and large the cause of accidents in India. Moreover, poor vision, old age, intoxicated driver also play important role in India. Adequate management of all above factors can reduce the number of accidents in India.

FINANCIAL IMPLICATION OF HEAD INJURY

Head injury involves young people in their productive part of their life. Loss of life and rehabilitation of severely disabled victims costs a lot of money and incurs a significant economic burden to the country. One of the WHO report mentioned 3.5 million deaths all over the world in a year, due to injury, among them 700,000 were due to road accidents. The same report mentioned, 1.5 million injured people required medical care. Nakajima in 1993,[21] reported 5000 billion US dollars being the medical bills and rehabilitation cost. This is a tremendous financial loss due to accidents.

In India and other developing countries increasing accidents not only results in loss of young life, but also damage to the family and financial burden. Currently number of deaths due to road accidents alone in India is over 60,000 and large number of deaths do occur due to various other injuries. Hence, it will not be an exaggeration if I say total number of deaths are around 100,000 in India, every year. Several years back, Ramamurthi,[12] quoted Rs. 350 crore financial loss per year, due to accidents. Presently, the figure must be higher.

CONCLUSION

Epidemiological studies show increasing incidence of head injury in developing countries. In India, incidence of head injury is much higher as compared to US, UK or Japan.

Children constitute 25 to 30 percent of all head injury victims. Mortality and morbidity due to head injury is high and cost over 5000 billion US dollar as medical bills and rehabilitation cost.

Prevention of head injury should be the aim and this can be achieved by improving the road condition, education of people and providing more safety measure in motorized vehicles.

REFERENCES

1. Kraus JF. Epidemiology: In NINS. Head Injury Clinical Management and Research Elizabeth Frost (Eds) AIREN-Geneva, Switzerland ISSN-1012-9871,1990:113-24.
2. Field JH. Epidemiology of Head Injury in England and Wales. Department of Health and Social Security. Her Majesty's stationery office, London 1976.
3. Jennett B, MacMillan R. Epidemiology of head injury. Br Med J 1982;182:101.
4. Selecki BR, Ring IT, Simson DA, et al. Injuries to head, spine and peripheral nerves. Report on a study. The Neurological Society of Australia and Health Commission of New South Wales 1981.
5. Klauber MR, Marshall LF, Barrett CE, Bowers SA. Epidemiology of head injury a prospective study of an entire community; San Diego County. Arne J Epidemiol 1981;9:236.
6. Edna TH, Cappelen J. Hospital admitted head injury: A prospective study in Tromdelag, Norway, 1979-80. Scan J. Sco Med 1984;12:7.
7. Kraus JF, Black MA, Hessol L, et al. The incidence of acute brain injury and serious impairment in defined population. Am J Epidemiol 1986;119:186.
8. Fife D, Faich G, Hollinshead W, et al. Incidence and outcome of hospital treated head injury in Rhode Island. Am J Public Health 1986;76:773.
9. Editorial: Head injuries: A neglected field in India. National Medical Journal 1991;4:44-53.
10. Report of Road Safety Cell: Ministry of Transport. Govt. of India 1993.
11. Sambasivan M. Epidemiology of Neurotraumic. Neurology India 1993;3(suppl):41.
12. Ramamurthi B. Road accidents, Epidemiology and Prevention. Neurology India 1995;(Suppl)43:9-15.
13. Mahapatra AK. Current management of head injury. Neuroscience Today 1997;1:197-204.
14. New York Times, 26th October 1986. Quoted In: Progress in clinical Neurosciences 1987;360.
15. Becker DP, Povlishock JT. Central Nervous System Trauma Status Report 1985. National Institute of Health and Communicative Disorders and Stroke, National Institute of Health, Bethesda, Md 1986.
16. Besse MD. Pediatric head injuries. Observations in pediatric surgery. 1019 cases, Anaesth Analg (Paris) 1980;37:181-5.
17. Kalyanaraman S. Organization of a head injury services. Ann Ind Aca Med, Sci 1971;7:1.
18. Mahapatra AK. Monitoring on pediatric head injury patients. Neurology India 1995;(Suppl):43:64-7.
19. Sambasivan M. Epidemiology Paediatric head injuries. Neurology India 1995;(Suppl)43:57-8.

20. Reverdin A. Head injury in children. In: NINS. Head injury, Clinical Management and Research. Elizabeth Frost (Eds), Airen Publisher, Geneva, Switzerland 1990; 193-204.
21. Nakajima H. Speech on World Health day 1993.
22. Mahapatra AK. Head injury a global Scenario. Asian Archivee of Anaesthesiology and Resuscitation 2002; 555-62.
23. Mahapatra AK, Jaiswal A. Epidemiology of Head Injury Neuroscience Today 2003;7:29-32.
24. Olson D. Head injury. E Medicine 2002.
25. Thurman DJ, Alverson C, Dunn KA, et al. Traumatic brain injury in the United States. A public health perspective. J Trauma Rehabil 1999;14:602-15.
26. Wagner AK, Sassere HC, Hammond PM, et al. International traumatic brain injury: Epidemiology, risk factors, and associated with Severity and Mortility. J Trauma 2000;49:404-10.
27. Wang CC, Schoenberg BS, Li SC, et al. Brain injury due to head trauma. Epidemiology in urban areas of People's Republic of China. Arch Neurol 1986;43:570-2.
28. Guerreo JL, Thurman DJ, Snievek JE. Emergency department visits associated with traumatic brain injury. US 1995-1996. Brain Injury 2000;14:181-6.
29. Thurman D, Guerrero J. Trends in hospitalization associated with traumatic brain injury. JAMA 1999;282:954-7.
30. Yates PJ, William WH, Harris A, et al. An epidemiological study of head injuries in UK population attending an emergency department: J Neurology, Neurosurgery and Psych 2006;77:699-701.
31. Williamson LM, Morrison A, Stone DH. Trends in head injury mortality among 0-14 years old in Scotland. J of epidemiol, and comm. Health in 2002;56:285-8.
32. Times of India (Delhi). No accused in 33% fatal mishaps 18th July 2010;2.
33. Times of India (Lucknow). Roads converted to killing mines, 29 Jan 2009.

3 Biomechanics of Head Injury

Raj Kamal, Raj Kumar

The mechanical forces directed to the head that results in the multitude of head injuries observed clinically is necessary for planning prevention strategies. The mechanical forces can be classified (Fig. 3.1) as static or dynamic in nature.[1] Dynamic loading is more common and is defined as input force applied to the cranium in very short-time usually less than 50 ms. Static loading is uncommon and is defined as input force applied to the load slowly in period greater than 200 ms. Typical examples of static loading are slowly moving vehicles, earthquakes that trap the head against rigid structures resulting in slow crushing of skull. Static loading will cause multiple comminuted fractures of vault or base of skull (Figs 3.2 and 3.3). Severe neurological deficits are uncommon and will be present only if the brain is distorted or compressed directly because of the static loading.

Impulsive and impact loading are two subtypes of dynamic loading. Impact loading is common type of dynamic loading usually a combination of contact forces and inertial forces. The quick impact force causes head to accelerate. In certain situation inertial effects are minimized when the head is immobilized following impact. Effects on intracranial structures and skull differ when head is allowed to accelerate or not in particular situation. The response of the skull to impact depends on the position of head and the object that strikes the head. For objects larger than 2 sq inch, local skull deformation of the skull immediately beneath the point of impact. This skull deformity will result in skull fracture if it exceeds the tolerance of skull.

Impulsive loading occurs when the head is set gap into motion or when the moving head arrested without its being struck or impacted. In impulsive loading there is no direct impact on the head hence no contact forces occur. The resulting head injuries are caused only by the inertial forces. A blow to the thorax or face can set head into violent motion without direct impact to the skull, e.g. fall from height or being thrown off a moving vehicle.

The primary injury to the brain occurs through two major mechanisms: Direct injuries due to skull distortion (contact injuries) and indirect that arise irrespective of skull deformation.[2,3]

Contact injuries and inertial injuries can explain most head injuries.

CONTACT INJURIES

Contact injuries result from the forces that occur during direct impact. The direct impact results in complex

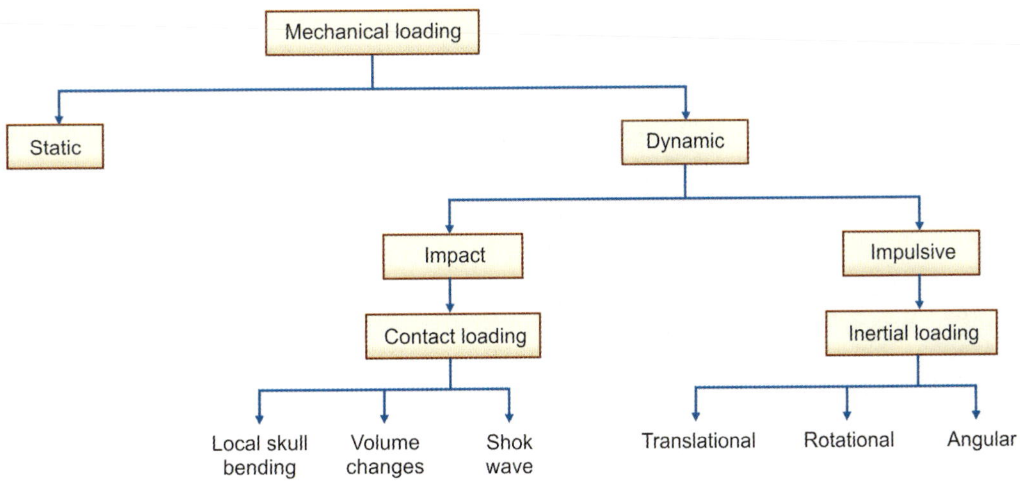

Fig. 3.1: Classification of the types of mechanical loading

mechanical events that occur both near and distant from the point of contact (Contact phenomenon).

Contact injuries typically causes focal injuries, they do not cause diffuse brain injury. Neural damage by this mechanism, therefore, is typically superficial and localized to the immediate vicinity of skull injury.[2,3] Since most impact set the head into motion, these injuries are associated with acceleration injuries. Contact forces have local and remote effects.

LOCAL EFFECTS

Effects of local contact include depressed fractures, linear fractures, basilar skull fractures, extradural hematoma and coup contusions.

Depressed skull fractures are the result of concentrated force immediately beneath the impacting object. The area of hitting object is small enough to cause concentration of stress and strain (Fig. 3.4). The momentum of object is bore by the localized area of skull and not to the remaining skull as in linear fractures. The momentum may be strong enough to penetrate completely through the skull.

Linear skull fractures[2] follows local skull bending occurring at the site of impact which exceeds the strain limit for the bone. The bone bends inwards like a cone and it breaks at inner table which forms the apex of cone. The inner table breaks first because of greater tensile strain on the inner table (Fig. 3.4).

Forces and strains, is weaker to the tensile forces on the inner table. The fracture tends to follow the path of least resistance and splits into components thus dissipating the energy into fracture. The linear fracture is complete when the energy in the impact process is dissipated completely.

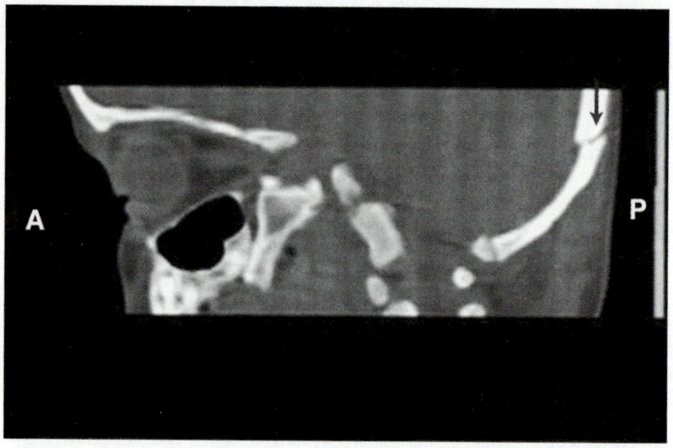

Fig. 3.3: CT shows fracture of occipital squama, basiocciput and clivus in a small child, atlantoaxial complex is intact

The direct impact to **mastoid** and **occiput** can produce basilar skull fractures in similar manner. A strong impact on facial bones can also result in basilar skull fracture (Figs 3.2 and 3.3).

Local bending of skull bones due to direct impact can lead to tear of dural vessels and injury to brain or pial vessels with or without fracture resulting in epidural hematoma and coup contusions.

High-negative pressure develops when the inbent skull rapidly snaps back to its normal position which puts brain and pial vessels to a very high-degree of tensile strain. This high-strain can lead to disruption of pial vessels and cortical vessels resulting in localized contusion of brain.

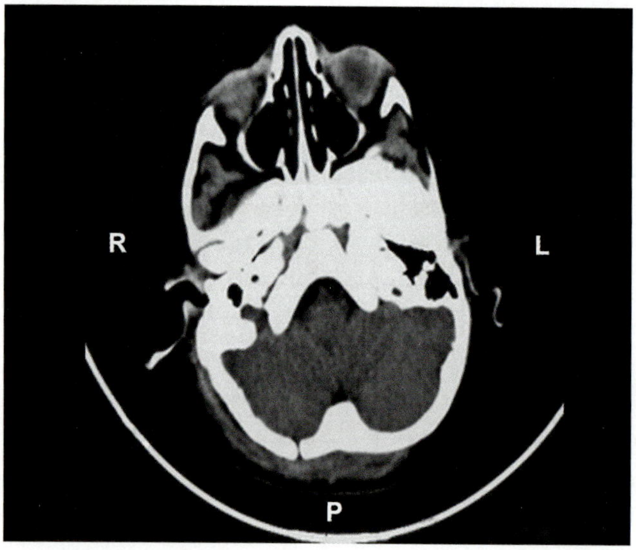

Fig. 3.2: CT shows fracture of right occipital squama

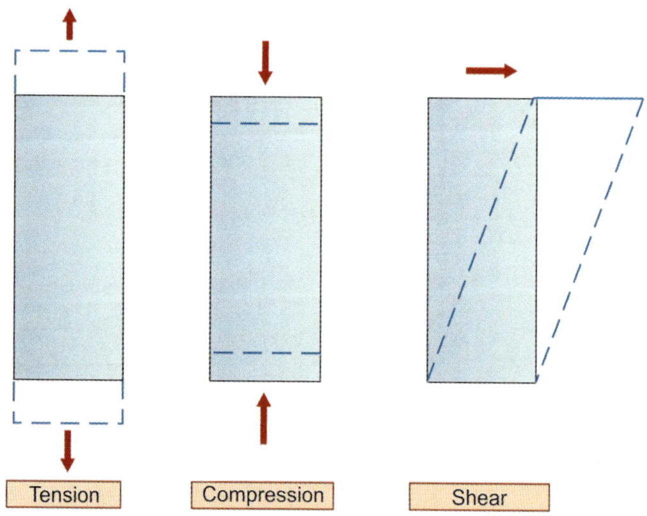

Fig. 3.4: Types of strains. Strain is the amount of deformation that tissue can undergo as a result of mechanical force

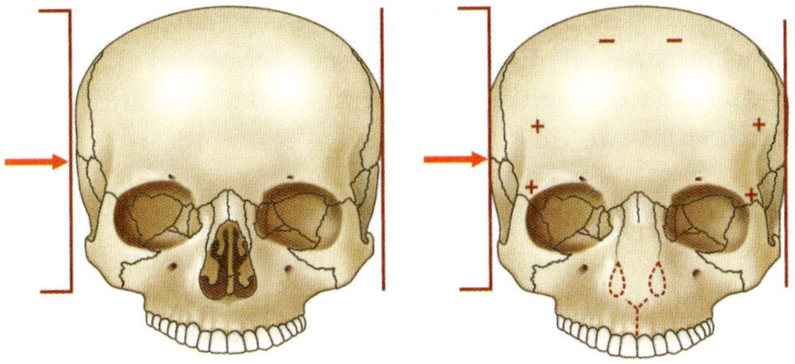

Fig. 3.5: Impact loading with no head motion. Note high-pressure at the impact site and negative-pressure at outward bending site

REMOTE CONTACT EFFECTS

Remote contact effects are the result of skull distortion and stress waves. If the impacting object is broad and the impact occurs over a thick portion of the skull, then the remote thinner position of skull will bend due to decreased tensile strength resulting in remote linear fracture.

Large broad impacts can lead to localized pressure changes and intracranial volume fluctuations. These changes are transient because of inherent elastic properties of the skull. Above mentioned events produce negative pressure at places where the skull has been pulled away from the brain (Fig. 3.5) which may result in contrecoup contusion. A sudden change in ICP can lead to brain herniations, e.g. tentorial herniation. The intracranial volume changes may explain part of distinct neurological and pathological observations found in infants and children with developing skulls that maintain a fair degree of flexibility.

Stress waves also account for the remote contact effects. Stress waves originate at the point of impact travelling at very high-speed in all directions producing remote vault fractures, basilar fractures, potential hemorrhages and intracerebral hematomas.

INERTIAL INJURIES

These are commonly called acceleration and deceleration injuries. The acceleration of the head causes either a functional or structural failure of neural and vascular structures, where the severity and extent of disruption are linked to magnitude, rate, duration and type of inertial loadings.[5]

Head motion will cause structural or functional damage by relative movement of brain in relation to dura and skull. Bridging vein's may tear if the strain exceeds the vascular tolerance. The relative movement of brain away from skull creates tensile strain causing contrecoup contusions.[6]

The head motion can produce strain in the brain parenchyma itself causing cerebral concussion, diffuse axonal injury, deep petechial hemorrhages.[6]

Three types of acceleration may occur (Figs 3.6A to C):

(1) Translational acceleration occurs when the brain moves in a straight line at its center of gravity, i.e. pineal gland, (2) Rotational acceleration occurs when brain tissue moves around its static center of gravity, (3) Angular acceleration occurs when there is movement of the center of gravity in an angular manner. Angular acceleration is combination of both translational and rotational acceleration.

Angular acceleration is most commonly encountered clinically. The center of angulation is usually mid-cervical to lower cervical region. Higher the center of angulation greater will be the rotational component. As the center of gravity becomes lower in cervical spine, proportionately translational component increases.

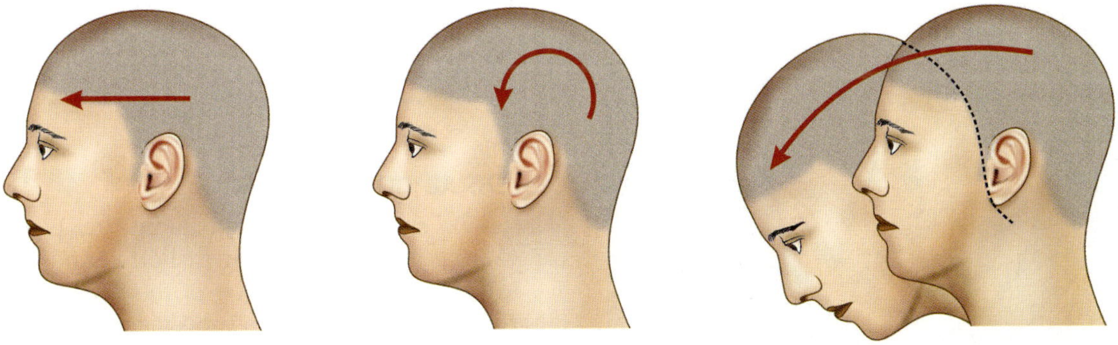

A, Translational

B, Rotational

C, Angular

Figs 3.6A to C: Types of acceleration

Angular acceleration is most injurious and the severity depends on the amount of acceleration, its rate and duration. Angular acceleration or deceleration causes shear strain deformation, which is characterized by a change in shape without change in volume.[2-4] Shear strain forces are maximum at the junction of tissues of different density and rigidity. Shear strain develops because of differential movement of one portion of brain with respect to another portion. Neurons are highly susceptible to the shear strain forces.

Three zones (surface, intermediate, deep) of interest are encountered as acceleration duration increases at a constant acceleration.[6] At short acceleration duration, brain experiences very little strain resulting in only surface zone injury.

At longer acceleration duration, inertial effects are maximum and the resulting strains are able to propagate deeper into the brain. This can cause deep diffuse axonal injury. Intermediate zone injury occurs with acceleration duration is intermediate. Strain rate also increases if the acceleration magnitude is increased resulting in vascular tissue intolerance.

Hence, structural damage to superficial vascular tissue (bridging veins and pial vessels) occurs in short acceleration duration with large acceleration magnitude whereas brain tissue injury occurs in longer duration and lesser acceleration magnitude.

MECHANISM OF INJURIES

Skull fractures, epidural hematoma coup contusion (Fig. 3.7). These are the result of contact injuries. In infants and children, sutural diastasis may occur. The mechanisms of linear fracture, depressed fracture, basilar skull fractures, epidural hematoma and coup contusions are described above.

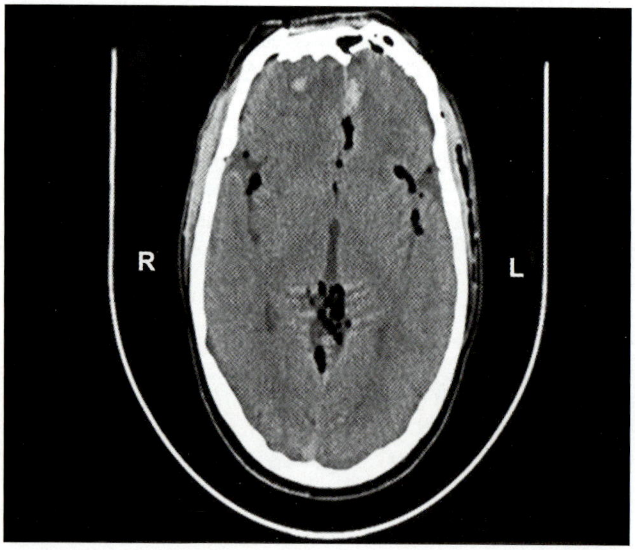

Fig. 3.7: CT shows multiple intracranial air pockets with basifrontal contusions following right frontal fracture in the region of frontal sinus

Contrecoup Contusions

The predominant mechanisms for contrecoup contusions is head acceleration (inertial effects). For contrecoup contusions impact is not necessary, hence the term is misnomer. In situations where the head undergoes impulsive loading, contrecoup lesions occur solely because of acceleration effects.[7]

A hard, small impact surface such as hammer blow tends to produce depressed fracture with underlying coup contusion with no contrecoup contusion. But, if the object has larger impact surface following fall then it results in a very little focal injury, more energy is converted into setting the head into motion, thus producing large contrecoup contusions.

INTRACEREBRAL HEMATOMA

Intracerebral hematomas are usually associated with extensive cortical contusion in which larger and deeper vessels have been disrupted. Smaller hematomas that are not associated with contusion occurs because of stress waves concentration due to impact or acceleration induced tissue strains. Small deep hemorrhagic tensions are due to areas of strain concentration due to acceleration effects.

SUBDURAL HEMATOMA

Acute subdural hematoma is due to disruption of surface vessels, usually bridging veins. Disruption of bridging vein occurs mostly from inertial and not from contact forces.

Subdural hematoma (SDH) results from head acceleration that produce short duration, high strain ratio loading.[8] Hence, subdural hematomas are usually associated with diffuse axonal injury (DAl). This explains those cases where SDH is small but associated brain damage is great.

CEREBRAL CONCUSSION

Concussion refers to an immediate but transient loss of consciousness associated with a short-period of amnesia. It occurs after deceleration of the frontal or occipital areas that creates sudden movement of brain within skull. Angular or rotational head motions cause transient electrophysiologic dysfunction of reticular activating system (RAS) in the upper midbrain, caused by rotation of the cerebral hemispheres on a relatively fixed brainstem.

In this type of injury, most of the strain is insufficient to cause structural damage but biochemical and ultrastructural changes such as mitochondrial ATP depletion and local disruption of the blood-brain barrier may occur. The physiological basis of amnesia is not yet clear.

DIFFUSE AXONAL INJURY

Diffuse axonal injury (DAI) considered to be severe form of concussion injury. Diffuse axonal injury is caused by angular acceleration or rotational acceleration. The extent of axonal damage depends upon magnitude, duration and rate of angular acceleration.[9] The extension of focal neuronal damage is centripetal from the cortex inward to the brainstem as the injury force increases. Almost all cases of severe DAI arise from vehicular accident in which acceleration is long. The direction of acceleration is important in the production of axonal injury. Sagittal acceleration only occasionally produces DAI of grade I. Angular acceleration is coronal plane has a high-incidence of severe form of DAI.

DELAYED EFFECT

Soldiers returning home from Iraq are experiencing an increased number of head injuries related to blasts and explosions compared to soldiers of previous conflicts. These injuries are often undetected until the soldiers return home and have difficulty functioning as they did prior to the war. It is therefore important for occupational workers and researchers to understand more about the blast injury, its pathophysiology, methods for detecting traumatic brain injury, and how these patients can be treated.[10]

CONCLUSION

The mechanical forces causing head injury can be classified into dynamic and static in nature. If the input force is applied to the cranium in short-time (less than 50 ms) then it is called dynamic loading. Dynamic loading is further subclassified into impact loading and impulsive loading. Direct impact results in contact injuries. Contact injuries cause skull fractures, extradural hematomas and coup contusions. Both impulsive and impact loading will result in acceleration injuries. Acceleration injuries are of three types: (i) Translational, (ii) Rotational, (iii) Angular. Acceleration produces different magnitude of strain in brain depending upon its rate and duration. Cerebral concussion, diffuse axonal injury and acute subdural hematoma are typical examples that occur following acceleration injuries.

REFERENCES

1. Gennarelli TA, Meaney DF. Cranial Trauma, Neurosurgery (Ed). Wilkins RH, Rengachary SS, Mc Graw Hill, 1996;2611-22.
2. Holbourn AHS. Mechanics of Head Injuries. Lancet 1943;2:438-41.
3. Holbourn AHS. The Mechanics of Brain Injuries. Br Med Bull 1945;3:147-9.
4. Rowbotham GF. The mechanism of injuries to the head. In: Rowbotham GF (Ed). Acute injuries of the head. 4th edn. Edinburg and London E & S. Livingstone 1964; 56-92.
5. Adams JH, Gennarelli TA, Graham DI. Brain damage in nonmissile head injury: Observation in man and subhuman primates. In: Smith W, Cavanal JB (Eds). Recent advances in Neuropathology, Edin: Churchill Livingstone 1982;165-90.
6. Gennarelli TA. Head injury in man and experimental animals: Clinical aspects. Acta Neurochir (Wien) [Suppl] 1983;32:1-13.
7. Ommaya AK, et al. Coup and contrecoup injury observations on the mechanics of visible brain injuries in the rhesus monkeys. J Neurosurg 1971;35:503.
8. Gennarelli TA, Thibault LE. Biomechanics of acute subdural haematoma, J Trauma 1982;22:680-6.
9. Adams JH, Graham DI, et al. Diffuse axonal injury due to non missile head injury in humans: An analysis of 45 cases: Ann Neurol 1982;12:557-63.
10. Zeitzer MB, Brooks. In the line of fire: Traumatic brain injury among Iraq War veterans. JMAAOHN J 2008; 56:347-53; quiz 354-5.

4 Pathophysiology of Traumatic Brain Injury

Raj Kamal, Raj Kumar

CELLULAR METABOLISM

Direct impact injury to brain produces parenchymal contusion and axonal injuries of brain. These primary injuries trigger a sequence of events which result in alterations in brain metabolism, disruption of cerebral blood flow (CBF) and brain edema.

These secondary alterations can produce increased intracranial pressure (ICP) and brain herniation. Many casualties can be prevented by early recognition and successful treatment of these secondary derangements. In a study from USA, Traumatic Coma Data bank, on 716 patients hypotensional and hypoxia was associated with 150% increase in mortality rate.[2a,2b] Accordingly, another recent study from US the death and disability correlate well with duration of systemic hypotension.[15-17]

These secondary changes ultimately produces cerebral ischemia and hypoxia.[2] Ischemia after head injury may result from: (1) Increased ICP, (2) Local brain distortion secondary to clot, (3) Vasoconstriction due to release of neurotransmitters. Hypoxia results from inadequate ventilation or problems of oxygen delivery.[1]

A study carried out to determine the statistical characteristics of blood pressure (BP) readings from large number of head injured patients revealed a near normal distribution of blood pressure reading that were skewed towards higher values. While the relationship between BP and ICP (Intracranial pressure) may be triphasic with a BP rising at 0.28 mm Hg/mm Hg of ICP, for ICP up to 32 mm Hg, and 0.9 mm Hg of ICP for ICP between 33 and 55 mm Hg, and falling sharply with rising ICP for >55 mm Hg.[19]

Ischemia or hypoxia will cause decrease in ATP level because of anaerobic glycolysis. In presence of oxygen, pyruvate is oxidized through the reactions of Kreb's cycle, generating a net 36 moles of ATP per mole of glucose by the reaction of oxidative phosphorylation. Anaerobic glycolysis produces only 2 moles of ATP per mole of glucose. The Na^+, K^+ pump uses ATP and pumps $2K^+$ into cell and $3Na^+$ out of cell across cell membrane. The Ca^{2+} pumps out $2Ca^{2+}$ out of cell per ATP.[3,4]

Acidosis

Failure of Na^+, K^+ pump and Ca^{2+} pump following nonavailability of ATP will result in: (1) increase in intracellular Na^+, (2) increase in intracellular accumulation of Ca^{2+}, (3) intracellular acidosis. Acidosis further inhibits glycolysis. Thus, a vicious cycle is established. Acidosis alters protein function displacing Ca^{2+} from intracellular binding sites. So, acidosis and Ca^{2+} pump failure leads to significant increase in intracellular Ca^{2+}, which activates Ca^{2+} dependent proteases causing proteolysis and breakdown of cell membrane. Phospholipases are also activated by intracellular Ca^{2+}, which causes release of FFA. Free fatty acids disrupt the lipid portion of cell membranes.

Free Radicals

Ischemia and hypoxia following head injuries produces free radicals. The oxygen-based free radicals, such as superoxide anion (O^{2-}), hydrogen peroxide (H_2O_2), hydroxyl (OH^-) are formed. Free iron can be released from the heme groups of hemoglobin after hemorrhage. These free radicals induce peroxidation of polyunsaturated fatty acids in cellular membranes and further generation of more free radicals.

Free radicals affect the enzyme glutamine synthetase, which converts toxic ammonia and glutamate to glutamine in astrocytes. This leads to higher-levels of ammonia and glutamate in brain and serum.

Transmitters

Head trauma results in high-levels of extracellular K^+, glutamate and adenosine. Massive release of K^+ and glutamate will lead to increased influx of Ca^{2+}, which will cause breakdown of cell membrane by activating Ca^{2+} dependent proteases causing proteolysis.[6]

Adenosine increases CBF and has neuroprotective role as it inhibits glutamate release.

CBF Regulation

The mean CBF obtained in an adult male by Kety was 54 ml/100 g/min.[7] Gray matter flows are considerably higher than those in white matter, with typical relative values of 70 and 20 ml/100 g/min, respectively. CBF values are higher in children and decrease after the age of 60 years.

Autoregulation is defined as the maintenance of a constant level of CBF in the presence of alterations in systemic arterial pressure. Cerebral autoregulation fails below 70 mm Hg and above 150 mm Hg.

Disordered autoregulation may occur following traumatic brain injury, causing CBF to become passively dependent on mean arterial pressure (hence cerebral perfusion or CPP). In absence of an autoregulatory response, moderate or transient hypotention can cause cerebral ischemia.

CBF is closely coupled with the metabolic rate as shown in Table 4.1. Following severe traumatic brain injury relationship between metabolism and cerebral blood flow (also called Metabolism-CBF coupling) has been found to be abnormal. CBF is often normal in presence of low metabolism (Relative hyperemia) or high CBF in relation to normal metabolism (Absolute hyperemia). Cerebral perfusion is an important factor. CPP between 60 and 70 is safe. CPP below 60 to 65 mm of Hg in adult or below 55 mm of Hg in child is consider critical, below which ischemic changes occur.[16,17] As autoregulation is disruptal in severe head injury, CBF is largely dependent an CPP.[17]

Continuous jugular venous bulb's oxygen saturation measurements have been used to estimate $CMRO_2$/CBF ratio.[9] Metabolic demands can be reduced by barbiturate induced coma by increasing the availability of O_2 in ischemic cortex provided mean arterial pressure is maintained.[10]

Table 4.1: Relationship between brain activity $CMRO_2$ and CBF[8]

		$CMRO_2$ ml/100 g/min	*CBF*
Unconscious	Epilepsy	9	150
		8	125
	Delirium	7	
	Anxiety	6	100
	Excitation	5	
Conscious			
	Alertness	4	75
	Sleep	3	50
		2	
Unconscious		1	25
	Death	0	0

BRAIN EDEMA AND ICP

Brain edema is defined as a net increased in the water content of cerebral tissue that leads to an increase in overall brain mass. Brain swelling refers to increase in brain volume caused by increased intracranial blood volume as well as brain edema.

According to mechanism of formation, brain edema is classified into vasogenic edema and cytotoxic edema. In vasogenic edema the blood-brain barrier (BBB) is opened up, resulting in net gain of water in extravascular-extracellular compartment. The fluid resultant from BBB disruption is usually protein rich, having more characteristics of blood ultrafilterate. Vasogenic edema extends preferentially through white matter. The spread of vasogenic edema compromises local microcirculation, adding further ischemic insult to edematous area. Clinically, vasogenic edema is demonstrated by hypodensity of the white matter on computed tomography (CT).

In cytotoxic edema cellular swelling occurs BBB remains intact. Following severe head injuries astrocytic swelling was seen three hours to three days after injury.[11]

Breakdown of cell membrane following traumatic brain injury is the cause of cytotoxic edema. Cell membrane breakdown results from ischemia which causes failure of Na^+-K^+ pump and Ca^{2+} pump, release of free fatty acids (FFAs) and free radicals.

Cellular swelling can produce numerous deleterious secondary effects in the cell, including: (1) membrane depolarization secondary to loss of intracellular K^+, (2) release and decreased uptake of excitatory amino acids, as seen in astrocytes.[5]

Intracranial Pressure

The intracranial volume of an adult is approximately 1500 ml, which is about 2 percent of total body weight. It contains three constituents: CSF, blood and brain parenchyma. The largest intracranial compartment is the incompressible brain parenchyma, which comprises about 80 percent of this compartment. The total CSF volume in normal conditions is about 120 to 140 ml; ventricular volume is about 40 ml, the spinal subarachnoid space contains about 30 ml, and the remaining CSF occupies the cranial subarachnoid space and cisterns.

The total cerebral blood volume is approximately 150 ml. Following traumatic brain injury several compensatory mechanisms can operate to keep intracranial pressure ICP low, initiating reduction in the volume of intracranial CSF. Further increase in ICP compresses veins, thus decreasing blood volume.

Till this phase, there is no change in ICP. Beyond this stage intracranial compliance decreases. Thus, producing comparatively higher increase in ICP with small increase in intracranial volume. This initial phase of decompensation can be rapidly controlled with mannitol and hyperventilation.

A principal strategy for managing head injury is to reduce the frequency and severity of secondary brain insult from raised intracranial pressure and low cerebral perfusion pressure (CPP). A critical threshold for CPP values in children aged 2 to 6, 7 to 10 and 11 to 15 years were 48, 54 and 58 mm Hg, respectively. The pressure time index (PTI) is first substantive pediatric index of total ICP and CPP following head injury. The insult thresholds generated are identical to age related physiological values. The management guidelines for pediatric head injuries should take account of these CPP thresholds to titrate appropriate pressure therapy.[14,18,20]

'Compliance' is defined as the ratio of the change in volume to the resulting change in pressure (dV/dP). High compliance means that large volume can be added without a much change in intracranial pressure. The pressure volume curve (Fig. 4.1) is exponential in shape.[12,13] Hence, the compliance and elastance, changes continuously, throughout. 'Elastance' is reciprocal of compliance (dP/dV).

Langfitt et al[12,13] used an inflatable epidural balloon in monkeys and simultaneously monitored pressure in the lateral ventricle and plotted the pressure volume curve (Fig. 4.1). Compliance is high till the line is horizontal (i.e. ICP remains low even when intracranial volume is increased). As volume increases further, threshold for compensation is reached, and even small increase in volume cause very high increase in ICP. At this stage compliance is low and elastance is high.

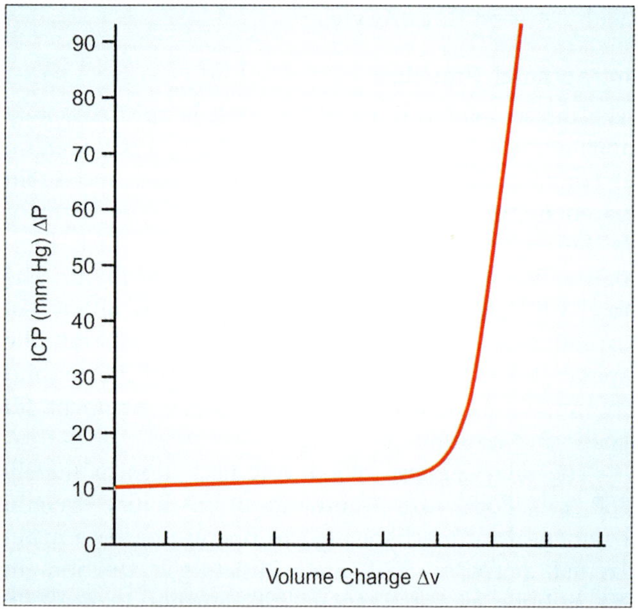

Fig. 4.1: Volume pressure relationship

If ICP continues to rise, compliance decreases further. At this stage plateau waves appear during continuous ICP monitoring. Vasomotor paralysis is the last stage in the decompensation of protective mechanisms. Brain swelling also increases the ICP following head injury.

A rapidly developing hematoma is poorly tolerated than a slowly developing mass lesion because adequate time should be available for compensatory mechanisms to act. This quantity is described as cerebral capacitance. This quantity represents the rate at which the brain can accomodate changes in intracranial volume and is determinded by the time dependent derivatives of the same variables determinning cerebral compliance.[13] Thus, traumatic intracranial hematomas that grow rapidly may result in rapid increase in intracranial pressure and fatal cerebral herniation, while a meningioma in a similar location may produce few symptoms.

SYSTEMIC MANIFESTATIONS OF HEAD INJURY

Systemic abnormalities to head injury may occur immediately, over hours or days. Trauma induces catecholamine release from adrenal medulla which may cause deleterious effects on the heart, the vascular system and on metabolism.

EFFECT ON CARDIOPULMONARY SYSTEM

Neurogenic pulmonary edema is relatively uncommon and is associated with diminished lung compliance. Alveoli are flooded by protein rich fluid. It results in decreased lung compliance. As a result severe hypoxemia develops. Endotracheal intubation with positive end expiratory pressure (PEEP) is helpful in preventing low PaO_2.

The neurogenic pulmonary edema may occur due to:

1. **Hyperdynamic state:** Increased left ventricular afterload occurs because of hypertension with increased peripheral vascular resistance. It causes increased pulmonary capillary pressure resulting in lung edema.
2. **Sympathetic stimulation:** Increased sympathetic stimulation on lung vasculature results in increased vascular permeability.
3. Release of platelet and fibrin microaggregates from injured lung vasculature.

CONCLUSION

The primary injury to the brain triggers a sequence of events, which results in alteration in brain metabolism, and cerebral blood flow. Cerebral ischemia results due to increased intracranial pressure (ICP), local brain distortion occurs secondary to clot and vasoconstriction. Hypoxia and cerebral ischemia will cause anaerobic glycolysis, intracellular acidosis, release of free radicals and high levels of extracellular K^+, glutamate, adenosine. All these factors will lead to tremendous increase in intracellular accumulation of Ca^{++}, causing breakdown of cell membranes by activating Ca^{++} dependent proteases and release of FFA.

Autoregulation is deranged following head injury. The relationship between metabolism ($CMRO_2$) and cerebral blood flow (CBF) has been found to be abnormal. Head trauma results in cytotoxic edema, brain swelling and hence intracranial hypertension.

REFERENCES

1. Popp AJ, Fenstel PI, Kimelberg HK. Pathophysiology of traumatic brain injury. In Neurosurgery 1997, Wilkins RH, Rengachari SS (Ed), 1997;2623-37.
2. Graham DI, Ford I, Adam JH, et al. Ischemic brain damage is still common in fatal non-missile head injury. J Neurol Neurosug Psychiat 1989;52:346-50.

2a. Olson OA. Head Injury Medicine 2002.

2b. Paul ME, Joseph V, Todd T. Management of Head Trauma (Critical review) Chest 2002;122:699-711.

3. Siesjo BK. Pathophysiology and treatment of focal cerebral ischemia Part I. Pathophysiology. J Neurosurg, 1992;77:169-84.
4. Siesjo BK. Pathophysiology and treatment of focal cerebral, ischemia. Part II Pathophysiology. J Neurosurg, 1992;77:337-54.
5. Faden AI, Demedink P, Panter SS, Vink R. Role of excitatory amino acids and NMDA receptors in traumatic brain injury. Science 1989;244:798-800.
6. Katayama Y, Becker DP, et al. Massive increases in extracellular potassium and the indiscriminate release of glutamate following concussive brain injury. J Neurosurg 1990;73:889-900.
7. Kety SS. Circulation and metabolism of the human brain in health and disease. Am J Med 1950;8:205-17.
8. Ingvar OH, Lassen NA. Regulation of cerebral blood flow. In: Himwich HE (Ed). Brain metabolism and cerebral disorders. New York: Spectrum Publication 1976;181-206.
9. Guz J, Miner ME, Allen SJ, et al. Continuous monitoring of cerebral oxygenation in acute brain injury: Assessment of cerebral haemodynamic reserve. Neurosurgery 1991; 29:743-9.
10. Fenstel PI, Ingvar MC, Severinghaus JH. Cerebral oxygen availability and blood flow during middle cerebral artery occlusion. Effects of pentobarbitol. Stroke 1981;12:850-63.
11. Bullock R, Maxwell WL, et al. Glial swelling following human cerebral contusion: An ultrastructural study. J Neurol Neurosurg Psychiat 1991;54:427-34.
12. Langfitt TW, Weinstein JD, Kassell NF. Cerebral vasomotor paralysis produced by intracranial hypertension. Neurology 1965;15:622-41.
13. Langfitt TW, Weinstem JD, Kassell NF, et al. Transmission of increased intracranial pressure within the craniospinal axis. J Neurosurg 1964;21:989-97.
14. Schweitzer JS, Bergsneider M, Becker DP. Intracranial Pressure Monitoring. In Cottrell JE, Smith OS (Eds). Anesthesia and Neurosurgery, 3rd edn, Mosby 1994;117-35.
15. Eisenberg HM, Gary HE, Aldrich EF, et al. Initial of finding in 753 patients with severe head injury. A report from the NIH Traumatic Coma Data Bank. J Neurosurg 1990;73:788-98.
16. Rosner MJ, Rosner RD, Johnson AH. Cerebral perfusion pressure: Management protocol and clinical results. J Neurosurg 1995;83:949-82.
17. Guidelines for cerebral perfusion pressure. J Neurotrauma 2000;17.507-11.
18. Initial assessment and management. Advanced trauma life support for doctors. Student Course Manual. Chicago II. American College of Surgeon 1997;21-46.
19. Michell P, Gregson BA, Piper IAN, et al. Blood pressure in head injury patients. J Neurol Neurosurg and Psychiat 2007;78:399-402.
20. Chambers IR, Jones PA, Lo Tym, et al. Critical thresholds of intracranial pressure and cerebral perfusion pressure related to age in pediatric head injury. J Neurol, Neurosurgery and Psychiat 2006;77:234-40.

5 Pathology of Head Injury

MC Sharma, Chitra Sarkar

INTRODUCTION

Cerebrospinal injury causing death or permanent disability remains single most important public health problem encountered in industrialized society. Injuries are still responsible for more years of potential life lost than cancer and cardiovascular diseases combined. In US, injuries accounted for about one-third of the total deaths in 1985.[1] The head injury rate varies among different population settings for urban and rural. The causes of head injuries are traffic and transport accidents in 50 percent, gunshot in 20 to 40 percent, fall in 10 percent, and assault in 5 to 10 percent.

Head injury is a major cause of mortality and morbidity at all ages. The death rate of head injury in children is about 10 per 100,000, five times the mortality rate of leukemia,[2] the next leading cause of death. The most common causes of head injury in childhood are, falls, recreational activities, traffic accidents and child abuse.[2]

A performance on neuropsychological tasks that are presumed to be related to temporal lobe, frontal lobe and white matter integrity is worse in patients with APOE e4 allele than in those without it. More neurobehavioral disturbances are observed in APOE e4 carriers than in APOE e2 and e3 carriers.[39]

For many years, pathologists have recognized the characteristic focal lesions found in fatal head injuries. In recent years the recognition of the diffuse lesions—diffuse axonal injury (DAI), ischemic brain damage and brain swelling—more fully explains the pathophysiologic abnormalities that accompany such injuries. The old concept that trauma induces immediate and irreversible injury of the central nervous system is questioned by recent studies.[3]

Types of head injuries are shown in Table 5.1.

SKULL FRACTURES

The presence of a skull fracture signifies that traumatic cranial injury had occurred. Skull fractures occur in up to 8 percent of fatal head injuries.[4] A number of variables will determine the case with which bone will fracture including the age, sex, race of the patient, any disease states and the anatomic location of the bone. Concomitant brain injuries also occur frequently, but they are by no means an invariable consequence of skull fractures.[5] Skull fractures are classified as follows:

A. *Linear fractures:* A linear fracture is a simple fracture line that tends to radiate outwards from the point of impact along with path of least resistance. A linear fracture is produced by a broadbased force such as traffic accidents and falls.
B. *Basilar skull fractures:* Basilar skull fracture may be linear, depressed or comminuted. Fracture of skull may be limited to the area of base or may spread into the base from the calvarium. Fractures of the base of skull are not reliably depicted by radiographic examination.[6] Hence, the routine removal of the dura mater from the skull is necessary to identify fractures at autopsy. Fracture line usually radiates from the impact point. Multiple interlacing fracture lines suggest that multiple blows produced the fractures.
C. *Depressed fractures:* This type of fractures are produced by forceful or heavy impacts striking the skull over a small surface area, resulting in a portion of the

Table 5.1: Classification of primary head injuries

Skull fractures	*Local injuries*	*Diffuse injuries*
Linear	Contusions	Concussion
Basilar	Coup	
	Contrecoup	
Depressed	Intermediate	
	Fracture	
Comminuted	Lacerations	Diffuse axonal injury
Compound	Hematomas	Mild
		Moderate
		Severe
Childhood	Epidural	Brain swelling
	Subdural	
	Subarachnoid	
	Intracerebral	
	Intraventricular	

bone, being pushed inwards to impinge on the brain. Occasionally, such fractures are referred to as bending fracture. If the fracture shows bending outward distal to the impact site, it is known as bursting fracture. When fracture separates the suture line they are called as diastatic fractures. These fractures may be closed or open type depending upon the nature of injuries of the overlying soft tissues and scalp.

D. *Comminuted fractures:* This type of fractures result from forceful and heavy impact striking the head over a wider area with bone breaking into multiple pieces.
E. *Compound fractures:* Compound fractures are those where overlying scalp is lacerated. They may occur with any other type of fractures.
F. *Childhood fractures:* Skull fractures of children present with a number of interesting cases. Most of the features of skull in children are due to abusive trauma, traffic accidents, falling from height and after devastating situations. Hobbs[7] suggested that skull fractures after the alleged minor accident indicated abuse, if one or more of the following were present.
   1. Multiple as complex fractures.
   2. Depressed fractures.
   3. Maximum fracture width greater than 3 mm.
   4. Growing fracture.
   5. Involvement of more than one cranial bone.
   6. Nonparietal fracture.
   7. Associated intracranial injury.

Another interesting lesion is growing fracture produced by an enlarging traumatically induced leptomeningeal cyst. This cyst is lined by fibrous connective tissue and is filled by CSF. It protrudes through a tear in the underlying dura mater, enlarges a linear fracture and erodes the bone along the fracture margins. The enlargement and erosion of the bone are believed to be caused by pulsation of the brains. Growing fractures usually occur in children less than 3 years of age and are not associated with significant injury to the brain.

Compound and basal skull fracture results in cerebrospinal fluid fistulae, CSF rhinorrhea, otorrhea and meningitis.

Lacerations: A laceration is a mechanical tear or rent in normal tissue. They result from greater force and appear at the same site as contusions. They may or may not be accompanied by skull fracture. Cerebral lacerations usually involve inferior surface of frontal lobe or temporal lobe tips. Lacerations, if associated with diffuse axonal injury commonly involve corpus callosum and the brainstem.

Tears, lacerations or brainstem avulsion of the pontomedullary junction and cerebral peduncles occur as a result of hyperextension.[14] They are usually seen in fatal road accidents, atlanto-occipital dislocations and high cervical fracture.

DIFFUSE AXONAL INJURY (DAI)

The diffuse axonal injury was first described by Strich[15] in 1956 as diffuse degeneration of the white matter and was thought to be essential component of post-traumatic dementia. Later on, some authors called it as inner cerebral trauma[16] and shearing injury.[17] The currently accepted name used to describe this entity is diffuse axonal injury (DAI).[18,19]

Axonal injury is a key feature of the post-traumatic encephalopathies and is an important determinant of the outcome in nonmissile head injury. DAI is an important cause of coma in the absence of an intracranial expanding lesion of the vegetative state and of disability after head injury.[20] DAI is a distinct clinicopathologic entity which may develop after mild concussion up to and including persistant post-traumatic case.[22,23]

DAI develops most frequently in patients who have been injured in vehicle accidents both occupants and pedestrians, after falls, after assaults and with child abuse. Compared with other head injury patients, patients with DAI have fewer skull fractures and a lower incidence of cerebral contusions, intracranial hematoma and raised intracranial pressure. Patients with moderate to severe diffuse axonal injury are rendered immediate unconscious by their injury and remain unconscious until their death. Those who survive for longer period are in vegetative states. These patients survive longer than severely diffuse head injured patients without axonal injury.[18]

In DAI, grossly brain may appear normal. But in most severe degree of DAI, focal lesions are seen in corpus callosum, one or both dorsolateral quadrants of the rostral brainstem. In the early stage of injury the lesions are hemorrhagic and appear as petechial size hemorrhages, streaks of hemorrhages or as small intraparenchymal hemorrhage.

Similar hemorrhages occur, in addition to corpus callosum and brainstem, in subcortical white matter, fornix, tela choroidea, walls of third ventricle, basal ganglia and hippocampal regions. In very severe cases larger streaks of hemorrhage are seen in the white matter. As the hemorrhagic lesions age, they become softened, granular and finally cystic. In the later stage there is dilatation of the ventricles because of reduced bulk of white matter.

On microscopic examination, the hallmark of DAI is axonal swelling (retraction balls) in the cerebral white matter, corpus callosum and upper brainstem. Axonal swelling becomes apparent within hours of the injury and may persist for a year or more. In patients who survive, microglial stars (clusters of microglial cells) develop at the site of injury and replace the swollen axons.

To diagnose DAI, evidence of axonal injury needs to be found independent of other lesions such as infracts and hematoma. The histologic appearance of axonal injury depends upon the length of survival after injury. Affected patients have a high mortality, and if they survive, a high morbidity, often improving into only a persistent vegetative state. Diffuse axonal injury can be diagnosed by diffusion-weighted MRI. If survival is from hours to a few days many irregular swellings of the axons and oval or rounded bulbs at the end of the axon are eosinophilic in H and E stain sections. Axons may appear tortuous or varicosed and show irregular thickening. These findings are better brought out in silver staining. Identification of axonal swelling can be augmented by staining for ubiquitin or amyloid precursor protein (APP). If patient survives for many months in vegetative state then Wallerian degeneration appear.

DAI appears to be a distinct clinicopathologic entity which may develop after mild concussion. The findings of occasional clusters of microglia in patients dying soon after a minor head injury suggested that axonal injury had occurred.[23] More recently axonal damage has been demonstrated in patients who died from unrelated causes after sustaining a mild injury by using antibody against amyloid precursor proteins.[24-26]

Possession of e4, allele of the apolipoprotein E gene (APOE e4) is associated with greater incidence of moderate/severe contusional injury and severe ischemic brain damage in fatal cases of TB1. This may be associated with poor outcome.[40]

Adams et al[27] proposed a grading system based on the severity of injury. In grade I DAI, the histological evidence of axonal damage is found in the white matter of the cerebral hemispheres; corpus callosum, brainstems and less commonly in the cerebellum. In grade II DAI, in addition to widely distributed axonal injury there is also focal lesion in the corpus callosum. Grade III, represents the most severe spectrum of DAI and takes the form of diffuse damage to axons and focal lesions in both corpus callosum and dorsolateral quadrant or quadrants of the rostral brainstem. These authors have shown correlation between the grade and level of consciousness.

Strich[28] proposed that axonal damage is produced by mechanical forces engendered at the moment of impact that physically disrupt axons. Some authors have suggested that the damage to white matter is a secondary event and is due to hypoxic brain damage, edema or herniation.[29] Gennarelli et al[19] experimentally produced diffuse axonal injury in monkeys using only controlled angular head accelerations in the sagittal, oblique or lateral direction without the necessity of impact to the head. Experimental studies by Porlishock and Coworkers[30,30a] had identified the axonal changes that produced the axonal retraction balls. The mechanism postulated to cause diffuse axonal injury is the shearing force generated by movements of the head, which physically tear the axons. Retraction balls formed from swelling of the axons, which resulted from accumulation of organelles as axoplasmic transport was impaired. The separation of proximal and distal segments did not occur until the reactive swelling was formed.

BRAIN SWELLING

Brain swelling is an increase in the size of one or both cerebral hemispheres. The extent of involvement depends on a number of features such as patient's age and nature of the injury. The term brain swelling includes both edema and cerebrovascular congestion.[31] Two closely related clinicopathologic syndromes of diffuse brain swelling were identified by CT scanning. These syndromes occur almost exclusively in children and adolescents.[32] In one, diffuse swelling is the result of edema which is of vasogenic nature. In vasogenic edema there is injury to the capillary endothelial junctions, site of blood brain barrier, leading to passage of plasma proteins and electrolytes into the brain extracellular space. Edema fluid flows from the site of capillary injury in the white matter towards the ventricles under hydrostatic pressure of circulation. In the gray matter, the edema fluid does not extravasate into the extracellular space and the astrocytes take in the fluid and swell. Edema fluids in the white matter move into the ventricles and enters CSF pathway. Presence of edema contributes to increase in the intracranial pressure and may depress cerebral blood flow and impair autoregulations.

The other type of diffuse brain swelling is due to increased blood flow and severe hyperemia. The clinical importance of these two types of diffuse brains swelling lies in the fact that in first type, patients often follow relentless course to death whereas in second type recovery follows without in sequelae.

Diffuse swelling causes flattening of gyri, narrowing of sulci and symmetrical collapse of the ventricular system. In localized swelling distortion and herniation occur. Minimal swelling may not be recognized early. Cerebral edema produces pallor of the myelin, distention of perivascular and pericellular spaces, rarefaction of subpial spaces, a vacuolar appearance of the neuropil; and pools of proteins rich fluid in the spongy looking areas. However, measurement of water content is the most reliable method of diagnosing cerebral edema.

HEMORRHAGE

In head injury patients hemorrhages develop in the epidural, subdural, subarachnoidal space and in the brain parenchyma. When such bleeds form mass lesions, they often produce devastating neurophysiologic effects and cause significant mortality and morbidity.

Epidural Hematoma

Epidural hematoma follows cranial trauma complicated by temporal bone fracture and result from laceration of middle meningeal artery branches that penetrate the skull in the regions of the pterion.[33] The accumulation of blood between calvarium and endosteal surface of the dura mater is rapid and is accompanied by rapid deterioration of consciousness. If not evacuated promptly, it leads to transtentorial herniation and compression of brainstem. Chronic subdural hematomas are usually of venous origin.

Subdural Hematoma

Normally the space between dura mater and arachnoid is closely opposed. Subdural hematomas result from the dissection of blood into this potential space. Most common location is over the cerebral convexities and supposed to be because of rupture of delicate bridging veins that traverse the arachnoid dura interface enroute to the superior segittal sinus. These vessels are susceptible to shearing forces generated by sudden angular acceleration of the head. Patients on anticoagulants are more prone to subdural hematoma. Subdural hematomas may be acute, subacute or chronic, depending upon the interval of injury and onset of symptoms. Acute hematoma becomes symptomatic within 3 days. When the symptoms develop between 3 and 21 days then subacute. If they become symptomatic after 21 days, they are chronic. However, these distinctions are arbitrary and some authors prefer to identify age of the lesion from its pathologic appearance.[34]

The pathology of subdural hematoma depends upon the age. If evacuated early it consist of clotted blood. In later stages organization start and hematoma gets surrounded by collagenous membranes leading to see formation. The membrane may attain thickness of several millimeters and are composed of proliferating spindle cells, loose connective tissue budding capillaries, siderophages and lymphocytes. In some cases a significant number of eosinophils are also seen.

Subdural Hygroma

A subdural hygroma is the accumulation of watery serious fluid in the subdural space. The other terminologies used for this condition are meningitis serosa series traumatica and traumatic subdural effusion. Hygroma may develop immediately after head injury or after sometimes. Hygroma occurs alone or concomitantly with other head and brain injuries. Symptoms depend upon the rate at which fluid collects. Tears of the arachnoid or impaired CSF absorption are likely to be etiological factors.

Subarachnoid Hemorrhage

Trauma is the most frequent cause of subarachnoid hemorrhage besides other nontraumatic causes. Injury of any magnitude can cause subarachnoid hemorrhage. Subarachnoid hemorrhage is found overlying contusions, spreading outwards from lacerations and around gunshot wounds. In subdural hemorrhage, if veins are teared in the subarachnoid space then hemorrhage lies under the subdural hematoma also. Traumatic basilary subarachnoid hemorrhage is a massive hemorrhage over the ventral surface of brainstem.

Within a few hours of bleeding into the CSF, fever and meningisms develop. There is polymorphonuclear response within 24 hours and becomes prominent by 48 hours. After 48 hours, lymphocytes and macrophages start replacing them. Macrophages phagocytose RBCs and such lipid laden in phagocytes may persist for years in the arachnoid meninges and Virchaow-Robin's spaces. Repeated episodes of CSF hemorrhage may impede the absorption of CSF and may produce hydrocephalus.[35]

Intracerebral Hemorrhage

Intracerebral hemorrhage vary in size from a small petechial hemorrhage of less than 0.5 cm to a large hematoma and may be single or multiple in number. An intracerebral hematoma may also occur along with epidural hematoma alone or combined with subdural hematoma.

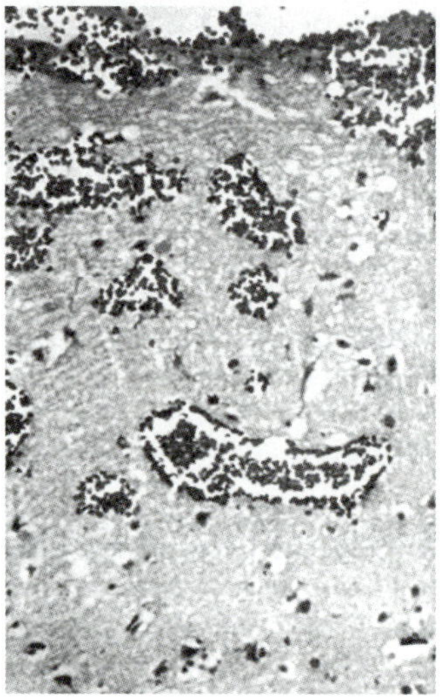

Fig. 5.1: Photomicrograph contused hemorrhages in the gray matter along with ischemic charges in the neurons. Some of the neurons show more eosinophilic cytoplasm

The large intracerebral hematomas are most commonly located in frontal and temporal lobes and are associated with adjacent contusions and lacerations.[36] Large parenchymal hemorrhages may extend into the ventricles, resulting in IVH.

The other subgroup of intracerebral hemorrhages is associated with diffuse axonal injury (Fig. 5.1). Small hemorrhage appears in the white matter and basal ganglia and probably due to tearing of small vessels by the same shearing force which damage axons. These small hemorrhages may enlarge over several days.

Delayed Traumatic Intracerebral Hematoma

A delayed traumatic intracerebral hematoma is one that arises in an area of brain that has been previously injured by impact usually in a contusion. Due to injury, vessels are weakened within the contused area and if autoregulation fails or systemic hypertension develops then bleeding occurs.

Burst Lobe

A burst lobe is severely contused frontal or temporal pole, whose cortical surface is pulped and lacerated with extension of hemorrhage through the arachnoid into subdural space. Burst lobe occurs most commonly in association with contrecoup contusions.

Intraventricular Hemorrhage (IVH)

Intraventricular hemorrhage is bleeding within the lateral ventricles that may extend into subarachnoid space. Traumatic intraventricular hemorrhage occurs commonly in association with other intracranial injury. The volume of blood varies from few ml to large hemorrhage of 40 to 60 ml.

Brain Damage Related to Trauma

Immediate impact injuries are traumatically caused lesions that are generated at the time of impact and are produced by the direct damage of the impact itself rather than as a complication of the traumatizing force.

CONCUSSION

A cerebral concussion (commotio cerebri) is a temporary, reversible neurologic deficiency caused by trauma, which results in immediate loss of consciousness which is temporary. Concussion is accompanied by retrograde and post-traumatic amnesia and duration of which depends upon the severity of concussion. When concussion lasts more than 24 hours or longer, diffuse brain injury is usually present. Experimental studies of concussion have shown minimal non-specific neuronal changes.[9,10] Neuropathology studies of classical cerebral concussion in humans have rarely been available to study. Concussion is usually accompanied by other injuries like contusions, skull fractures and multiple brain injuries. The morbidity and mortality of cerebral concussion depends on the severity of the associated brain injuries.

CONTUSIONS

A contusion is a bruise of the cortical surface of the brain which results as a hemorrhage around the blood vessel (Fig. 5.2). The overlying pia mater always remains

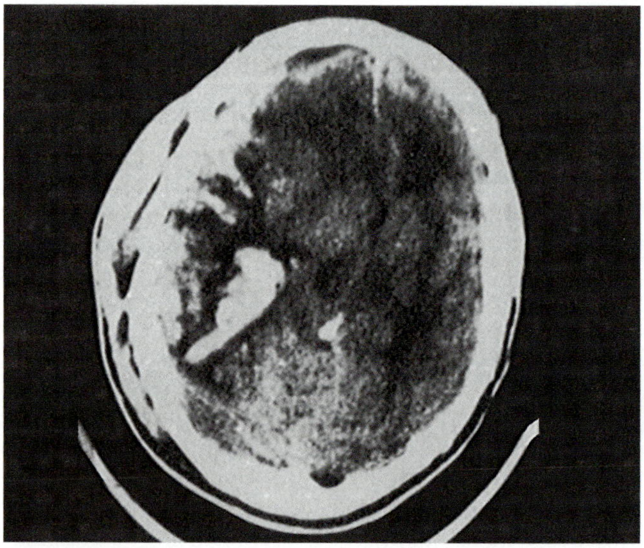

Fig. 5.2: CT head shows right hemispheric extradural hematoma with multiple contusions and intraparenchymal hematoma, note subgaleal collection on right side

intact. Contusions are usually result of mechanical injury and extent depends upon the forcefulness of the impact which results in contusions. They may occupy part or all of the cortical layers. Contusions tend to be wedge-shaped with base towards the surface and may cause full towards the surface and may cause full thickness necrosis of the cortex. Continuous bleeding within a contusion results in contusion bleeding which may extend into the white matter or cortical surface and CSF. Contusions are focal damage (Fig. 5.3) and even in severe cases, there may be complete recovery, clinically if there is no accompanying diffuse axonal injury.

Contusions tend to be large and more hemorrhagic in hypertensive, alcoholic or who have bleeding diathesis. Adams et al[11] developed a contusion index in which the depth and extent of the contusions were graded in frontal, temporal, parietal and occipital lobes and in the cortex above and below the Sylvian fissures and the cerebellum. The indices that reflected the severity of contusion at each site and their mean were used to assess other types of head injury such as skull fractures or diffuse axonal injury.

Contusions formed at the site of cranial impact are coup contusions; those opposite the cranial impact, contrecoup contusions; and those at the margins of brain herniation, herniation contusions. Herniation contusions are most frequently located along the margin of the falx cerebri, tentorium or foramen magnum. Bruises found along the edges of skull fractures are fracture contusions. Gliding contusions are deep parenchymal injuries that may or may not be comparable to surface contusions.

Contusions form in certain locations depending upon the position and motion of the body at the time of impact which has been supported by experimental studies.

A number of theories have been proposed to explain the phenomenon of contusion.

Houlbourn's rotational shear force theory to some extent explains the contrecoup contusions.[12,13] This theory suggests that rotational movements of the brain generate shearing forces that produce contusion in a distribution referred to as contrecoup.

As the contusion ages, the necrotic cortical tissue is removed, leaving behind a shrunken orange brown scar. Some contusions are large enough to produce subcortical head injuries. Spinal cord may be contused over an extended area or may show hemorrhagic necrosis. Evolution of damage to the cord includes gliosis and cavitation of the spinal cord adjacent to a transection. Ascending and descending wallerian degeneration of injured fiber tracts evolve. Traumatic neuroma and post-traumatic syringomyelia may develop.

SECONDARY COMPLICATIONS

Increased intracranial pressure: Increased intracranial pressure is the most common cause of death in head injury. Pressure necrosis in one or both parahippocampal gyri at autopsy may be used as a criterion of whether intracranial pressure had been raised to a significant level. The common causes of increased intracranial pressure are intracranial hematomas and brain swelling.

Hypoxic brain damage: In patients who die from head injury, the ischemic change is a frequent finding (Fig. 5.3). Ischemic damage is more common in patients who have had a clinical episode of hypoxia, either as hypotension or hypoxemia, and in patients who have had elevated intracranial pressure. In addition, vascular spasm contribute to the etiology of ischemia. Ischemic damage is more common in the watershed

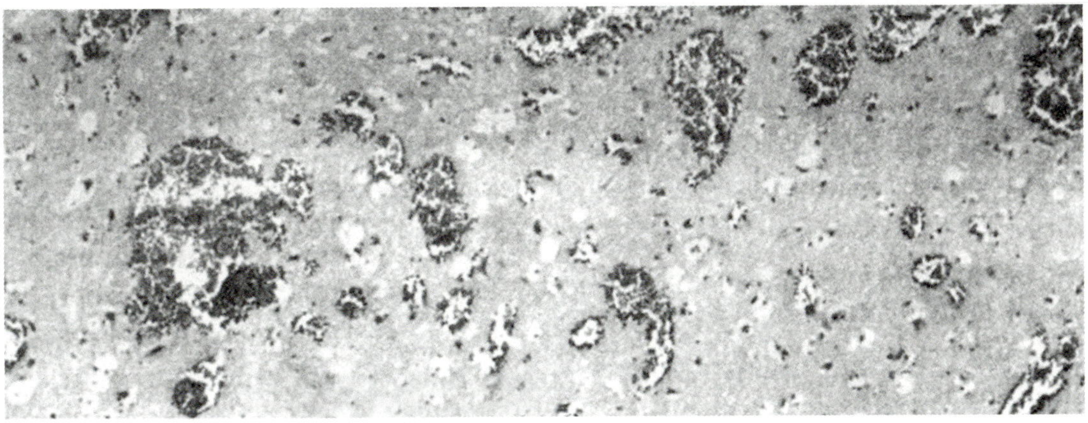

Fig. 5.3: Photomicrograph showing contused brain, i.e. petechial hemorrhages around the small vessels in the cerebral cortex

zones or throughout the cerebral cortex, basal ganglia and cerebellum.

Pathology of head injury is increasingly well understood. Mechanical forces result in shearing and compression of neuronal and vascular tissue at the time of impact. A series of pathological events may then ensue leading to further brain injury. This secondary injury may be amenable to intervention and is worsened by secondary physiological insults. Some preventive factors to hault the secondary insult such as hypotension and hypoxia are potential areas of medical intervention. A prompt specialist neurocritical case is hence associated with improved outcome.[38]

REFERENCES

1. Centres for disease control: Estimated years of potential life lost before age 65 and cause specific mortality, by cause of death: US, 1985, Morbid Mortal Weekly Rep 1987;36-447.
2. Kraus JF, et al. Incidence, severity and external causes of pediatric head injury. Am J Dis Child 1986;140:687.
3. Povilshock JT, Jenkins LW. Are the pathobiological changes evoked by traumatic brain injury immediate and irreversible? Brain Pathology 1995;5:415.
4. Adams JH. The neuropathology of head injuries. In: Vinken PJ, Bruyn GW (Eds). Handbook of clinical neurology Vol. 23, Amsterdam: North-Holland 1975;35.
5. Servadei F, Giucci G, Morchetti A, et al. Skull fracture as a factor of increased risk in minor head injuries. Indication for a broader use of cerebral computed tomography scanning. Surg Neural 1988;30:364.
6. Ehler E, Ivankievicz D, Schomachar GH. Diagnosis of skull fractures by autopsy and radiology. Acta Morphol 1980;28:291.
7. Hobbs CJ. Skull fracture and the diagnosis of abuse. Arch Dis Child 1984;56:246.
8. Taveres J, Ransokoff J. Leptomeningeal cysis of the brain following trauma with erosion of the skull. A study of seven cases treated by injury. J Neurosurg 1953;10:233.
9. Adams JH, Graham DI, Gennarelli TA. Acceleration induced head injury in the monkey. Acta Neuropathol 1991;7 (Suppl):26.
10. Groat RA, Windle WF, Magoun HW. Functional and structural changes in the monkey's brain during and after concussion. J Neurosurg 1994;2:26.
11. Adams JH, Doyle D, Graham Dr, et al. The contusion index: A reappraisal in man and experimental non-missile head injury. Neuropathol Appl Neurobiol 1985;11:299.
12. Holbourn AHS. Mechanics of head injuries. Lancet 1943;2:438.
13. Holbourn AHS. Mechanics of head injuries. Brit Med Bull 1945;3:147.
14. Lindenberg R, Freytag E. Brainstem lesions characteristics of traumatic hyperextension of the head. Arch Pathol 1970;90:509.
15. Strich SJ. Diffuse degeneration of the cerebral white matter in severe dementia following head injury. J Neurol Neurosurg Psychiat 1956;19:163.
16. Greevic N. Topography and pathogenic mechanisms of lesion in "inner cerebral trauma". Rad Acad Sci 1982;402:265.
17. Peerless SJ, Rewcastle NB. Shear injuries of the brain. Can Med Assoc J 1967;96:577.
18. Adam JH, Graham Dr, Murray LS, Scott G. Diffuse axonal injury due to non-missile head injury in human. An analysis of 45 cases. Ann Neurol 1982;12:557.
19. Gennarelli TA, Thibault LE, Adams JH, et al. Diffuse axonal injury and traumatic coma in the primate. Ann Neurol 1982;12:567.
20. Adams JH. Head injury. In: Adams JH, Duchen W (Eds). Greenfield's Neuropathology, 5th edn. London: Arnold 1992;106.
21. Blumbergs PC, Jones R, North JB. Diffuse axonal injury in head trauma. J Neurol Neurosurg Psychiatr 1989; 52:838.
22. Clerk JM. Distribution of microglial clusters in the brain after head injury. J Neurol Neurosurg Psychiatr 1974; 37:467.
23. Oppenheimer DR. Microscopic lesions in the brain following head injury. J Neurol Neurosurg Psychiatr 1968;31:299.
24. Blumbergs PC, Sçott G, Manavis J, Wainwright H, Simpson DA, Mclean AJ. Staining of amyloid precursor protein to study axonal damage in mild head injury. Lancet 1994;344:1055.
25. Grady MS, McLaughlin MR, Christman CW, Valadka AB, Flinger CL, Povlishock JT. The use of antibodies targeted against the neurofilament submits for the detection of diffuse axonal injury in humans. J Neuropathol Exp Neurol 1993;52:143.
26. Gultekin SH, Smith TW. Diffuse axonal injury in craniocerebral trauma: A comparative histologic and immunohistochemical study. Arch Pathol Lab Med 1994;118:168.
27. Adams JH, Doyle D, Ford I, Gennarelli TA, Grahm Dr, McLellan DR. Diffuse axonal injury in head injury: Definition, diagnosis and grading. Histopathology 1989; 15:49.
28. Strich SJ. Shearing of nerve fibres as a cause of brain damage due to head injury. Lancet 1961;2:443-8.
29. Jellinger K, Seiterberger F. Protracted post-traumatic encephalopathy: Pathology, pathogenesis and clinical implications. J Neurol Sci 1970;10:51.
30. Povlishock JT, et al. Axonal change in minor head injury. J Neuropathol Exp Neurol 1983;42:225.

30a. Buki A, Povlishock JT. Evidence for Calpain-Mediated spectin protrolysis in the pathoguries of traumatically induced axoval injury. J Neuropath Exp. Neurol 1999; 58:365-75.

30b. Povlishock JT, Erb DE, Astrue J. Reactive axonal change, deafferentation and Neuropathology. J Neurotrauma 1992;9:5189-5200.
31. Klagzo L. Neuropathological aspects of brain oedema. J Neuropath Exp. Neurol 1967;26:1.
32. Graham DI, Ford I, Adams JH, Doyle D, Lawrence AE, Mc Clellan DR. Fatal head injury in children. J CIin Pathol 1989;42:18.
33. Hardman JM. Cerebrospinal trauma. In Davis RL, Robertson DM (Eds). Textbook of neuropathology Baltimore. Williams and Wilkins 1991;973-4.
34. Fogetholm R, Heiskanen O, Waltimo O. Chronic subdural haematoma in adults. Influence of patient's age on symptoms, signs and thickness of haematoma. J Neurosurg 1975;42:43.
35. Gilles FH, Shilliot J Jr. Infan tile hydrocep halus Retrocerebellar subdural hematoma. J Pediatric 1970;76:529.
36. Gurdigian ES. Cerebral contusions: Re-evaluation of the mechanism of their development. J Trauma 1976;16:35.
37. Liu AY, Maldjian JA, Bagley LJ, et al. Traumatic brain injury diffusion: Weighted MR imaging findings. AINR 1999;20:1636-41.
38. Moppett IK. Traumatic brain injury assessment, resuscitation and early management. Brit J of Anaesthesia 2007;99(1):18-31.
39. Ariza M, Pueyo R, Martin Mdelm, et al. Influence of polymorphism on cognitive and behavioral outcome in moderate and sever traumatic brain injury. J Neurol, Neurosurgery and Psychiat 2006;77:1191-3.
40. Smith C, Graham D1, Murray LS, et al. Association of APOE e4 and cerebrovascular pathology in traumatic brain injury J Neurol, Neurosurgery and Psychiat 2006; 77:363-6.

6 Traumatic Brain Edema

AK Mahapatra, Raj Kumar

Edema is a condition, where there is accumulation of fluid in extracellular spaces. Traumatic brain edema is a distinct condition 1 to 4 which can be present alone or in association with other focal pathological processes like contusion, laceration or intracerebral hematoma. The traumatic brain edema is one of the most undesirable pathology, associated frequently, and difficult to treat. Unfortunately, edema is the cause of death in large number of head injury patients, in whom intracranial pressure persistently remains high, leading to widespread damage. In young children, edema behave very differently and may lead to death more often, hence, recently termed as malignant brain edemas. This chapter deals with some aspects of traumatic brain edema.

PATHOPHYSIOLOGY OF BRAIN EDEMA

Brain edema is a dynamic process in which a series of changes occur in endothelial cells in blood vessel, blood brain barrier and cell membrane, leading to biochemical changes which ultimately result in fluid extravasation. However, the process is very complex and involves a large number of neurotransmitters.[6-10] Generally, edema is a secondary pathology in the brain following head injury, and may be of vasogenic or cytotoxic in origin. More often the edema may be of mixed type. Due to injury, there is breakdown in blood-brain barrier (BBB), and exudation of fluid. This process sets in around the focal brain lesions like contusion, intracerebral hematoma and give rise to focal brain edema.[8] Thus, vasogenic edema, is the result of a vascular insult leading to increased permeability of endothelial cells to macromolecules, which includes protein and other molecules. The extravasated fluid accumulate in extracellular space of the white matter. Cytotoxic edema occurs due to metabolic dysfunction in cell causing intracellular accumulation of fluid.

Penfield and Cone 1938[12] proposed involvement of oligodendroglia in the process of acute brain swelling. However, recent clinical and experimental studies have shown wide range of chemical neurotransmitter changes following head injury which leads to brain edema (Table 6.1).[12-15] Some authors have shown the role of vasogenic amine in increase permeability of endothelial cells[16,17] giving rise to vasogenic edema. Cytokines, capsain mediated spectrin proteolytic enzymes capase activation also induces post-traumatic edema.[18a,18b]

Most important in production in brain edema is ischemia which alters the membrane permeability, which on the other hand leads to: (a) vasogenic edema because of opening of tight junction in endothelial cells and (b) cytotoxic edema due to cellular membrane damage leading to abnormal fluid accumulation in cells.[15] The combination of cytotoxic and vasogenic edema increases the brain volume and decreases perfusion to brain tissue causing more damage.

Cell membrane damage plays an important role in pathological manifestations in head injury. Neuronal membrane damage causes efflux of K^+ into extracellular space and intracellular Ca^{++} increases. There is increase in extracellular glutamate. Glutamate also damages the cell membranes and causes further K^+ efflux,[9-18] leading to the disturb feedback between K^+ and glutamate liberation. This also leads to damages of calcium homeostasis. Large number of membrane receptor such as N-Methyl-D-Aspartate (NMDA) and Alpha-amino-3-hydroxy-3-methyle-4 isoxasol (AMP A) and kinate receptors also play an important role in membrane breakdown. Phospholipase C, and inositol triphosphate (IP_3) enhance the intracellular calcium liberation. Activation of AMP A and kinate receptor helps in sodium and chloride influx leading to cellular edema and cell death. Sodium influx depolarize the Neuronal membrane rapidly by operating through voltage operated channel (VOC). While sodium influx is rapid, calcium influx is mediated through NMDA receptor and relatively slow process[8] (Table 6.2). Recently, cytokine and calpain-mediated spectrin proteolysis is postulated in the pathogenosis of traumatically induced axonal injury.[18a,18b]

Recently, calcium bind Calmodulin (Cam) and Nitric oxide synthetase (NOS) are reported to be important in formation of edema. NOS is a very important factor giving rise to edema in not only head injury but also in brain tumors.[20] These chemicals, damage DNA and

Table 6.1: Potential cellular mechanism of damage

a. Phospholipid metabolism abnormality lipid peroxidation
  - Prostaglandin, leukotrienes
  - Platelet activating factors (PAFs)

b. Biberation of oxygen free radicals (OFRs) – Free iron catalysis

c. Excitatory mechanism
  - Glutamate increased

d. Neuropeptides raised
  - Endorphin
  - Thyrotropin releasing hormone

e. Calcium and magnesium metabolism abnormality

f. CNS lactic acidosis

Table 6.2: Mechanism of edema

In head injury
Focal contusion/Laceration
Raised intracranial pressure
Impaired cerebral blood flow and ischemia
Neuronal anoxia → Axonal flow fails
Glutamate accumulation
Release of free radical
Impaired lipid peroxidation
Failure of ion pump
Ca^{++} and K^{+} leakage
Cytotoxic edema
Vasogenic edema

inhibit mitochondrial function leading to more free radical release. In head injury, Lipid peroxidation can also be directly activated by the presence of ferrous ion. Intracellular calcium influx activates Phospholipase A_2 lipoxygenase and Cyclo-oxygene. The above substances degrade arachidonic acid into large number of metabolites like thromboxane A_2 prostaglandins and leukotrienes, oxygen and hydroxyl free radical.[21] Superoxide radicals are also increased in extracellular space and also involved in membrane damage and enhances the edema (Table 6.3).

Overall cerebral function is dependent on adequate and continuous supply of blood and oxygen. The regulated blood flow and intact blood brain barriers are general requirements for maintenance of microenvironment of the brain. Damage in the mechanism of maintenance of microenvironment leads to chemical changes, cell death and edema (Table 6.4).

Table 6.3: Superoxide radicals enhancing the edema

- Head injury® Raised ICP® Fall of cerebral Perfusion + platelet aggregation
- Damage to BBB Hypoxia
- Edema® Impaired® Membrane function substances and free radicals

Table 6.4: Chemical changes leading to brain damage

a. Ischemia–hypoxia (Basic cause)
b. Lactic acidosis—vasospasm
c. Ca^{2+} and Na^{+} into cells, K^{+} comes out of the cells
d. Activation of phospholipase A_2
e. Liberation of arachidonic acid
f. Membrane damage–leading edema formation
g. Further compromise in glucose and oxygen supply:

Vascular damage	Reoxidation
Prostaglandins and other free radicals	Neurotransmitter dysfunction

Oxidation of arachidonic acid by cyclo-oxygenase and Lipoxygenase

BRAIN DAMAGE

Pathology and Natural Course of Brain Edema

Microscopically, astrocytes are specially vulnerable for damage in brain edema. Astrocytes look swollen and pale. In the initial phase, neurons look normal. Subsequently, because of cytotoxic effect neuron may get swollen. Most remarkable changes do occur in white matter. However, oligodendroglia and myelin do not get affected. Maximum damage is seen in pericapillary area. Vascular damage and ischemic changes are invariably observed histologically. Few days later, macrophages appear and try to engulf the debris. Subsequently, gliosis sets in 3 to 4 weeks time.

Resolution of edema is well-studied in human and experimental animals. Edema increases over a period of 3 to 4 days then reach the peak. Within a period of 7 to 10 days, edema subsides.[5] However, with stimulating factor for edema, such as low-perfusion, hypoxia, metabolic or electrolyte disturbances and hyperpyrexia can prolong the resolution of edema. By and large the time period for resolution of edema is unpredictable.[5] With the advent of CT scan the onset, progress and the resolution of edema are easily evaluated.[4,22,23] Bruce et al[22] had shown malignant brain swelling in children. CT scan has proved that the edema is a dynamic process and is influenced by large number of factors. CT scan also differentiate edema from brain swelling.[4,21]

Treatment of Brain Edema

Large number of substances like 20 percent mannitol, hypertonic saline, 50 percent glucose, Furosemide and glycerol are used routinely in brain edema with success. Use of corticosteroids has been proved ineffective in patients with severe head injury. It is surprising, that the steroid which works like magic in brain edema of nontraumatic origin does not work in edema due to head injury. Barbiturate has a limited role in head injury. While hyperventilation is not only useless but also can prove hazardous as it may wash out CO_2 and induce cerebral vasospasm, which can lead to further ischemia and edema.

Recently, free radical scavengers like vitamin E is widely used. Glutamate is one of the most important factor in ischemia and production of brain edema. NMDA receptor antagonist like Phencyclidine, MK-801 and dextromethorphan have been tried in animal models[14] of traumatic brain injury. MK-801, phencyclidine and ketamine have a lot of side effects in man. However, dextromethorphan may be useful in future. Vitamin E, Selenium and superoxide dismutase can reduce the free radicals and reverse or stop lipid peroxidation.[25,26]

Calcium influx into the cells can be prevented by calcium channel blockers. Few years back, expectation was raised regarding the role of Nimodipine in reducing ischemic, hypoxic damage and brain edema in head injury. Surprisingly, however, multicentric European trial with Nimodipine was not encouraging.[27]

Hypothermia, has long been known to reduce cerebral metabolism and protect brain. Recently, mild hypothermia is proved to be helpful in head injury. In a randomized trial, Marion et al[28] had shown lowering of brain temperature and reduction of CBF with a 40 percent drop of ICP by using cooling blankets and cold saline gastric perfusion. Thus, it may be possible to get a beneficial effect by mild hypothermia of 33 to 34°C.

CONCLUSION

Brain edema is an important secondary pathology in brain following head injury. Edema is a complex and dynamic process mediated through large number of chemicals and neurotransmitters. Basic trigger points are ischemia and hypoxia. Liberation of free radicals and damage to all membranes are probably two important steps in formation of edema. Availability of CT scan has helped us in studying brain edema in patients. Corticosteroids are of no value in traumatic brain edema. Mild hypothermia, adequate oxygenation, perfusion and free radical scavengers can reduce brain edema and change the out look of head injury patients.

The recent imaging studies using CT and or MRI clearly demonstrate that traumatic brain edema is a combination of vasogenic and cellular, with the cellular component predominating and that cerebral blood volume is reduced in the most cases with severe brain swelling, although these result suggest that ischemic brain damage is closely involved in trauma induced brain edema. The mechanisms underlying the edema formation can not be fully explained by ischemia alone. Cerebral blood flow decreases but still exists in traumalized brain suggesting that water supply from the blood vessels is not completely interrupted. In cerebral contusion, diffusion MR imaging demonstrates that cells in central area of contusion undergo shrinkage, disintegration and homogenization, whereas cellular swelling is predominant in the peripheral area of contusion. It appears that the capacitance for edema fluid accumulation increases in central area, and the edema third propagation decreases in peripheral area.[29]

REFERENCES

1. Brock M. Basic concept of brain oedema. In: Traumatic brain oedema. F Cohadon, A Baethman, JD Miller (Eds). Liviana Press, Padova 1987;123-7.
2. Clasen RA, Penn RD. Traumatic brain swelling and oedema. In: Head Injury. PR Cooper (Ed). William and Wilkins, Baltimore 1987;285-312.
3. Long DM. Traumatic brain oedema. Clinical Neurosurgery 1982;29:174-202.
4. I to U, Tometa SH, Yamazaki Y, Takada Y, et al. Brain swelling and brain oedema in acute head injury. Acta Neurochir (Wien) 1986;79:120-4.
5. Bruce DA, Ter Weeme C, Kaiser G, et al. Mechanism and time course for clearance of vasogenic cerebral edema. In: Neuronal Trauma. AJ Popp, et al (Eds). Raven Press, New York, 1979.
6. Long DM, Maxwell RE, French LA. (i) The effect of glucosteroids upon cold induced oedema. (ii) Ultrastructure evaluation. J Neuropath Exp Neurol 1971; 30:680-97.
7. Astrop J. Energy-requiring cell function in the ischaemic brain. J Neurosurg 1982;56:482-97.
8. Choic DW. Ionic dependance of glutamate neurotoxicity. Neurosciences 1987;7:379-83.
9. Klatzo I, Piraux A, Laskowski E. The relationship between oedema, blood-brain barrier and tissue element in local brain injury. J Neuropath 1958;17:548-63.

10. Katayama Y, Becker DP, Tamara T, et al. Increase in extracellular glutamate and associated ionic influx following concussion brain injury. J Neurosurg 1990;73:889-900.
11. Galbraith S, Cardoso E, Patterson J. The water content of white matter after head injury in man. In: Recent progress in the study and therapy of brain oedema. Gok G, Bethman A (Eds) New York 1984;323-29.
12. Penfield W, Cone W. Acute Swelling of the oligodendroglia. Arch Neurol Psychiat 1938;20:1.
13. Kontos HA, Wei EP. Superoxide production in experimental brain injury. J Neurosurg 1986;64:803.
14. Faden A, Demediuk P, Panter S, Vink R. The role of excitatory amino acids and NMDA receptors in traumatic brain injury. Science 1989;244:298.
15. Suguru I, Marmarou A, Clarke GD, Andersor BJ, et al. Production and clearance of lactate from brain injury. J Neurosurg 1988;69:736.
16. Fishman R, Chan PH. Metabolic basis of brain oedema. In: Advances in neurol 28: Cervos-Navarroj, Ferszt XR (Eds) Brain oedema, Raven Press, New York 1980.
17. Mohanty S, Dey PK, et al. Role of histamine in traumatic brain oedema. An experimental study in rat. J Neurol Sci 1989;90:87-97.
18a. Shohami E, Gallily R, Mechoulam R, et al. Cytokine production in brain following closed head injury: Dexanabinol is a novel TNF (Alpha) inhibitor and effective neuroprotectant. J Neuroimmunol 1997;72:169-177.
18b. Buki A, Povlishock JI. Evidence for calpin-mediated spectrin proteolysis in pathogenesis of traumatically induced axonal injury. J Neuropathol Exp Neurol 1999; 58:365-75.
19. Nicholls D, AHwell D. The release and uptake of excitatory amino acids. Trends in Pharmacological Science 1998;11:462-8.
20. Bakshi A, Nagi C, Wadhwa S, Mahapatra AK, Sarkar C. The expression of nitric oxide synthetase in human brain tumour and peritumoural areas. J Neurological Sci 1998;155:196-203.
21. Wolfe L. Eicosanoids, Prostaglandins, thromboxane leukotrienes and other derivatives of carbon-20, unsaturated fatty acids. Neurochem 1982;38:74.
22. Bruce DA, Alavi BK, Dolinskas L, et al. Diffuse cerebral swelling following head injuries in children. The syndrome of malignant brain oedema. J Neurosurg, 1981;54:170-8.
23. Lobato RD, Sarabia R, Cordabe F, Riivas JJ. Post-traumatic cerebral hemispheric swelling. Analysis of 55 cases studied with CT. J Neurosurg 1988;68:417-23.
24. Zimmerman RA, Bilaniuk LT, Bruce O, et al. Computerized tomography of pediatric head trauma: Acute general cerebral swelling. Radiology 1978;126:403-8.
25. Muizelaar JP, Marmarou A, Young HF, et al. Improving the outcome of severe head injury with oxygen radical scavenger polyethylene glycol conjugated superoxide desmutase. A phase II trial. J Neurosurg 1993;78:375-82.
26. Anderson D, Saunders Ra, Deme dink P, et al. Lipid hydrolysis and peroxidation in injured spinal cord. Partial protection with Methyle prednisolone, Vito E and Selenium. CNS Trauma 1985;2:257-67.
27. Cohadon F. Brain protection. In: Advances in technical standard in Neurosurgery. L Symon (Ed). Springer Verlag (Wien), Vol 21, 1994.
28. Marion OW, Gbrist WD, Carlier PM, et al. The use of moderate therapeutic hypothermia for patients with severe head injuries. A preliminary report. J Neurosurg, 1993;79:354-62.
29. Tatsuro K, Yochi K. Traumatic brain edema in diffuse brain injury, advances in Neurological Sciences 2006;50 (2):241-7.

7 Role of Abnormal Calcium Homeostasis in Head Injury

P Sarat Chandra, AK Mahapatra

INTRODUCTION

Clinical recovery after central nervous system (CNS) trauma, to a great extent affected by a neural injury process that is triggered and perpetuated at the cellular level, and is more than a surgically curable operable lesion. It is widely thought that one such process, (a fundamental pathological mechanism initiated by CNS injury) is the disruption of cellular Ca^{2+} homeostasis. Because of the critical role of Ca^{2+} ions in regulating innumerable cellular functions, this major homeostatic disturbance is thought to trigger neuronal and axonal degeneration and produce clinical disability. The following chapter will review the normal and pathological Ca^{2+} homeostasis in neurons that relate to traumatic brain injury and the possible role of neuroprotective strategies. Of interest particularly is the contribution of Ca^{2+} permeable ionic channels, Ca^{2+} pumps, intracellular Ca^{2+} stores, intracellular Ca^{2+} buffering systems, and the roles of secondary, Ca^{2+} dependent processes in neurodegeneration. A number of hypotheses linking Ca^{2+} ions and Ca^{2+} permeable channels to neurotoxicity are discussed with an emphasis on strategies for lessening Ca^{2+} related damage. A number of these strategies may have a future role in the treatment of traumatic brain injury.

Although, there exist multiple mechanisms by which the central nervous system (CNS) tissue may be damaged. It is now widely accepted that one of the important underlying common factors in the above mentioned cellular disturbances is the disruption of intracellular calcium ion homeostasis. A lot of recent cellular and molecular research has focussed on the study of normal and abnormal Ca^{2+} signaling in neurons. The knowledge gained forms the basis for rational design of the therapeutic interventions aimed at reducing the Ca^{2+} induced neurotoxicity in CNS injury. In addition, the new informations may explain why past attempts at lessening neuronal injury by pharmacological means have failed in clinical settings. Unfortunately, it is impossible in this Chapter to cover comprehensively all the potentially relevant aspects of neuronal Ca^{2+} homeostasis. The purpose of this article, therefore, is to review some of the issues that may have relevance to the pharmacotherapy of neurosurgical patients presently and in the future. It is highly likely that, some of the newer therapeutic strategies that are now in process of evaluation and development will be added to the existing clinical armamentarium.

A BRIEF REVIEW OF NORMAL CALCIUM HOMEOSTASIS

All mammalian cells use calcium ions as signals to perform innumerable vital functions such as, the control of cell-growth and differentiation,[1] the maintenance of cytoskeletal structure,[2] membrane excitability,[3] exocytosis and synaptic activity.[4,5] Because of the pivotal role of Ca^{2+} ions as regulators of normal neuronal function, neurons have evolved homeostatic mechanisms to tightly bind this crucial ion within the intracellular organelles and thus strictly monitor the free cytoplasmic concentration of Ca^{2+} ions. These mechanisms consist of a complex interaction between four general categories of events: Ca^{2+} influx, Ca^{2+} buffering, internal Ca^{2+} storage, and Ca^{2+} efflux. A fifth process, intracellular Ca^{2+} diffusion, links the aforementioned events and is also crucial to Ca^{2+} homeostasis. Together, these mechanisms maintain Ca^{2+} at extremely low levels intracellularly (100 nmol/L or 105 times lower than extracellular Ca^{2+}), so that relatively small or localized increases in Ca^{2+} can be used by the cell as a signal to trigger a physiological effect, such as the activation of an enzyme or an ion channel. From a physiological standpoint, the delicate interplay between these five processes allows multiple Ca^{2+} dependent processes to be regulated smoothly independently within the same cell. Maintaining this balance is the goal of all clinically relevant pharmacotherapeutic strategies aimed at lessening Ca^{2+} related neurotoxicity in brain injury.

CALCIUM INFLUX

This is chiefly governed by ionic channels. Ion channels are the gates on the cell membrane by which ions gain access into the intracellular space. These specialized pores in the cell membranes are classified physiologically by their specific selectivities for certain ions (Ca^{2+}, K^+, Na^+, or cn and by their gating mechanism. Some ion channels are sensitive to membrane voltage and change their conformation between a number of open and closed states, depending on whether the cell membrane is depolarized or repolarized (voltage-gated channels). Other ion channels are associated with receptors that when activated by a specific ligand, induce conformational changes in the ion channel pores, which cause the pore to open. These ionic channels are frequently named according to their specific ligands (for example, "nicotinic" acetylcholine receptor channels). Voltage-gated ionic channels frequently contain binding sites for certain ligands, and ligand-gated channels may exhibit certain forms of voltage dependence. There exist many types of voltage and ligand-gated ion channels that are either Ca^{2+} permeable or that cause Ca^{2+} to rise through a second-messenger pathway.

CALCIUM BUFFERING

Another strategy to regulate the spread of Ca^{2+} ions within neurons is by Ca^{2+} buffering. As calcium ions diffuse into the cell, they are rapidly buffered by a number of cytoplasmic proteins, such as calmodulin, calbindin, and parvalbumin.[6] Approximately 95 to 99 percent of Ca^{2+} ions entering the cell under physiological conditions are buffered.[7,8] Although the precise role of Ca^{2+} buffering substances remains poorly understood, recent evidence indicates that they may act to keep Ca^{2+} at high levels in localized areas within cells, to limit those high Ca^{2+} levels to those specific areas, and to rapidly dissipate the Ca^{2+} gradients and thus limit the time course of activation of Ca^{2+} dependent processes.[9,10]

Ca^{2+} Sequestration and Storage

The Ca^{2+} buffering capacity of cytosolic Ca^{2+} binding proteins is limited. Therefore, neurons also possess mechanisms for sequestering Ca^{2+} ions into organelles, situations in which Ca^{2+} loads exceed the ability of Ca^{2+} buffers to maintain Ca^{2+} at tolerable levels. These include, the smooth endoplasmic reticulum, mitochondria, and synaptic vesicles. These organelles can sequester large quantities of Ca^{2+} under a variety of conditions, using active and passive Ca^{2+} transport mechanisms, similar to those found in the plasma membrane. Although, Ca^{2+} storage in the organelles is an efficient mechanism for controlling cytoplasmic Ca^{2+}, this Ca^{2+} "lowering" system operates at a much slower time scale than cytoplasmic Ca^{2+} binding proteins. Therefore, it is incapable of modulating rapidly changing or highly localized changes in Ca^{2+}.[11]

CALCIUM EXTRUSION

All the cells must expend metabolic energy to extrude Ca^{2+}. The large extracellular-to-intracellular Ca^{2+} ion concentration gradient and the electrical driving force propelling the positively charged Ca^{2+} ions toward the negatively charged inner plasma membrane necessitate the presence of efficient Ca^{2+} extrusion mechanisms. Neurons have at least two such mechanisms, **adenosine triphosphate (ATP)-driven** Ca^{2+} **pumps** (Ca^{2+} **ATPases)** and a Na^+/Ca^{2+} **exchange transport** mechanism.[12-14]

Both the above systems are heavily dependent of ATP, which rapidly depletes in head injuries, thus producing a state of Ca^{2+} excess. Thus, Ca^{2+} influx may easily overwhelm cytoplasmic Ca^{2+} buffering mechanisms, resulting in an uncontrolled rise in the concentration of unbound intracellular Ca^{2+} ions, that are then free to activate numerous secondary Ca^{2+} dependent cascades, which ultimately result in cell death.

INTRACELLULAR CALCIUM DIFFUSION

Ca^{2+} concentration profiles within the cytoplasm are determined by the type and the subcellular distribution of Ca^{2+} entry sites (Ca^{2+} channels) and depend on Ca^{2+} buffering and sequestration systems and by Ca^{2+} extrusion mechanisms. These modulators have marked effects on the ability of Ca^{2+} ions to diffuse into the cell. For example, Ca^{2+} ions bound to Ca^{2+} binding proteins possess markedly different diffusion characteristics from free Ca^{2+} ions.[8,15] Also, Ca^{2+} influx sites may be coupled with Ca^{2+} binding sites within the cell (e.g. Ca^{2+} dependent enzymes).[16] These mechanisms serve to selectively couple Ca^{2+} entry with specific intracellular targets of Ca^{2+} ions. Thus, any process that modifies cytoplasmic Ca^{2+} diffusion may disrupt this coupling process and prevent Ca^{2+} ions from reaching their sites of intracellular action. This concept has recently been extended to the use of Ca^{2+} chelating agents, to uncouple Ca^{2+} ion entry and Ca^{2+} neurotoxicity both *in vitro*[17] and in experimental settings, thus producing a potentially useful future clinical therapeutic strategy.[18]

How Does Calcium Ions Cause Cell Damage?

Disturbances in Ca^{2+} homeostasis as a "final common Pathway" of neurodegeneration:

A significant step towards the understanding of the mechanisms that trigger cellular injury was initiated in non-neuronal tissues, when pathologists noted the calcium deposited in areas of tissue necrosis.[19] Thereafter, Schanne et al[20] observed that the cultured hepatocytes could be killed when exposed to various toxins in the presence, but not in the absence, of extracellular Ca^{2+}. They inferred that Ca^{2+} entry into cells was an absolute requirement for the expression of toxicity and termed this process the "final common pathway of cell death". In neurons, early studies in tissue cultures showed that amputated axons degenerated only if Ca^{2+} ions were present in the culture medium.[21] More recently, neurodegeneration induced by neurotoxins such as, capsaicin and the excitatory amino acid (EAA) glutamate was shown to be associated with increases in tissue Ca^{2+}.[22] Further investigations on the toxicity of EAAs in cultured neurons and in brain slice preparations also confirmed an association between the observed toxicity and the presence of Ca^{2+} in the extracellular medium.[23,24]

Currently, studies both *in vitro* and *in vivo* support the association between Ca^{2+} influx and damage to neural tissues. For example, experimental spinal cord injury may produce significant Ca^{2+} accumulation in white matter axons,[25,26] possibly as a consequence of white matter anoxia/ischemia. Thus, although the idea that Ca^{2+} is a final common pathway of cell death has not gone unchallenged.[27] Ca^{2+} triggered injury seems to play a major role in the mammalian nervous system.

CALCIUM IONS, GLUTAMATE RECEPTORS AND "EXCITOTOXICITY"

A mechanistic link between cell destruction and Ca^{2+} excess was made by physiologists studying the actions of glutamate, the major excitatory neurotransmitter in the CNS.[28] Glutamate acts on neurons and glia via a number of cell membrane receptors. These are classified into two groups, ionotropic and metabotropic receptors, based on pharmacological, electrophysiological, and biochemical studies.[28] The ionotropic receptors are subdivided into the N-methyl-D-aspartate (NMDA) receptors and α-amino-3-hydroxy-5-methyl-4-isoxazolepropio-nattokainate receptors, identified according to their selective agonists. Activation of these receptors leads to the opening of their associated ion channels, which are typified by their permeabilities to Na^+, K^+, and Ca^{2+}. After the channel open, these receptors may desensitize, causing the ion channel to close again. Thus, the actions of glutamate, via a variety of membrane receptors, affects intracellular Ca^{2+} through several distinct mechanisms. Recently, recombinant deoxyribonucleic acid (DNA) techniques have revealed that many glutamate receptor subtypes exist within each receptor family.[29] The functional consequences of this diversity are incompletely understood and remain under intense investigation.

Under physiological conditions, the synaptic release of glutamate is thought to mediate rapid neuronal excitation, plasticity, and possibly processes involved in learning and memory.[28,30] However, glutamate excess can be toxic. This was noted even before the realization that cellular Ca^{2+} accumulation may be critical in neurotoxicity. This notion was strengthened when glutamate receptor antagonists, such as 2-amino-7-phosphonoheptanoic acid and MK-801, were found to attenuate ischemic neuronal injury *in vivo*.[31] Thereafter, the term "excitotoxicity," initially coined by Olney,[32] came to indicate the process by which excessive synaptic release of excitotoxic amino acids (BAAs) resulted in neurotoxicity.

Several key experiments have shown mechanisms by which glutamate excess triggers toxicity. In brief, the activation of every glutamate receptor subtype has, at some point, been implicated in mediating hypoxic/ischemic neuronal death.[33,34] Current views suggest that the activation of distinct glutamate receptor subtypes may produce distinct types of neurodegeneration. However, there is general agreement that the NMDA glutamate receptor plays a key role in mediating many aspects of glutamate neurotoxicity because of its high Ca^{2+} permeability, as compared with non-NMDA ionotropic glutamate receptors.[35,36]

Consequently, ever since NMDA and other EAAs were found to produce calcium influx into neurons,[37] the link between synaptic over-activity, extracellular glutamate excess, and Ca^{2+} overload has been considered as the fundamental phenomenon in triggering intracellular neurodegeneration.[34,38-40] Recently, increased levels of EAA have been hown to occur after traumatic head injury,[41] lending further credence to the clinical relevance of the excitotoxicity hypothesis.

MECHANISM OF Ca^{2+} NEUROTOXICITY

Mechanisms leading to Ca^{2+} neurotoxicity can be classified into two stages. The first consists of the pathological mechanisms that trigger and sustain intracellular Ca^{2+} excess (Flow chart 7.1), whereas the second consists of the secondary phenomena thought to be precipitated by intracellular Ca^{2+} excess (Flow chart 7.2). This two-stage concept is relevant therapeutically, because most pharmacotherapeutic strategies for trauma may be classified under one of these categories. Thus, certain drugs are aimed at blocking Ca^{2+} influx into cells (e.g. Ca^{2+} channel blockers), whereas others are targeted at the consequences of this Ca^{2+} excess (e.g. free radical scavengers).

Flow chart 7.1: Depicting mechanisms by which trauma and ischemia produce intracellular Ca^{2+} elevations. VSCC-voltage-gated calcium channel

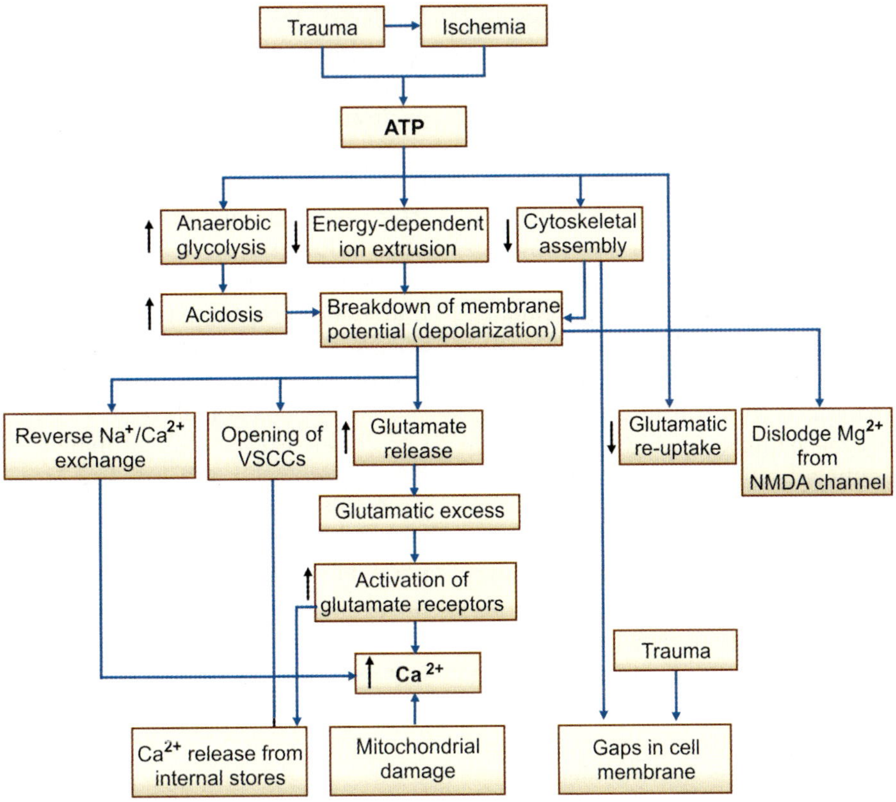

Flow chart 7.2: Depicting mechanisms by which intracellular Ca^{2+} trigger the secondary Ca^{2+} dependent phenomena which result in neurotoxicity

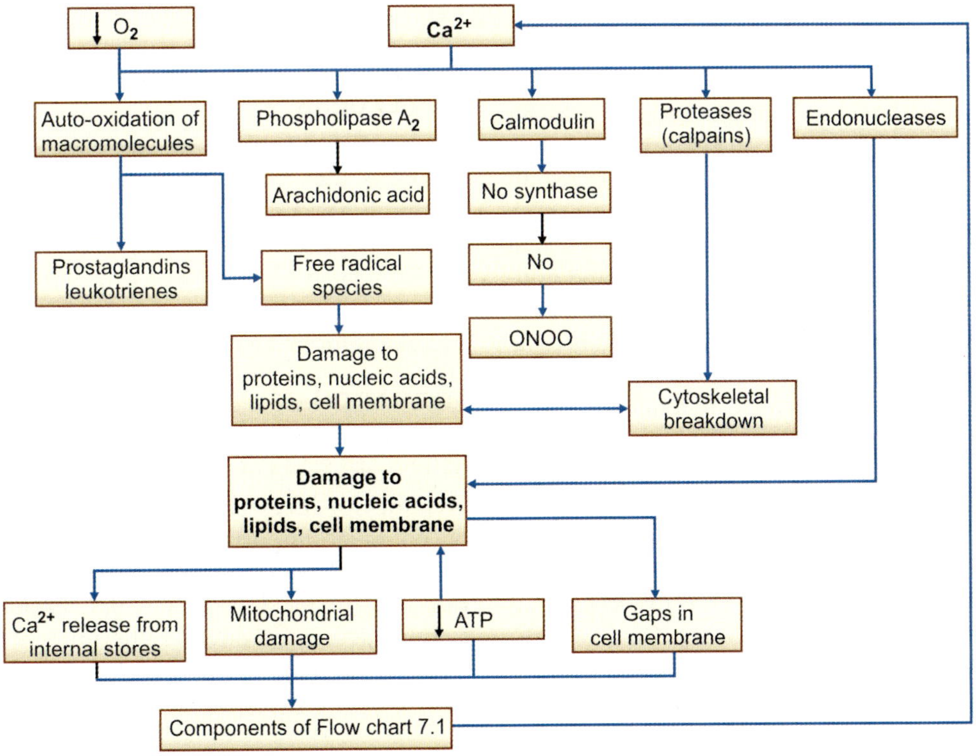

MECHANISM TRIGGERING AND SUSTAINING INTRACELLULAR Ca^{2+} EXCESS

Central to the process traumatic neurodegeneration is the concept of cellular energy failure in neurons and axons after the interruption of blood flow, nutrients, and oxygen[42,43] (Fig. 7.1). Inadequate synthesis of ATP has several consequences, in addition to causing a loss of Ca^{2+} homeostasis. It is thought to produce cellular acidosis through the stimulation of anaerobic glycolysis, a disruption of ion homeostasis caused by the loss of energy-dependent ion transport mechanisms, and a loss of cytoskeletal integrity as a consequence of decreased synthesis of macromolecular assemblies required for maintaining cell structure. Cellular energy failure is also hypothesized to result in Ca^{2+} overload through a number of mechanisms, including increased Ca^{2+} influx, decreased Ca^{2+} efflux, and altered internal Ca^{2+} buffering and sequestration.

The increase in Ca^{2+} influx, during the energy failure, occurs by several mechanisms. First, as transmembrane ionic gates breakdown because of the failure of energy-dependent ionic pumps (e.g. Na^+ - K^+ ATPase), the plasma membrane depolarizes, causing the opening of voltage-operated Ca^{2+} channels. In traumatic injuries, the disruption of cell membranes causes an efflux of potassium ions, contributing further to ionic gradient collapse and membrane depolarization in the remaining cells. Depolarization also dislodges positively charged magnesium cations from the NMDA channel pores, where they normally prevent ion fluxes. This facilitates the activation of NMDA currents and Ca^{2+} influx by EAAs.[44,45] Depolarization also increases glutamate release from synaptic terminals, this being coupled with a decline in energy-dependent glutamate reuptake in neurons and glia.[46-48] The resulting rise in the extracellular concentrations of glutamate and other EAAs is thought to trigger neurodegeneration both *in vitro* and *in vivo*, by activating both the NMDA and non-NMDA glutamate receptors.[49,50] Finally, an additional mechanism of Ca^{2+} influx during energy failure is through the Na^+/Ca^{2+} exchanger. The normal operation of this exchanger depends on the maintenance of a normal extracellular-to-intracellular Na^+ concentration. When the transmembrane Na^+ gradients collapse, during the energy failure, the exchanger operates in reverse, i.e. pumping Ca^{2+} in and Na^+ out instead of pumping Ca^{2+} out and Na^+ into the cells.[12,51]

Another important process is mitochondrial Ca^{2+} sequestration, which begins when Ca^{2+} rises to micromolar levels.[12,52] Although this temporarily aids in keeping Ca^{2+} low, the process of Ca^{2+} transport across the mitochondrial membrane is ATP dependent and occurs at the expense of energy production, which is already hindered by anoxia. Excessive Ca^{2+} sequestration in mitochondria may render them permanently inactive. Ca^{2+} sequestration by mitochondria during excitotoxicity also adds to cytoplasmic acidosis.[55] A further mechanism contributing to Ca^{2+} homeostatic failure and neurodegeneration may be Ca^{2+} release from intracellular stores. This is presumably because of a failure of Ca^{2+} sequestration mechanisms or to the activation of Ca^{2+} release either by metabotropic glutamate receptor activation or by Ca^{2+} induced Ca^{2+} release. All of the above mechanisms seriously limit the ability of neurons to extrude or buffer nonphysiological Ca^{2+} loads,[51] leading to an eventual deregulation of Ca^{2+} homeostasis and ultimately to an uncontrolled rise in both total and free Ca^{2+} ion concentrations.[40]

Additional mechanisms of Ca^{2+} influx probably exist. For example, in CNS trauma, Ca^{2+} ions may permeate into the cytoplasm through gaps in the cell membrane, produced by the mechanical insult. It is very clear that there exist multiple pathways by which excessive Ca^{2+} loading may occur in traumatized axons and neurons. Thus, from a clinical perspective, it is increasingly apparent that blocking a single pathway of Ca^{2+} influx may not suffice to protect neurons against Ca^{2+} neurotoxicity. This may explain why studies using single Ca^{2+} channel blockers in CNS trauma and ischemia have yielded conflicting and of ten contradictory results *in vitro* and *in vivo*.

SECONDARY PHENOMENA PRECIPITATED BY Ca^{2+} EXCESS

A complete discussion of all Ca^{2+} dependent cellular processes that may contribute to neuronal damage is beyond the scope of this chapter. However, a number of specific processes are thought to contribute significantly to Ca^{2+} related neuronal and axonal injury. It is expected that pharmacological agents targeted at these processes will be useful in the clinical management of CNS trauma.

FORMATION OF FREE RADICAL SPECIES

A free radical is any molecule, atom, or group of atoms with an unpaired electron in its outmost orbital, which accounts for its extreme reactivity. Free radical species of potential importance in cerebral trauma include superoxide (O^{2-}) and hydroxyl (OH^-) radicals. Free radicals are produced in small amounts by normal cellular processes, such as the mitochondrial electron transport system, reactions catalyzed by prostaglandin hydroperoxidase, and the auto-oxidation of small molecules, such as catecholamines, and by the microsomal cytochrome P-450 reductase system. Free radicals may play physiological roles, such as the modulation of a number of membrane receptors, including NMDA receptor function.

Free radicals are formed in excess during traumatic and hypoxic injuries, because insufficient O_2 is available to accept electrons passed along the mitochondrial electron transport chain, leading to the reduction of other components of the system, such as flavin adenine dinucleotide and coenzyme Q. These molecules then auto-oxidize to produce free radical species. Also, during reperfusion, reactive oxygen radicals may form as by-products of the reactions of arachidonic acid metabolism to produce prostaglandins and leukotrienes. Arachidonic acid, particularly abundant during ischemic conditions, is released from membrane phospholipids during this time. Free radicals can react with and damage proteins, nucleic acids, lipids, and other classes of molecules, such as extracellular matrix glycosaminoglycans. Sulfur-containing amino acids and polyunsaturated fatty acids are particularly vulnerable. The latter are found at very high concentrations in the CNS as components of the plasma membrane. Thus, EAA release and free radical formation may act synergistically in lipid peroxidation and the production of ischemia-induced neuronal membrane damage.[27]

The Formation of NO

NO, first identified as an endothelium-derived relaxing factor, is a short-lived, diffusible, highly reactive gas that has recently gained wide attention as a member of a newly discovered class of messenger molecules. NO serves a variety of functions in different tissues, including vascular endothelium, immune cells, neurons, smooth muscle, and cardiac muscle. NO produced in one cell can diffuse and produce biological effects in neighboring cells. In the brain, it is produced by both vascular endothelium and neurons. NO produced in vascular endothelium has major effects on governing cerebral blood flow and acts as a potent vasodilator. A deficiency or inhibition of NO production is postulated as one of the mechanisms of cerebral vasospasm after aneurysmal subarachnoid hemorrhage. In neurons, NO has been implicated in modulating a number of biological phenomena related to synaptic plasticity, including the NMDA receptor function and long-term potentiation.

NO production occurs at low levels during physiological function and is governed by NO synthase. Its synthesis is regulated by the Ca^{2+} dependent regulatory enzyme, calmodulin, which is induced by the influx of Ca^{2+} ions through NMDA receptors. NO production can affect intracellular Ca^{2+} pools in neurons and adjacent cells by modulating Ca^{2+} release from intracellular stores through a cyclic guanosine monophosphate kinase-mediated mechanism. NO in itself is not highly toxic but can lead to the formation of toxic species by reacting with free oxygen radicals, particularly superoxide. NO reacts with superoxide to form the powerful oxidant peroxynitrite ($ONOO^-$), which directly oxidizes sulfhydril groups, lipids, DNA, and proteins thus leading to breakdown of the cell structure. Excessive NO production has been postulated as a causative mechanism in neurotoxicity presumably via Ca^{2+} overload leading to the ultimate overexpression of the mechanisms described above.[20,68]

ENDONUCLEASES, APOPTOSIS AND NECROSIS

Ca^{2+} overload also activates endonucleases, a series of Ca^{2+} dependent enzymes that degrade DNA and that may play role in two well-recognized forms of cell death, necrosis and apoptosis. Apoptosis is a form of programmed cell death, which occurs during fetal development as well as during adult life. The physiological function of apoptosis in the CNS seems to be to remove those neurons of which the processes have failed to find their targets during development or regeneration. Apoptosis is pathologically distinct from necrosis, involving compaction of the cell body, nuclear fragmentation, and the formation of surface blebs. Apoptosis can also be identified by a characteristic DNA fragmentation resulting from the cleavage of cell chromatin into oligonucleosome-length fragments seen as a "ladder" pattern on electrophoretic gels.[20,40,71]

MITOCHONDRIAL DAMAGE

Mitochondria serve as the energy generators of the cell. Considerable evidence indicates that they buffer Ca^{2+} ions during physiological and pathological states.[12,52] Work from several laboratories suggests that mitochondrial dysfunction is a common event in cell injury caused by mechanical trauma.[53] Anoxia causes the transmitochondrial membrane potential to collapse, and then impairment of ATP production ensues. In addition to anoxia, the act of Ca^{2+} buffering by mitochondria also causes the transmembrane potential to decrease, resulting in intramitochondrial Ca^{2+} accumulation and a further collapse of ATP production. This process is accompanied by a concomitant release of H^+ ions from mitochondria. It is likely that extreme Ca^{2+} overload irreversibly damages mitochondria and that this event commits the cell to die.

ACIDOSIS

CNS trauma, and excitotoxicity produce acidosis. Ample evidence indicates that this occurs both at the tissue[6,54] and at the cellular levels.[55,56] Several mechanisms of acidosis production are in effect during neuronal injury. First, an obligatory shift from aerobic to anaerobic metabolism results in lactate production and the release of two H^+ atoms for every two molecules of ATP produced. However, protons are also released during many other reactions, such as phospholipid hydrolysis. Particularly, Ca^{2+} influx causes a rapid intracellular acidification[55] through a number of mechanisms, including a number of membrane exchangers ($Ca^{2+}/2H^+$ exchange at the cell and organelle membranes, Na^+/H^+ exchange to restore Na^+ gradients), the displacement of bound H^+ by Ca^{2+} at negative groups intracellularly, and the release of H^+ from mitochondria during Ca^{2+} buffering as a consequence of $Ca^{2+}/2H^+$ exchange.

The mechanism by which acidosis induces cell damage is possibly due to excess accumulation of Ca^{2+}, enhancing free radical production,[57] or accelerating the DNA damage. At present, although experimental rials with agents such as trimethamine have been encouraging,[58] clinical trials in patients with head injuries have failed to reveal a beneficial effect of acidosis treatment.[59]

STRATEGIES FOR THE TREATMENT OF Ca^{2+} NEUROTOXICITY

The above described cellular and molecular mechanisms of Ca^{2+} related damage constitute the foundation for the recent expansion in a number of potential pharmacological treatments for CNS injury. A number of these treatments have been validated *in vitro* and *in vivo* and are approaching tests in clinical trials.

GLUTAMATE ANTAGONISTS

Antagonists of glutamate receptors are currently among the most widely investigated potential treatments of CNS injury. Studies aimed at characterizing the role of glutamate receptor-mediated mechanisms in traumatic cell death (see Sections above) have produced a number of agents of potential clinical usefulness. For example, antagonists of NMDA receptors, such as dizocilpine maleate (MK-801), aminophosphonoheptanoic acid and its analogs, and other agents (e.g. CGS 19755 and CPP), are able to markedly attenuate glutamate toxicity *in vitro*[34,39] and hypoxic/ischemic cell death in a number of models of CNS trauma. Much of the effectiveness of these agents has been ascribed to their ability to reduce cellular Ca^{2+} loading during periods of cerebral metabolic compromise.

DRUGS THAT ATTENUATE EXCITATORY NEUROTRANSMISSION

Another approach has been to use agents that attenuate the excessive release of *EAAs* altogether presynaptically, thereby attenuating the consequent neuronal damage.[60] Experimental agents, such as nizofenone,[61] BW1003C87,[62] and phenytoin,[63] probably act by blocking sodium channels and preventing the propagation of action potentials to synaptic terminals, where glutamate is released. These agents have been shown to reduce hypoxic/ischemic damage *in vitro* and *in vivo* and may represent a suitable alternative strategy to glutamate antagonists.

Nimodipine, an antagonist of dihydropyridine-sensitive (L-type) Ca^{2+} channels, reduces the incidence of ischemic sequelae of vasospasm after aneurysmal subarachnoid hemorrhage. Although the precise mechanism of this action is uncertain, the action may be caused by the drug's effect on Ca^{2+} channels in cerebrovascular smooth muscle, rather than on neurons.[64] Thus, nimodipine has been successful in ameliorating outcome from ischemic CNS injury in which the primary defect is thought to lie in the cerebral vasculature rather than in the neuron.

To date, however, dihydropyridine class antagonists of voltage-gated Ca^{2+} channels have not been highly effective in reducing other forms of traumatic/ischemic CNS injury.

AGENTS THAT ACT DIRECTLY ON INTRACELLULAR Ca^{2+} IONS

A recent approach to protect neurons against Ca^{2+} neurotoxicity *in vitro* and *in vivo* has been the use of cell-permeant Ca^{2+} chelating agents, such as 1,2-bis-(2-aminophenoxy) ethane-N,N,N', N'-tetra-acetic acid (BAITA) acetoxymethyl ester. BAIT A acetoxymethyl is a lipophilic compound capable of crossing cell membranes, but it does not bind Ca^{2+} ions and does not alter extracellular Ca^{2+} concentrations. However, once the compound has crossed the neuronal membrane, intracellular esterases cleave the acetoxymethyl ester moiety, thereby forming the ionized Ca^{2+} binding compound, BAPTA, which remains trapped within the cells.[65]

DRUGS THAT ATTENUATE THE SECONDARY PROCESSES TRIGGERED BY Ca^{2+} EXCESS

A comprehensive review of the many approaches aimed at attenuating the secondary sequelae of Ca^{2+} excess cannot be achieved in the present review. However, a few strategies are approaching clinical applicability and will be mentioned briefly.

Considerable efforts are being extended to develop and test clinically tolerable free radical scavenging agents. For example, glucocorticoid and nonglucocorticoid steroids having free radical scavenging activity are currently in clinical trials for a variety of neurosurgical disorders, including stroke, head trauma and spinal cord injury, of which methylprednisolone is one already in clinical use. Other free radical scavenging agents, such as polyethylene glycol congugated SOD[66] and vitamin E,[67] may also have a role in certain forms of Ca^{2+} dependent tissue injury.

Other strategies currently under investigation include the use of protease inhibitors to block Ca^{2+} dependent proteolysis and cytoskeletal degradation after excitotoxic or hypoxic/ischemic injuries,[68] anti-DNA fragmentation drugs to retard or abolish apoptosis,[69] and a variety of genetic and environmental manipulations of neurons to render them more resistant to hypoxic/ischemic damage.[70]

Central nervous system trauma produce a deregulation of cellular Ca^{2+} homeostasis by numerous mechanisms, including energy depletion, cell membrane depolarization, excessive synaptic activity, and organelle dysfunction. This pathological increase in intracellular Ca^{2+} ions, which normally regulate numerous intracellular cascades, triggers further injury to neuronal and axonal elements. A key feature of Ca^{2+} neurotoxicity is that Ca^{2+} ions must rise in specific, nonrandom subcellular sites to trigger secondary cascades, which cause neurodegeneration. In some forms of injury, these sites may be located near NMDA receptors.

Considerable advances have been made in recent years in the study and understanding of neuronal Ca^{2+} homeostasis, resulting in the advent of numerous novel neuroprotective strategies. It is hoped that these strategies will find clinical applicability in the next decade. Basic research into the cellular and molecular mechanisms of CNS damage is essential and must continue for further understanding.[71]

Calcium has been implicated in pathophysiology of TBI induced neuronal death and other forms of brain injury including strok and status epilepticus. However, the potential role of long-term changes in neuronal calcium (Ca^{2+}) dynamics after TBI has not been evaluated till recent past. The studies evaluating the mechanism underlying the altered Ca^{2+} homeostasis in TBI indicated that necrotic or apoptotic cell death and abnormalities in Ca^{2+} influx and efflux mechanism could not account for these changes. It was suggested that long-term changes in Ca^{2+} bufferians/sequestration/release mechanism underline thsese changes in Ca^{2+} homeostasis after TBI. Further elucidation of mechanism of altered Ca^{2+} homeostasis in traumatized surviving neurons in TBI may offer novel therapeutic interventions that may contribute to the treatment and relief of some of morbidity associated with TBI.[71]

REFERENCES

1. Kater SB, Mattson MP, Guthrie PB. Calcium-induced neuronal degeneration: A normal growth cone regulating signal gone awry. Ann NY Acad Sci 1989;568:252-61.
2. Schlaepfer WW, Zimmerman UJ. Mechanisms underlying the neuronal response to ischemic injury: Calcium-activated proteolysis of neurofilaments. Prog Brain Res 1985;63:185-96.
3. Kure S, Tominaga T, Yoshimoto T, Tada K, Narisawa K. Glutamate triggers internucleosomal DNA cleavage in neuronal cells. Biochem Biophys Res Comm 1991;179:39-45.
4. Augustine GJ, Charlton MP, Smith SJ. Calcium entry into voltage-Iamped presynaptic terminals of squid. J Physio 1985;367:143-62.
5. Brose N, Petrenko AG, Sudhof TC, Jahn R. Synaptotagrnin: A calcium sensor on the synaptic vesicle surface. Science 1992;256:1021-5.
6. Baimbridge KG, Celio MR, Rogers JR. Calcium-binding proteins in the nervous system. Trends Neurosci 1992; 15:303-8.
7. Neher E, Augustine GJ. Calcium gradients and buffers on bovine chromaffin cells. J Physiol 1992;450:273-301.
8. Zhou Z, Neher E. Mobile and immobile calcium buffers in bovine adrenal chromaffin cells. J Physiol 1993;469:245-73.
9. Chard PS, Bleakman D, Christakos S, Fullmer CS, Miller RJ. Calcium buffering properties of calbindin D28k and parvalbumin in rat sensory neurons. J Physiol 1993;472:341-57.
10. Kasai H, Peterson OH. Spatial dynamics of second messengers: IP3 and cAMP as long-range and associative messengers. Trends Neurosci 1994;17:95-101.
11. Balentine JD, Paris DU, Dean DL. Calcium-induced spongiform and necrotizing myelopathy. Lab Invest 1982;47:286-95.
12. Blaustein MP. Calcium transport and buffering in neurons. Trends Neuro Sci. 1988;11:438-43.
13. Carafoli E. The Ca^{2+} pump of the plasma membrane. J Bioi Chern 1992;267:2115-18.
14. Lwe VL, Tsien RY, Miner C. Physiological [Ca^{2+} level and pump-leak turnover in intact red cells measured using an incorporated Ca chelator. Nature 1982;298:478-81.
15. Benveniste H, Drejer J, Schousboe A, Diemer NH. Elevation of the extracellular concentrations of glutamate and aspartate in rat hippocampus during

transient cerebral ischemia monitored by intracerebral microdialysis. J Neurochem 1984;43:1369-74.
16. Kitamura Y, Miyazaki A, Yamanaka Y, Nomura Y. Stimulatory effects of protein kinase C and calmodulin kinase II on N-methyl-D-aspartate receptor/channels in the postsynaptic density of rat brain. J Neurochem 1993; 61:100-109.
17. Tymianski M, Charlton MP, Carlen PL, Tator CH. Properties of neuroprotective cell-per meant Ca^{2+} chelators: Effects on Ca^{2+} and glutamate neurotoxicity *in vitro*. J Neurophysiol 1994;267:1973-92.
18. Mianski M, Spigelman I, Zhang L, Carlen PL, Tator CH, Charlton MP, Wallace MC. Mechanism of action and persistence of neuroprotection by cell permeant Ca^{2+} chela tors. J Cereb Blood Flow Metab 1994;14:911-23.
19. McLean AEM, McLean E, Judah JD. Cellular necrosis in the liver induced and modified by drugs. lnt Rev Exp Pathol 1965;4:127-57.
20. Schanne FAX, Kane AB, Young EA, Farber JL. Calcium dependence of toxic cell death: A final common pathway. Science 1979;206:700-702.
21. Schlaepfer WW, Bunge RP. Effects of calcium ion concentration on the degeneration of amputated axons in tissue culture. J Cell Biol 1973;59(2):456-70.
22. Jancso G, Karcsu S, Kiraly E, Szebeni A, Toth L, Bacsy E, Joo F, Parducz A. Neurotoxin induced nerve cell degeneration: Possible involvement of calcium. Brain Res 1984;295:211-6.
23. Choi DW. Glutamate neurotoxicity in cortical cell culture is calcium dependent. Neurosci Lett 1985;58:293-7.
24. Garthwaite G, Garthwaite J. Neurotoxicity of excitatory amino acid receptor agonists in rat cerebellar slices: Dependence on calcium concentration. Neurosci Lett 1986;66:193-8.
25. Balentine JD. Spinal Cord Trauma. In search of the meaning of granular axoplasm and vesicular myelin. J Neuropathol Exp Neurol 1988;47:77-92.
26. Balentine JD, Paris DU, Dean DL. Calcium-induced spongiform and necrotizing myelopathy. Lab Invest 1982;47:286-95.
27. Cheung JY, Bonventre N, Malis CD, Leaf A. Calcium and Ischemic Injury. N Engl J Med 1986;314:1670-76.
28. Dingledine R, Boland LM, Chamberlin NL, Kawasaki K, Kleckner NW, Traynelis SF, Verdoorn TA. Amino acid receptors and uptake systems in the mammalian central nervous system. CRC Crit Rev Neurobiol 1988;4:1-97.
29. Nakanishi S. Molecular diversity of glutamate receptors and implications for brain function. Science 1992;258:597-603.
30. Collinridge GL, Singer W. Excitatory amino acid receptors and synaptic plasticity. Trends Pharmacol Sci 1990;11:290-96.
31. Ozyurt E, Graham DI, Woodruff GN, McCulloch J. Protective effect of the glutamate antagonist MK-801 in focal cerebral ischemia in the cat. J Cereb Blood Flow Metab 1988;8:138-43.
32. Olney JW. Brain lesion, obesity and other disturbances in mice treated with monosodium glutamate. Science 1969;164:719-21.
33. Choi DW, Maulucci-Gedde M, Kriegstein AR. Glutamate neurotoxicity in cortical cell culture. J Neurosci 1987; 7:357-68.
34. Garthwaite J, Garthwaite G. The mechanism of kainic acid neurotoxicity. Nature. 1983;305:138-40.
35. Gilbertson TA, Scobey R, Wilson M. Permeation of calcium ions through non-NMDA glutamate channels in retinal bipolar cells. Science 1991;251:1613-5.
36. Hollman M, Hartley M, Heinemann S. Ca^{2+} permeability of KA-AMPA-gated glutamate receptor channels depends on subunit composition. Science 1991;252:851-3.
37. MacDermott AB, Mayer ML, Westbrook GL, Smith SJ, Barker JL. NMDA-receptor activation increases cytoplasmic calcium concentration in cultured spinal cord neurons. Nature 1986;321:519-22.
38. Choi OW. Ionic dependence of glutamate neurotoxicity. J Neurosci 1987;7:369-79.
39. Choi OW, Maulucci-Gedde M, Kriegstein AR. Glutamate neurotoxicity in cortical cell culture. J Neurosci 1987; 7:357-68.
40. Eimrel S, Schramm M. The quantity of calcium that appears to induce neuronal death. J Neurochem 1994; 62:1223-6.
41. Baker AI, Moulton RI, MacMillan VB, Shedden PM. Excitatory amino acids in cerebrospinal fluid following traumatic brain injury in humans. J Neurosurg 1993; 79:369-72.
42. Astrup J, Siesjo BK, Symon L. Thresholds in Cerebral Ischemia: The Ischemic Penumbra. Stroke 1981;12:723-5.
43. Ozawa K, Seta K, Araki H, Handa H. The effect of ischemia on mitochondrial metabolism. J Bioi Chern 1966;61:512-14.
44. Cox JA Lysko PG, Henneberry RC. Excitatory amino acid neurotoxicity at the N-methyl-D-aspartate receptor in cultured neurons: Role of the voltage-dependent magnesium block. Brain Res 1989;499:267-72.
45. Nowak L, Bregestovski P, Ascher P. Magnesium gates glutamate-activated channels in mouse central neurones. Nature 1984;307:462-5.
46. Abele AE, Scholz KP, Scholz WK, Miller RJ. Excitotoxicity induced by enhanced excitatory neurotransmission in cultured hippocampal pyramidal neurons. Neuron 1990; 4:413-19.
47. Rosenberg PA, Aizenman E. Hundred-fold increase in neuronal vulnerability to glutamate toxicity in astrocyte-poor culture of rat cerebral cortex. Neurosci 1989;103: 162-8.
48. Rosenberg PA, Arnin S, Leitner M. Glutamate uptake disguises neurotoxic potency of glutamate agonists in cerebral cortex in dissociated cell culture. J Neurosci 1992;12:56-61.
49. Choi OW. Cerebral hypoxia: Some new approaches and unanswered questions. J Neurosci 1990;10:2493-2501.

50. Kiedrowski L, Brooker G, Costa E, Wroblewski JT. Glutamate impairs neuronal calcium extrusion while reducing sodium gradient. Neuron 1994;12:295-300.
51. De Erausquin GA, Manev H, Guidotti A, Costa E, Brooker G. Gangliosides normalize distorted single-cell intracellular free Ca^{2+} dynamics after toxic doses of glutamate in cerebellar granule cells. Proc Natl Acad Sei USA 1990;87:8017-21.
52. Vlessis AA, Widener LL, Bartos D. Effect of peroxide, sodium, and calcium on brain mitochondrial respiration in vitro: Potential role in cerebral ischemia and reperfusion. J Neurochem 1990;54:1412-8.
53. Gadian DC, Frackowiak RSJ, Crockard HA, Proctor E, Allen K, Williams SR, Russell RWR. Acute cerebral ischemia. Concurrent changes in cerebral blood flow, energy metabolites, pH and lactate measured with hydrogen clearance and 31p and lH nuclear magnetic resonance spectroscopy-I: Methodology. J Cereb Blood Flow Metab 1987;7:199-206.
54. Hartley Z, Dubinsky JM. Changes in intracellular pH associated with glutamate excitotoxicity. J Neurosci 1993;13:4690-99.
55. Irwin RP, Paul SM. Glutamate exposure rapidly decreases intracellular pH in rat hippocampal neurons in culture. Sac Neurosci Abstr 1992;18:118-10.
56. Siesjo BK, Katsura K, Tibor K. Acidosis related brain damage, in Siesjo BK, Wieloch T (Eds): Advances in Neurological Cellular and Molecular Mechanisms of Ischemic Brain Damage. New York, Raven Press.
57. Gaab MR, Seegers K, Smedema RJ, Heissler HE, Goetz C. A comparative analysis of THAM (Tris-buffer) 41 trauatic brain oedema. Acta Neurochir Suppl (Wien) 1990;51:320-23.
58. Wolf AL, Levi L, Marmarou A, Ward JD, Muizelaar JP, Choi 5, Young H, Rigamonti D, Robinson WL. Effect of THAM upon outcome in severe head injury: A randomized prospective clinical trial. J Neurosurg 1993;78:54-9.
59. Eimrel S, Schramm M. The quantity of calcium that appears' to induce neuronal death. J Neurochem 1994;62: 1223-6.
60. Matsumoto Y, Kamata T, Goto N. The suppression by niz of enone of the release of glutamate and lactate as a mechanism of its neuroprotective effect: An *in vivo* brain microdialysis study. J Cereb Blood Flow Metab 13 [Suppl 1]:S742,1993.
61. Graham SH, Chen J, Sharp FR, Simon RP. Limiting ischemic injury by inhibition of excitatory amino acid release. J Cereb Blood Flow Metab 1993;13:88-97.
62. Boxer PA, Cordon IT, Mann ME, Rodolosi LC, Vartanian MG, Rock DM, Taylor CP, Marcoux FW. Comparison of phenytoin with noncompetitive N-methyl-D-aspartate antagonists in a model of focal brain ischemia. Stroke 1990;21 [Suppl 11]:1147-51.
63. Tymianski M, Tator CH. The direct effects of nimodipine on intracellular calcium in spinal neurons in explant culture. Drugs Dev 1993;2:337-47.
64. Tsien RY. New calcium indicators and buffers with high selectivity against magnesium and protons: Design, synthesis, and properties of prototype structures. Biochemistry 1980;19:2396-2404.
65. Tombaugh GC, Sapolsky RM. Mechanistic distinctions between excitotoxic and acidotic hippocampal damage in vitro model of ischemia. J Cereb Blood Flow Metab 1990;10:527-35.
66. Fariss MW, Pascoe GA, Reed OJ. Vitamin E reversal of the effect of extracellular calcium on induced toxicity in hepatocytes. Science 1985;227:751-4.
67. Iadecola C, Pelligrino DA, Moscowitz MA, Lassen NA. State of the art review: Nitric oxide inhibition and cerebrovascular regulation. J Cereb Blood Flow Metab 1994;14:175-92.
68. Roberts-Lewis JM, Marcy VR. Zhao Y, Vaught JL, Siman R, Lewis ME. Aurintricarboxylic acid protects hippocampal neurons from NMDA- and ischemia-induced toxicity *in vivo*. J Neurochem 1993;61:378-81.
69. Rodorf G, Koroshetz WJ, Bonventre V. Heat shock proteins protect cultured neurons from glutamate toxicity. Neuron 1991;7:1043-51.
70. M Tymianski, Tator CH. Normal and abnormal calcium homeostasis in neurons: a basis for the pathophysiology of traumatic and ischemic central nervous system injury. Neurosurgery 1996;38:1176-95.
71. Sun DA, Deshpande LS, Sombati S, Baranova A, et al. Traumatic brain injury causes a long lasting Ca^{2+} plateau of elevated intracellular ca level and altered Ca^{2+} homeostatic mechanisms in hippocampal neurons surviving brain injury. Europ J of Neurosciences 2008; 7:1659-72.

8 Ischemic Damage in Brain Following Head Injury

AK Mahapatra

INTRODUCTION

Head injury is a growing public health problem in India, as well as all over the world with an overall incidence ranging from 200 to 300/100,000 population. Over last decade, the incidence has steadingly increased in Indian metropolies and in 2008, over 2276 fatal head injuries were reported from Delhi and over 10,000 had minor injuries. No doubt, prevention of head injury is ideal. However, in best of the circumstances it may not be possible. Thus, early diagnosis, timely surgery and adequate protection of brain are probably the main objectives of modern treatment of severe head injury. The ultimate outcome of severe head injury depends on several factors. Secondary damage such as edema, ischemia and necrosis play an important role in ultimate outcome. Graham and his colleague have demonstrated ischemic damage in fatal head injury.[1-3] However, sometimes it is possible to prevent the secondary pathological process which are almost invariably present following injury[4-9] and more harmful than primary damage. These are edema, ischemia and necrosis. In this chapter attempt has been made to highlight the role of the ischemic brain damage following head injury.[2,4,10-13] In fatal head injury, ischemic damage is reported in 85 to 90 percent cases.[1-3]

PATHOPHYSIOLOGY OF ISCHEMIC INJURY

Pathological changes in head injury is the widespread which affect brainstem, cerebellum and cerebrum. Primary pathology following injury are the various intracranial hematomas, cerebral contusion and laceration. However, with the advent of the CT scanning it has been very well observed that a significant number of severe head injury patients may die or remain vegetative even in absence of demonstrated hematomas in brain.[14,15] Recently, MRI, SPECT studies and cerebral perfusion parameters have demonstrated widespread cerebral ischemia following head injury,[10,16-19] SPECT studies have shown reduction of blood flow in frontal and temporal lobe even in minor head injured patients with postconcussion syndrome.[19a] The histopathological studies by Graham and his colleague[1-3,9] had proved beyond doubt the widespread ischemic injury in brain, in patients with head injury. In 1977 Graham[3] described the pathological changes in brain, in patients with head injury, secondary to hypoxia and ischemic damage in 91 percent cases of 151 fatal nonmissile head injury. Recent autopsy studies have also shown ischemic brain damage in over 85 percent patients with fatal closed head injury.[2,16] Low cerebral perfusion is also recorded around focal contusion, and acute SDH.[16a,16b]

FAILURE OF MICROCIRCULATION

Basic reason leading to the development of ischemic lesions in head injury is raised RCP, compromising cerebral perfusion. Systemic blood pressure remaining constant, when intracranial pressure increases the cerebral perfusion pressure (CPP) falls. However, the perfusion is maintained till the perfusion pressure is above 70 mm Hg. When EPP reduced below 70 mm Hg, there is likelihood of cerebral ischemia. There is selective vulnerability of different part of the brain to the ischemic insult, which is also of varying degree at different areas of the brain. Graham et al in 1989 reported almost equal incidence of ischemic injury in brain in patients between 1968-72 and 1981-82. Ischemic damage is observed more frequently in Hippocampus. Basal ganglia (Fig. 8.1) than cerebral cortex and cerebellum. As ischemic damage is related to high rep and low perfusion pressure, this condition is reported in all the age groups.[1,3,17,20] The available evidences suggest that in majority cases ischemia occurs fairly early after injury.[1,3,8,9,13] Moeschier et al[8] reported systemic insults occurring either prior to hospital admission or within hospital, during the emergency procedures. They also reported short episodes of hypotension may involve marked cerebral ischemia, which even persists after adequate systemic hemodynamic restoration. Sahuquillo et al[13] analyzed the risk factors for early post-traumatic ischemia and concluded that the ischemia is highly prevalent in the early period after severe head injury.

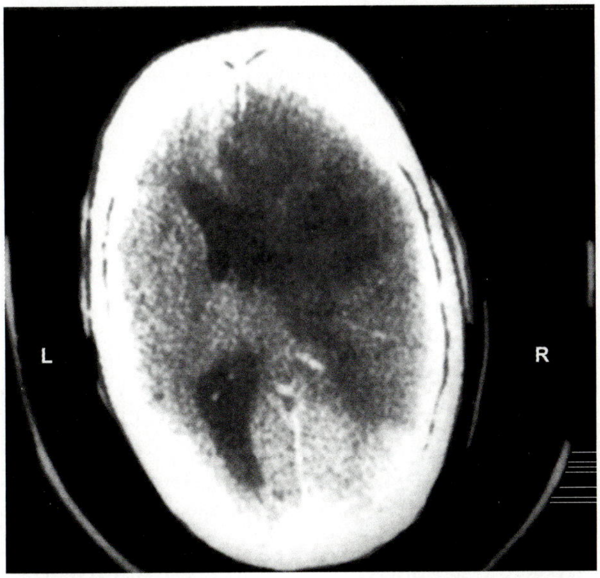

Fig. 8.1: NCCT showing right hemispheric infarct

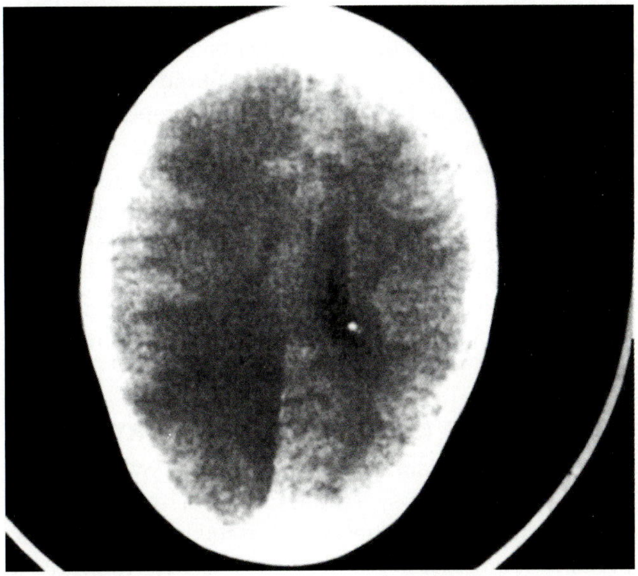

Fig. 8.2: NCCT head shows left sided basal ganglia infarct in a patient with head injury

FACTORS RESPONSIBLE FOR ISCHEMIA

Evidences from the clinical studies show that the ischemic brain damage is the major factor for bad outcome in severe head injury. Laboratory studies and animal experiments indicate that the excitatory amino acids are important mediators causing brain damages.

The mechanisms involved in ischemic brain damage is primarily due to calcium overload, acidosis and liberation of free radicals. In ischemia there is anaerobic metabolism leading to lactic acidosis. The presence of glutamate and increased intracellular calcium the calcium channel opens up.

The early post-traumatic blood flow mapping and small vessel ultrastructure studies at different points reveals a zone of ischemic brain, invariably present around the contusion. Ischemic damage also occurs in acute subdural hematoma.[6]

Ischemia results due to increase in extracellular glutamate concentration. Hence, the drugs which act at N-Methy 1-0 Aspartate, (NMOA)/receptor, which is a subtype of glutamate, have been shown to reduce ischemic brain damage. Inglis et al[6] in an experimental study in rats assessed the cerebral glucose utilization and CBF, by using double lable autoradiography. They found a hypermetabolic state and increase glucose utilization in the Hippocampus.

Sahuquillo et al[13] studied severe head injured patients to detect early ischemia. They analyzed arteriojugular venous differences of oxygen ($AVDO_2$) and arterior jugular lactate-oxygen $AOOL/AVDO_2$. They divided patients into ischemic group and non-ischemic group. They observed that the arterial hemoglobin and the ischemia score were significantly different in both groups.

Ischemia can develop due to large artery involvement.[11,12,21] Post-traumatic occlusive vascular problem is more frequent in children than adult. Occlusion may involve internal carotid or MCA (Fig. 8.2) artery. In a study of 220 pediatric head injury Walia[22] noticed 4 children with hemispheric (Fig. 8.3) infarcts. Rarely ischemia does involve the basal ganglia area.[20] In infants ischemia can also result due to hemoconcentration, resulting from the use of osmotic diuretics and restricted fluid intake. Thus, the microcirculation gets involved leading to ischemic damage. Post-traumatic

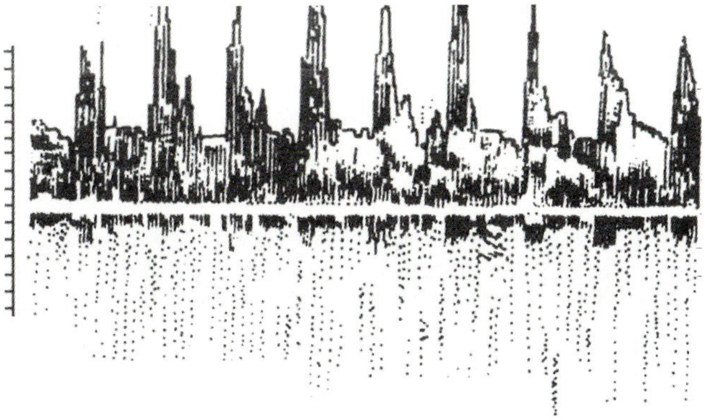

Fig. 8.3: TCD, right MCA shows normal flow velocity in patient with severe head injury

vasospasm can lead to ischemic brain damage, reported up to 20 percent patients.[11,12,23,24] Marshall and Gautille 11 reported subarachnoid hemorrhage in 491 patients with head injury and reported small and large area of infarct as seen in CT scan. Marshall et al[23] 1978, reported vasospasm leading to clinical deterioration between 5th and 9th day. Recently, Bakshi and Mahapatra[24] have demonstrated high blood flow velocity in basilar artery, in 40 percent patients severe head injury. Very very rarely venous sinus thrombosis can lead to venous infarct in brain following head injury.

DIAGNOSIS OF ISCHEMIC BRAIN INJURY

Ischemic brain damage in head injury was initially diagnosed in autopsy studies.[1,3] Even recent studies have shown the presence of ischemia in over 85 percent fatal cases.[2,4] With routine ICP monitoring and CBF study it is possible to find out the time of onset of ischemia.[6,10,17,25] With the advent of CT, MRI and SPECT the ischemia is well visualized and can be graded (Table 8.1).[10,18,25] SPECT helps in assessing regional cerebral blood flow using (HMPAO) or mTC Ethylene Cyteine Dimer (ECD). The tomographic image obtained with Gamma camera provides cerebral perfusion in different cortical areas. Normally, there is bilateral symmetrical cortical uptake of HMPAO.

Use of TCD is helpful in assessing blood flow velocity[24-26] (Fig. 8.3). Czosnyka et al[25] in 1994, studied ICP, blood flow velocity (FV) and pulsatility index (PI). They estimated cerebrovascular resistance (CVR= CPP/FV). Their results showed CPP lower than 55 mm Hg means failure of autoregulation and onset of cerebral ischemia. Chan et al[16] performed TCD in head injury patients, and the blood flow velocity in MCA was recorded. They concluded that TCD can provide an alternative mean to identify cerebral ischemia. Bakshi and Mahapatra[24] for the 1st time studied the basilar artery blood flow velocity in 16 severe head injury patients. They observed abnormally high flow velocity in 7 patients.

Table 8.1: Ischemic brain injury as seen in CT or autopsy	
Focal	a. With focal lesion
	b. Without focal lesion
Hemispheric	a. With focal lesion
	b. Without focal lesion
Diffuse	

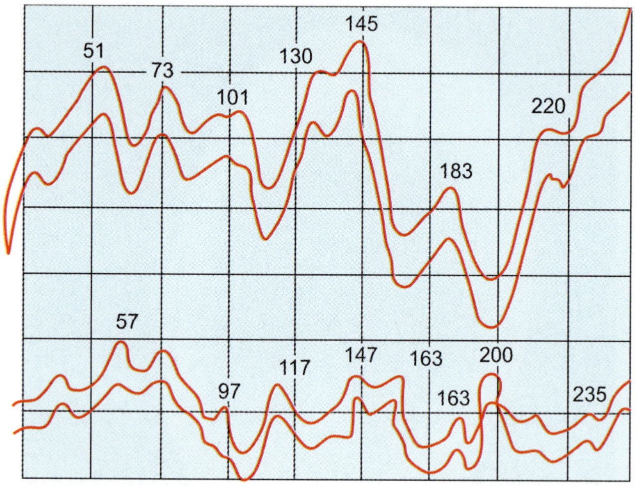

Fig. 8.4: Brainstem auditory evoked potential

Evoked potentials (EPs) are (Fig. 8.4) helpful to assess cerebral cortical and brainstem function in head injury patients.[14,19] In absence of detectable CT pathology abnormal BAEP or SEP mean impaired function most likely due to ischemia. Lesnick et al[19] reported altered sensory evoked potential (SEP) in patients with global cerebral ischemia.[19a] Thus, indicating usefulness of SEP (Fig. 8.5).

Excitotoxicity and oxidative stress mediate neuronal death after hypoxic ischemic brain injury. 2-hydroxy-5-2 (2,3,5,6-tetrafluoro-4-trifluoromethyl-benzylamino)-benzoic acid (Neuro 2000) derived from aspirin and sulfasalazine was used to prevent both NMDA neurotoxicity and oxidative stress in experimental animals. Neuro 2000 may be novel therapy in preventing neuronal death from ischemia and may offer profound neuroprotection.[28]

PREVENTION OF ISCHEMIC INJURY

Ischemic injury to brain is one of the most important preventable cause of death, even today.[2,5,9,13] In a study conducted by Bullocks it was observed that in a third

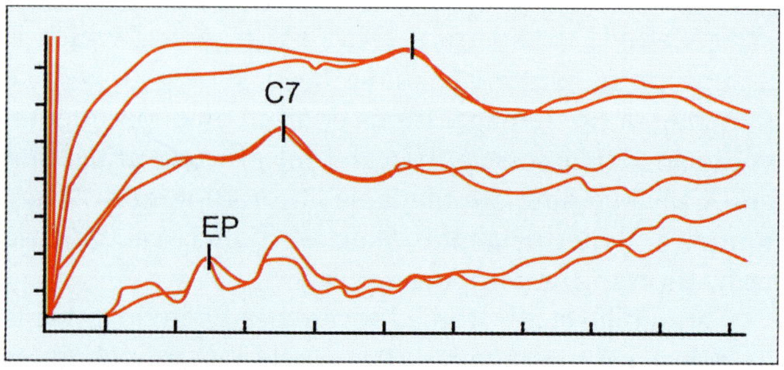

Fig. 8.5: Sensory evoked potential (SEP) in a patient with severe head injury shows normal wave

Table 8.2: Protection from ischemia
Prevention of hypoxia by timely intubation
Reduction of ICP
Maintenance of systemic blood pressure and CPP
Role of steroid
Role of hypervolemia
Raising hemoglobin contain of blood

of the cases, death could have been prevented and among them 88 percent were due to hypoxic ischemic damage.

Factors included in preventable cause of death are, failure to prevent hypoxic brain damage by timely intubation and quick resuscitation (Tables 8.2 and 8.3). This happens mostly prior to arrival in a specialized center. Delay in referral and inadequate control of raised ICP are the most important causes. Systemic insults can occur even before the patients reach the hospital, during intrahospital transport or at the time of embergery management. Recent studies have indicated that the short episodes of hypotension may result in severe ischemic brain damage, that will persist even after complete hemodynamic restoration. Hence, the treatment of the episodic hypotension should be quick and aggressive. Heros and Kotosne[27] suggested hemodilution to increase the cerebral blood flow, which is likely to reduce ischemic damage. Thus, one important key to prevent the ischemic brain damage is to maintain the oxygenation and systemic blood pressure, which can prevent perfusion defect and anaerobic metabolism.

Adequate prevention of raised ICP is important. Raised ICP reduces cerebral perfusion pressure. Hence, it is necessary to continuously monitor ICP for 2-3 days and adequately control ICP to maintain cerebral perfusion. Intravenous mannitol is one of the widely used method to reduce ICP (Table 8.3). However, prolonged use is sometime harmful and ineffective. Recently, methylprednisolone is a widely used neuroprotective drug.[28] Glucocorticoids and nonglucocorticoid steroids exert free radicae scavanging activity and are tried in neurosurgical disorders including head injury. Methylprednisolone is already in common clinical use in spinal for injury and is also used as neuroprotective agent in the management of subarachnoid hemorrhage and severe head injury. Chen et al[28] studied the cellular uptake and transport of methylprednisolone (MP) at the level of blood-brain barrier, in guinea pigs. MP has a membrane stabilizing effect by binding to cytoplasmic endothelial glucocorticoid receptors.

Table 8.3: Mode to increase cerebral perfusion
a. By reducing ICP
Mannitol
High dosage steroid
Ventricular drainage
b. By increasing systemic pressure
Maintaining blood pressure
Increasing circulating volume
Reducing viscosity of blood
c. By preventing dehydration
Adequate treatment of fever, electrolyte disturbance and infection

Recently, calcium channel blockers have been tried. In a multicentric study no beneficial effect was noticed using calcium channel blocker. As the hypoxia leads to acidosis, it is most important to treat acidosis. Tris-hydroxymethyl aminothane (THAM) is widely used to raise the cellular pH and combat acidosis. Recently, NMDA antagonists are used to reduce ischemic damage.[5,6] In an experimental study Bullock[5] reported dramatic reduction of ischemic damage in cats pretreated with NMDA antagonist, prior to MCA occlusion. Similar results were observed in rats with experimental subdural hematoma. Identical observations were made by Inglis et al in 1990[6] in an experimental study in rats. MK 801, a potent NMDA blocker helps in reducing ischemic injury to brain. However, these agents are not widely used in clinical practice.

NEWBORN ENCEPHALOPATHY (NE)

The term hypoxic-ischemic encephalopathy (HIE) of newborn and perinatal asphyxia have been used loosely. Clinical sigus–of HIE are often wrongfully considered to result from intrapartum asphyxia. In reality, establishing a clear relationship between perinatal brain injury and HIE is often different. The term newborn encephalopathy (NE) was hence proposed as an alternative. In immediate newborn period many factors can produce symptoms like HIE including prepartum and postpartum ischemia, genetic factors, metabolic diseases and maternal and fetal drugs.[29]

The other features of NE includes decreased activity after first day of life, need for incubator for more than 3 days, feeding problems, poor suck and respiratory difficulties and static motor deficits (cerebral palsy) epilepsy and mental retardation. Low Apgar score neonatal seizure stupor and coma, etc. In fetal life these disturbances are primarily due to hypoperfusion because the arterial partial pressure of O_2 (PaO_2) normally is low. Despite this sever hypoxia can occur leading to myocardial dysfunction, cerebral hypoperfusion and failure of autoregulation. Hypoperfusion may lead to neuronal ischemia.[30]

CONCLUSION

Ischemic brain damage is one of the most important secondary change that occurs following head injury. Ischemia is noticed over 85 percent patients with fatal head injury. Very often it is preventable. **Hypoxia** and **hypotension** are the two most important causes which lead to ischemic brain damage. Adequate prevention to **hypoxia** and **hypotension** will significantly reduce the ischemic brain lesion and increase the chance of survival and recovery in patients with severe head injury.

REFERENCES

1. Graham DI, Adam JH, Doyle D. Ischaemic brain damage in nonmissile head injury. J Neurol Sciences 1978;39:213-34.
2. Graham DI, Ford I, Adam JH, Doyle O, Teasdale GM, Lawrence AE, Mclellan DP. Ischaemic brain damage is still common in fatal non-missile head injury. J Neurol Neurosurg Psychiat 1989;52:346-50.
3. Graham DR. In: Pathology of hypoxic brain damage in man, hypoxia and Ischemia. BC Mirson (Ed). J of Clin Pathol (Suppl) Royal College of Pathology 1977;11:170-80.
4. Bennett M, O'Brien DP, Phillips JP, Farrell MA. Clinicopathological observation in 100 consecutive patients with fatal head injury admitted to a neurosurgical unit. Irs Med J. 1995;88:168-68.
5. Bullock R. Introducing NMDA antagonist into clinical practice. Why head injury trials? Br J Clin Pharmacol 1992;34:396-401.
6. Inglis FM, Bullock R, Chen MH, Graham DI, Miller JD, McCulloch J. Ischaemic brain damage associated with tissue hypermetabolism is acute subdural haematoma, reduction by a glutamate antagonist. Acta Neurochir Suppl (Wien) 1990;51:277-9.
7. Kriger AI, Adler RJ. Advances in the prevention and treatment of secondary brain injury. In: Modern Trend in the Management of Neurotrauma. PS Ramani and Alok Sharma (Eds), Lavanya Prints, Bombay 1994;29-32.
8. Moeschler O, Boulard G, Ravussin P. Concept of secondary cerebral injury of systemic origin. Ann Fre Anaesth Reavin 1995;14:114-21.
9. Siesjo BK. Pathophysiology and treatment of focal cerebral ischemia. Part II Mechanism of damage and treatment. J Neurosurg 1992;77:337-53.
10. Bullock R, Sakas D, Patterson J, et al. Early post-traumatic cerebral blood flow mapping. Correlation with structural damage after focal injury. Acta Neurochir Suppl (Wien) 1992;55:14-17.
11. Marshall LF, Gaotille TH. Large and small "Holes in the brain, reversible or irreversible change in head injury. Acta Neurochir (Suppl) 1990;51:300-1.
12. MacPherson P, Graham Dr. Correlation between angiographic findings and the ischemia of head injury. J Neurol Neurosurg Psychiat 1978;41:122-7.
13. Sahuquillo J, Pica MA, Garnacho A, Robles A, Coello F, Godot C, Triginer C, Rubio E. Early ischaemia after severe head injury. Preliminary result in patient with diffuse brain injury. Acta Neurochir (Wien) 1993;122:204-14.
14. Mahapatra AK, Tandon PN. Brainstem auditory evoked response and vestibulo-occular reflex in severe head injury. A prospective study of 60 cases. Acta Neurochir (Wien) 1987;87:40-3.
15. Mahapatra AK, Tandon PN, Bhatia R, Banerji AK. Bilateral decerebration in head injury patients. An analysis of 62 cases. Surg Neurol 1985;23:36-40.
16. Chan KH, Dearden NM, Miller JD. Transcranial Doppler sonography in severe head injury. Acta Neurochir Suppl (Wien) 1993;59:81-5.

16a. McLaughlin MR, Marion DW. Cerebral blood flow and Vasoresponsibility within and around cerebral contusion. J Neurosurg 1996;85:871-6.

16b. Salvant JB, Muizelaar JP. Changes in cerebral blood flow and metabolism related to subdural haematoma Neurosurg 1993;33:387-93.

17. Jenkin A. The importance of cerebral perfusion pressure maintenance in severe head injury. In: Modern Trend in the management of Neurotrauma. PS Ramani and Alok Sharma (Eds), Lavanya Print, Bombay 1994;33-4.
18. Lele YR. Single photon emission computed tomography (SPECT) studies in head trauma. In: Modern trend in management of Neurotrauma. Lavanya Prints, Bombay 1994;27-8.

18a. Agrawal D, Naveen K, Bala CS, Mahapatra AK. Post Concussion. Syndrome in the Pediatric Population. Is medial temporal damage is responsile ? Correlation with Brain SPECT. A prospective controlled study. Child's Nerves Syst. IT : 628, 2003 (Abstract).

19. Lennick JA, Michele JJ, Simeone FA, Defeo S, Walsh FA. Alteration of somatosensory evoked potentials in response to global ischaemia. J Neurosurg 1984;60:490-94.

19a. Cater GB, Butt W. Review of the use of somatosensory evoked potential in the prediction of outcome after severe brain injury. Crit Care Med 2001;29:178-86.

20. Dharkar SR. Traumatic ischaemic lesion in children. Neurology Ind (Suppl) 1995;43:61-5.

21. Willkin RH, Odoms GL. Intracranial arterial spasm associated with craniocerebral trauma. J Neurosurg 1970;32:626-33.
22. Walia B. Head Injury in Pediatric age group. M Ch. Thesis submitted AIIMS 1996.
23. Marshall LF, Bruce DA, Bruno L, Langfit TW. Vertebrobasilar spasm, a significant cause of neurological deficit in head injury. J Neurosurg 1978;48:560-4.
24. Bakshi A, Mahapatra AK. Basilar artery vasospasm in severe head injury. A preliminary transcranial Doppler study. NMJI 1998;113:220-21.
25. Czosnyka M, Guazzo E, lyre V, Kirkpatrick P, Smielewski P, et al. Testing of cerebral autoregulation in head injury by waveform. Analysis of blood flow velocity and cerebral perfusion pressure. Acta Neurochir Suppl (Wien) 1994;6:468-71.
26. Yang BO, Feng Z, Zhang Z, Sun H. A transcranial Doppler study of drainage of CSF and intracranial haematoma. In modern trends in the management of Neurotrauma. PS Ramani and Alok Sharma (Eds), Lavanya Prints, Bombay, p-36, 1994.
27. Heros RC, Kotosne K. Haemodilution for cerebral ischaemia. Curr Concept Cerebrovas Dis Stroko 1988; 23:31-6.
28. Chen TC, Mackie JB, Mccomb JG, et al. Cellular uptake and transport of methylprednisolone at the blood-brain barrier. Neurosurgery 1996;38:348-61.
29. Gwag BJ, Lee YA, Kosy, Lee MJ, et al. Marked prevention of ischemic brain injury by Neuro 2000, an NMDA antagonist and antioxidant derived from aspirin and sulphasalazine: J Cerebral Blood Flow Metab 2007;(6): 1142-51.
30. Menezes MS, Shaw DWW. Hypoxic ischemic brain injury in newborn in medicine specialities, 2006.

9 Neurological Examination of Head Injured Patients

Raj Kamal

INTRODUCTION

The neurological evaluation of the patient with head injury remains the single most comprehensive process in the diagnostic evaluation. Thorough and careful examination provides an index of generalized and focal dysfunction of the nervous system which is not provided by CT scanning, ICP monitoring or any other modern technology. Repeated good, reliable thorough examination indicates the ongoing neurological state and the progress or failure of treatment rendered. The clinical value of neurological examination thus remains prominent in the initial assessment and subsequent management of head injured patients.

Also, careful general examination must define associated injuries, any source of internal bleeding or any other clinical problem requiring prompt therapy.

The major goals in the evaluation of patients with head injury are:

1. To define the presence of intracranial mass lesion requiring operative removal.
2. To determine abnormal intracranial mass lesion in order to guide and direct appropriate operative or nonoperative therapy.
3. To diagnose associated serious injuries.

In patients who are conscious, the initial examination is as thorough as possible. In patient with altered consciousness, emphasis is given to certain critical aspects that will guide immediate treatment.

HISTORY

Information regarding precise time of injury and mechanism of injury should be obtained. Acceleration injuries as a result of vehicular accidents and falls is associated with serious diffuse brain injury and polar contusion. Impact injuries such as blow to cranial vault result in underlying focal brain damage.

A history of the patient's neurological function at the scene of the accident and during transport to the hospital should be sought from police, relatives or witnesses. Any history of loss of consciousness and seizures should be obtained. A report from a referring hospital of the patient's condition should also be sought and recorded.

Information regarding drug or alcohol intake and the past medical history is also valuable.

INITIAL EXAMINATION

Vital Signs

Pulse rate, blood pressure and respiration should be assessed and given top priority in the management of traumatic brain injury. **Hypertension** associated with bradycardia suggests severely increased intracranial pressure from increasing intracranial clot. Unexplained hypotension with bradycardia points towards a possibility of cervical injury. **Hypotension** associated with tachycardia usually indicates presence of visceral injury elsewhere such as abdominal or thoracic injury.

Hypertension + Bradycardia ~ Intracranial clot

Hypotension + Bradycardia ~ Cervical injury

Hypotension + Tachycardia ~ Abdominal/Thoracic injury

Shallow and deep respirations in a cyclical fashion known as Cheyne-Stokes breathing.[2] It occurs in diffuse, bilateral cortical dysfunction, sufficient to result in drowsiness. Cheyne-Stokes breathing result in hypoventilation and hypercarbia leading to increased intracranial pressure, secondary to vascular stasis and blood pooling. Spontaneous hyperventilation with deep respiration may occur in injury at pontine level often leading to hypocarbia from hyperventilation. Ataxic or irregular respiration occurs in medullary or pontomedullary injuries resulting in hypercarbia.

General Examination

Scalp wounds include small lacerations, perforating lacerations, contused lacerations and massive avulsions. Scalp wounds may be associated with underlying skull fracture (compound injury).

Bleeding from the nose and ear should be recorded. Associated CSF leak from nose (CSF rhinorrhea) and from ear (CSF otorrhea) are usually secondary to basal skull fractures. Fractures of the orbital roofs (Fig. 9.1) result in bilateral periorbital hematomas (raccoon eyes). Associated bleeding beneath the pericranium over the mastoid (Battle's sign) is clinically apparent after 2 or 3 days. Facial paresis or paralysis can occur in patients

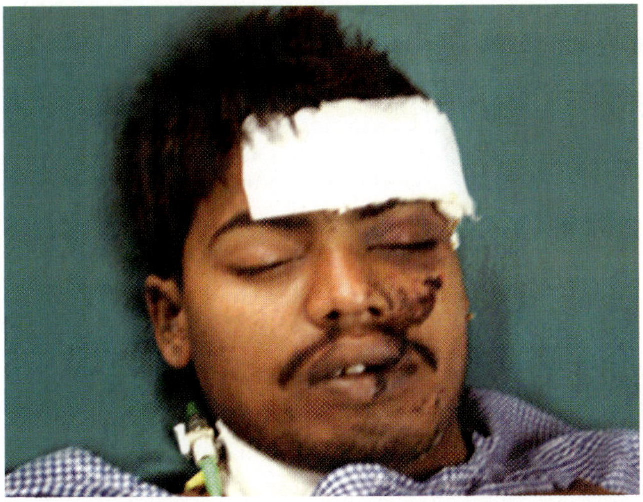

Fig. 9.1: Clinical print of a patient showing periorbital ecchymosis of left eye, multiple abrasions (and cut on lip) over face and dressed forehead wound

with fracture of the petrous bone. The forehead should be palpated for signs of depressed fracture or frontal sinus injury. Asymmetry or irregularity of orbital margins and nose should be checked. Dental occlusion should be checked to rule out mandibular fracture. Cervical injury should be suspected in all severe head injuries and should be ruled out radiologically.

LEVEL OF CONSCIOUSNESS

Level of consciousness is the single most important parameter in a patient of head injury. Many pathological process may impair conscious level and numerous terms have been employed to describe the various clinical states which result, including stupor, semicoma and deep coma. These term result in ambiguity and inconsistency when used by different observers. Teasdale and Jennetr proposed that the degree of coma after severe head injury is the most reliable clinical indicator of the severity of brain damage and present a scale to assess the depth and duration' of impaired consciousness and coma. Coma was defined as the inability to Obey commands, to speak, or to open the eyes, and these three behavioral aspects were incorporated into the Glasgow coma scale[3,4] first introduced in 1974 and then revised by the addition of another motor response level in 1978 (Table 9.1). The sum of the E + M + V value indicates the level of consciousness. Fully conscious patients will have a GCS of 15. GCS of 8 or less is found in coma. Deterioration or improvement can thus be made out at subsequent examinations.

Table 9.1: Glasgow coma scale

Eye opening	
Spontaneous	E4
To Speech	3
To pain only	2
No eye opening	1
Best motor response	
Obeys command	M6
Localizes to stimulation	5
Withdraws from stimulation	4
Abnormal flexion	3
Abnormal extension	2
No motor response	1
Best verbal response	
Oriented and appropriate	V5
Confused	4
Inappropriate words	3
Incomprehensible sounds	2
No verbal response	1

Glasgow coma scale has been adopted by neurosurgical units throughout the world to evaluate their patients with head injuries. Despite its wide acceptance GCS has numerous valid drawbacks.

GCS has been criticised on following points:

1. GCS does not take account of pupillary size and reactivity, pulse rate, respiration, BP.
2. Eye movements and other brainstem reflexes are not included in the scale.
3. Inaccurate recording in patients with bilateral ecchymosis of the eyelids (cannot open his eyes even though fully conscious), aphasia or dysphasia.

The Persistent Vegetative State, Locked-in Syndrome, Akinetic Mutism

The patient who appears to be asleep and is at the same time incapable of being aroused by external stimuli and inner needs is in a state of comas. There are various degrees of coma. In deep coma no reaction of any kind is obtainable: Corneal, pupillary, pharyngeal, tendon and plantar reflex are all absent. With lesser degrees of coma, pupillary reactions, reflex ocular movements and other brainstem reflexes are preserved, and there may be signs of decerebration.

Following modern treatment of severe cerebral injury more and more patients survive for indefinite periods without regaining any meaningful mental function. For the first week or two after the cerebral injury these patients are in a state of deep coma. Then they start opening their eyes spontaneously. The patient

Table 9.2: Neurologic conditions that produce unresponsiveness

Condition	*Self-awareness*	*Motor function*	*Experiences suffering*	*Respiratory function*	*Prognosis*
Persistent vegetative state	Absent	No purposeful movements, no visual tracking	No	Normal	One year outcome in traumatic cases: Died 33% Severely disabled 28% Mod. disabled 17% Good recovery 7% Persistent vegetative state 15%
Locked-in syndrome	Present	Quadriplegia, pseudobulbar palsy, preserved vertical eye movements	Yes	Normal	Recovery unlikely, remains quadriplegic prolonged survival possible
Akinetic mutism	Present	Paucity of movement	Yes	Normal	Recovery unlikely
Brain death	Absent	Absent	No	Absent	None

may blink eyes spontaneously. However, the patient remains inattentive, shows no signs of awareness of the environment or the inner need; responsiveness is limited to primitive postural and reflex movements of limbs. The EEG may approach normality, even showing alpha rhythm and sleep patterns. If lasting, this syndrome referred to as the persistent vegetative state. Neurologic conditions that produce unresponsiveness are given in Table 9.2.

The locked-in state is due most often to a lesion of the basis pontis in which there is a little or no disturbance of awareness but only an inability to respond adequately. Such a lesion interrupts corticospinal and corticobulbar pathways sparing the ascending neuronal systems and somatosensory pathways which are responsible for arousal and wakefulness.[5,7]

Akinetic mutism refers to a partially or fully awake patient who is immobile and silent. The state may result from large bilateral lesion both frontal lobes or in cingulate gyrus.

MEMORY FUNCTION

Memory is usually divided into three categories: Immediate, recent and remote. Immediate memory has a finite capacity and information remains in the store for relatively brief period of time (seconds to minute). This type of store would hold a telephone number for a short time. Immediate recall is tested by forward and backward repetition of digit spans (Seven digits forward and six backwards). Immediate memory is mostly related to attention and consciousness.

Recent memory is assessed at the bedside by telling the patient to remember four different words or objects. After ten minutes the patient is requested to recall from memory the four original objects. Known anatomical substrates for recent memory are located within Hippocampal fornicial mamillothalamic pathways. The exact pathophysiology accounting for loss of recent memory in head trauma is not yet correctly known.

Recent memory typically refers to memories in hours to days, in duration and remote memory refers to distant past memories of many years. These memories are thought to be retained in cerebral cortex.

Memory loss for events prior to injury is termed retrograde amnesia. With recovery, retrograde amnesia shrinks from several hours to several minutes. Hence in retrograde amnesia the problem is in retrieval not in registration. Antegrade amnesia is an inability to lay down new memories following the head injury.

In severe head injuries, antegrade amnesia may persist indefinitely. Post-traumatic amnesia (PTA) refers to the time from injury until the return of a full, ongoing memory process. It is same as antegrade amnesia. Russell and Collaborators[8] have established a direct correlation between severity of the head injury and duration of post-traumatic amnesia (PTA). They established the following scale:

PTA
0-1 hour ~ Mild head injury
1-24 hours ~ Moderate head injury
1-7 days ~ Severe head injury
>7 days ~ Very severe head injury

Studies have shown a close correlation between neurosurgical estimation or post-traumatic amnesia and neuropsychological deficits.

EYES

Pupils

Pupillary size is determined by balance of tonic forces consisting of the pupilloconstrictor parasympathetic and pupillodilator sympathetic controls.

Pathway of pupillary constriction and the light reflex (parasympathetic).

A stimulus, such as bright light shown in the left eye will send an efferent from the retinal ganglion cell through the optic nerve, chiasma, and tract, terminating medially in the pretectal nuclear area, here a second order fiber (intercalated neurons) passes to the Edinger-Westphal nucleus (a IIIrd nerve nucleus) on the same and opposite side via the posterior commissure (Fig. 9.2). The efferent limb of the arc consists of preganglionic parasympathetic neurons joining the oculomotor nerve. The pupillomotor fibers are superficially located in IIIrd nerve. At the level of the superior orbital fissure of the oculomotor nerve divides and the parasympathetic fibers follow the branch to the inferior oblique muscle to synapse in the ciliary ganglion. Postganglionic short ciliary fibers penetrate the globe.

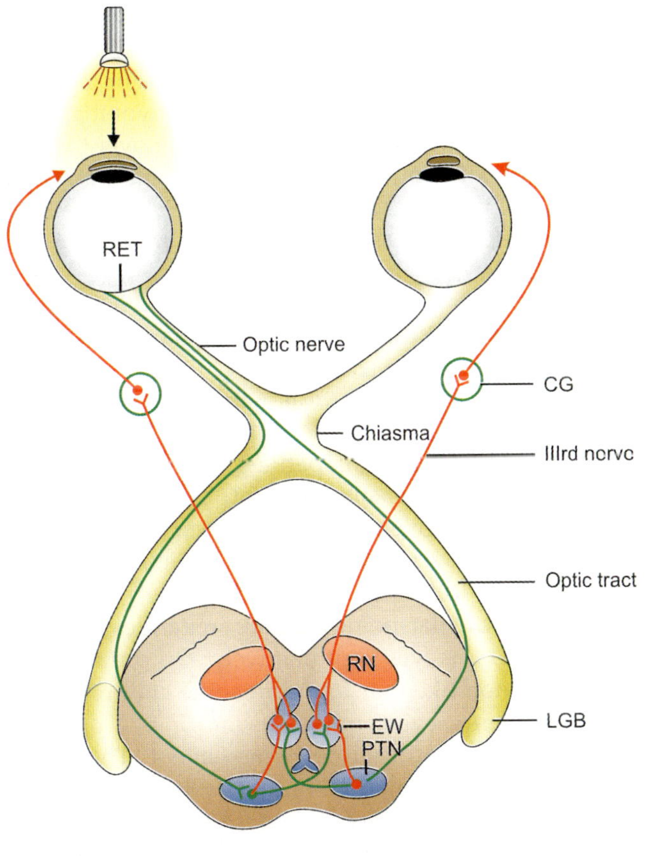

Fig. 9.2: Pupillary light reflex: Parasympathetic pathway stimulation of the retinal photoreceptors, results in excitation of ganglion cells whose axon travel within optic nerve partially decussate in the chiasma, then leave the optic tract and pass through brachium of the superior colliculus (SC) before synapsing at the pretectal nucleus. This structure connects bilaterally within oculomotor nuclear complex at Edinger-Westphal (EW) nuclei, parasympathetic fibers that travels through inferior division of third nerve and end at the ciliary ganglion (CG) in the orbit, RN—Red nucleus, PTN—Pretectal nucleus, LGB—Lateral geniculate body

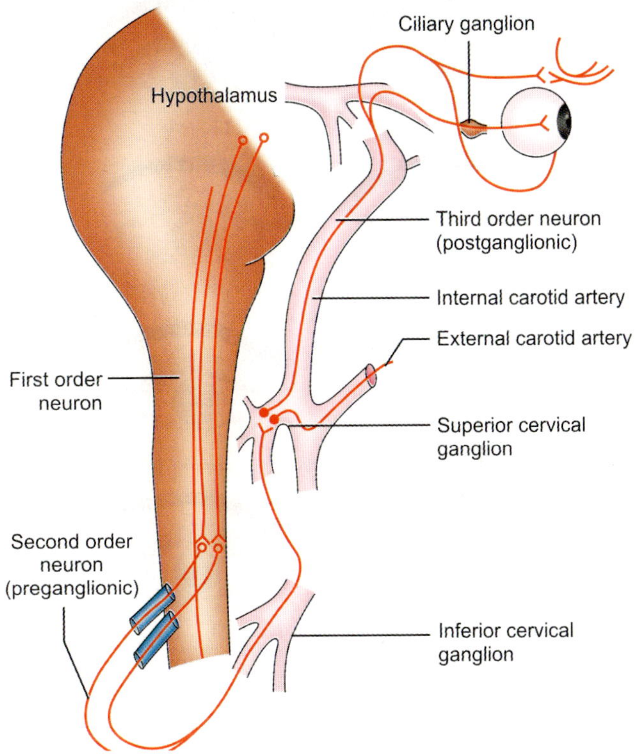

Fig. 9.3: Sympathetic pathways to the eye

Sympathetic fibers descend from hypothalamus through the lateral aspect of brainstem into the spinal cord. The pupillary fibers emerge through the ventral roots of C8, and TI, enter the sympathetic chain and, in the superior cervical ganglion (Fig. 9.3). The postganglionic fibers, arise in the superior cervical ganglion, ascend on the wall of internal carotid artery to enter the cranium. The sympathetic plexus around the internal carotid artery sends branch through the ciliary ganglion, and these postganglionic fibers reach the eyeball through the short ciliary nerves; but some sympathetic fibers may travel through the long ciliary nerves to reach the eyeball. Sudomotor fibers (concerned with sweating) passes through the external carotid artery to the dermis of the face.

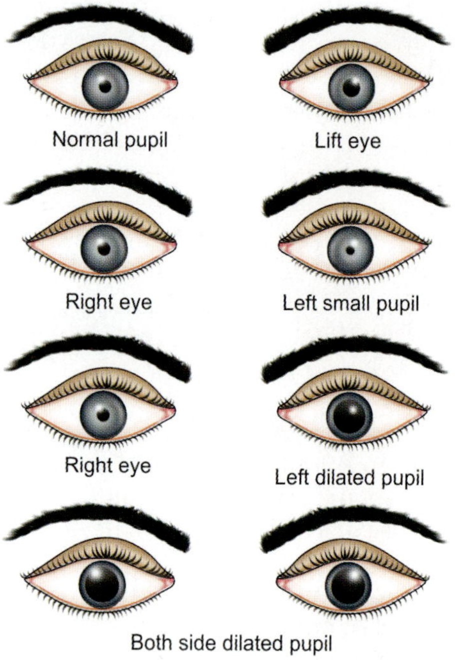

Fig. 9.4: Hutchinson's pupil: Stages

Unilateral, nonreactive dilatation of pupil indicates of transtentorial herniation secondary to an expanding hematoma. Initially, pupil on the side of injury contracts due to irritation of the oculomotor nerve, the opposite pupil remains normal size. In the next stage, the ipsilateral pupil dilates due to paralysis of oculomotor nerve. Finally the pupils of both sides become dilated and fixed, not reacting to light (Hutchinson's pupil) (Fig. 9.4). The light reflex is also excellent for assessment of midbrain function, assuming that the efferent arc is intact.

Direct and Consensual Light Reflexes[9]

If a light is shone into an eye, the pupils of both eyes normally constrict. The constriction of the pupil on which the light is shone is called the direct light reflex; the constriction of the opposite pupil even though no light fell on that eye is called consensual light reflex.

Unilateral dilated, nonreactive pupil with absent consensual reflex will point to an optic nerve injury. When the light is directed to the unaffected eye, both pupil will react normally.

Marcus Gunn Pupil

During swinging flash light test, when the light is directed to the abnormal eye with relative efferent pupillary defect (say partial optic nerve injury), both pupil will dilate because of the comparatively weaker pupillary constriction. Apparently, light signals transmitted to the Edinger-Westphal nucleus in the midbrain through the injured optic nerve are insufficient to maintain the constriction induced by illumination of the unaffected or normal eye. The paradoxical pupillary dilation observed as the light is moved from the normal to the abnormal eye, is termed efferent pupillary defect.

Horner's Syndrome

Interruption of any oculosympathetic neurons may result in Horner's syndrome, characterized by unilateral miosis, facial anhidrosis, ptosis. The eyelid abnormality may give a false impression that the eye is set back in orbit (Pseudoenophthalmos).

Lesion of the third order neuron distal to the carotid bifurcation results in loss of sweating on forehead, whereas more proximal lesion, including those of first and second order neurons involve the whole one half of face (Fig. 9.3).

The Horner's syndrome can occur in the trauma patient from interruption of the sympathetic pupillodilator pathways anywhere between the hypothalamus and upper thoracic cord. Loss of sweating over the face occurs with disruption of the sympathetic pathways prior to the bifurcation of the common carotid artery, the point at which sweat fibers course with external carotid artery.

The diagnosis of Horner's syndrome associated with brachial plexus injury, or spinal cord trauma is important.

Brainstem hematoma following traumatic brain injuries may produce pin point pupils.

In metabolic encephalopathies, the pupils may be small but remains reactive to light.

Extraocular movements in an unconscious patient may be tested by rotating head in various directions (provided cervical injury is ruled out). The eyes will be fixed at a particular point in space, regardless of head rotation, and the eyes kept passively at a certain gaze, a phenomenon like that found in some children dolls, i.e. the patient's eye tend to deviate in the opposite direction to the induced head movement. The movement depends on intact vestibular reflex mechanisms. This oculocephalic reflex is a test of the peripheral sense organs, the labyrinths and otoliths, and their central connections in brainstem, including the vestibular nuclei, the MLF (medial longitudinal fasciculi) and the efferent pathway through oculomotor, trochlear and abducent nerves and their nuclei.

CALORIC REFLEXES

Brainstem function can be assessed by oculocephalic reflex (Doll's head ocular movement) and oculovestibular reflex (caloric response). The patient lies supine with head flexed 30° so that the horizontal semicircular canal lies in the vertical plane, with ampullae at the highest point. The ears are irrigated first with water at 30°C then at 44°C for 40 seconds. In the comatose patient irrigation of the external auditory meatus (after excluding perforation of tympanic membrane) on one side with at least 20 ml of ice-cold water induces slow conjugate derivation towards the irrigated side after few seconds delay.[10] The irrigation of cold water causes ampullofugal endolymph flow; this reduces the vestibular output from one side, creating an imbalance, resulting in conjugate deviation of eye towards irrigated side (Fig. 9.5). Rapid corrective movements result in nystagmus away from the stimulated ear. Nystagmus is absent in unconscious patient.

DISORDERS OF GAZE OF TRAUMATIC BRAIN INJURY

Two cortical centers of ocular control are recognized:

1. Middle gyrus of frontal lobe (area 8) for conjugate saccadic movements.
2. Occipital cortex for pursuit movements.

Fronto-mesencephalic and occipito-mesencephalic pathways traverse the genu of internal capsule, descend and decussate in the lower midbrain and upper pons to terminate in PPRF (Paramedian pontine reticular formation) which represents the brainstem center for ipsilateral conjugate gazeh (Fig. 9.6).

Medial longitudinal fasciculus (MLF) interconnects oculomotor, trochlear and abducens cranial nerve nuclei (see legend of Fig. 9.6) with vestibular and cerebellar complex. MLF provides the basis for normal oculocephalic and oculovestibular reflexes described above.

Supranuclear Gaze Palsies

An irritative lesion in frontal area (small hematoma causing seizures) will cause contralateral gaze deviation. Large frontal contusion hematoma (destructive lesion) will cause ipsilateral conjugate gaze deviation. The patient looks towards his lesion.

If the lesion is in the pons involving pontine paramedian reticular formation (PPRF) which represents the brainstem center for ipsilateral conjugate gaze there will be conjugate deviation of the eyes to the opposite side.

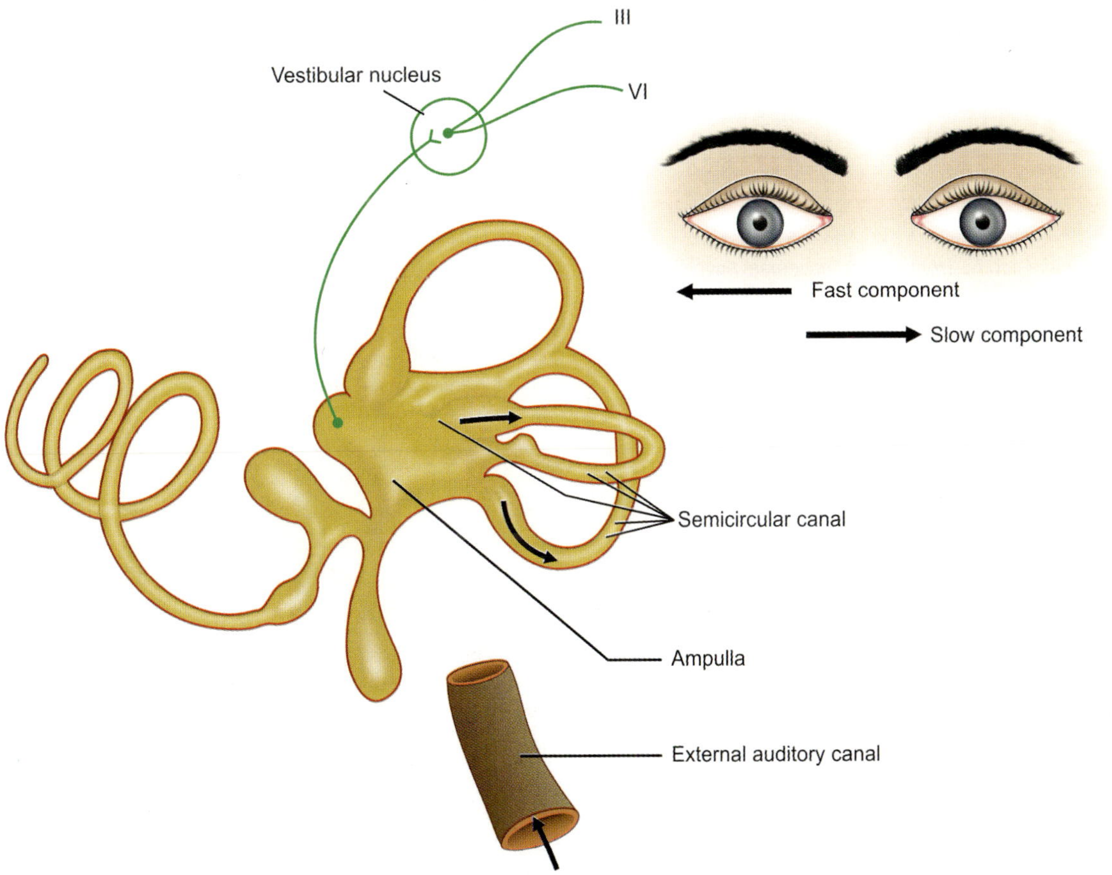

Fig. 9.5: Caloric response

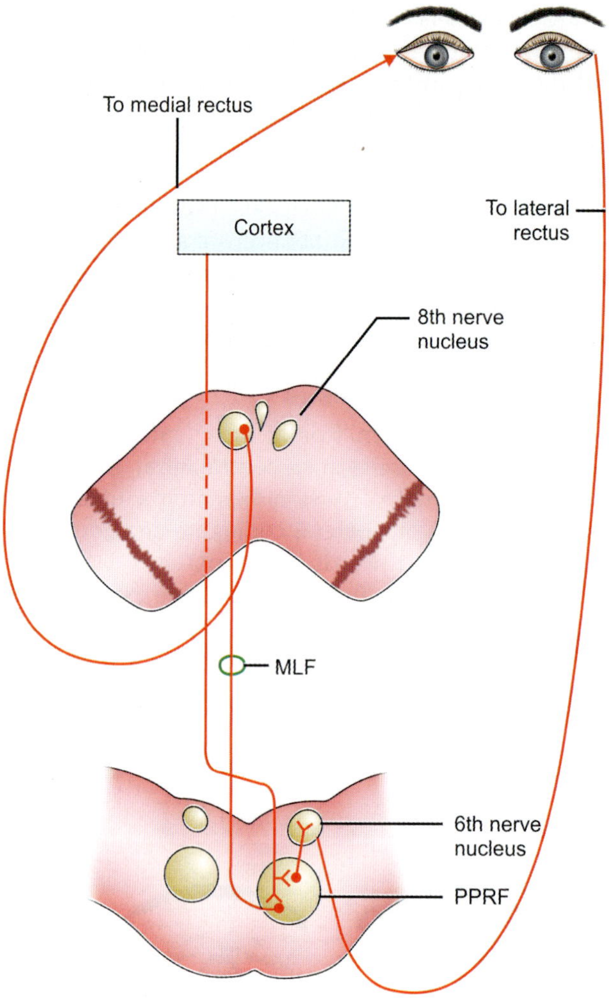

Fig. 9.6: Pathways for horizontal eye movement involving PPRF (Paramedian pontine reticular formation), MLF (Median longitudinal fasciculus), IIIrd and IVth cranial nerves. Stimulation of PPRF causes stimulation of ipsilateral lateral rectus and contralateral medial rectus (i.e. gaze toward ipsilateral side). Right MLF lesion will cause (a) Paresis of right adduction, (b) Nystagmus in left abducting eye. Left PPRF lesion will cause left lateral gaze palsy

Internuclear ophthalmoplegia is due to lesion in MLF in the midbrain (Fig. 9.6). It will cause impaired adduction of ipsilateral eye with nystagmus of the abducting opposite eye during attempted lateral gaze to opposite side.

In 'one-and-a-half syndrome' a lesion involving both PPRF and MLF on the same side will cause ipsilateral gaze paresis with impairment of adduction of ipsilateral eye and nystagmus on abduction of the opposite eye.

Upward gaze paresis occurs in compressive or destructive lesions involving the pretectal area of the midbrain, posterior commissure, and dorsal midbrain tegmentum.

Skew deviation of the eyes—in which one eye is directed upwards and the other downwards reflect lesions involving the brachium pontis or dorsolateral medulla.

Infranuclear Palsies

Trochlear nerve is difficult to assess in unconscious patient. Sixth cranial nerve paresis will cause unilateral esotropia and decreased lateral excursion of that eye upon oculocephalic testing. Bilateral sixth nerve paresis will cause convergence of both eyes. Bilateral sixth nerve paresis occurs in increased ICP.

A unilateral exotropia with limited medial, superior or inferior movements associated with dilated pupil points to oculomotor nerve paresis.

Other Cranial Nerves

The olfactory nerve is impossible to examine in unconscious patient. Unilateral or bilateral anosmia may be associated with anterior cranial fossa fractures with or without CSF rhinorrhea exclusive frontal lobe contusion. CSF leak if present should be recorded.

The Optic Nerve

Anatomy: From the retina, the fibers of the optic nerve pass back to the optic chiasm. At the chiasm, fibers from nasal retina cross, and the most ventral axons from the inferior nasal retina bend through the contralateral optic nerve (von Willebrand's knee), whereas fibers from temporal retina remain ipsilateral (Fig. 9.7).

Ipsilateral temporal fibers and contralateral nasal fibers join to form optic tracts. At the lateral geniculate body, the ganglion cell axons in optic tract synapse

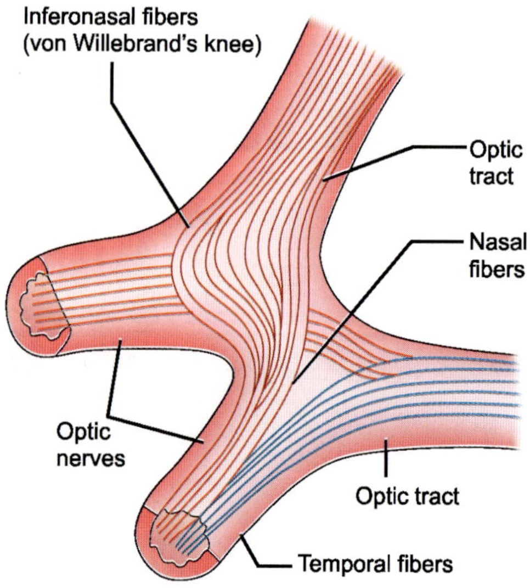

Fig. 9.7: von Willebrand's knee

with neurons to become the optic radiation. Some fibers called Meyers loop course through the temporal lobe anterior to the inferior horn of lateral ventricles, subserve visual information from the lower retina and connect to the inferior bank of calcarine cortex.

The parietal portion of the optic radiation relays information from the upper retina to the superior bank of the calcarine cortex. Broadmann area 17 is the end organ of the different visual system and is located in the calcarine cortex in the occipital lobe.

In a conscious patient visual acuity should be recorded carefully. Complete blindness is termed as no light perception (NLP).

Optic nerve injury should be suspected in a patient of head injury who has periorbital ecchymosis or complained of loss of vision.

In unconscious patient optic nerve injury should be suspected in all patients with unilaterally dilated pupils. Optic nerve injury should be differentiated from oculomotor paresis due to transtentorial herniation. In optic nerve injury ipsilateral direct pupillary reflex and consensual reflex in the opposite eye will be absent whereas in oculomotor paresis ipsilateral direct pupillary reflex will be absent but consensual reflex in opposite eye will be present. Progressive opposite or central herniation compresses parasympathetic neurons in the upper midbrain and causes dilatation of the pupil and paralysis of light response. With full mydriasis (6 to 8 mm pupil), ptosis and paresis of the medial rectus and other ocular muscles innervated by the oculomotor nerves appear. Ophthalmoscopic examination should be done to rule out hemorrhage or distortion of the retina.

Visual field are useful in diagnosing various types of field defects involving optic tracts or geniculocalcarine pathways.

In occipital contusions, transient cortical blindness can occur. Some of these patients with acute cortical blindness are unaware of visual loss due to coincidental involvement of parietal connections (Anton's syndrome).

The trigeminal and facial nerves may be tested with corneal responses to a light cotton wisp or response to more severe facial stimuli, to assess for facial grimace and eye closure. Facial nerve injury is apparent by widened palpebral fissure and sagging facial muscles.

The seventh and eighth cranial nerves are often injured in the basal fractures involving petrous bone.

It is impossible to test auditory components of eighth nerve directly in unconscious patient (except by evoked potential using audiometric inputs). Vestibular component of eighth nerve can be tested by caloric testing.

Assessment of gag, swallowing and vocal cord function will partially evaluate the glossopharyngeal and vagus nerves. This can be observed in manipulating the endotracheal tube in a comatose patient.

MOTOR RESPONSE

In alert patients, muscle tone can be evaluated by passive range of movement of upper and lower limb, muscle power can be treated by voluntary movement against resistance:

The Medical Research Council Scale is used to grade muscle functions:

- Grade 0: Complete paralysis
- Grade 1: Flicker of contraction
- Grade 2: Muscle contracts, but cannot overcome gravity
- Grade 3: Muscle contraction against force of gravity only
- Grade 4: Some degree of weakness, can be overcome with resistance
- Grade 5: Normal power.

In an unconscious patient evaluation of the motor abilities of the uncooperative or unresponsive patient consists of observing the characteristics and strength of the skeletal muscle responses to painful stimuli. Painful stimulus is given by nibbing thumb nail in supraorbital groove thus giving painful stimuli to supraorbital nerve. In GCS the motor responses are grouped as:

- M6 Follows command
- M5 Localizing to pain
- M4 Withdraws from stimulation
- M3 Abnormal flexion
- M2 Extension
- M1 No response

Limb weakness in an unconscious patient can be determined by comparing the response in each limb to painful stimuli. The most frequently recognized combination is dilatation of pupil on one side with contralateral hemiparesis or hemiplegia (Figs 9.8A and B). The dilated and non-reactive pupil can be associated with ipsilateral hemiplegia. This is due to indentation of the contralateral cerebral peduncle by the edge of the tentorium cerebelli (Kernohan's notch).

Abnormal flexion response is characterized by adduction and internal rotation of shoulder, relatively slow flexion of the elbow, wrist, and fingers with flexion or extension of lower extremeties. This type of response is commonly described as decorticate posture which indicates severe supratentorial damage.

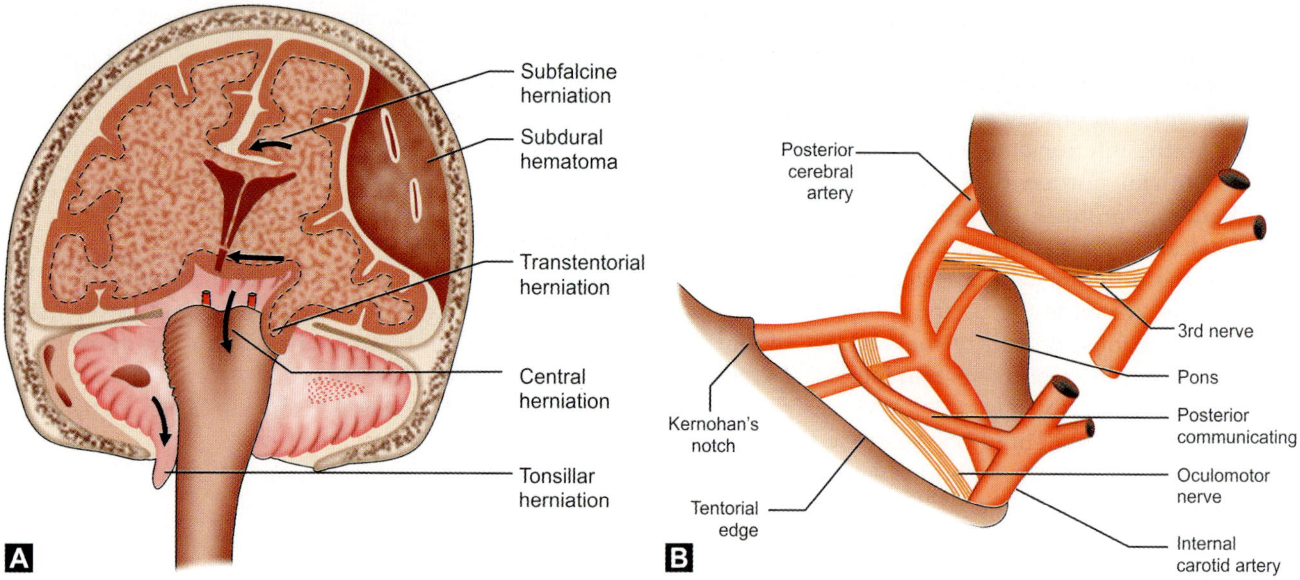

Figs 9.8A and B: Herniation and Kernohan's notch

Decorticate rigidity signifies lesion in cerebral white matter or internal capsules and thalamus.

In extensor motor response the head is thrown back with extension of all limbs with internal rotation of arms and opisthotonos position (decerebrate rigidity). In decerebrate rigidity the lesion is in midbrain between superior and inferior colliculus. While abnormal extensor posturing is generally assumed to occur solely in comatose patients, alert patients with decerebrate rigidity have been described. This is because of different anatomical locations which regulate consciousness and which are concerned with motor functions.

Deep tendon reflexes and superficial reflexes should be examined. Tendon reflexes include bicep jerk, supinator jerk, triceps jerk, knee jerk and ankle jerk. Abnormal tendon reflexes can be exaggerated, diminished or absent.

Superficial reflexes include plantar reflex, superficial abdominal reflex and corneal reflex.

Babinski's response (extensor plantar) is found in patients with corticospinal tract lesions. In conscious patients coordination, involuntary movements and gait should be included in the motor examination. Sensory examination includes examination of pain temperature touch, vibration, position sense.

Neck stiffness should be seen carefully after excluding cervical injury.

Neurological examination should conclude by detailed 'local examination'.

ADJUNCT DIAGNOSTIC MODALITIES

Radiological investigation, X-ray films, CT scan, MRI, scanning, etc. are discussed elsewhere in this book.

BRAIN DEATH EXAMINATION

Patient with severe head injury may develop irreversible untreatable high intracranial pressure but without a focal mass lesion or he may develop severe herniation syndrome as a result of large contusion or hematoma before treatment. The herniation may progress rapidly to an irreversible state and decompression after this time may not result in any functional improvement because of irreversible brainstem changes. The intracranial swelling and initial damage may lead to cessation of all valuable brain function, termed brain death.[11] The lack of brain function includes dilated unreactive pupils, no caloric response, no oculocephalic response, no spontaneous respiration and no motor or sensory response. While testing for brain function one should ensure that patient has not received any sedatives, paralytic drugs. Clinically, Apnea test must be done for brain function. Apnea test is performed with 100 percent O_2 cannula in the endotracheal tube for oxygenation and end PCO_2 should be at least 60 mm Hg. Patient should be re-examined at 6, 12 or 24 hours before declaring brain dead. A number of test have also been suggested, including an angiographic study showing no cerebral blood flow and silent EEG.

The value of declaring brain death is for possibility of viable organ donation. Brain death must be declared before the organs are harvested.

MINOR HEAD INJURY

In cases of minor head trauma following needs to be assured:

- Corroborate and record the history from witnesses. Ascertain why the patient was injured (was there a seizure or sudden weakness?) and rule out particularly dangerous types of head trauma. (A blow by a brick or hammer is more likely to produce a depressed skull fracture).
- Perform and record a physical examination of the head, looking for signs of a skull fracture, such as hemotympanum or bony depression, and examine the neck for spasm, bomy tenderness, rage of motion, and other signs of associated injury.
- Perform and record a neurological examination, with special attention to mental status, cranial nerves, strength, and tendon reflexes to all four limbs.
- If the history or physical examination suggests there could be a clinically significant intracranial injury, obtain a noncontrast computed tomography (CT) scan of the head. Criteria for obtaining a CT scan include: documented loss of consciousness, amnesia, cerebrospinal fluid leaking from nose or ear, blood behind the tympanic membrane or ever the mastoid (Battle's sign), stupor, coma, or any focal neurological sign.
- If the history or physical examination suggests there could be a clinically significant skull fracture, obtain skull X-rays. Criteria for obtaining skull X- rays include: a blow by a heavy object, suspected skull penetration and palpable depression.
- If there is no clinical indication for CT scan or skull films, explain to the patient and concerned family and friends why X-ray images are not being ordered. Many patients expect X-rays, but will gladly forego them once you explain they are of little value.
- Explain to the patient and responsible family or friends that the more important possible sequelae of head trauma are not diagnosed with X-rays, but by noting certain signs and symptoms as they occur later. Make sure that they understand and are given written instructions that any abnormal behavior, increasing drowsiness or difficulty in rousing the patient, headache, neck stiffness, vomiting, visual problems, weakness, or seizures are signals to return to hospital immediately.[11-13]

CONCLUSION

The clinical value of the neurological examination in the initial assessment and subsequent management of head injured patient is very important. Glasgow coma scale has been widely accepted for evaluation of head injured patients despite its certain drawbacks. Neurologic conditions that produce unresponsive are akinetic mutism, locked in syndrome, persistent vegetative state and brain death. Most of the cranial nerves can be examined even in unconscious patient. Direct and consensual reaction of pupil can diagnose optic nerve and third nerve injuries. Unilateral, nonreactive dilatation of pupil with deteriorating consciousness indicates of an expanding hematoma. Gaze paresis and caloric response are good parameters for evaluation of brainstem reflexes in unconscious patient. One should do all bedside tests several times before declaring brain death.

REFERENCES

1. Selhorst John B. Neurological examination of head injured patients in textbook of head injury: Becker DP, Gudeman SK (Eds) 1989;82-101.
2. Levy DE. The comatose patient, Rosenberg RN (Ed). Comprehensive Neurology Raven Press 1990;817-32.
3. Teasdale G, Jennett B. Assessment and prognosis of coma after head injury. Acta Neurochir (Wien) 1976;34:45-55.
4. Teasdale G, et al. Observer variability in assessing impaired consciousness and coma. J Neural Neurosur Psychiatry 1978;41:603-10.
5. Adams RD, Victor M. Coma and related disorders of consciousness. In Principles of Neurology. McGraw Hill 1993;300-18.
6. Symonds C. Concussion and its sequelae. Lancet 1962; 1:1-5.
7. Victor M. The amnestic syndrome and its anatomical basis. Can Ked J 1969;100(2):1115-25.
8. Russell WR, Smith A. Post-traumatic amnesia in closed head injury. Arch Neurol 1961;5:1-17.
9. Sambasivan M, Ramamurti B. Assessment, Head Injuries in Textbook of Neurosurgery, Second edn, Tandon PN, Ramamurti B (Eds) 1996;259-64.
10. Jadhav WR, Sinha A, Tandon PN, et al. Cold calorie test in altered state of consciousness. Laryngoscope 1971; 81:391.
11. Shackford SR, Wald SL, Ross SE, et al. The clinical utility of computed tomographic scanning and neurologic examination in the management of patients with minor head injuries. J Trauma 1992;33:385-94.
12. Mitchell KA, Fallat ME, Raque GH, et al. Evaluation of minor head injury in children. J Ped Surg 1994;29:851-4.
13. Staffeld L, Levitt A, Simon, et al. Identification of ethanol-intoxicated patients with minor head trauma requiring computed tomography scans. Acad Emerg Med 1993;1:227-34.

10 Imaging in Head Injury

Raj Kamal, AK Mahapatra

Computed tomography (CT) remains the imaging study of choice in the investigation of the head injured patients. CT reliably demonstrates midline shift, acute hemorrhage, intracranial masses, and fractures. CT scanners provide direct and accurate images rapidly and noninvasively. The early and accurate diagnosis of intracranial pathologies have led to lower mortality and morbidity rate because one can quickly and reliably take a decision whether it is amenable to surgical evacuation or not. CT scan can be repeated easily. It can be done in intubated patients who are on mechanical ventilatory support.

Non-hemorrhagic parenchymal injury is difficult to diagnose on CT. Nonhemorrhagic contusions are better visualized on MRI. MR is sometimes helpful for trauma patients with severe neurological deficits unexplained by CT scan results.

CT scan is also necessary to evaluate minor head injury. In the past, CT scan was considered unnecessary investigation. Recently there are reports suggesting need for CT in minor head injury.[1a-1c] About 3 to 5 percent patients of minor head injury may have clot in brain and 33 to 40 percent them ultimately need surgery. Patients of minor head injury with severe headache, CSF leak, repeated vomiting and focal deficit need early CT scan.

MRI IN HEAD INJURY

MR is a superior imaging modality, however, it is rarely used in acute head injury. MRI is more sensitive in identifying non-hemorrhagic contusion and diffuse axonal injury. MRI also demonstrate deep lesions in thalamus, brainstem and cerebellum. In chronic state MR scan demonstrate corpus callosum degeneration following severe head injury with diffuse axonal injury (Fig. 10.1). Furthermore increased total volume of contusion in FLAIR image has been demonstrated to have poor clinical outcome.

DTI is a clinically relevant biomarker in TBI, which may have prognostic value and might serve as a tool for revealing changes in neural tissue during recovery.[27]

Diffusion tensor imaging (DTI) in diffuse axonal injury revealed that white matter region with reduced anisotropy is detected in first 24 hours after traumatic brain injury. This imaging hence may become a powerful technique in detection of diffuse axonal injury.[28]

Advantages

1. Better evaluation of nonhemorrhagic contusion.
2. Evaluation of stage of parenchymal hemorrhage.
3. Useful in CT isodense subdural hematoma.

Disadvantages

1. Longer scan time.
2. Difficult to manage life-support and monitoring equipment at a distance from patient within strong magnetic field.

Normal, fresh whole blood is hyperdense [50 to 100 Hounsfield units (HUs)] relative to normal brain (20 to 35 HU). This density is proportional to the protein moiety of hemoglobin.

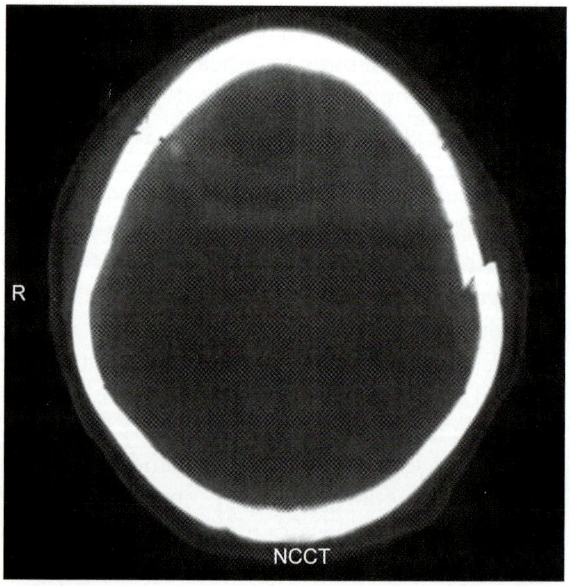

Fig. 10.1: Plain CT showing left parietal fracture on bone window

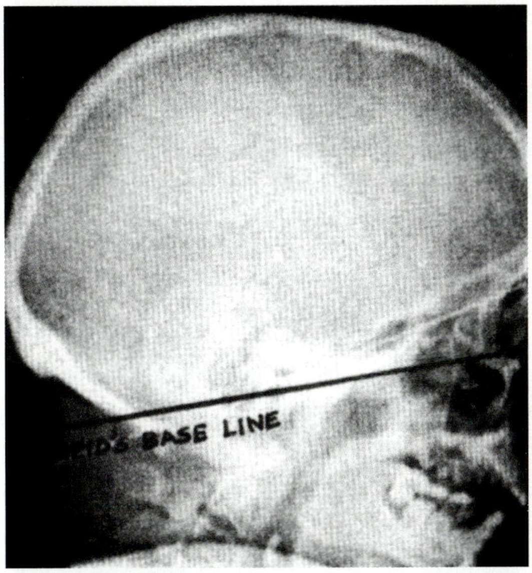

Fig. 10.2: Reid's baseline in a topogram to delineate precisely anatomical areas that are to be scanned

Owing to clot formation and retraction, the density of acute hematoma usually increases in density by 20 to 30 HU in first 48 hours and then passes through an isodense to a hypodense phase, approaching the density of cerebrospinal fluid.[2]

A cranial CT examination consists of a topogram followed by series axial sections, 5 to 10 mm thick, are obtained in plane parallel to Reid's baseline (Fig. 10.2). Reid's baseline is drawn from the lower margin of the orbit to the superior border of the external auditory meatus. Orbitomeatal line is drawn from the outer canthus to the center of meatus.

SKULL FRACTURES

Skull fractures often occur without significant brain injury and many patients with severe brain injury do not have skull fractures. Skull fractures can be classified as **linear (Table 10.1), comminuted, depressed or basilar.** On routine skull X-rays, linear fractures are typically well defined, and appear as fine lines of decreased density. They sometimes branch, and must be distinguished from the vascular markings. The fracture appears thinner and more lucent than vascular grooves. A fracture passing through a sinus or air cell is **internally compound** (Fig. 10.3) and of great clinical significance. Fractures associated with widening (diastasis) of one or more sutures, particularly lambdoid. CT scan head may not detect linear fractures that lies parallel to plane of CT image. Routine CT (Fig. 10.4) examination of the head in axial projection, as many as 30 to 40 percent of fractures are not seen.[3]

Table 10.1: Time taken for linear fractures to heal

1. Infancy and early childhood	3 to 6 months
2. Children 5 to 12 years	~ 1 year
3. Adolescence	Months to years
4. Adult	Throughout life

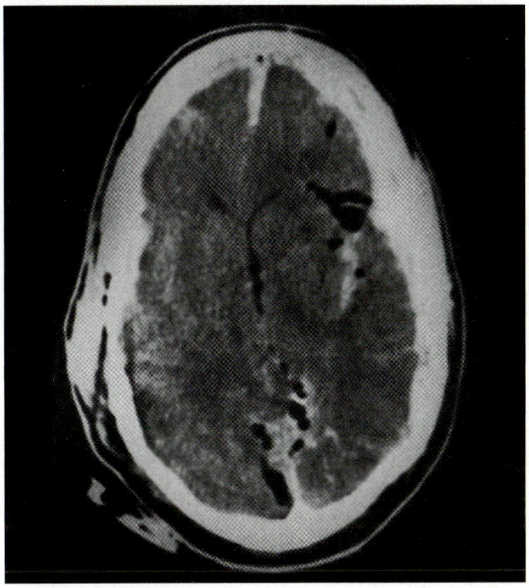

Fig. 10.3: Planning of CT with bullet in maxillary region

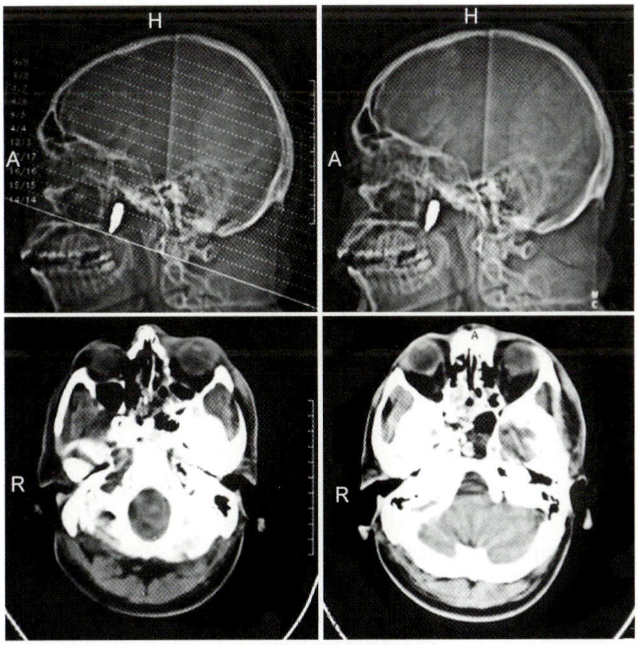

Fig. 10.4: CT shows multiple cisternal and parenchymal bleeds and air pockets suggestive of compounding

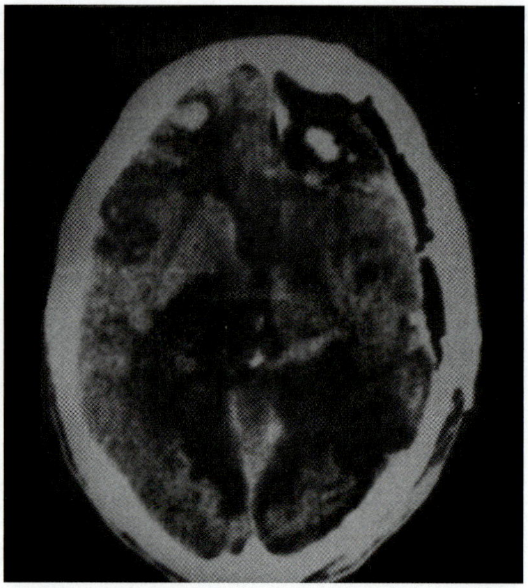

Fig. 10.5: CT showing multiple hematomas and multiple focal brain swelling and ventricular dilatation

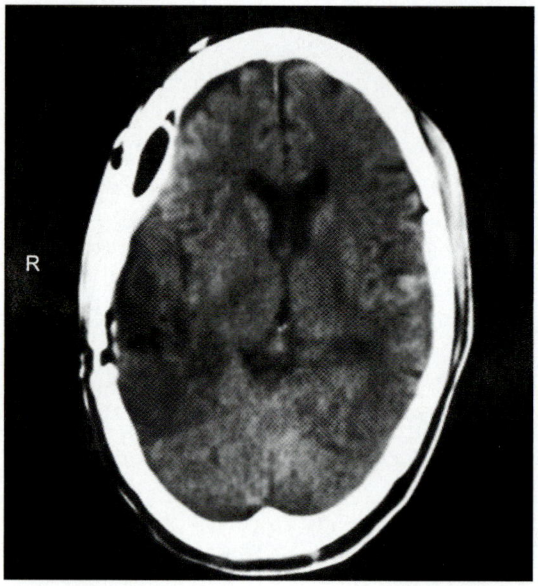

Fig. 10.6: CT showing right temporal contusion and intradural air

Depressed fractures may be diagnosed by plain films but are usually diagnosed by CT (Fig. 10.3), which also shows any associated intracranial lesion. On plain X-rays, **depressed fractures** often appear as comminuted fracture with areas of overlap in some projections and inward displacement in others.

Basilar skull fractures are often missed in routine X-rays. Basilar skull fracture (Fig. 10.5) are best demonstrated by high resolution, thin section of CT in both axial and coronal planes.[4]

Growing skull fractures (leptomeningeal cyst) usually occur after head injury in young children. The dura underlying a linear fracture is torn, sometimes intact **arachnoid** gets trapped in the fracture which transmits the brain pulsations. There is progressive widening, eversion and smoothening of bone edges, owing to pulsation of cyst like collection of fluid in the partially walled off subarachnoid space. CT scan is a good investigation for the diagnosis of growing fractures as it shows the changes in the underlying brain, which is seen to herniate through the skull defect.

CSF Rhinorrhea

It results from the rupture of basal dura and arachnoid, where it connects with the paranasal sinuses. CT is the procedure of choice.

CT scan with thin coronal cuts, occasionally augmented by **cisternography** using water soluble contrast such as **metrizamide** demonstrated defect in the anterior cranial fossa in majority of cases.[6] Presence of fluid levels in the **ethmoid sinus or frontal sinus** indicate bony defect anteriorly in cribriform plate whereas fluid level in sphenoid sinus indicates defect in sphenoid bone.

Radionuclide can be injected into the lumbar spinal canal and recovered with cotton pledgets inserted on each side of nose to detect minimal CSF leak.

MR cisternography using fast spinecho technique has demonstrated defect in the dura at appropriate level.[5] Post-traumatic CSF rhinorrhea usually has an abrupt onset within 48 hours of the trauma with spontaneous remission in 70 to 80 percent of patients within a week. Up to 50 percent of those cases that do not remit develop meningitis.[17] **Pneumocephalus** is often present in these cases.

Extradural Hematoma

Extradural hematoma is seen on CT sections as a biconvex dense area immediately beneath the skull vault (Fig. 10.6). Because of the dural attachments at the sutures, EDH forms focal biconvex collections.[7] The temporoparietal convexity is the most common site (about 65%), in which lesions are easily detected on axial sections.[8] Skull fractures are present in as many as 90 percent of patients with extradural hematoma (Fig. 10.7). This type of fracture frequently disrupts middle meningeal artery and its branches. Extradural hematoma may result from rupture of dural sinus or a venous tributary of **diploic veins**. Hence, EDH may cross midline (due to rupture of superior sagittal sinus) but does not cross suture line.

Posterior fossa extradural hematoma accounts for 3 to 13 percent of all cranial traumatic extradural

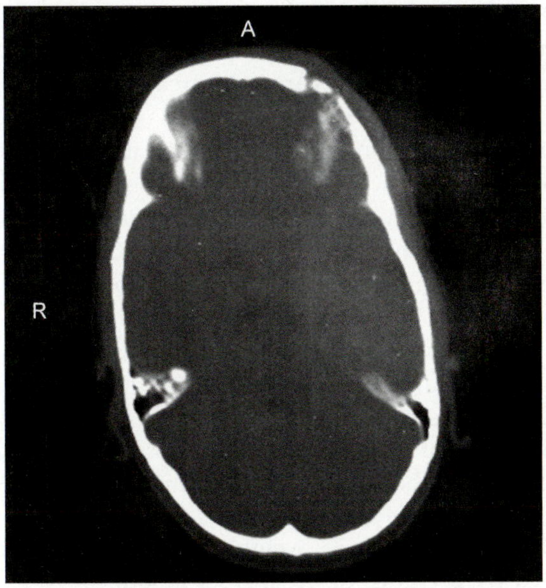

Fig. 10.7: CT bone window showing left frontal fracture in compound head injury

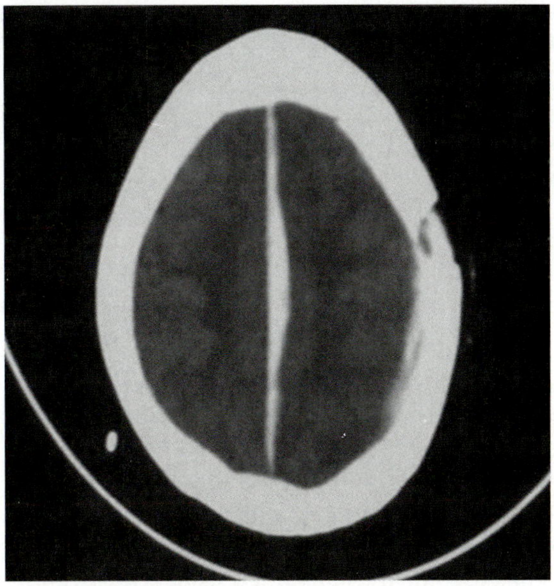

Fig. 10.8: CT showing post-traumatic bleed along the falx, note a left frontal fracture

hematomas. CT study is carried low enough to adequately assess posterior fossa. CT findings include **biconvex, hyperdense** collection just beneath the occipital bone, which can extend above tentorium. Posterior fossa extradural hematoma results from injury to the transverse or sigmoid sinuses and the torcular herophili. It can be associated with occipital skull fracture invariably crossing venous sinuses.[9,10]

Indications for immediate surgical evacuation:

1. Large extradural hematoma.
2. Local mass effect on brain.
3. Presence of significant midline shift.
4. Signs of herniation.
5. Increase in size on repeat CT even without clinical deterioration.

Subdural Hematoma

Acute Subdural Hematoma

Acute subdural hematomas (SDHs) 'are crescentic, hyperdense collections adjacent to calvarium (Fig. 10.8). They differ from extradural lesions in being crescentic, i.e. concave towards brain. They may be localized to one or both lobes or may be hemispheric. Acute SDH are sometimes isodense in anemic patients or when subdural hematoma is diluted by CSF.[11,12] The high morbidity of these lesions, particularly in the aged, is due in large part to the associated swelling, contusion or laceration of the underlying brain. It is often evident that midline displacement is greater than would be accounted for by the mass of the hematoma alone. The interhemispheric subdural hematoma extends along the falx cerebri and may spread onto tentorium, giving a characteristic comma shape on axial CT sections. MRI has limited role in acute SDH.

Chronic Subdural Hematoma

CT is the investigation of choice for evaluation of chronic SDH (Fig. 10.9). The density of the subdural hematoma decreases with the passage of time. A

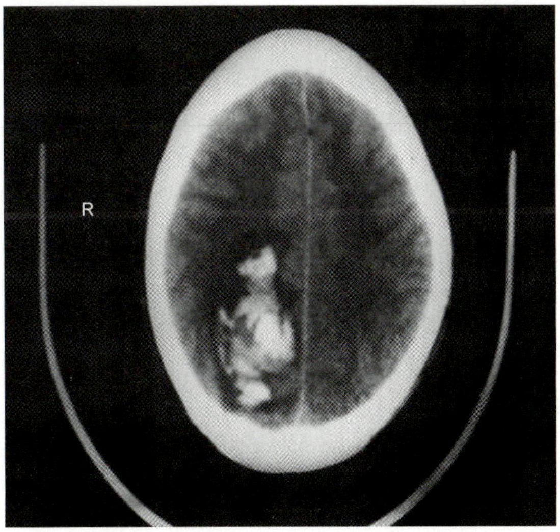

Fig. 10.9: CT shows right parietal bleed and edema dominantly present anterior to blood clot

Table 10.2: Changes in MRI on hematoma evolution

Hematoma	T_1	T_2
Hyperacute (few hours)	Hypo	Hyper (oxy Hb)
Acute	Iso to Hypo	Hypo (due to deoxy Hb)
Subacute	Hyper	Hypo (intracellular meth Hb)
Chronic	Hyper	Hyper (Release of meth Hb after lysis of RBC)

chronic subdural hematoma is hyperdense in first week after injury. It becomes isodense in about ten days to 2 weeks and thus could be overlooked on the CT scan examination. After 3 weeks, chronic subdural hematoma usually appears hypodense on CT. It is often difficult to distinguish isodense chronic SDH from cerebral parenchyma. Isodense SDH displaces surface sulci of the brain away from inner table. They have been often misdiagnosed as cerebral swelling or tumor. Chances of missing bilateral isodense subdural hematoma is still higher.

Subdural hematoma (1-2 weeks) have high signal on both T_1 and T_2 weighted images due to presence of extracellular methemoglobin (Table 10.2).

Subacute subdural hematomas are hyperintense on T_1 weighted images and hypointense (i.e. dark) relative to brain (Table 10.2) and CSF due to presence of intracellular methemoglobin.

MRI can also demonstrate acute hemorrhages within chronic SDH. MRI is more sensitive than CT in identifying isodense SDH.

SUBARACHNOID HEMORRHAGE (SAH)

Subarachnoid hemorrhage is seen better with CT than with MRI. A subarachnoid hemorrhage forms isodense to hyperdense collections in cisterns and sulci. Normally cisterns have hypodense appearance, which is similar to the density of CSF. The subarachnoid hemorrhage may be focal, in the area of a fracture, and may indicate that there has been trauma to the surface vessels.

CEREBRAL CONTUSION AND EDEMA

A cerebral contusion consists of perivascular hemorrhages surrounded by necrotic brain involving crests of gyri and tend to be wedge-shaped (Fig. 10.5). The piaglial membrane is intact. In cerebral lacerations there is disruption of piaglial membrane.

On CT, a contusion manifests as hyperdensity mixed with hypodensity (salt pepper appearance). A contusion may also appear as an area of low attenuation.

Existing contusion or hematoma can increase in size between two scans. This possibility is higher, if the initial CT is done very early following trauma. Study done, from our department showed changes in CT finding in 48 percent patients between initial and repeat CT. In 36 percent cases CT scan worsened, while in 12 percent cases CT scan showed resolution of hematoma.[12a]

Post-traumatic edema can be focal or generalized. Focal edema is more common.

On CT, focal edema is seen as uniform hypodensity. In focal injuries both edema and contusion can produce mass effect. On MRI, contusion is hypointense on T_1 and hyperintense on T_2 weighted images, which are affected by presence or absence of blood.[13]

Diffuse cerebral edema can be diagnosed on CT on the basis of:

1. Decreased gray/white matter differentiation.
2. Decrease in size of ventricles.
3. Decrease in size of perimesencephalic, quadrigeminal cisterns.

In severe head injury, there can be loss of autoregulation causing high cerebral blood flow, which causes very high intracranial pressure (ICP) resulting in severe cerebral, brain edema. Severe cerebral ischemia produces acute cerebral edema.

Bruce et al[14] described the syndrome of diffuse cerebral edema in children and concluded that the etiology was related to increased blood volume, not edema, since the Hounsfield values were significantly higher.

INTRACEREBRAL HEMATOMA

Traumatic intracerebral hematomas may result from the coalescence of the hemorrhages within a contusion, or they may develop *de novo*. The margins of such hematoma tend to be more irregular and ill defined than those of hematomas due to hypertension or aneurysmal rupture.[15] A thin rim of edema usually surrounds post-traumatic hematoma. These hematomas can be multiple. Midline shift and evidence of herniation should be looked for.

DIFFUSE AXONAL INJURY (DAI)

Diffuse axonal injury is a form of brain damage associated with a severe rotational injury to the cranium, causing tearing of nerve fibers in specific areas of the brain, notably at the junction of gray and white

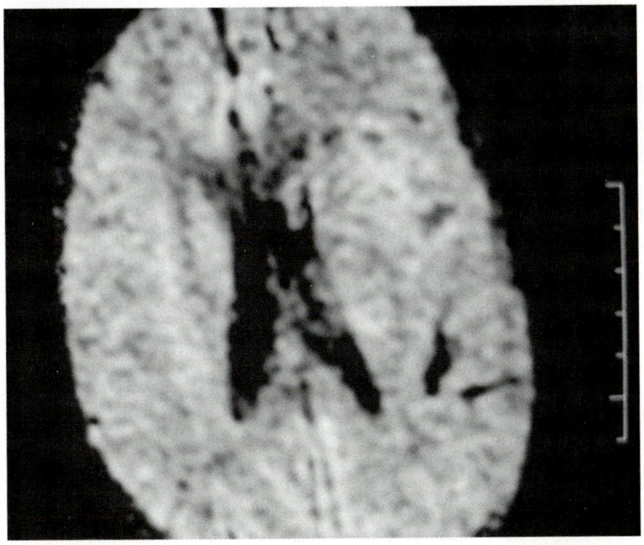

Fig. 10.10: Perfusion weight images of child with diabetes insipidus showing changes in anterior corpus callosum

matter, brainstem, corpus callosum, internal capsule. Such damage reflects widespread white matter injury, often with devastating effect in neurologic function. Many patients remain permanently in vegetative state. Diffuse axonal injuries are described in detail elsewhere in this book.

The CT findings include scattered small hemorrhages in cerebral white matter, **basal ganglia, corpus callosum**, or dorsal part of **brainstem**.[13,16] The two most common location for these hemorrhages are corpus callosum and dorsolateral quadrant of the rostral brainstem in the region of cerebral peduncle. Occasionally, hemorrhage is seen in the structures making up the walls of the third ventricle (thalamus, column of the fornices, anterior commissure).[15]

The vast majority (80%) of DAI lesions are nonhemorrhagic and only about 20% of lesions contain small central areas of petechial hemorrhage.

For diagnosing diffuse axonal injury MRI is superior to CT (Fig. 10.10).

Nonhemorrhagic contusions are seen as isointense or hypointense on T_1 weighted images and hyperintense on T_2 weighted images.

PRIMARY BRAINSTEM INJURY

Primary brainstem injury usually are non-hemorrhagic and, therefore, are better diagnosed by MR than by CT. These brainstem injuries should be differentiated from Duret hemorrhages (caused by downward transtentorial herniation.[18,18a] Primary brainstem lesions are usually localized to the dorsolateral midbrain and upper pons. Primary brainstem injuries are those that result from the initial trauma, while secondary brainstem injuries are those that develop later. The most common type of primary brainstem injury, by far, is that associated with widespread DAI. DAI lesions of the brainstem are almost invariably associated with macroscopically and microscopically similar lesions in the corpus callosum and deep cerebral white matter.

ANGIOGRAPHY

Cerebral angiography is indicated in patients of head injury in whom there is suspicion of vascular complications. Vascular complications following head trauma are post-traumatic aneurysms, traumatic dissection of the internal carotid or vertebral arteries, arterial spasm, thrombosis, CCF (caroticocavernous fistula) and dural sinus laceration.[19]

Catheter angiography remains the definitive method of diagnosing vascular injury. However, **MR angiography** may be used for noninvasive evaluation.

Traumatic intracranial aneurysms are less than 1 percent of reported aneurysm in large series.[20,21] Traumatic aneurysms are located on the distal middle cerebral artery, distal anterior cerebral artery, basal internal carotid artery.[22,23] Basal skull fractures may be associated with cavernous internal carotid artery aneurysm.[24] Post-traumatic aneurysms can be false or true aneurysm.

False aneurysm occurs when the full thickness of vessel is lacerated and the apparent wall is actually organized hematoma. "True" aneurysm occurs following limited damage to the wall and persistence of all layers.[24] Penetrating injuries can be associated with traumatic aneurysms.

Indications for cerebral angiography after trauma include a penetrating or perforating injury, an unexplained prominent collection of subarachnoid blood.

Conventional cerebral angiography, often with digital subtraction, is the best method for detecting traumatic aneurysms. Traumatic aneurysms are usually more peripherally situated than are berry aneurysms and typically do not occur at branching sites. A post-traumatic aneurysm is irregular in contour, may be fusiform or lobulated, often has no definable neck, and may fill and drain slowly.[24]

Magnetic resonance angiography or three dimensional CT may eventually be able to detect traumatic aneurysms.

Traumatic dissection of internal carotid artery can occur following sudden severe sketch of the internal carotid artery over upper cervical spine when the neck is hyperextended. Other causes of traumatic dissection includes direct injury to artery, by compression between the angle of mandible and upper cervical vertebrae. Dissection of internal carotid artery leads to thrombosis and embolus formation.

The angiographic abnormalities following dissection are localized narrowing of the upper cervical carotid artery or aneurysmal outpouching between C2 and the skull base.[25,26]

CONCLUSION

CT scan remains the investigation of choice in head injured patients. CT scan can be repeated easily and can be done in patients on ventilator. CT scan can accurately diagnose extradural hematoma, acute and chronic subdural hematoma, contusion, post-traumatic intracerebral hematoma. However, there are some conditions, such as diffuse axonal injury, non-hemorrhagic contusion, for which MRI may be required to make the diagnosis. MRI can help by demonstrating the age of the chronic subdural hematoma.

Catheter angiography is indicated in post-traumatic aneurysms, traumatic dissection of internal carotid or vertebral arteries and caroticocavernous fistula. However, routine carotid angiography has now become investigation of the past with historical significance.

REFERENCES

1. New P, Aronow S. Attenuation measurements of whole blood and blood fractions in computed tomography. Radiology 1976;121:635-40.
1a. Stein SC, Ross SE. Mild head injury: A Plea for routine early scanning. J Trauma 1992;33:11-3.
1b. Stiell IG, Well GA, Vandem heen IC, et al. The Canadian CT head rule for patients with minor head injury. Lancet 2001;35:1391-6.
1c. Jevet JS. Minor head injury and CT Scanning-Letter. J Trauma 1993;35:490-1.
2. Scotti G, Terbrugge K, et al. Evaluation of the age of subdural haematomas by computed tomography. J Neurosurg 1977;47:311-5.
3. Taveras JM. Head Injuries and their Complications. Neuroradiology, 3rd edn, Williams & Wilkins 1996;327-64.
4. Johnson D, Hasso A, et al. Temporal bone trauma: High resolution computed tomographic evaluation. Radiology 1984;151:411-5.
5. El Gammal T, Brooks BS. MR Cisternography: Initial experience in 41 cases. AJNR 1994;15:1647-56.
6. Ozgen T, Tekkok IH, et al. CT cisternography in evaluation of cerebrospinal fluid rhinorrhoea. Neuroradiology 1989; 32:481-4.
7. Dublin AB, French BN, Rennick JM. Computed tomography in head trauma. Radiology 1977;122:365-9.
8. Zimmerman RA, Bilaniuk LT. Computed tomography staging of traumatic epidural bleeding. Radiology 1982; 144:809-12.
9. Cooper PR. Post-traumatic intracranial mass lesions. In Cooper PR (Ed). Head injury. 2nd edn. Baltimore: Williams & Wilkins 1987;238-84.
10. Tsai FY, Teal JS, et al. Computed tomography of posterior fossa trauma. J Comput Assist Tomogr 1980;4:291-305.
11. Johnson MH, Lee HS. Computed tomography of acute cerebral trauma. Radiol Clin North Am 1992;30:325-51.
12. Moeller A, Erikson K. Computed tomography of isoattenuating subdural haematomas. Radiology 1979; 130:149-52.
12a. Dubey AK. Role of repeat CT scan in head injury. A prospective study of 146 patients. MCh thesis submitted. Deptt of Neurosurgery, AIIMS, New Delhi.
12b. Lobato RD, Rivas JJ, Gomez PA, et al. Head injured patient who talk and deteriorated into coma. Analysis of 211 cases studied with computed tomography. J Neurosurg 1991;75:256-61.
13. Kelly AB, Zimmerman RD, Snow RB, et al. Head trauma: Comparison of MR and CT—experience in 100 patients. AJNR 1988;699-708.
13a. Paterakis K, Karantanas AH, Komnos A, et al. Outcome of patients with diffuse axonal injury: The significance of prognostic value of MRI in the acute Phase. J Trauma 2000;49:1071-5.
13b. Pierallini A, Pantano P, Fantozzil LM, et al. Correlation between MRI findings and long-term outcome in patients with severe head trauma. Neuroradiol 2000;42:860-67.
14. Bruce DA, Alavi, et al. Diffuse cerebral swelling following head injuries in children: The syndrome of "malignant brain edema." J Neurosurg 1981;54:170-78.
15. Graeb DA. Intracranial trauma. In: Pulamen CE, Ravin CEo (Eds). Textbook of Diagnostic imaging, 2nd edn, WB Saunders 1994;185-202.
16. Gennarelli TA, Jhibault LE, Adam JH, et al. Diffuse axonal injury and traumatic coma in primate. Ann Neurol 1982;12:564-74.
17. Manelfe C, Cellerier P, et al. Cerebrospinal fluid rhinorrhea: Evaluation with metrizamide cisternography. AJNR 1982;3:25-30.
18. Gentry LR, Godersky JC, Thompdon BH. Traumatic brainstem injury: MR imaging. Radiology 1989;171:177-87.
18a. Bhatoe IH. Primary brainstem injury: Benign course and improved survival. Acta Neuro-Chirurg (Wien) 1999; 141:315-19.
19. Taveras JM. Head Injuries and their complications, Neuroradiology, 3rd edn. Williams and Wilkins, Baltimore 1995;327-63.

20. Benoit BG, Wortzman G. Traumatic cerebral aneurysms: Clinical features and natural history. J Neurol Neurosurg Psychiatry 1973;36:127-38.
21. Kassell NF, Torner JC, et al. The international cooperative study on timing of aneurysm surgery. Part 1. Overall management results. J Neurosurg 1990;73:18-36.
22. Fleischer AS, Patton JM, Tindall GT. Cerebral aneurysms of traumatic origin. Surg Neurol 1975;4:233-9.
23. Kieck CF, de Villiers JC. Vascular lesions due to transcranial stab wounds. J Neurosurg 1984;60:42-6.
24. Crowell RM, Ogilvy CS. Traumatic Intracranial Aneurysms. In: Ojemann RG, Ogilvy Cs Crowell RM, Heros RC (Eds). Surgical Management of Neurovascular disease. Williams and Wilkins 1995;377-84.
25. Stringer WL, Kelly DL. Traumatic dissection of the extracranial internal carotid artery. Neurosurgery 1980; 60:123-30.
26. Zelenock GB, Kazmers A, et al. Extracranial internal carotid artery dissections: Non-iatrogenic traumatic lesions. Arch Surg 1982;177:425-32.
27. Arfanakis K, Haughton VM, Carew JD, Rogers BP, et al. Diffusion tensor imaging in diffuse axonal injury. AJNR 2002;23:794-802.
28. Sidaros A, Engberg AW, Sidaros K, et al. DTI during recovery from severe TBI and relation to clinical outcome, brain 2008;131(2):559-72.

11 Role of Intracranial Pressure (ICP) Monitoring in Head Injury

AK Mahapatra

INTRODUCTION

The outcome of patients with head injury depends upon several factors, and most important among them is the raised intracranial pressure (ICP). Moreover, raised ICP is the most common cause of death, in patients with head injury. Uncontrolled intracranial hypertension produces secondary damage by reducing cerebral blood flow. However, surprisingly routine ICP monitoring in head injury is still continues to be a subject of controversy.[1-6] Lundberg[7] was the first person to introduce ICP monitoring. Today, ICP monitoring has gained a place in neurosurgical ICU management and become an integral part of ICU care. ICP monitoring is extensively studied in head injury patients in last two decades[1,3,4,8-10] either to establish its practical value for therapy or as a prognostic factor.[4,5,9,10] Surprisingly, however, there are neither clear cut guidelines for ICP monitoring nor there is uniform policy for duration of ICP recording. Increased ICP has been defined as pressure more than 20 mm Hg for more than 5 minutes.[9,9a] Several studies linked high level of ICP with high mortality and morbidity. Persistent raised ICP has a direct effect on the brain tissue inspite of cerebral perfusion pressure being normal. We at the AIIMS regularly performing ICP monitoring since last 12 years as and when necessary following our indications (Table 11.1).

Table 11.1: Indications for ICP monitoring in head injury

a. All severe head injury patients.
b. Patients with good coma scale, CT scan showing multiple small hematoma not meriting surgery.
c. Patients with good coma scale with single large intracranial hematoma diagnosed in CT scan.
d. Patients with diffuse brain swelling those who need aggressive management.
e. Postoperative ICP monitoring following evacuation of hematoma.

INDICATIONS FOR ICP MONITORING

Indications for ICP monitoring have changed in last 15 years since routine CT scans are available worldwide. Virtually all major head injury centers use ICP monitoring in the management of head injury. There are few key questions in ICP monitoring. They are: (a) Which are the patients at high-risk for ICP elevation? (b) How do ICP data help in patient management? and (c) Does ICP monitoring improve the ultimate outcome? Dealing with above points, till 1996 there are a total of 146 published articles on ICP monitoring in head injury, forty-one publications on head injury and ICP monitoring. More importantly, 27 articles have dealt with indications for ICP monitoring.

Which Patients are at High-risk of Raised ICP?

Severe Head Injury

The correlation between high ICP and poor outcomes has been well reported by many authors.[2,6,8,9,13,13a] It is clearly established that by lowering elevated ICP, the risk of transtentorial herniation is also reduced and cerebral perfusion improves.[4,14] In 1982, Narayan et al reported 53 to 63 percent raised ICP in severe closed head injury patients with abnormal CT scan. In contrast severe head injury patients with a normal CT had 13 percent incidence of raised ICP. There were three adverse factors in normal CT scan group, those were: (a) patients above 40 years of age, (b) unilateral or bilateral posturing: and (c) patients with systolic BP lower than 90 mm Hg. The risk of raised ICP was similar to those patients with abnormal CT.

Minor and Moderate Head Injury

It is an accepted belief that the patients with mild or moderate head injury, risk of raised ICP is low. The incidence of raised ICP in minor head injury is three percent and in moderate head injury 10 to 20 percent. Thus, routine ICP monitoring not indicated in mild head injury.[14a,14b] However, sometimes patients with minor head injury may need repeated CT scan and ICP monitoring.

Considering all above points and availability of facilities, one can decide his own indications. However, I feel the rational indication of ICP monitoring in head injury as follows:

a. All patients with severe head injury with mass lesion with midline shift or compression of the ventricles or cisterns.
b. Patients with good coma scale with hematomas diagnosed in CT scan.
c. Patients with multiple small intracranial hematoma and not meriting a surgical evacuation.
d. Patients with diffuse swelling, who needs aggressive management.
e. Patients with multiple hematomas of which the only largest one is being removed.
f. Postoperative ICP monitoring after evacuation of hematoma.

US Guidelines for ICP Monitoring[15a]

a. Severe head injury patients with abnormal CT scan. Abnormal CT scan is one that reveals hematoma, contusion, edema or compression of basal cisterns.
b. ICP monitoring is also indicated in severe head injury with a normal CT scan when a patient is above 40 years of age, unilateral or bilateral motor posturing, and when systolic blood pressure is less than 90 mm Hg.
c. ICP monitoring is not routinely indicated in patients with minor or moderate head injury. However, ICP monitoring may be indicated with mass lesion, when a clinician feels the need.

Methods of Monitoring ICP

There are three methods of ICP monitoring by using: (a) Richmond subarachnoid screw, (b) Leed's bolt, (c) Intraventricular or intracavitary catheter. Richmond screw is inserted by making a twist drill hole at a site, 3 cm lateral to midline and 1 cm in front of coronal suture (Fig. 11.1). Dura and arachnoid are coagulated and cut, allowing the CSF to flow, then the bolt is tightened in the hole, after proper hemostasis. Intraventricular catheters are placed through a drill hole at the same site and the catheter is placed in the right frontal horn. In the operated cases, a catheter can be left at the operation cavity for ICP monitoring. Both intracavitary and intraventricular catheters are taken out at least 5 cm always from the main wound, through a subcutaneous tunnel. This is basically to prevent infection.

After placement of the catheter or a screw, all the devices are connected through a fluid filled line

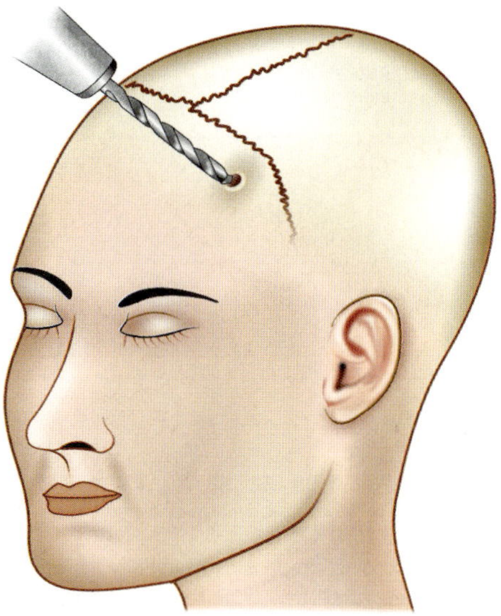

Fig. 11.1: Site of placement of bolt

(containing antibiotic and saline solution) to a strain gauze transducer, zeroed at the level of external auditory meatus. The recording are made using monitor which provides waveform, as well as 24 hours trends and absolute values at an adjustable present time interval. ICP is monitored 24 to 48 hours. The patients are prescribed systemic antibiotics to reduce the risk of infection.

A subdural transducer tipped catheter (CMS) can be used as first time equipment for monitoring of ICP in patients with severe head injury. The clinical results remain similar with other studies.[28]

It is difficult to decide the optimum duration of ICP monitoring in head injury. Sometimes, the ICP can remain high for a long duration, as many systemic factors can give rise to brain swelling and prolong the duration of raised ICP. Thus, duration of raised ICP is unpredictable, and there is phenomenon of secondary rise of intracranial pressure. Most of the reports indicate ICP monitoring 48 to 72 hours[3,12,16] (Fig. 11.2). ICP monitoring for longer period increases the risk of infection. However, in patients with moderate to severe brain swelling and sustained raised ICP (Fig. 11.3), the duration of ICP monitoring may extend a longer period. The rationale of monitoring ICP for five to six days is due to well accepted clinical experience, that the intracranial hypertension is maximum between 48 and 72 hours following trauma. In few patients, secondary raised ICP can occurs, between 7 and 10 days after trauma.[15] We at AIIMS usually record the

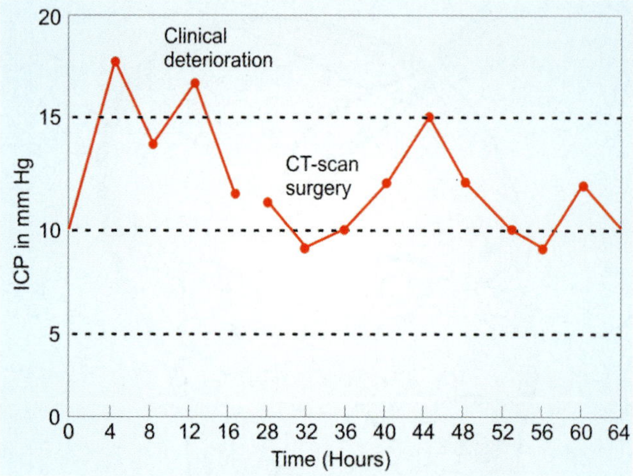

Fig. 11.2: ICP recording graph shows initially 12 hours ICP was midly elevated then ICP remained normal

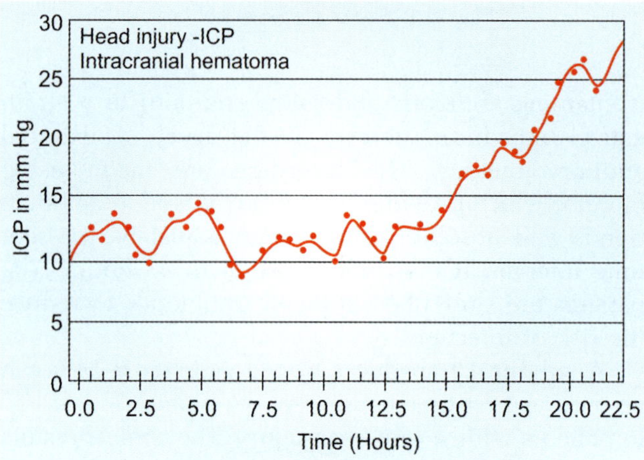

Fig. 11.3: ICP recording graph shows initially normal ICP followed by persistently high ICP

ICP for 24 to 48 hours, and the minimum duration is 24 hours[10] (Table 11.2). We routinely monitor ICP in head-injured patients according to our protocol and ICP is frequently monitored in patients following evacuation of hematoma.

How does ICP Monitoring Influence Head Injury Management?

Intraventricular pressure monitoring helps in assessing the level of ICP and also allows CSF drainage. However, primarily may guide the therapy.[8,17,18] It is a well known fact that one cannot ascertain level of ICP just looking at the clinical state, or pupillary size. On the other hand, all the therapeutic modalities to control raised ICP are double-edged sword. For example, prolonged use of I/V mannitol creates problem and

Table 11.2: ICP monitoring—an experience at AIIMS number of head injury trials

	Year	*Number of patients*	*Type of monitoring*
1.	1979–1980	12	Leeds Bolt
2.	1981–1983	20	Leeds Bolt
3.	1987–1990	59	Leeds Bolt and Richmond Screw
4.	1994–1995	51	Richmond Screw
	Total	142	

prolonged hyperventilation has been conclusively shown to worsen the outcome in severe head-injured patients. Hyperventilation reduces the CO_2, leading to vasoconstriction and causes ischemic damage.[10-21] Surprisingly, hyperventilation is still liberally used in the management of head injury to reduce ICP.[22] The role of mannitol is also unpredictable, both the extent and the duration of action.[23,24] ICP recording not only helps in guiding therapy, but also helps in predicting the outcome.[1,8-10,25]

ICP and Outcome

Intracranial pressure monitoring improves the mortality from head injury. In 1977 Jennett et al[26] reported mortality in severe head injury around 50 percent. Subsequently other authors reported lower mortality with aggressive treatment.[1,3,8,9,13a,27] The aggressive management means ICU care, ventilation and ICP monitoring. Saul and Ducker[27] treated two groups of severe head injury patients, with mannitol and CSF drainage. In the patients in whom ICP was between 20 and 25 mm Hg had a 46 percent mortality as compared to 28 percent mortality in patients in whom ICP was 15 mm Hg. In our study,[10] 65 percent patients had raised ICP. Only 26 percent patients with mass lesion had a normal ICP as compared to 67 percent normal ICP when CT scan did not reveal mass lesion. In 12 patients ICP was more than 30 mm Hg. Overall 52 percent patients with raised ICP had poor outcome and only 15 percent had a good outcome (Table 11.3). The improved outcome of patients with severe head injuries in US has been ascribed to aggressive management protocol, which includes ICP monitoring and drainage of CSF to control ICP.[9a,15a,28]

Table 11.3: Outcome of head injury correlated to ICP

Authors	*No. of patients*	*ICP in mm of Hg*	*Good moderate disable*	*Outcome % dead*
Becker et al[8] 1977	160	> 20/40	60	30
Miller et al[3] 1977	225	> 25	56	34
Narayan et al[4] 1982	207	> 25	57	34
Smith et al[16] 1986	37	> 25	54	35
Paul & Ducker[27] 1982	127	> 25	-	46
Chajar et al[22] 1993	34	> 15	59	12

Limitations of ICP Monitoring

There is a little doubt about the beneficial role of ICP monitoring in head injury. However, the routine ICP monitoring use has not been widely used in India. Except half a dozen centers, ICP monitoring is not used in the management of head injury. The basic problem is that the ICP monitoring is an invasive method and require a good ICU care. The complication of ICP monitoring is not infrequent. The frequent problem is the blocking of the device or dampened tracings. Infections and hematoma formation are two other complications. Narayan et al[4] in 1982 reported 6.3 percent infection and 1.4 percent intracranial hemorrhage in patients undergoing ICP monitoring. In our study at AIIMS, we observed 6 percent infection in patients who had an ICP monitoring. Luckily, we did not encounter intracranial hematoma in our patients, in whom ICP monitoring was carried out.

There is wide range (0–15.3%) in literature of reported incidence of intracranial hemorrhages following placement of ICP monitoring devices. In one study complication rate was 9.7 percent with no grade 3 hemorrhages. Although most common grade 1 hemorrhage seemed to be unimportant in this study. It may have a chance of false reading of high ICP with subsequeal therapeutic interventions. The incidence of grade 3 hemorrhage was 0.15 percent (1 in 684 procedures) for a general neurosurgical population including trauma, tumor and cerebrovascular. Even with utmost precautions, hemorrhagic complications may occur.[28]

CONCLUSION

ICP monitoring helps in early detection of intracranial mass, limits the indiscriminate use of therapeutic modalities to reduce raised ICP can reduce ICP by allowing the CSF drainage, and helps in prognosticating the outcome. Routine ICP monitoring is not indicated in minor or moderate head injury, except in patients with large intracranial hematoma, when the treating neurosurgeon feels the possibility of raised ICP. Blockage is the most frequent cause for discontinuing ICP monitoring, while infection such as meningitis is the most dangerous complication. Even with all above, ICP monitoring deserve a special place in the management of head injury.

REFERENCES

1. Marshall LF, Smith RW, Shapiro HM. The outcome with aggressive treatment in severe head injury. Part 1. The significance of intracranial pressure monitoring. J Neurosurg 1979;80:20-5.
2. Johnston IH, Johnston JA, Jennett WB. Intracranial pressure following head injury. Lancet 1970;2:433-6.
3. Miller JD, Becker CD, Ward JD, et al. Significance of intracranial hypertension in severe head injury. J Neurosurg 1977;47:563-76.
4. Narayan RK, Kishore PR, Becker DP, et al. Intracranial pressure to monitor or not to monitor? A review of our experience with severe head injury. J Neurosurg 1982;56:650-9.
5. Miller JD. ICP monitoring-current states and future direction. Acta Neurochir 1987;85:80-6.
6. Marmarou A, Anderson RL, Ward JD, et al. Impact of ICP instability and hypotension on outcome in patients with severe head trauma. J Neurosurg 1991;75:559-66.
7. Lundberg N. Continuous recording and control of ventricular fluid pressure in neurosurgical practice. Acta Psychiatr Neurol Scand (Suppl) 1960; 36:1-193.
8. Becker DP, Miller JD, Ward JD, et al. The outcome from severe head injury with early diagnosis and intensive management. J Neurosurg 1977;47:491-502.
9. Miller JD, Butterworth JF, Gudeman SK, et al. Further experience in management of severe head injury. J Neurosurg 1981;54:289-99.

9a. Bullock MR, Chestnut RM, Clifton GL, et al. Intracranial pressure treatment threshold. J Neurotrauma 2000; 17:493-5.

10. Mahapatra AK, Bansal S. Role of ICP monitoring in head injury. A prospective study. Neurology India 1998; 46:109-14.

11. Ostrup RC, Luerssen TG, Marshall LF, Zornow MH. Continuous monitoring of intracranial pressure with a miniaturized fibreoptic device. J Neurosurg 1987;67: 206-9.
12. Jane JA, Luerssen TG, Marmarou A, Foulkes MA. The outcome of severe closed head injury. J Neurosurg 1991; 1991;75(Suppl):528-36.
13. Marshall LF, Gautille T, Klauber MR, et al. The outcome of severe closed head injury. J Neurosurg 1991;75:528-36.
13a. Lane PL, Storetz TG, Doig G, et al. Intracranial pressure monitoring and outcome after traumatic brain injury. Can J Surg 2000;43:442-8.
14. Eisenber HM, Gary HE Jr, Aldrich EF, et al. Initial CT findings in 753 patients with severe head injury. A report from the NIH Traumatic coma data Bank. J Neurosurg 1990;73;688-98.
14a. Stein SC, Ross SE. Mild Head Injury: A plea for routine early CT scanning. J Trauma 1992;33:11-3.
14b. Jevet JS. Minor Head Injury and CT Scanning. Letter J Trauma 1993;35:490-1.
15. Unterberg A, Kiening K, Schmiedek P, Lanksch W. Long-term observation of intracranial pressure after severe head injury. The phenomenon of secondary rise of intracranial pressure. Neurosurg 1993;32:17-24.
15a. Bullock MR, Chestnut RM, Clifton GL. Indications for ICP monitoring. J Neurotraum 2000;17:474-91.
16. Smith HP, Kelly DL Jr, Mc Whorter JM, et al. Comparison of mannitol regimens in patients with severe head injury undergoing intracranial pressure monitoring. J Neurosurg 1986;65:820-4.
17. Chesnut RM, Crisp CB, Klauber MR, et al. Early routine paralysis for intracranial pressure control in severe head injury: Is it necessary? Crit Care Med 1994;22: 1471-6.
18. Feldman Z, Narayan RK. Intracranial pressure monitoring. Techniques and pitfalls. In: Cooper PR (Ed). Head injury, 3rd edn, Williams and Wilkins, Baltimore, 1993.
19. Muizelaar JP, Marmarou A, Ward JD, et al. Adverse effects of prolonged hyperventilation in patients with severe head injury. A randomized clinical trial. J Neurosurg, 1991;5:731-9.
20. Robertson CS, Contant CF, Gokaslan ZL, et al. Cerebral blood flow, arteriovenous oxygen difference and outcome in head injured patients. J Neurol Neurosurg Psychiatr 1992;55:594-3.
21. Gopinath SP, Robertson CS, Contant CF, et al. Jugular venous desaturation and outcome after head injury. J Neurol Neurosurg and Psychiat 1994;57:717-23.
22. Ghajar JB, Brown R, Narayan RK, et al. Survey of critical care management of comatose head injured patients in the United States: Crit Care Med 1995;23:560-7.
23. Marshall LF, Smith RW, Ranscher IA, et al. Mannitol dose requirements in brain injured patients. J Neurosurg 1978;48:169-72.
24. Mendelow AD, Teasdale GM, Russell T, et al. Effect of mannitol on cerebral blood flow and cerebral perfusion pressure in human head injury. J Neurosurg 1985;63: 43-8.
25. Narayan RK, Greenberg RP, Miller JD, et al. Improved confidence of outcome prediction in severe head injury: A comparative analysis of clinical examination, multimodal evoked potentials, CT scanning and intracranial pressure. J Neurosurg 1981;54:751-62.
26. Jennett B, Teasdale G, Galbraith S, et al. Severe head injury in three countries. J Neurol Neurosurg Psychiat 1977;40:291-5.
27. Goldstein B. Power ICS head trauma in children. Peditr Rev 1994;15:213-9.
28. Bullock MR, Chernut RM, Clifton GL, et al. Critical pathways for treatment of established intracranial hypertension. J Neurotrauma 2000;17:537-47.

12 Monitoring in Head Injury

AK Mahapatra, Raj Kumar

As the outcome of head injury is multifactorial, the factors influencing the outcome have to be carefully assessed time-to-time, to assess the progress of the patients. Over the years, monitoring system has improved, this is because of advances in the knowledge of understanding of the mechanism of brain damage, along with technological explosion. In spite of all diagnostic and monitoring facilities, large percentage of severe head injury patients die or fair poorly. Even in US, not all centers perform ICP monitoring, as many level I centers manage a significant number of severe head injury. Only 28 percent centers frequently use ICP monitoring,[1] while 7 percent centers never use ICP monitoring. Thus, there is a great deal of variation in head injury management protocol. Hence, there is a need for uniform management protocol to compare the data.

There are large number of parameters that can be monitored (Table 12.1) depending on facility available and interest of the management team.[1,3] Hence, multimodality monitoring is important and should be used more frequently to achieve a good result.

CLINICAL MONITORING

Head injury is a dynamic process, and the changes occurring at cellular, biochemical and molecular level are continuous. However, the starting point of these changes is the point of trauma. As the changes keep on progressing or regressing, the patients may show deterioration or improvement. Hence, the importance of clinical monitoring cannot be over emphasized. The clinical parameters which need to be monitored are: (a) level of consciousness: (b) cranial nerve function: (c) Doll's eye movement: (d) vestibulo-ocular response. These parameters are vital and have tremendous prognostic value. Level of consciousness must be analyzed on the Glasgow coma scale (GCS) which is easy to follow. Even, the nurses must be trained in monitoring patients neurological state and respiration. GCS provides the idea of patient's improvement or deterioration. If carefully evaluated, clinical monitoring will indicate in what stage patient needs surgery and further observation and waiting may risk the patient's life or may lead to irreversible brain damage. Hence, clinical monitoring is vital in head injury management.

Table 12.1: Various monitoring in head injury

A. Clinical monitoring
  - Conscious state
  - Focal deficit
  - ICP, pulse, BP
  - Cold caloric response

B. ICP monitoring
C. Evoked potential monitoring
D. CT scan monitoring
E. Blood gas, jugular oxygen monitoring
F. Transcranial Doppler monitoring
G. Metabolic monitoring with emission tomography
H. Microdialysis of the brain

Cerebral dysfunction in head injury is reflected in myotactic reflex abnormalities, which can be measured at bed side with greater reproducibility, reflex measurement may assist monitoring of patients with head injury. For evaluation of this reflex, a phasic stretch reflex of biceps brachii is illicited by a servo-positioned tendon hammer. Antagonistic inhibition is evoked by vibration to the triceps. Using surface EMG, the amplitude of an unconditioned bicep reflex and percentage antagonistic inhibition is measured. The unconditioned reflex was found to be absent in most patient with GCS less than 5, otherwise it varied little across the patient group in one study. The conditioning lest interval fell progressively with lower GCS, although patients individuals could not be assessed with single measurement. Both reflex indices correlate with GCS.[46]

Among the clinical monitoring, most important is close observation of Glasgow coma scale (GCS). GCS is internationally accepted as a standard method of assessing the conscious state, which include: (a) eye opening, (b) best motor response: and (c) best verbal response. The details of GCS is described elsewhere. However, over the years the limitations of GCS are well recognized. In children under 5 years of age where assessing the verbal response is difficult, GCS is of limited value. This is particularly so in infants where assessment of best motor and best verbal response is also difficult.

Eye opening is sometimes difficult due to gross eye swelling or black eyes. Similarly, patient may be conscious and may not be able to speak because of damage to speech area, giving rise to dysphasia. Answering also depends on language that the patient understands. It is particularly so in country like India, where people speak different languages. In motor scoring, abnormal flexon is sometime over looked, hence likely to under estimate the motor scoring. Another point also confuses the motor scoring, when a patient has multiple limb fractures or injury when performing a motor movement is difficult, except facial and neck muscles. Amongst the all factors motor scoring is probably most prognostic.[5-5b] Moreover, GCS does not include vital parameters like respiration, blood pressure, pupillary state and other associated problems, which significantly contribute to the ultimate outcome. Shippy et al,[5a] in 1984, had highlighted role and limitation of blood volume estimation in critically sick patients.

MONITORING OF VESTIBULO-OCULAR REFLEX (COLD CALORIC RESPONSE)

Vestibulo-ocular reflex (VOR) is a reliable test of assessing brainstem function.[6-8] Medial longitudinal fasciculous (MLF) in the brainstem, is connected to vestibular apparatus in inner ear, vestibular nuclei and nuclei of 3rd, 4th and 6th cranial nerves on the both sides. Thus, VOR provides a very good physiological substrate for studying brainstem function. In a normal situation, by stimulating the external ear, one can stimulate vestibular apparatus and induce a conjugate eye movement, which is otherwise called VOR. VOR is also utilized to establish the brain death, when it is absent in association with other parameters.

Over last few decades, VOR is utilized as a reliable bed side test to establish the integrity of brainstem function, in various neurological disorders, and more importantly, in head injury, to prognosticate the outcome. As early as 1969, Jadav, et al,[8] analyzed the role of VOR in patients with altered conscious state. Bruce et al,[9] in 1982, reported VOR as a good predictor of outcome in pediatric head injury. Mahapatra et al,[6] reported good outcome in decerebrating head injured patients with normal outcome. In another study Mahapatra and Tandon[7] compared VOR with brainstem auditory evoked potential (BAEP) and found that, VOR was as good or even better than BAEP in predicting outcome in severe head injury patients. BAEP is more difficult to perform than VOR, which is a simple bed side test. It can be repeated as and when necessary, without much problem.

Table 12.2: VOR and outcome in severe head injury[3]

VOR findings	*Total No. of patients*	*Good outcome %*	*Poor outcome %*
Normal	70	88	12
Abnormal	36	30	70
Absent	18	–	100

Normal VOR indicates a very good outcome.[3,7,8] In a study Mahapatra reported[3] good outcome in 85 percent patients, when VOR was normal, while 100 percent patients with an absent VOR had a poor outcome (Table 12.2).

EVOKED POTENTIAL MONITORING

Evoked potential monitoring provides the functional assessment of neuronal structures in a tested pathways.[10,16,16a] Functional or physiological monitoring can be performed through EEG, sensory evoked potential (SEP) and auditory brainstem evoked potential (ABEP) (Figs 12.1A to C). Over last 3 decades, considerable interest has been shown in studying evoked potential in head injury patients, to predict the outcome. Greenberg and his colleagues[12,13,17] were the first to perform multimodal evoked potential studies in severe head injury and established the predictive value. They graded, evoked potentials into four different grades. Grade I was normal, Grade II mild abnormality, Grade III severe abnormality and Grade IV was absent response. Mahapatra and Tandon[7] and Mahapatra classified EP into normal, abnormal and absent.

Sensory evoked potentials (SEPs) represent minute electrical responses generated in sensory pathway in response to stimuli. The responses are quantified according to amplitude, latency and conduction time. Unlike EEG, SEP monitoring is relatively resistant to artifact. Overall, SEP has a better predictive value as compared to BAEP.[2,14] Humes and Cant[14] in 1981, emphasized the role of central conduction time (CCT), which essentially means, time taken by the stimuli to reach from lower medulla to sensory cortex. Greenberg et al[12,13] concluded that the SEP is of greater predictive value than that of BAEP. Seales et al[6]

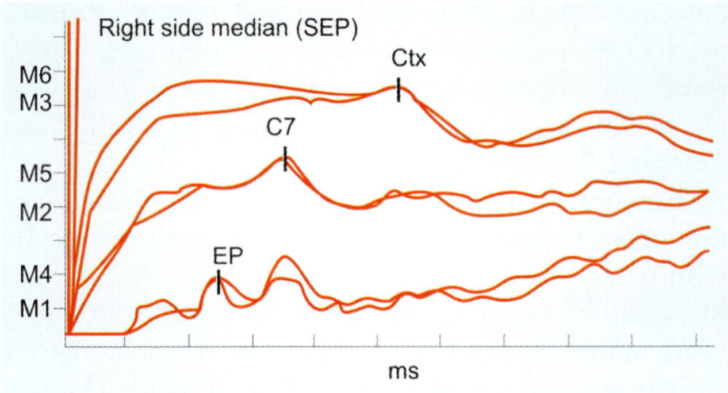

Fig. 12.1A: Sensory evoked potential (SEP) in a patient with severe head injury shows normal response

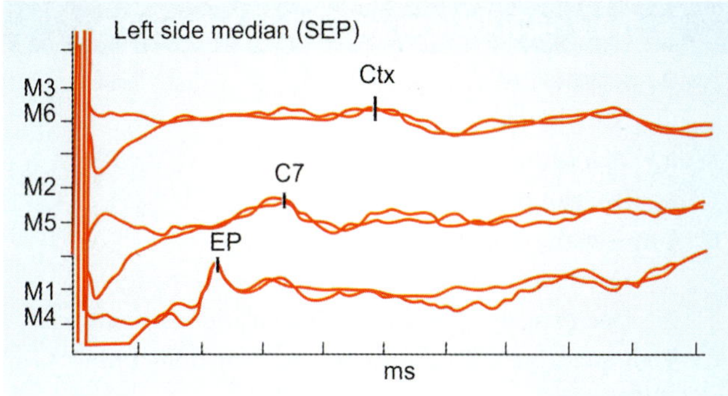

Fig. 12.1B: SEP in a patient with severe head injury shows low amplitude cortical wave

find out a 100 percent correlation between abnormal BAEP and death. Moultan et al in 1994[18] reported good correlation between SEP findings and poor outcome. In those patients in whom SSEP deteriorated, an increased arteriovenous desaturation of oxygen ($AVDO_2$) was recorded. Mahapatra in 1990[15] reported a good outcome in 87 percent and 83 percent patients with normal BAEP and normal SEP, respectively. When both BAEP and SEP were normal, good recovery was recorded in 93 percent patients. Uniformly poor outcome was observed when both BAEP and SEP were absent. Greenberg et al[12] reported a 71 percent good recovery in head injury patients with normal BAEP. In another study, Mahapatra and Tandon[7] had observed 81 percent good recovery in patients with normal BAEP. Surprisingly, 2 out of 7 patients with absent BAEP had good outcome, emphasizing the limitation of BAEP. This limitation can be avoided by repeating the study 2 to 3 times, which can provide 100 percent predictive value.

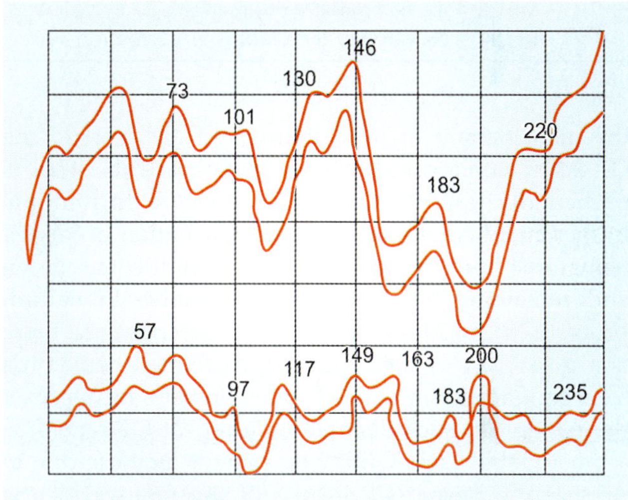

Fig. 12.1C: Brainstem auditory evoked potential (BAEP) shows low amplitude cortical wave

CT SCAN MONITORING

CT scan is the gold standard in diagnosis of intracranial pathology in head injury. However, over the years the limitation of CT scan has been well recognized.[19,21] Neurological deterioration can be due to acute focal or generalized brain swelling[22] or even expanding mass lesion, either extra-axial or intra-axial.[19] This only means CT scan performed in early post injury period is likely to worsen over 24 hours. Brain swelling is difficult to see in CT, initially as brain shows an homogeneous isodensity or fairly hyperdense appearance in early post-trauma period. CT done within 24 hours may show small ventricles and compression or obliteration of cisterns. It is well accepted that edema progress 3 to 5 days to reach the peak. Ito et al[23] used planimetric sequence CT scan and reported diffuse hyperemic swelling within 2 to 4 hours, while first sign of edema developed only 24 hours later. According to their experience brain swelling subsided within 3 to 5 days, but edema reached the peak on 6 to 8th days.

Hematoma can develop or the existing hematoma can increase in size between two scans. This possibility is higher in the initial CT done very early following trauma. Labato et al[19] reported extracerebral and intracerebral mass lesions expanding progressively over several hours. Study done, from our department showed change in CT finding in 48 percent patients between initial and repeat CT.[21] In 36 percent cases CT scan worsened, while in 12 percent cases CT scan showed resolution of hematoma. Interestingly, in patients undergoing ICP monitoring, when ICP remained high or increased over a period of time, repeat CT almost always revealed worsening of intracranial pathology. This observation has become an important factor in

Table 12.3: Role of RPT CT in head injury

A. Appearance of
  i. New hematoma
  ii. Worsening of edema
  iii. Development of infarction

B. Improvement of CT finding
  i. Decrease in size of hematoma or contusion
  ii. Decrease in edema and visualization of ventricle

C. Postoperative CT scan (when patient does not improve)
  i. May show improvement of scan
  ii. May show increase in size of small hematoma
  iii. Recollection of blood at operation site
  iv. Appearance of brainstem hematoma or occipital infarct secondary to transtentorial herniation

the management of head injury and has lead to the CT scan monitoring of head injury patients. This is particularly important, when a patient with multiple intracranial hematomas undergo evacuation of largest hematoma, presuming that ICP would come down and remaining hematoma would resolve in natural process, in few days time. In such a situation, there is a possibility of increase in size of small hematoma to a significant size, which may prevent recovery of the patient. In such a situation, a repeat CT scan(s) is a must (Table 12.3). Otherwise patient may die due to persistently raised ICP inspite of the removal of the largest hematoma. Thus, the monitoring of CT scan has become absolute important in the management of severe head injury.

TRANSCRANIAL DOPPLER MONITORING

It was generally believed that the vasospasm never occurs in traumatic subarachnoid hemorrhage. Over the years it has been proved wrong, not only by carotid angiography[24,25] which showed focal or generalized narrowing of vessel, but also CT scan may show appearance of an infarct which may not be present in the initial scan. This finding in CT scan did confirm the focal vasospasm leading to focal infarction.

Over last two decades, transcranial Doppler sonography (TCD) has been routinely used to evaluate the blood flow in intracranial vessel. Intracranial blood flow velocity (BFV) can be repeatedly studied in head injury patient.[10] It also helps in finding pulsatility index (PI) by finding out difference in systolic and diastolic flow velocity.[26] By monitoring flow velocity in ICA and MCA through TCD, post-traumatic vasospasm can be detected.[1,5] In a study by Matz and Pitts they measured BFV on consecutive days, post-traumatic vasospasm was diagnosed when MCA, flow velocity was above 120 cm/sec. In some patients increased BFC was observed 5-15 days after injury.[25]

Cerebral vasospasm was also confirmed by Lindegaard ratio[24] by comparing MCA flow velocity with extracranial ICA blood flow velocity. Bakshi and Mahapatra[27] observed basilar artery spasm in severe head injury. Thus, TCD can be used to demonstrate vasospasm and predict cerebral compliance changes in head injury, using portable TCD machine. However, the limitation of TCD is that, it only provides qualitative estimation of regional CBF.

TCD can be helpful in preventing secondary brain damage due to ischemia.[28,30] In some patients, there may be unilateral increase in BFV, and these patients are likely to develop focal infraction, supplied by the vessel having vasospasm. Maneuvers to increase CPP will prevent ischemic damage. Martin et al[25] reported elevated MCA, BFV in 27 percent patients. In 17 percent patients elevated MCA velocity was associated with traumatic subarachnoid hemorrhage. Thus, a combination of traumatic SAH and vasospasm lead to a poor outcome.[25,30] Generally raised BFV reduces in few days time (5-15 days), the pattern is exactly similar to spontaneous SAH. Increased BFV may also be associated with cerebral hyperemia,[31] depending on vascular resistance. Both hyperemia and vasospasm are associated with impaired autoregulations. Over the years, the role of ischemic damage is well established. The ischemia is due to traumatic SAH and vasospasm, demonstrated in TCD. Thus, TCD monitoring has become an important ICU parameter in the management of severe head injury.

JUGULAR VENOUS SATURATION MONITORING

The utilization of oxygen by the brain is critical for normal brain function. In head injury patients, this function becomes more important. Continuous monitoring of jugular venous bulb oxygen saturation ($SJVO_2$) provides valuable information regarding cerebral oxygen metabolism ($CMRO_2$). The $SJVO_2$ monitoring is carried out by fiberoptic catheter inserted into the internal jugular vein, and placed at jugular bulb. $SJVO_2$ helps in calculating Arteriovenous desaturation of oxygen ($AVDO_2$) which is equal to 1.39 x Hb x arterial oxygen saturation (SAO_2) minus $SJVO_2$.[32-33a] Sheinberg et al[33a] reported the useful value of continuous monitoring of jugular venous oxygen saturation in head injured patients.

The catheter is placed in jugular bulb.[34] A skull film is used to confirm that the catheter is at the right position. The monitoring is based on fiberoptic reflectance spectrophotometry. The $SJVO_2$ represents the ratio of actual to potential saturation of venous blood Hb and is a percent.

Some authors have used 5.5 french dual lumen balloon tipped catheter, with a integral thermistor.[35] Episodes of $SJVO_2$ 50 percent for 15 min are considered desaturation. It has been observed that even a single desaturation correlates closely with poor outcome. Multiple episodes of desaturations is a good predictor of poor outcome.[35-37] Unfortunately, artifacts are common with $SJVO_2$ monitoring, 5 to 55 percent[37,38] and usually occurs when fiberoptic catheter get occluded, by blood or breakage of the optical fibers. Episode of early desaturation was observed in 39.6 percent[1] usually within 24 hours of injury.[37] Generally, venous desaturation in severe head injury increase the mortality.[32,34,37,38] Cruze in 1996, reported the relationship between early patterns of cerebral extraction of oxygen and outcome from severe acute traumatic brain swelling and cerebral ischemia with impaired cerebral viability.

Venous desaturation from various pathologies reduce oxygen flow to the brain. Desaturation can occur with reduced arterial oxygen as a result of hypotension of hypoxia, or due to increased cerebrovascular resistance of vasospasm. Finally, cerebral hypoperfusion due to low CPP also results in desaturation. Desaturation is immediate due to systemic hypotension, while desaturation due to raised ICP is delayed.[36]

Limitations of $SJVO_2$

Even though $SJVO_2$ is a good predictor or outcome in moderate or severe head injury, the method only provide global oxygen consumption. The $SJVO_2$ is dependent on BP, ICP, hemoglobin and more importantly the affinity of Hb for oxygen. One of the drawback is the procedure is invasive and required experience.

METABOLIC MONITORING IN HEAD INJURY

Cerebral ischemia is one of most important causes of secondary brain insults following acute brain injury. While intracranial pressure monitoring does not reflect the state of oxygenation of injured brain. The holy grail of neuromonitoring is modality that would reflect accurately real time. The status of oxygenation in tissue of interest, artifact free to provides information that can be used for therapeutic interventions to improve outcome.[47]

Cerebral blood flow (CBF) and $CMRO_2$ can be measured, by using radionuclide tracers.[32,39,40] Positron emission tomography (PET) can be used to measure $CMRO_2$ by using emission CT, during inhalation of $C^{15}O_2$ and $^{15}O_2$.[39] Cerebral oxygen utilization can be evaluated in brain slices cerebral metabolism of glucose can be measured by utilizing (18°F) Fluorode oxyglucose. Thus, by using PET scan one can assess $CMRO_2$ and cerebral metabolic rate of glucose. However, PET scanning is not routinely used in head injury due to various reasons.

Recently, SPECT scanning is used to assess the regional cerebral blood flow. The agents used are HMPAO or 99mTc ethylene cysteine dimer (ECD). These two substance cross the blood-brain barrier and distributed in cerebral cortex, in proportion to the cerebral perfusion. Images obtained by gamma Camera (SPECT) demonstrates cerebral perfusion at different areas. Cerebral contusion and hematoma show hypometabolic state. SPECT also detect the cerebral perfusion abnormalities earlier than that of CT scan. In acute head injury, SPECT detect more lesions than seen on CT scans. Rarely, SPECT may fail to detect contusion seen as CT scans. This is possible that these are normal flow contusion, may simply indicate luxury perfusion, dissociating flow from metabolic activity. In traumatic brain injury SPECT is not extensively used, this is basically due to poor resolution and difficulties in qualification of flow. SPECT scan is also helpful in predicting the degree of permanent damage and those patients likely to develop post concussion syndrome.

BRAIN MICRODIALYSIS

Over last 2 decades, the neurochemical and neurotransmitter changes in acute head injury is well recognized. Hypoxia and hypoperfusion results in anaerobic glycolysis and accumulation of lactate and pyruvate. There is also a significant rise of glutamate, glycine and 'Y amino butyrate. It leads to acidosis. Recently, it has become possible to monitor these chemicals in experimental and clinical set up by microdialysis of the brain.[40-44] Bullock et al[45] reported 60 head injury patients in whom brain O_2, CO_2, pH, temperature, glutamate, aspartate, potassium, lactate and glucose was monitored. Elevated excitatory amino acid level most closely correlate to elevated potassium level and raised ICP. Surprisingly, they did not find any correlation between elevated lactate, cerebral perfusion or poor outcome. Brain oxygen monitoring appeared to be most useful in guiding therapy and predicting the outcome.

Microdialysis is used in head injury with SAH. Langemann et al[43] monitored glucose, lactate and pH in the dialysate in head injury patients and reported glucose lactate ratio to some extent correlated with clinical course. Interestingly, Bullock et al[45] reported elevated excitatory amino acids for a longer period in head injury patients than that observed in experimental animals. Persson et al[44] utilized microdialysis and reported, that the persistently elevated lactate. Pyruvate ratio and glutamate level well correlated with the outcome. Thus, the present experience suggests that the microdialysis is a promising tool for monitoring various amino acids and response to the treatment.

REFERENCES

1. Matz PG, Pitts L. Monitoring in traumatic brain injury In: Clinical Neurosurgery. Editor-in-chief S Grandy, Williams and Wilkins, Baltimore 1996; vol 44: p. 267-94.
2. Ghajar J, Har RJ, Narayan RK, et al. Survey of critical care management of comatose, head injured patients in US. Crit Care Med 1995;23:560-7.
3. Mahapatra AK. Monitoring in Paediatric Head injury patients. Neurology India, (Supp!) 1995;43:64-7.
4. Jordan KG. Neurophysiologic monitoring in the neurosciences intensive care unit. Neurol Clin 1995;13:579-625.

4a. Silverston P. Pulse oximetry at road side: a study of pulse oximety in immediate care. BM J 1989;298:711-3.

5. Colohan AR, Alves WM, Gross CR, et al. Head injury mortality in two centres with different emergency medical services and intensive care. J Neurosurg 1989; 71:202-7.

5a. Shippy CR, Appel PL, Shoemaker WC. Reliability of clinical monitoring to assess blood volume in critically ill patients. Crit Care Med 1984;12:107-12.

5b. Initial assessment and management. Advanced trauma life support for Doctors: students course manual. Chicago II American College of Surgeon 1997;21-46.

6. Mahapatra AK, Tandon PN, Bhatia R, Banerji AK. Bilateral decerebration in head injury patient. An analysis of 62 cases. Surg Neurol 1985;23:536-40.
7. Mahapatra AK, Tandon PN. Brainstem auditory evoked potential and vestibulo-ocular reflex in severe head injury. A prospective study of 60 cases. Acta Neurochirurgi (Wien) 1987;87:40-3.
8. Jadav SR, Sinha A, Tandon PN, et al. Cold caloric test in altered state of consciousness. Laryngoscope 1971;8:391-7.
9. Bruce DA, Alavi A, Balaniwk LT, et al. Diffuse cerebral swelling following head injury in children. The syndrome of malignant brain oedema. J Neurosurg 1981;54:170-8.
10. Jordan KG. Neurophysiologic monitoring in the neurosciences intensive care unit. Neurol Clin 1995;13:579-626.
11. Solan TB. Electrophysiologic monitoring in head injury. New Horiz 1995;3:431-8.
12. Greenberg RP, Becker DP, Miller JD, et al. Evaluation of brain function in severe head trauma with multimodality evoked potential Part II. Localisation of brain dysfunction and correlation with post-traumatic neurological condition. J Neurosurg 1977;47:163-77.
13. Greenberg RP, Newlong PG, Hyatt MJ, et al. Prognostic implication of multimodal evoked potential in severe head injury patients. A prospective study. J Neurosurg 1981;55:227-36.
14. Humes AL, Cant BR. Central Somatosensory conduction time after head injury. Ann Neurol 1981;10:411-9.
15. Mahapatra AK. Evoked potentials in severe head injury. A prospective study of 40 patients. J Ind Med Asso 1990; 88:217-20.
16. Seals DM, Rossiter VS, Weinstein ME. Brainstem auditory evoked responses in patients comatose as a result of blunt head trauma. J Trauma 1970;19:347-53.

16a. Guerit JM. Usefulness of EEG exogenous evoked potentials, and cognitive evoked potentials in the acute stage of postanoxic and post-traumatic coma. Acta Neurol Belg 2000;100:229-36.

17. Seelig JN, Becker DP, Miller JD, et al. Traumatic acute subdural haematoma. Major mortality reduction in comatose patients treatment within 4 hours. New Engl J Med 1981;304:1511-8.
18. Moulten RJ, Shedden PM, Tucker WS, et al. Somatosensory evoked potential monitoring following severe closed head injury. Clin Invest Med 1994;17:187-95.
19. Labato RD, Rivas JJ, Gomez P Castanedam. Head injury patients who talk and deteriorated into coma. Analysis of 211 cases studied with CT. J Neurosurg 1991;75:256-61.

19a. Stiell IG, Wells GA, Vandemheen K, et al. The Canadian. CT head rule for patients with minor head injury. Lancet 2001;357:1391-6.

20. Labato RD, Sarabia R, Cordaes F, Rivas JJ. Post-traumatic cerebral hemisphere swelling. Analysis of 55 cases studied with CT. J Neurosurg 1988;68:417-23.

20a. Jevet JS. Minor head injury and CT Scanning (Letter) J. Trauma 1993;35:490-1.

21. Dubey AK. Role of repeat CT scan in head injury. A prospective study of 146 patients. MCh. Thesis submitted to AIIMS 1991.
22. Bruce DA, Alavi BL, Dolinskas C, et al. Diffuse cerebral swelling following head injury in children. The syndrome of malignant brain oedema. J Neurosurg 1981;54:170-8.
23. Ito U, Yamazaki Y, et al. Brain swelling and brain oedema in acute head injury. Acta Neurochir (Wien) 1986;79:120-4.
24. Lindegaard KF, Nornes H, Bakke SJ, et al. Cerebral vasospasm diagnosed by means of angiography and blood velocity measurements. Acta Neurochir (Wien) 1989;100:12-24.
25. Martin NA, Doberstein C, Zane C, et al. Post-traumatic cerebral arterial spasm: Transcranial Doppler ultrasound, cerebral blood flow, and angiographic findings. J Neurosurg 1992;77:575-83.

26. Coraj B, Rifkinson-Mann S, Leslie DR, et al. Correlation of intracranial pressure and transcranial Doppler resistine index after head trauma. Am J Neuro Radio 1994;15:1333-9.
27. Bakshi A, Mahapatra AK. Basilar artery vasospasm in severe head injury. A preliminary TCD study. NMJI 1998;113:220-1.
28. Chan KH, Deardan NM, Miller JD. The significance of post-traumatic increase in cerebral blood flow velocity. A transcranial Doppler ultrasound study. Neurosurg 1992; 30:697-700.
29. Shigemori M, Kikuchi N, Tokutomi T, et al. Monitoring severe head injury patients with transcranial Doppler ultrasonography. Acta Neurochir Suppl (Wien) 1992; 55:6-7.
30. Steiger HJ, Aaslid R, Stooss R, et al. Transcranial Doppler monitoring in head injury. Relations between injury, flow velocity Vasoreactivity, and outcome. Neurosurg 1994;34:79-85.
31. Romner B, Bellner J, Kongstad P, et al. Elevated transcranial blood flow velocities after severe head injury: Cerebral vasospasm or hyperemia? J Neurosurg 1996;85:90-7.
32. Martin NA, Dobertein C. Cerebral blood flow measurement in neurosurgical intensive care. Neurosurgia Clin North Ame 1994;5:607-18.
33. Ritter AM, Robertson CS. Cerebral metabolism. Neurosurg Clin N Ame 1994;5:633-45.
33a. Sheinbergin, Kanter MI, Robertson CS, et al. Continuous monitoring of jugular oxygen saturation in head injured patients. J Neurosurg 1992;76:212-7.
34. Andrews PJ, Dearden NM, Miller JD. Jugular bulb cannulation. Description of a cannulation technique and validation of a new continuous monitor. Br J Anaesth 1991;67:553-8.
35. Villanueva PA. Jugular venous bulb saturation ($SJVO_2$) monitoring in head injury. In: Modern Trends in the management of neurotrauma. PS Ramani, Alok Sharma (Eds). Lavanya Print, Bombay 1994;79-81.
36. Sheinbreg M, Kanter M, Robertson CS, Contant CF, et al. Continuous monitoring of jugular venous oxygen saturation in head injured patients. J Neurosurg 1992; 76:212-7.
37. Copinath SP, Robertson CS, Contant CF, et al. Jugular venous desaturation and outcome after head injury. J Neurol Neurosurg, Psychiat 1994;57:717-23.
38. Lewis SB, Myburgh JA, Reilly PI. Detection of cerebral venous desaturation by continuous jugular bulb oximetry following acute Neurotrauma. Anaesth Intensive Care 1995;23:307-14.
39. Franckowiak RS, Lenzi GL, Jones T, et al. Quantitative measurement of regional cerebral blood flow and oxygen metabolism in man using ^{15}O and positron emission tomography. Theory, procedure and normal values. J Comput, Assist Tomogr 1980;4:727-36.
40. Hill TC, Magistretti PL, Holman BL, et al. Assessment of regional cerebral blood flow (rCBF) in stroke using SPECT, and N-isopropyl (I-123) P-iodoam phetamine (IMP) Stroke 1984;15:40-5.
41. Landolt H, Langemann H, Mendlowitsch A, et al. Neurochemical Monitoring and on-line pH measurements using brain microdialysis in patients in intensive care. Acta Neurochir Suppl (Wien) 1994;60:475-8.
42. Kanthan R, Shuaib A. Clinical evaluation of extracellular amino acids in severe head trauma by intracerebral *in vivo* microdialysis. J Neurol Neurosurg Psychiatry 1995; 59:326-7.
43. Langemann H, Mandelowitsch A, Landolt H, et al. Experimental and clinical monitoring of glucose by microdialysis. Clin Neurol Neurosurg 1995;97:49-115.
44. Persson L, Valtysson J, Enblad P, et al. Neurochemical monitoring using intracerebral microdialysis in patients with subarachnoid haemorrhage. J Neurosurg 1996; 84:606-16.
45. Bullock R, Zanner A, Myseros JS, et al. Evidence for prolonged release of excitatory amino acids in severe human head trauma. Relationship to clinical events. Ann NY Acad Sci 1995;765:260-97.
46. Cozens JA, Miller S, Chambers IA, Mandelow AD. Monitoring of head injury by myotactic reflex evaluation. J Neurol Neurosurgery & Psychiat 2000;68:581-8.
47. Ng I, Lee KK, Wong J. Brain tissue oxygenation monitoring in acute brain injury. Acta Neurochir 2005; [Suppl] 95:447-51.

13 Management of Severe Head Injury

Raj Kamal, AK Mahapatra

INTRODUCTION

Initial management of acute closed head injury at the accident site and during transit.

Life-saving measures should be started at the site of the accident. The aims of this emergency service are: (1) Resuscitation, (2) Prevention of second accident, (3) Preparation of the injured for transport and (4) Maintenance of optimum condition possible during transport until the patient is taken care of in the hospital.

The "ABC" system, where A = Airway, B = Breathing, and C = Circulation, is aimed at rapidly assessing and initiating the life supports urgently needed, followed by more detailed diagnostic examination and adjustment of treatment. Usually the head injured patients come quickly under the care of police and sometime under the ambulance services. Until the patient arrives at hospital care must be taken to see that the airway is clear. It is reported that approximate 50 percent severe head injury patients are hypoxic at the site of injury, which is associated with an increased mortality.[1,1a] A control study had suggested prehospital intubation was associated with significant reduction of mortality.[1a]

INITIAL MANAGEMENT OF AIRWAY

Initial management of airway involves clearing the upper airway of vomitus, blood, secretions, and foreign bodies such as false or loose teeth. If possible an airway should be placed and oxygen should be given by mask. Where multiple injuries are suspected and particularly in the case of fractures of the spine, the pelvis, a femur or a tibia, transport by stretcher is advised. Some authors have advised pulse oximetry during transport of patient.[2a]

It is reported that approximately 50 percent severe head injury patients are hypoxic at the site of injury, which is associated with an increased mortality.[1,1a] A control study had suggested prehospital intubation was associated with significant reduction of mortality.[1a]

MANAGEMENT IN THE CASUALTY ROOM

In emergency room, the patient should be examined carefully and quickly. The airway patency and blood pressure should be checked. Associated injuries should be identified and recorded. If a patient airway cannot be obtained with simple oral or nasopharyngeal tubing, the patient should be intubated. In patients suspected to have cervical injury, intubation should be performed cautiously. Intubation should be done preferably by an anesthetist or by a qualified doctor to do so. If due to any reason intubation is not possible or delayed, an immediate tracheostomy should be done in patient who are having respiratory obstruction.

The neurological evaluation includes neurological evaluation of the level of consciousness as determined by the Glasgow coma scale (Table 13.1), pupillary examination for size and reactivity, to assess potential or impending herniation. External evaluation of the head may reveal signs of basal skull fracture, such as mastoid ecchymosis (Battle's sign), periorbital ecchymosis (racoon eyes), and CSF otorrhea or rhinorrhea. Head injury can be classified as mild, moderate and severe according to Glasgow coma scale (GCS).

Table 13.1: Glasgow coma scale

A.	**Eye Opening**	
	Spontaneous	4
	To speech	3
	To pain	2
	No eye opening	1
B.	**Best Motor Response**	
	Obeys command	6
	Localizes to pain	5
	Withdraws from stimulation (Flexion)	4
	Abnormal flexion	3
	Extension	2
	No motor response	1
C.	**Best Verbal Response**	
	Oriented	5
	Confused	4
	Inappropriate words	3
	In comprehensible sounds	2
	No verbal response	1

Mild Head Injury – GCS Score 13 to 15
Moderate Head Injury – GCS Score 9 to 12
Severe Head Injury – GCS Score < 8

A CT scan is indicated immediately in all patients with moderate and severe head injury to rule out any intracranial mass lesion (Flow chart 13.1). The primary approach to a large extradural hematoma or subdural hematoma with significant midline shift is surgical removal. In contrast, for patients with diffuse head injury and compressed cisterns should be treated in an ICU with a systematic protocol that includes ICP (Intra-cranial pressure) monitoring and control, management of respiratory and cardiovascular parameters and cerebral metabolic control.[1]

If CT scan is unavailable, burr hole exploration is performed. Most extra-axial, intracranial lesions can be localized, and the rate of false negative results after six-hole exploration appears to be small.[2]

As stated earlier systematic arterial blood pressure should be monitored and kept in normal range to maintain cerebral perfusion pressure (CPP). Crystalloid solution should be infused through a good intravenous line. Hypotonic solutions should not be used as they can produce or aggravate brain edema by lowering serum osmolality. Any patient presenting with hypotension, the source of internal bleeding must be sought. In unconscious patients with hypotension, hemopneumothorax, abdominal trauma, pelvic fracture should be carefully ruled out.

Abdominal paracentesis is useful for diagnosing hemoperitoneum, but a negative tap does not exclude the diagnosis. Diagnostic peritoneal lavage may be done for diagnosing hemoperitoneum.

Subsequently CT scan of abdomen should be planned in doubtful abdominal injury. X-ray films of the chest, pelvis may determine pneumohemothorax and fractured pelvis respectively. Cervical injury may also lead to hypotension. A failure to detect these injuries in an unconscious patient can result in drastic consequences.

Miller et al[3] found additional systemic injuries in 49 percent cases of severe head injuries, the most common being limb fracture (30%). Chest injury occurred in 29 percent, abdominal injuries in 17 percent and spinal injuries in 6 percent of cases.[3a]

The practical essential steps to be taken when a patient of severe head injury arrives in casualty.[26,26a]

1. Maintenance of airway
   - Nasopharyngeal tube
   - Intubation or
   - Tracheostomy.
2. Breathing (Ventilation)

Flow chart 13.1: Management of severe head injury

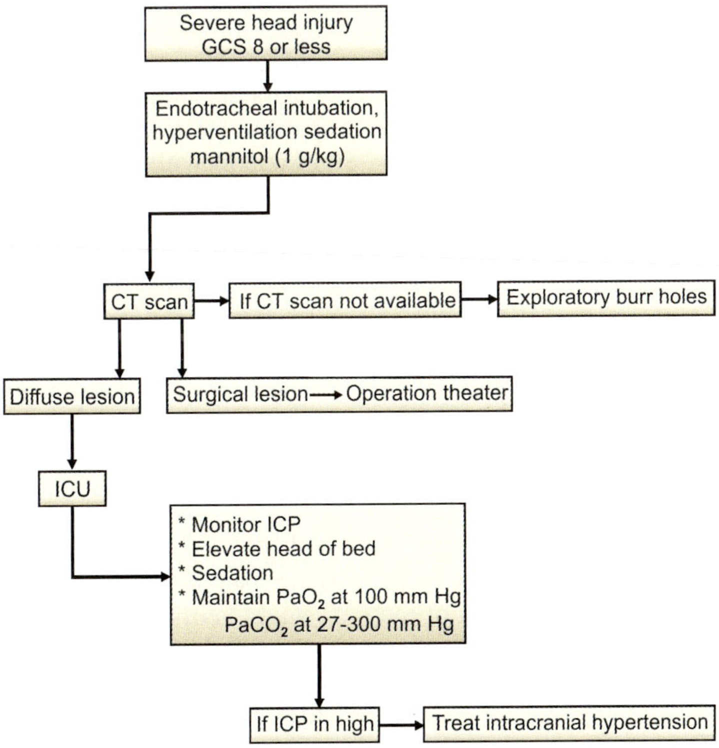

3. Circulation
   - Maintenance of systematic BP
   - Good intravenous line
   - CVP line
   - Crystalloid infusion
   - Blood transfusion, if required.
4. Foley's catheterization and nasogastric intubation
5. Neurological assessment
   - GCS score
   - Pupillary size reaction
   - External injuries.
6. Investigation
   - X-ray skull AP/Lat.
   - X-ray chest
   - X-ray cervical spine AP/Lat.
   - CT scan head.

If required, X-ray pelvis, X-ray abdomen, or CT abdomen.

Arterial blood gases (ABGs).

INTENSIVE CARE UNIT MANAGEMENT

Intensive care unit management of both surgically treated and non-surgical patients is similar. Potentially treatable factors such as hypoxia, hypercapnia, hypotension and intracranial hypertension should be identified and treated accordingly. The outcome from severe head injury to a large extent depends on recognition and early treatment of the preventable secondary damage.

In the ICU following parameters can be monitored:

1. Neurological assessment
2. Intracranial pressure monitoring
3. Cerebral perfusion pressure monitoring
4. Systemic physiologic monitoring—heart rate, BP, temperature, fluid intake and output.

These parameters will guide in proper medical and surgical management.

Neurological Monitoring

Periodic good neurological assessment will help in detecting early deterioration, improvement or static nature during therapy. No investigation can substitute for good neurological assessment.

Intracranial Pressure Monitoring

Normally, resting ICP is 0 to 15 mm. Transient elevations of ICP occurs normally with straining, coughing or the Trendelenburg position. A sustained ICP greater than 20 mm Hg is clearly abnormal. An ICP between 20 and 40 mm Hg is considered moderate intracranial hypertension. An ICP greater than 40 mm Hg represents severe, usually life-threatening intracranial hypertension.[4] About 50 percent of the patients with severe head injury will develop increased intracranial pressure. Increased ICP occurs in 50-70 percent of patients even after evacuation of intracranial hematoma. The incidence of intracranial hypertension is greater after evacuation of an intracerebral hematoma, 71 percent compared with 39 percent after evacuation of a subdural or epidural hematoma.[5]

The association between the severity of intracranial hypertension and a poor outcome after severe head injury is well recognized. Miller[3] reported that mortality rate increased from 18 to 92 percent and the frequency of good outcomes decreased from 74 to 3 percent in patients with normal ICP compared with patients who had intracranial hypertension that could not be reduced below 20 mm Hg. Saul and Dicker reported a 69 percent mortality rate in patients with an ICP greater than 25 mm Hg, compared with a mortality rate of 15% if ICP remained less than 25 mm Hg.[6]

Measurement of intracranial pressure in the ICU:

A. Indications for ICP monitoring in head injury
B. Methods
C. Management of raised ICP.

Indications for ICP Monitoring in Head Injury Patients

1. Patients with GCS score > 8, in whom the decision to surgically evacuate the hematoma is equivocal.
2. Inability to monitor serial neurologic examination in a patient undergoing elective ventilation, e.g. patients undergoing elective ventilation for traumatic brain swelling.
3. Patients with multiple small intracranial hematoma not meriting surgical evacuation.
4. Patients with good coma scale with hematoma diagnosed on CT scan.
5. Patients with multiple hematomas of which the only largest one is being removed.
6. Postoperative patients who are paralyzed and being electively ventilated require ICP monitoring.
7. Postoperative patients, who are not on elective ventilation, in whom brain was not lax or inadequate hemostasis at operation.

Methods

Two types of ICP monitoring devices are available:

1. Fluid coupled
2. Non-fluid coupled

The fluid coupled devices are placed in ventricles, subarachnoid space or the subdural spaces and are connected to a pressure transducer through a fluid filled line. The ventriculostomy catheter remains the standard against which all of the newer monitors are compared. Ventricular catheter also allows cerebrospinal fluid drainage for therapeutic purposes. It can be placed easily and quickly in most patients with head trauma, even those with mass effect. Disadvantages of ventricular catheter include infection rate of 8 to 10 percent and 1 to 2 percent risk of intracranial hemorrhage.[7] Subdural bolt (Richmond screws) which is placed in subdural space is less invasive. Subdural and epidural devices are comparatively less reliable and higher rate of blockage.

Non-fluid coupled system such as the Camino intraparenchymal monitor is placed within the parenchyma and therefore is not subjected to the discontinuities of pressure transmission afforded by the subarachnoid or dural layers and it is not prone to clogging. This system is expensive and the risks involved are similar to the fluid coupled systems.

Management of Raised ICP (Flow chart 13.2)

Treatment of raised ICP should only start after removal of all other remediable factors, e.g. any intracranial hematoma significant enough for surgical evacuation. Most investigators report improved outcome with treatment of raised ICP at levels from 15 to 20 mm Hg.[8]

Intracranial pressure more than 20 minutes for an interval more than 20 mt should be treated because of increased possibility of transtentorial herniation.

Patients with head injury not requiring ICP monitoring: Patients less than 40 years without evidence of abnormal motor activity, with normal pupillary examinations, with no significant history of secondary brain insults, and with CT scans showing no pathology and open basilar cisterns. These patients may be managed without ICP monitoring if they can undergo continuous neurological observation in the intensive care unit.[9]

The Monro-Kellie doctrine states that the total intracranial volume will remain essentially constant; therefore, if anyone of the primary intracranial components, i.e. brain parenchyma, blood, or CSF is increased (e.g. cerebral edema or tumor), or if another process (e.g. intracranial hematoma) occupies space, one of the primary components must be displaced or ICP will increase.

Hence, therapeutically, reducing cerebral blood volume (head-up positioning, hyperventilation and barbiturates); reducing CSF volume (CSF drainage) and reducing brain tissue volume (osmotic diuretics and glucocorticoids). Other conventional treatments, such as neuromuscular blockage, sedation and analgesia exert less specific effects.

Flow chart 13.2: Management of raised intracranial pressure

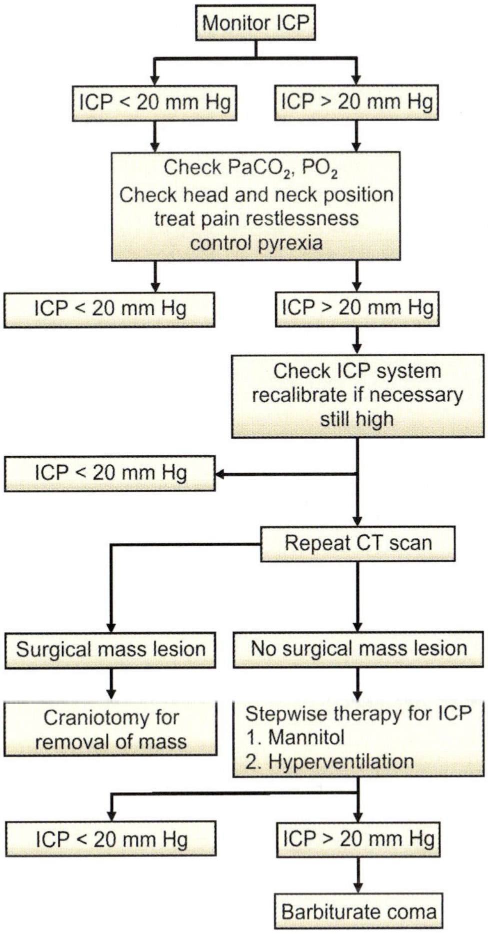

Position of the patient's head: Ventilated head injured patients should be nursed with 15 to 30 degrees from horizontal and the head should be maintained in neutral position. This enhances cerebral venous drainage. This is an effective method of decreasing ICP and also may decrease the likelihood of subsequent ICP spikes. Care should be taken to note the level of the external auditory meatus, which is the zero reference point for the calibration of ICP monitors.

Hyperventilation: Hyperventilation to produce an arterial PCO_2 of 25 to 30 mm Hg will reduce ICP by promoting cerebral vasoconstriction and subsequent reduction of cerebral blood flow (CBF). The onset of action is within 30 seconds and peaks within 8 minutes after PCO_2 drops to desired range.[10] In most patients hyperventilation lowers the ICP by 25 percent; if the patient does not rapidly respond, the prognosis for survival is generally poor. Prolonged hyperventilation probably loses its effectiveness and therefore, is of limited value beyond acute phase.[11,12] The partial pressure of carbon dioxide should not fall below 25 mm Hg because this may cause profound vasoconstriction and ischemia in normal and injured areas of brain. The major difficulty with managing hyperventilation is the difficulty in assessing its effect on CBF metabolism matching. One useful approach to this problem is the use of jugular venous saturation monitoring.

Gopinath et al[13] found that hypocapnia (30 mm Hg) increased the incidence of cerebral desaturation [decreased jugular bulb oxygen saturation ($SJVO_2$)]' Current data supports the concept of optimized hyperventilation ($PaCO_2$ 30-35 mm Hg).

SEDATION

Sedation is often indicated in agitated or uncontrollable patient movement resulting form pain related to trauma, diagnostic or therapeutic maneuvers resulting in increased ICP. A variety of different sedating agents have been used to facilitate ventilation, e.g. diazepam, midazolam, opiates and more recently propofol.

OSMOTIC AGENTS

Mannitol is commonly used to reduce ICP.

In the face of deepening coma, pupillary inequality, or other deterioration of the neurologic examination, mannitol may be life saving. Mannitol (0.25 to 1.0 gm/kg) can effectively reduce cerebral edema by producing an osmotic gradient that draws tissue water into the vascular space. In effect, this reduces brain volume. The effect of mannitol depends on the dose, rate of infusion, serum osmolality and patient's state of hydration. The upper limit of serum osmolality is 320 mosmol/L.

The osmotic effects of mannitol occur within minutes of its administration and peak at about 60 minutes after the bolus has been administered. The ICP-lowering effects of a single bolus may last for 6 to 8 hours. Mannitol has neuroprotective properties.

Mannitol is an effective free radical scavenger, reducing the concentration of oxygen free radicals that may promote cell membrane lipid peroxidation. Mannitol also promotes CBF by reducing blood viscosity and microcirculatory resistance. It reduces RBC deformity and, therefore, improves oxygen carrying capacity.

Mannitol can induce hypovolemic hypotension. Repeated doses of mannitol increases serum osmolality. This reduces the effectiveness of mannitol, may cause dilutional hyponatremia, and may precipitate acute renal failure. Also repeated episodes of diuresis may wash out the renal medullary concentration gradient and thereby interfere with the ability of the kidneys to concentrate the urine. As mannitol enters areas of damaged blood brain barrier (BBB), mannitol may concentrate within brain tissue, producing reverse osmotic effect. By reducing brain volume, tamponade of extra-axial hematoma may be decreased or lost, allowing more bleeding into traumatic lesion.

Doses of 0.25 g/kg appear to be equally effective as 1 gm/kg in terms of effect on ICP. Serum osmolality should not be allowed to increase beyond 320 mosmol/liter).

Furosemide is a loop diuretic often used in patients with head injury. It also can lead to significant dehydration and hypokalemia. Evidence exists that furosemide works synergistically with mannitol in lowering ICP.[14]

BARBITURATES

Barbiturates are effective in lowering ICP.

Second tier therapy with barbiturates is required in select group of patients with refractory intracranial hypertension.[15,16]

Barbiturates have a potent depressant effect on cerebral electrical activity and metabolism, with the degree of depression being related to the anesthetic depth.[17] Barbiturates decrease cerebral metabolism and thus the need for oxygen delivery. They are vasoconstrictors thereby decreasing cerebral blood flow (CBF) and ICP. In patients with intracranial hypertension, barbiturates caused the greatest reduction in ICP in those patients whose initial ICP was abnormally high. This decrease in ICP is often associated with an increase in cerebral perfusion pressure (CPP).

Barbiturates: Beneficial effects

- Decreases $CMRO_2$ and CBF
- Vasoconstriction
- Inhibits free radicals

Side effects:

- Hypotension
- Myocardial depression

Thiopental, a short acting barbiturate, is most commonly used to control intracranial hypertension.

Thiopental should be given only in patients admitted to an intensive care unit capable of intensive neurosurgical care. Barbiturate therapy should be accomplished with a loading dose of 10 mg/kg of thiopental given during 30 minutes. This dose should be followed by an infusion of 5 mg/kg/hr during the next 3 hours. The maintenance dose should be started on a 1 mg/kg/hr infusion.

During administration of loading dose, if the patient's blood pressure decreases, the intravascular volume should be increased and pressures such as dopamine should be started.

PROPOFOL

Propofol is a relatively new sedative-hypnotic with a very rapid onset and short duration of action. The intravenous anesthetic agent propofol has many advantages as an agent for treating raised ICP. It reduces $CMRO_2$ and CBF. It also reduces systemic BP usually results in net decrease in cerebral perfusion pressure (CPP). This decrease is usually not significant. At least two studies have shown a beneficial effect on ICP in head injury patients treated with this agent.[18-19a] Other drugs which reduce ICP (action similar to propofol) are: **Etomidate and Lidocaine**.

SEIZURE PROPHYLAXIS

Up to 9 percent of all patients sustain blunt head trauma suffer from early post-traumatic seizures.[20] The incidence of early post-traumatic seizure approaches 42 percent in patients who have sustained penetrating head trauma.[21] Although the occurrence of seizures in the immediate post-trauma period has no predictive value for future epilepsy, early seizures can cause hypoxia, hypercarbia, release of excitatory neurotransmitters and increased ICP, which can worsen secondary brain injury. Therefore, all paralyzed head injured patients should have prophylactic anticonvulsant therapy in the acute phase. If the patient is actively seizuring, benzodiazepines are effective rapidly acting anticonvulsants.

Diazepam: 0.1 mg/kg, up to 5 mg IV, every 5 minutes up to a total of 20 mg.

For a long-term anticonvulsant activity, phenytoin is given:

Loading dose: 15 mg/kg IV is given slowly @ 50 mg/minute.

Maintenance dose: 5 mg/kg.

CSF drainage: When ICP monitoring is carried out by a ventricular catheter, the option exists to treat raised ICP by draining off CSF. In presence of large ventricles, this procedure can be very useful in treating intracranial hypertension. The major disadvantages are infection and hemorrhage.

Corticosteroids and control of ICP: Steroids are highly effective in controlling brain edema when it is tumor associated, but there is no convincing evidence of their efficacy in head injury, intracerebral hematoma or stroke.[22-22b] However, further evaluation is necessary.

Hypothermia: Recent studies[25] in severe head injury utilizing mild hypothermia has shown beneficial effect. Hypothermia reduces cerebral metabolism and hence prevents hypoxic and ischemic damage.

CEREBRAL PERFUSION PRESSURE MONITORING

When ICP monitoring is used as a guide to the therapy of acutely brain injured patients, its main value is in preserving cerebral perfusion pressure (CPP).

Cerebral perfusion pressure (CPP) represents the pressure gradient across the intracranial compartment and is defined as the mean arterial pressure (MAP) minus the ICP. The major role of ICP monitoring lies in determination of CPP.

$$CPP = MAP - ICP$$

Recent work suggested that CPP should be kept above 60 mm Hg. If CPP is sustained above 60 mm Hg then long-term outcome improves significantly[23,24] while attempting to reduce ICP. Hence, mean arterial pressure (MAP) should be maintained. Rosner et al in 1995,[23a] had laid down the protocol for CPP management and reported good outcome when CPP was more than 70 mm Hg. However, CPP management can be possible following proper guidelines.[23b]

MEASURES TO MAINTAIN MAP

1. Administration of crystalloid, colloids and blood products to maintain euvolemia.
2. Administration of inotropes:
   - Dopamine
   - Dobutamine
   - Phenylephrine HCl.

Nutritional Support to Severely Head Injured Patients

Severe head injury results in a hypercatabolic state. Starting early enteral nutrition helps in establishing integrity of gastric mucosa, which has a beneficial effect on immunocompetence and helps in metabolic response to stress.[27,28,30] Some meta-analysis have shown the comparison of initiation of enteral nutrition within 36 hours and beyond. Early enteral nutrition showed 55 percent reduction in risk of infection. Parenteral nutrition must be avoided, as it is associated with profound metabolic immunologic and GI changed and increases the mortality. There is increased gastric emptying time in head injured patients.[29] Immune enhancing nutrition formula through nasogastric tube 20-30 ml per hour is started to achieve the nutritional goal.[28,30] Well planned and balanced nutritional replacement reduces the mortality by reducing risk of infection.

CONCLUSION

The management of severe head injury should aim toward prevention of secondary brain damage and maintenance of an optimum condition for adequate neuronal recovery. Prevention of secondary brain damage can help to reduce mortality and morbidity.

To prevent secondary brain insult, especially ischemia and brain swelling, the victim of TBI needs 3 to 4 weeks of vigilant supportive care in intensive care unit.[34]

Factors which ultimately play a role in outcome are hypoxia, hypotension, timely decompression of an intracranial hematoma, ICP > 20 mm Hg, level of cerebral perfusion pressure and associated medical problems. Any effort to maintain the above factors within normal limits will prevent secondary damage, hence outcome.

The preventive strategies are very important in lowering the social burden of severe traumatic brain injury. It is evident from dataset that transporting patients to large volume trauma centers with neurosurgical care improves the outcome of these cases.[31]

A study to examine the variations in care of patients with severe head injury in academic trauma centers across 45 revealed a considerable national variation in care of these cases. An aggressive management strategy is associated with decreased mortality rate for patients with severe head injury with no significant difference in functional status at discharge among survivors.[32]

An introduction of evidence based protocol to guide ICU management of patients with severe head injury has been associated with significant reduction in both ICU and hospital mortality.[33]

REFERENCES

1. Stocchetti N, Furlan A, Volta F. Hypoxemia and arterial hypotension at the accident scenie in head injury. J Trauma 1996;40:764-7.

1a. Witchall RJ, Hoyt DB. Endotracheal intubation in the field improves survival in patients with severe head injury. Arch Sury 1977;132:592-7.

1b. White RJ. Programmed management of severe head injuries revisited. J Trauma 1975;15:779-84.

2. Andrew BT, Pitts LH, et al. Is computed tomographic scanning necessary in patients with tentorial herniation? Results of immediate surgical exploration without computed tomography in 100 patients. Neurosurgery 1986;19:408-14.

2a. Silverston P. Pulse oximetry at the road side a study of pulse oximetry in immediate care. BMJ 1989;298:711-3.

3. Miller JD, Butlerworth IF, Gudeman SK, et al. Further experience in the management of severe head injury. J Neurosurg 1981;54:289-99.

3a. Michael DB, Guyot DR, Darmody WR. Coincidence of head and cervical spine injury. J Neurotrauma 1989; 6:177-89.

4. Lundberg N, Troupp H, et al. Continuous recording of the ventricular fluid pressure in patients with severe acute traumatic brain damage. J Neurosurg 1965;22:581-90.

5. Miller JD, Becker DP, et al. Significance of intracranial hypertension in severe head injury. J Neurosurg 1977; 47:501-16.

6. Saul TG, Ducker TB. Effect of intracranial pressure monitoring and aggressive treatment on mortality in severe head injury. J Neurosurg 1982;56:498-503.

7. Luerssen T, Chestnut R, et al. Post-traumatic cerebrospinal fluid infections in the Traumatic Coma Data Bank: The influence of type and management of ICP monitors. In: Avezaat C, Van Eyndhoven J, Mass A (Eds), et al. Intracranial pressure VIII. Berlin: Springer-Verlag 1963; 157-63.

8. Marshall LF, Smith RW, Shapiro HM. The outcome with aggressive treatment in severe head injury. The significance of intracranial pressure monitoring. J Neurosurg 1979;50:20-25.

9. Mendelow AD, Teasdale G, Jennett B, et al. Risks of intracranial hematoma in head injured adults. Br Med J 1983;287:1173-6.

10. Greenberg MS. Head trauma. In handbook of neurosurgery. Fla, Greenberg Graphics, 1994.

11. Muizelaar JP, Marmaror A, Ward JD, et al. Adverse effects of prolonged hyperventilation A randomized clinical trial. J Neurosurg 1991;75:731.

12. Michelle H Biros. Head Trauma. In Rosen P, Barkin R (Eds): Emergency Medicine, Concepts and Clinical Practice, 4th edn, Mosby, 1998.

13. Gopinath SP, Robertson CS, et al. Jugular venous desaturation and outcome after head injury. Neurol Neurosurg Psychiatry 1994;57:717-23.

14. White PF, Schlobohm RM, et al. A randomized study of drugs for preventing increases in intracranial pressure during endotracheal suctioning. Anesthesiology 1982; 57:242-4.

15. Marshall LF. Treatment of brain swelling and brain edema in man. Adv Neurol 1980;28:459-69.

16. Rea G, Rockswold G. Barbiturate therapy in uncontrolled intracranial hypertension. Neurosurgery 1983;12:401-4.

17. Michen felder JD. The interdependency of cerebral functional and metabolic effects following massive doses of thiopental in the dog. Anaesthesiology 1974;41:231.

18. Farling PA, Johnston JR, et al. Propofol infusion for sedation of patients with head injury in intensive care: a preliminary report. Anaesthesia 1989;44:222-6.
19. Hartung HJ. Intracranial pressure after propofol and thiopental administration in patients with severe head trauma. Anesthetist 1987;36:285-7.
19a. Moss E, Powell D, Gibson RM. Effect of etomidate on intracranial pressure and cerebral perfusion pressure. Br J Anaesth 1979;51:347-51.
20. Kennedy CR, Freeman JM. Post-traumatic seizures and post-traumatic epilepsy in children. J Head Trauma Rehab 1986;1(4):66.
21. Temkin NR, Dikmen SS, Winn HR. Post-traumatic seizures. Neurosurg Clin North Am 1991;2:425.
22. Todd NY, Teasdale GM. Steroids in human head injury. In: Capildeo R (Ed). Steroids in Diseases of the Central Nervous system. John Wiley 1989;151-9.
22a. Knietowicz Z. Trial of steroids for treating head injury begins. BMJ 1999;318:1441.
22b. Bullock MR, Chestnut RM, Clifton GL, et al. Role of steroids. J Neurotrauma 2000;17:531-5.
23. Chan KH, Miller JD, et al. The effects of changes in cerebral perfusion pressure upon middle cerebral artery blood flow velocity and jugular bulb venous oxygen saturation after severe brain injury. J Neurosurg 1992; 77:55-61.
23a. Rosner MJ, Rosner SD, John Son AH. Cerebral perfusion pressure. Management protocol and clinical results. J Neurosurg 1965;83:949-62.
23b. Guidelines for cerebral perfusion pressure. J Neurotrauma 2000;17:507-11.
24. Nordstrom CH, Messeter K, et al. Cerebral blood flow, vasoreactivity, and oxygen consumption during barbiturate therapy in severe traumatic brain lesions. J Neurosurgery 1988;68:424-31.
25. Shiozaki T, Sugimoto H, Taneda M, et al. Effect of mild hypothermia on uncontrolled intracranial hypertension after severe head injury. J Neurosurg 1993;79:363-8.
26. Initial assessment and management. Advanced trauma life support for doctors: Students course manual Chicago II American College of Surgeon 1997;21-46.
26a. Airway and ventilatory management. Advanced trauma life support for doctors: Students course manual Chicago II American College of Surgeons 1997;59-85.
27. K lodell CT, Carroll M, Carrillot, et al. Routine intragastric feeding following traumatic brain injury is safe and well tolerated. Am J Surg 2000;179:168-71.
28. Marik PE, Zaloga GP. Early enteral nutrition in acutely ill patients: A systemic review. Crit Care Med 2001;29: 2264-70.
29. Kao CH, Changlai SP, Chieng PU, et al. Gastric emptying in head-injured patients. Aue J Gastroenterol 1998;93: 1108-12.
30. Zaloga CP, Marik P. Promotality agents in the intensive care unit. Crit Care Med 2000;28:255-59.
31. Patel HC, Bouamra O, Woodford M, et al. Trauma audit and research network, trend in head injury outcome from 1989 to 2003 and effect of neurosurgical care: an observational study. Lancet 2005;366:1538-44.
32. Bulger EM, Nathen AB, Rivera FP, Moore M, et al. Management of severe head injury: institutional variation in care and effect on outcome. Crit Care Med 2002;30(8): 1927-9.
33. Clayton TJ, Nelson RJ, Manara AR. Reduction in mortality from severe head injury following introduction of protocol for intensive care management. Brit Journal Anaesthesia 2004;93(6)761-7.
34. Avabi B, Mehta R, Eisenberg HM. Management of severe head injury. Neurosurgery Principle and Practice 2007; 369-78 Springer link.

14 Minor Head Injury

Deepak Agarwal, AK Mahapatra

INTRODUCTION

'Minor head injury', also known as 'Mild traumatic brain injury' or 'concussion' has been the subject of intense investigation in recent years as it is being increasing realized that in spite of an apparently normal CT head, there might be subtle organic brain damage, which may be associated with distressing neuropsychological sequelae in these patients.[1]

EPIDEMIOLOGY

Head injuries are amongst the most common types of trauma seen in developing as well as developed countries. Minor head injuries in turn, form the bulk of these head injuries ranging from 80 to 90 percent. A typical review of head injured patients admitted to a neurosurgical service found that 5 percent were 'severe' (GCS score < 8), 11 percent were 'moderate' (GCS score 8 to 12) and 84 percent were 'minor' (GCS score 13 to 15).[2]

In United Kingdom some 500,000 children attended accident and emergency after head injury and about 50,000 were admitted. The death rate was 5.3 per 100000 children.[26]

CLINICAL FEATURES

The most widely used definition of minor head injury is a set of criteria published by the members of the Mild Traumatic Brain Injury Interdisciplinary Special Interest Group (BISIG) of the American Congress of Rehabilitation Medicine (Handbook 16)[3] which states that:

1. Loss of consciousness should not exceed 30 minutes.
2. After 30 minutes the initial GCS score should be between 13 and 15.
3. Post-traumatic amnesia does not exceed 24 hours.

Following minor head injury, a syndrome called the **postconcussion syndrome** has been reported to occur in up to 80 percent of the patients.[4] This syndrome includes symptoms such as headache, irritability, poor concentration, memory disturbances, dizziness, anxiety and depression. *Persistent postconcussion syndrome, defined as persistence of symptoms of postconcussion syndrome beyond three months*, is seen in more than 30 percent of the patients, and up to 15 percent may have persistent, disabling symptoms beyond six months.[5] To assist with the diagnosis of postconcussion syndrome, the International Statistical Classification of Diseases and Related Health Problems, 10th edition (ICD-10),[6] published a set of guidelines based on epidemiological studies in several countries and regions. Here *postconcussion syndrome was defined as history of head trauma with loss of consciousness that precedes symptom onset by a maximum of four weeks with three or more symptoms of the following*:

- Headache, dizziness, malaise, fatigue, noise intolerance.
- Irritability, depression, anxiety, emotional liability.
- Subjective concentration, memory or intellectual difficulties without neuropsychological evidence of marked impairment.
- Insomnia.
- Reduced alcohol tolerance.
- Preoccupation with above symptoms and fear of brain damage without hypochondriacal concern and adoption of sick role.

Rarely a hemorrhage into pre-existing arachnoid cyst may render an asymptomatic cyst symptomatic following minor head injury.[27]

PATHOPHYSIOLOGY

The clue to suspected structural damage in minor head injuries might be found in experimental studies, in which pathological evidence of damage to the medial temporal lobes after mild or moderate head injury has been documented. Smith et al[7] *found that bilateral dentate hilar neuron loss was a consistent finding two weeks after minor head injury* and was uniformly associated with memory dysfunction. In a related study, Kotapka et al,[8] delivered mild acceleration type experimental head injuries to nonhuman primates and found hippocampal lesions in virtually all animals injured in the lateral plane. The hippocampus, a key structure in the medial temporal lobe, is located within the hippocampal formation, a collection of cytoarchitecturally distinct subdivisions that also includes the dentate gyrus, subicular complex, and entorhinal cortex.[9] The hippocampus is especially vulnerable to mechanically induced head injury and to other types of insults such as ischemia, hypoxia, and seizures,[10] and the extent of hippocampal damage may be correlated with severity of memory impairment.[11]

Even more revolutionary is the study by Nakatomi et al[12] which provides the first evidence of functional neurogenesis. Using a rat model of transient forebrain ischemia, the authors evaluated whether they could manipulate and enhance ischemic injury induced endogenous neurogenesis. They administered fibroblast growth factor-2 (FGF-2) and epidermal growth factor (EGF) intraventricularly and found that it resulted in an increased repopulation of CA 1 hippocampal neurons lost following ischemic insult. *More importantly, growth factor treated rats demonstrated improved functional outcome as compared to control ischemic rats.* It is tempting to speculate that humans may similarly be affected with neuronal loss in hippocampus after minor head injury, which in future may be reversible. However, as practical considerations preclude histopathological analysis in this group of patients, newer investigative modalities such as SPECT and PET due to their high sensitivity appears as an attractive proposition for studying structural damage in such patients. At a study conducted at AIIMS using SPECT in children with persistent postconcussion syndrome and abnormal SPECT brain (unpublished data), all children showed medial temporal (86%) or frontal (13%) hypoperfusion, and no patient showed hyperperfusion. This finding of areas of hypoperfusion in minor head injury has been described previously[17-19] and may result from vasospasm, direct vascular injury and perfusion changes due to alterations in remote neuronal activity (diaschisis).[3] There is evidence to show that brain is more vulnerable to ischemic injury after minor head injury[14] and it has been hypothesized that SPECT findings representing hypoperfusion may in fact lead to secondary ischemic injury.[13] TCD study also shows defect in blood flow velocity (Fig. 14.1).

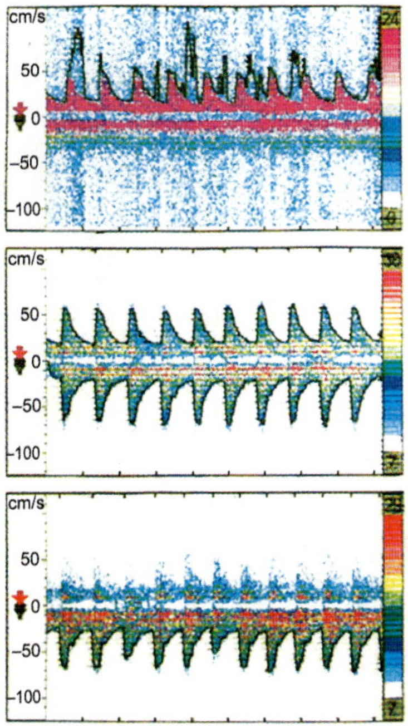

Fig. 14.1: Transcranial Doppler showing blood flow pattern in minor head injury

INVESTIGATIONS

In the recent years, with its widespread availability, the use of CT for minor head injury has become increasingly common. However, there is considerable disagreement in the literature as to the indications for CT in the large number of head trauma cases classified as 'minor'.[15] Some studies have tried to derive algorithms to identify a subset of patients in whom CT may be avoided.[15,16] These studies fail to address the basic issue of CT having a abysmally low sensitivity of less than 10 percent in the so called 'minor head injuries'.[17,18] Because of this, various modalities ranging from neuropsychological testing, evoked potential and P_{300} testing, to newer radiological techniques such as PET, SPECT and MRI have been investigated as tools to correlate cerebral dysfunction with symptoms in cases of minor head injuries.[19] Umile et al[19] tried to correlate dynamic imaging (PET and SPECT) findings with static imaging (CT and MRI) as well as with neuropsychological testing in 19 patients with minor head injury and postconcussion syndrome and found that 90 percent had abnormal findings on PET or SPECT imaging. Though PET is slightly superior to SPECT in terms of spatial resolution however, SPECT is much more affordable and widely available making it attractive as a cost-effective investigative and diagnostic tool in postconcussion syndrome. In our study SPECT has shown a sensitivity of 80 percent which is excellent when compared to abysmally poor sensitivities of 9 percent for CT and 46 percent for MRI scan recorded by others.[17,18] As our own studies show, perfusion abnormalities seen on SPECT do not correct spontaneously over a long time in a significant number of patients, and changes in cerebral perfusion have been found to persist for as long as one year following mild traumatic brain injury.[18,20]

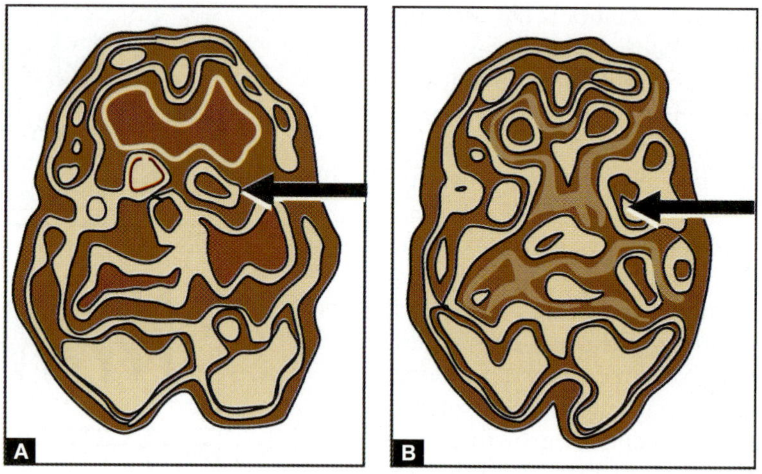

Figs 14.2A and B: (A) SPECT scan showing temporal hypoperfusion (arrow) in a patient with postconcussion syndrome; (B) SPECT scan of the same patient showing improvement in perfusion following six weeks treatment with piracetam

MANAGEMENT

Management of minor head injury revolves around two broad issues: Firstly, the use of investigative procedures such as SPECT, PET and neuropsychological testing as a means of prognostication and secondly, treatment strategies for postconcussion syndrome.

Investigative tools such as SPECT, PET and neuropsychological assessment help in prognostication, especially in preschool children (less than five years of age) as there is good evidence that even minor head injury, if occurring at an age that is critical for the development of a certain skill, may cause persisting deficits.[21] Wrightson et al[21] prospectively studied the effect of minor head injury on preschool children using neuropsychological tests and found that injury in the preschool years seemed to affect the process of learning to read. The authors stressed that if early identification and diagnosis of these children could be made, teachers could be made aware of this and remedial teaching could be made available to them.

Despite new insights gained in the pathophysiology of mild traumatic brain injury and the realization that there may be profound brain perfusion abnormalities existing behind a seemingly normal CT head of such 'minor' head injury patients with postconcussion syndrome, most neurosurgeons can do little except giving reassurance and prescribing analgesics and antivertigo medication. Recently, a neurotropic agent, piracetam has been tried in such patients. Piracetam has a unique mode of action that though not entirely clear, may be explained by its neuroprotective properties, mediated through effects on the cell membrane.[22] Piracetam improves membrane bound cell functions including ATP production[23,24] and secondary messenger activity.[23] It also has been shown that piracetam has beneficial effects on the cerebral blood flow, by decreasing the adhesivity, aggregation, and deformability of erythrocytes along with flow thrust tension of the blood.[25] We conducted a randomized controlled trial found that low dose of piracetam *successfully* reversed cerebral perfusion deficits and resulted in accelerated symptomatic *improvement* in patients with postconcussion syndrome (Figs 14.2A and B). However, as the study number was small, before recommending piracetam for clinical use in postconcussion syndrome, placebo controlled trials using larger number of patients are required.

REFERENCES

1. Watson MR, Fenton GW, McClelland RJ, Lumsden J, Headley M, Rutherford WH. The postconcussion state: Neurophysiological aspects. Br J Psychiatry 1995; 167:514-21.
2. Miller JD. Minor, moderate and severe head injury. Neurosurg Rev 1986;9:135-9.
3. Mild Head Injury Interdisciplinary Special Interest Group of the American Congress of Rehabilitation Medicine. Definition of mild traumatic brain injury. J Head Trauma Rehabil 1993;8:86-8.
4. Hugenholtz H, Stuss DT, Stethem BA, Richard MT. How long does it take to recover from a mild concussion? Neurosurgery 1995;22:853-58.
5. Alexander MP. Mild traumaic brain injury: Pathophysiology, natural history, and clinical management. Neurology 1995;45:1253-60.
6. World Health Organization: International Statistical Classification of Diseases and related Health Problems, 10th edn. Geneva, Switzerland, World Health Organization, 1992.

7. Smith DH, Lowenstein DH, Gennarelli DI, McIntosh TK. Persistent memory dysfunction is associated with bilateral hippocampal damage following experimental brain injury. Neurosci Lett 1994;168:151-4.
8. Kotapka MJ, Gennareli TA, Graham DI, et al. Selective vulnerability of hippocampal neurons in acceleration-induced experimental head injury. J Neurotrauma 1991; 8:247-58.
9. Zola-Morgan S, Squire LR, Amaral DC. Human amnesia and the medial temporal region: Enduring memory impairment following a bilateral lesion limited to field CAT of the hippocampus. J Neurosci 1986;6:2950-67.
10. Hicks RR, Smith DH, Lowenstein DH, Saint Marie R, McIntosh TK. Mild experimental brain injury in the rat induces cognitive deficits associated with regional neuron loss in the hippocampus. J Neurotrauma 1998; 10:405-15.
11. Rempel-Clower NL, Zola SM, Squire LR, Amaral DC. Three cases of enduring memory impairment after bilateral damage limited to the hippocampal formation. J Neurosci 1996;16:5233-55.
12. Nakatomi H, Kuriu T, Okabe S, et al. Regeneration of hippocampal pyramidal neurons after ischemic brain injury by recruitment of endogenous neural progenitors. Cell 2002;110:429-41.
13. Hofman PAM, Stapert SZ, van Kroonenburgh MJPG, Jolles J, de Kruijk Jelle, Welmink JT. MR imaging, Single-photon emission CT, and neurocognitive performance after mild traumatic brain injury. AJNR 2001;22:441-9.
14. Jenkins LW, Lu Y, Johnston WE, Lyeth BG, Prough DS. Combined therapy affects outcomes differentially after mild traumatic brain injury and secondary forebrain ischemia in rats. Brain Res 1999;817:132-44.
15. Steill IG, Lesiuk H, Wells GA, et al. The Canadian CT head rule study for patients with minor head injury: rationale, objectives and methodology for phase I (derivation). Ann Emerg Med 2001;38:160-9.
16. Haydel MJ, Preston CA, Mills TJ, et al. Indications for computed tomography in patients with minor head injury. N Eng J Med 2000;343:00-5.
17. Kant R, Smith-Seemiller L, Isaac G, Duffy J. Tc-HMPAO SPECT in persistent postconcussion syndrome after mild head injury: Comparison with MRI/CT. Brain Inj 1997; 11:115.
18. Jacobs A, Put E, Ingels M, Bossuyt A. One year follow-up of technitium-99m-HMPAO SPECT in mild head injury. J Nucl Med 1996;37:1605-09.

18a. Jain KC, Mahapatra AK, Walia BS. Objective assessment of post minor head injury syndrome. A P_{300} and blood flow velocity study. Clinical Neurology and Neurosurg 1997;99:574 (abstract).

18b. Jain KC, Mahapatra AK. Central blood flow velocity P_{300} studies in patients with minor head injury: A preliminary study. In: Brain protection and Neural Trauma. VK Khosla, VK Kal and BS Sharma (Eds). Narosa-publishers, New Delhi-2000;298-305.

19. Umile EM, Sandel E, Alavi A, Terry CM, Plotkin RC. Dynamic imaging in mild traumatic brain injury: Support for the theory of medial temporal vulnerability. Arch Phys Med Rehabil 2002;83:1506-13.
20. Agrawal D, Naveen K, Bal CS, Mahapatra AK. Postconcussion vertigo: Is the cause central? Correlation with single photon emission computed tomography. Neurosciences Today 2003;7:33-36.
21. Wrightson P, McGinn V, Gronwall D. Mild head injury in preschool children: Evidence that it can be associated with persisting cognitive defect. J Neurol Neurosurg Psychiatry 1995;59:375-80.
22. Peuvot J, Schanck A, Deleers M, et al. Piracetam-induced changes to membrane physical properties: A combined approach by 31P nuclear magnetic resonance and conformational analysis. Biochem Pharmacol 1995; 50:1129-34.
23. Nickolson VJ, Wolthuis OI. Effect of acquisition-enhancing drug Piracetam on rat cerebral energy metabolism: Comparison with naftidrofuryl and metamphetamine. Biochem Pharmacal 1975;25:2241-4.
24. Benzi G, Pastoris O, Villa RF, et al. Influence of aging and exogenous substances on cerebral energy metabolism in posthypoglycemic recovery. Biochem Pharmacol 1985; 34:1477-83.
25. Vernon E. Piracetam a nootropil analogue. In: Gouliaev AH, Seening A (Eds): Piracetam and other structurally related neurotropic. Brain research reviews 1991;19:180.
26. Geijerstam JL, Oredssons, Britton M. Medical outcome after immediate CT or admission for observation after mild head injury, randomized controlled trial. BMJ 2006; 333:455-6.
27. Goyal D, Sharma S, Thakur R, et al. Arachnoid cyst haemorrhage, a serious complication of minor head trauma Ind J. Radiol Image 2006;16(2):167-8.

15 Fluid and Electrolyte Imbalance in Head Injury

RR Sharma, Sanjay Pawar, RV Devadas

INTRODUCTION

The past few years have witnessed important advances in our understanding of the etiology and pathogenesis of acute head injury as well as development and use of new novel treatment strategies to improve overall outcome in such cases. Of particular note amongst these advances are active resuscitative measures as used in primary survey of acute trauma life support (ATLS), the introduction of GCS for initial and subsequent clinical evaluations, controlled ventilation, use of computed tomography (CT scan) to study intracranial status on periodic basis, emergency neurosurgical interventions, neurointensive care unit (NICU) care and intracranial pressure (ICP) and cerebral perfusion pressure (CPP) monitoring for physiologic management. However, arterial blood gases, coagulation profile, fluid and electrolyte balances are also of paramount importance in the day-to-day management of these patients. The field of acute head injury research is moving rapidly. In order to keep abreast of new discoveries and current thinking, we review our experiences in the area of fluid and electrolyte imbalance in head injury patients including therapeutic options.

GENERAL CONSIDERATIONS

In severe head injury patients, maintenance of precise fluid balance is of paramount importance in preventing hypovolemia, electrolyte imbalance and intravascular coagulation. Inadequate fluid therapy results in hypotension and underperfusion of the vital organs, whereas excessive fluid therapy results in cerebral, pulmonary and peripheral edema. The body's mechanisms for fluid balance will compensate for most inappropriate fluid therapy, but in the critically ill patients, the mechanisms are usually compromised.

Normal homeostatic mechanisms maintain intracellular fluid (ICF) and extracellular fluid (ECF) volume, tonicity and composition in healthy individuals (Table 15.1). However, in patients with acute head injury, alterations in fluid volume, tonicity and composition occur due to an emergent neuroendocrine surge antidiuretic hormone (ADH) to retain water, renin-angiotensinogen II-aldosterone to retain sodium, and catecholamines to support vascular system which is mainly aimed at maintaining an effective intravascular volume for adequate cerebral blood flow at the expense of ICF and ECF fluid tonicity and composition (Na^+, K^+, HCO_3^- and H^+).[1-4] Disturbances of ICF/ ECF fluid tonicity and composition are often associated with a worsening neurological status. Excessive capillary leakage in the brain is well recognized for acute cerebral swelling and its association with high mortality and morbidity. Inappropriate fluid therapy is therefore potentially harmful in such patients with acute cerebral trauma. The maintenance of a stable ionic concentration in the body fluids is necessary for normal cellular metabolism.[5,6] Many of these potentially serious complications due to improper fluid therapy are largely preventable and therefore should be recognized early and treated in time.

Serum electrolyte imbalances in patients with severe head injury more often present with diagnostic dilemma and therefore a list of diagnosis is resolved by investigations. A 70 Kg person has 42 liters of body water; 28 liters (66%) in intracellular space (ICF) and 14 liters in extracellular space (ECF). 10.5 liters in interstitial space and 3.5 liters in plasma. Water is obtained from the diet (1.5 to 2.1 L/day) and oxidative metabolism (400 ml/day) and is lost (2-2.5 L/day) through the kidneys (sensible loss of 1.5 L/day), lungs, gut and skin (sum total insensible loss of 1 L/day). Its distribution in ICF and ECF is determined by the osmolalities of these compartments. Normally, ICF and ECF are isotonic. Any change in osmolarity of a compartment results in the net to and fro movement of water between the ECF and ICF to restore isotonicity. The minimum volume of urine necessary for normal excretion of metabolic waste products is about 500 ml/day (20 ml/hr) and minimum daily dietary water intake is about 1100 ml.

Majority of exchangeable sodium is extracellular: The normal ECF sodium concentration is 135-145 mmol/L. while that of the ICF is only 4-10 mmol/L, Most cell membranes are permeable to sodium and the gradient is maintained by active pumping of sodium

Table 15.1: Composition of ECF and ICF compartments (mmol/L)

Sr. No.		Ion	ECF (plasma)	ECF (ISS)	ICF
Cations	1.	Na^+	135-145	135-140	5-10
	2.	K^+	4.5-5.5	4.5-5.5	156-160
	3.	Others	2-3	2-3	14
Anions	1.	Cl^-	101-105	115-120	3-4
	2.	HCO_3^-	26-28	26-28	10
	3.	$-PO_4$ and others (nondiffusible)	1	1	106
	4.	Protein (nondiffusible)	15-17	0	64-66
		Total	292	302	368

from ICF to ECF by Na^+, K^+ ATPase pump. The normal daily intake of sodium is about 100-200 mmol/ day. But daily obligatory loss is less than 10 mmol/ day. Sodium balance is maintained by regulations of its renal excretions, 70 percent of glomerular filtrate is absorbed in the proximal convoluted tubule, 25 percent in the loop of Henle and 5 percent in the distal convoluted tubules and collecting ducts **(renin-angiotensin II-aldosterone mechanism)**.[1-5]

Na^+ requirement is usually calculated by the following equation:

0.6 × body wt × serum Na^+ deficit = mmol of sodium × 0.05 = gm of salt required.

1 gm of NaCl gives 44 mmol of Na^+.

Na^+ deficit in mmol × 2 = ml of 3 percent saline.

One mL of 3 percent saline provides 0.5 mmol of Na^+.

The osmolarities of the ECF is normally maintained in the range 280-295 mmol/kg of water. Increase in ECF osmolality in comparison to ICF osmolality causes three main effects:[3-7]

1. Stimulation of hypothalamic thirst center promoting dietary water intake.
2. Movement of water from ICF to ECF in order to maintain isotonicity.
3. Stimulation of hypothalamic osmoreceptors causing the release of ADH for effective renal water reabsorption and minimizing urinary water output and therefore resulting in a concentrated (low water and high solute) urine.

Osmoreceptors are highly sensitive to increased ECF osmolality even by 1 percent more than the ICF osmolarity resulting in release of ADH in the circulation.[4-9] They are located outside the blood-brain barrier in the anteroventral region of the third ventricle in the hypothalamus. If the ECF osmolality falls, there is no sensation of thirst; ADH secretion is inhibited (and a dilute urine is produced) allowing renal water loss to restore ECF osmolality (by raising it) to a normal level. If an increase in ECF osmolality occurs as a result of a solute such as urea, which readily diffuses across cell membranes, the ICF osmolality is also increased. In such cases, the ECF and ICF remain isotonic and therefore osmoreceptors are not stimulated.

A significant hypovolemia (10%), is a powerful stimulus (via angiotensinogen, arterial and venous baroreceptors and volume receptors) to ADH release to restore effective ECF volume even though there is a decrease in osmolality.[2-4,7-10] Maintenance of volume takes precedence over the maintenance of serum osmolarity. ADH is synthesized in the supraoptic nuclei of the hypothalamus and pass down the nerve axons into the posterior pituitary from where it is released into the circulation.[2-5]

Antidiuretic hormone (ADH) is essential for life as it maintains serum osmolarity by enhancing renal water reabsorption as it increases the permeability of the renal collecting tubules to water in response to increase in ECF osmolarity (above 285 mmol/kg), however, if ECF osmolarity is below 285 mmol/kg, ADH secretion is strongly inhibited.[3-5,11-13]

Mechanism of action of ADH on renal tubules is interesting.[11,14] ADH attaches to a specific vasopressin receptor on the contraluminal side of the renal medullary tubular cell. This attachment activates renal (medullary tubular) cellular adenyl cyclase. The latter stimulates production of cyclic AMP. Abundant cellular cyclic AMP then activates a protein kinase on the luminal side of the cell causing phosphorylation of membrane protein leading to an increased permeability of the tubular cell to water, facilitating its transport into the renal medullary circulation and then back into

Table 15.2: Clinical manifestations of Na^+ imbalance

Sr. No.	*Organic systems/Clinical state*	*Hyponatremia*	*Hypernatremia*
1.	Neurological	Cerebral edema, disorientation, lethargy, apathy, impairment of consciousness, seizures, coma, Chyne-Strokes respiration, hypothermia	Cerebral dehydration restlessness, irritability, disorientation, ataxia, seizures, coma, hemorrhage, intracranial
2.	Muscular	Cramps, hypotonic weakness, depressed reflexes, rhabdomyolysis	Increased muscle tone hyperreflexia
3.	Renal	Oliguria, concentrated urine or hypertonic urine	Polyuria diluted urine or hypotonic urine
4.	Gastrointestinal	Loss of appetite, nausea, vomiting	Thirst

the general circulation. Steroid replacement therapy lowers plasma ADH to normal and inhibits the secretary activity of the supraoptic neurons, and therefore has some role in SIADH (syndrome of inappropriate ADH secretion).

ADH plays a vital role in the control of the tonicity of the ECF[8-14] and hence indirectly of the ICF and therefore overall of water balance. Excessive secretion results in dilutional hyponatremia (SIADH) with a risk of water intoxication while decreased secretion results in excessive renal water loss (diabetes insipidus-01) causing hypernatremia with a risk of severe dehydration (Table 15.2).

In head injury, SIADH occurs when there is no direct damage to the pituitary gland, whereas DI is commonly due to hypothalamopituitary axis disturbance/damage.[2-7,15,16] Damage to the posterior pituitary may also cause temporary failure of ADH secretion.

In head injury patients, ADH is released in response to the clinical status (raised ECF osmolarity, raised ICP, hypovolemia, nociceptive stimuli, emotional stress), drug therapy (barbiturates, morphine, carbamazepine, chlorpropamide, angiotensin, thyroxin, glucocorticoids, cholinergic and beta adrenergic stimulation) and mechanical ventilation (positive airway pressure); whereas ADH is suppressed by phenytoin, ethanol, anticholinergics, atropine alpha adrenergic stimulation, reserpine, chlorpromazine besides increased plasma volume (hypervolemia) and reduced plasma osmolarity.[3-5,8-11,13-15] Steroid replacement therapy lowers plasma ADH to normal and permits the normal diuretic response to hydration by inhibiting the secretory activity of the supraoptic neurons (a weak response).[3-5] Antinatriuretics [catecholamines, renin angiotensin-II-aldosterone, cortisol] attempts at volume restitution or expansion following trauma.

Atrial natriuretic peptide (ANP) and brain natriuretic peptide (BNP) (largely of cardiac ventricular origin) have similar biological effects on the control of blood volume, blood pressure and electrolyte composition. ANP/BNP induces natriuresis through direct tubular effects or by inhibition of the renin-angiotensin-aldosterone mechanism.[16-18]

Hypervolemia is also kept under check as there is no appreciable ADH secretion in such circumstances and the excess of water is therefore lost from the kidneys. It is routinely measured by central venous pressure monitoring. Moreover, natriuretic peptide hormone (ANP, a 28-amino acid peptide) is produced by the cardiac atria when hypervolemia exerts excessive stretch on the sensitive atrial stretch receptors. It antagonizes renin-angiotensin II-aldosterone mechanism and causes natriuresis and hypovolemia.[18-20]

Table 15.3: Characteristics of parenteral fluid therapy

Sr. No.	Name	Concentration	Na^+	Cl^-	K^+	HCO	Ca^{+2}	Calculated mmol/L
1.	Normal saline	NaCl 0.9%	150	150	–	–	–	300
2.	Hartman's solution (Ringer lactate)	Saline + K^+ + HCO_3^-	131	111	5	29	–	280
3.	5% glucose	5% dextrose	–	–	–	–	–	280
4.	Dextrose saline	4% glucose, 0.18% saline.	30	30	–	–	–	286
5.	Half normal saline	NaCl 0.45%	75	75	–	–	–	150
6.	Human plasma protein fraction	HPPF mol. wt. 69,000	150	150	5	–	2	314 or more
7.	Hemaccel polygeline	Degraded gelatin mol. wt. 24,500	145	145	5	–	6.25	310 or more
8.	Succinylated gelatin	Gel of using mol. wt. 22,600	154	154	0.4	–	0.4	310
9.	Hetastarch	Hydroxyethyl starch 6% in saline mol. wt. 70,000	154	154	–	–	–	310 or more
10.	Blood	Whole blood constituents.	140	102	4	26	2.4	285

In clinical practice the serum osmolarity is routinely measured using following equation:

Osmolarity = 2 × [Na^+] + [urea] + [Glucose] mmol/L. Osmolality is a measure of solute concentrate per kilogram of solvent; whereas osmolarity is a measure of solute concentrate per liter of solution.[4] In clinical practice, the difference between osmolality and osmolarity is negligible (Table 15.3).

In head injury patients abnormalities of serum sodium (<125 or >150 mEq/L) and serum osmolality (<260 or >320 mOsm/L) should be avoided. Overhydration per se will not cause brain edema if the serum sodium value is normal (135-145 mEq/L); however, it can cause brain edema at brain injury sites only when it is combined with hyponatremia (<130 mEq/L) because ECF water shifts to ICF compartment in an attempt to maintain ECF/ICF isotonicity.

The loss of fluid and electrolytes without protein loss will cause rise in the hematocrit and plasma protein concentration.[1-6,9-12] These two parameters provide a good guide to ECF losses. For example, an initial albumin (Pr1) goes up (Pr2) following dehydration then the percent fall in ECF volume can be calculated as follows:

Percent fall in ECF volume = (1 – Prl /Pr2) × 100.

A fall in plasma volume can be more precisely calculated with the initial (Hct 1) and subsequent (Hct 2) hematocrit readings:

Percent fall in plasma volume: 100 [l – (Hct 1/100 – Hct 2 × 100 – Hct 2/Hct 2)].

Hematocrit and plasma albumin are therefore more useful in the assessment of plasma and ECF losses than the Na^+ (measurements) which although being lost does not change in its serum concentration (CSWS).[2-6,14,20]

By invasive hemodynamic monitoring, a low pulmonary capillary wedge pressure (mm Hg) or low CVPc (<6 mm Hg) implies volume depletion. Clinical evidence of dehydration, weight loss, orthostatic hypotension, CVP <6 mm Hg and negative water balance are noted in CSWS. Moreover, elevation of hematocrit, the serum creatinine and serum protein concentration point to dehydration in CSWS. Increased natriuresis and elevated serum K^+ also suggest CSWS.[15-18,21]

Using isotope dilution techniques, a decreased plasma volume (<35 ml/kg) and a decreased total blood volume (<60 ml/kg) are central features of CSWS.[17]

In water loading test, an increased free water reabsorption suggests increased ADH secretion.[14,17,22] Appropriate or inappropriate ADH secretion can be differentiated from one another by examining the urine

Table 15.4: Clinical characteristics of common causes of Na^+ imbalance in head injuries

Sr. No.	Clinical features	Hyponatremia SIADH	Hyponatremia CSWS	Hypernatremia Solute diuresis	Hypernatremia DI
1.	Intravascular volume	Hypervolemia	Hypovolemia	Hypervolemia	Hypovolemia
2.	Dehydration features	Absent	Present	Absent	Present
3.	Body weight	Increased	Decreased	Increased	Decreased
4.	CVP	Increased	Decreased	Increased	Decreased
5.	Hematology				
	i. PCWP	Decreased	Increased or Normal	Variable	Increased
	ii. Hematocrit	Decreased	Increased	Decreased	Increased
6.	Biochemical Parameters				
	i. S. osmolarity	Decreased	Inc./normal	Increased	Increased
	ii. S. protein conc.	Decr./normal	Increased	Variable	Increased
	iii. BUN/creatinine	Decreased	Incr./normal	Variable	Incr./normal
	iv. S. uric acid	Decreased	Normal	Decr./normal	Normal
	v. S. Na^+	Decreased	Decreased	Increased	Increased
	vi. Urine Na^+	Incr./normal	Increased	Increased	Decreased
	vii. Urine osmolarity	Increased	Increased	Increased	Decreased
7.	Management	Fluid restriction, salt replacement, loop diuretics, phenytoin, demeclocycline, lithium, fludrocortisone, diuretics, hemodialysis	Fluid replacement with isotonic fluid therapy, blood transfusions, fludrocortisone	Fluid replacement with hypotonic fluid, treatment of cause	Fluid replacement with hypotonic fluids, vasopressin, chlorpropamide clofibrate, thiazide Carbamazepine, steroids, Hemofiltration

volume, creatinine clearance, osmotic clearance and fractional water excretion.[17] If overall results suggest dehydration, then the increased free water reabsorption points to an appropriate ADH secretion. On the other hand, the increased free water reabsorption in the absence of dehydration suggests an inappropriate ADH secretion in SIADH. Normal or reduced free water reabsorption, with dehydration (reduced creatinine clearance, polyuria, high fractional or osmotic diuresis) and inappropriate natriuresis (sodium excretion of > 0.001 mmol hour which is inappropriate in the presence of severe hyponatremia) are central features of CSWS. Disproportionate fractional water clearance relative to the free water clearance suggests an osmotic diuresis. In DI there is a disproportionate free water clearance.[12-15,17,21-24]

It is essential that appropriate fluid and electrolyte studies be done early in the course of management of the head injured patient. Therapy is directed primarily towards the underlying cause of the fluid and electrolyte abnormality. In the potentially salvagable patient optimal correction may occur spontaneously or may require cautious use of medical therapy to achieve a good outcome (Table 15.4).

MAINTENANCE OF VOLUME IN HYPONATREMIC STATES

Hyponatremia (a low serum sodium concentration) is a common finding in NICU as a secondary phenomenon reflecting the presence of dysregulation of hypothalamo-hypophyseal axis, metabolic response to trauma or a sick cell syndrome requiring principally the management of underlying cause.[1-6,13-16,23-26] It is commonly due to water excess than to sodium loss. Significant hyponatremia is relatively common after the head injury occurring in about 8 to 15 percent of patients with moderate and severe head injuries. Hyponatremia is divided into three categories: mild (Na^+ < 135 to 125 mEq/L); moderate (Na^+ 120-124 mEq/L) and severe (Na^+ >120 mEq/L).

Etiopathogenesis: The risk of developing hyponatremia increases in the presence of severe head injuries, fracture of skull base and subdural hematoma.[13,22,25,26]

Following acute injury, the body retains water and sodium as a consequence of an acute neuroendocrine surge in an attempt to maintain an effective extracellular volume and thereby intravascular volume. As the water content of ECF increases as compared to its solute concentration, a dilutional hyponatremia results.

Hyponatremia lowers the seizure threshold, exacerbates cerebral edema and causes impairment of the level of consciousness.[4,13,27] However, the degree of brain dysfunction depends upon the rapidity of the development of hyponatremia; the serum sodium level of 115 mmol/L may be asymptomatic if developing slowly over a period whereas rapidly developing serum sodium level of 120-130 mmol/L may have severe neurological disturbance. In the setting of hypervolemia with hyponatremia, initially the brain cells (glia and neurons) swell due to an increase in cell volume due to movement of ECF water to ICF compartment because of the fall in ECF osmolality as compared to ICF osmolarity. Later, a gradual adaptive down regulatory volume reduction is achieved by loss of intracellular ions such as K^+, Cl^-, taurine, phosphocreatine and amino acids including excitatory neurotransmitters (glutamine, glutamate); with consequent neurologic impairment.[1-6] Hyponatremia ultimately lead to cerebral edema and raised ICP with their deleterious consequences.

Water retention (not the natriuresis) is a marked feature of ADH excess whereas natriuresis (not the water retention) is a prominent feature of ANP excess therefore the volume expansion is a prominent feature of SIADH, and the concomitant volume depletion with natriuresis is a marked feature of CSWS (cerebral salt wasting syndrome). ANP can suppress ADH secretion while ADH may itself stimulate ANP secretion.

In SIADH water retention (hyponatremic hypervolemia) inhibits aldosterone secretion and therefore relative natriuresis continues. In SIADH and CSWS, there is an increase in ADH secretion. In SIADH, water retention occurs due to high ADH. Whereas CSWS have high natriuresis due to high ANP/BNP and a low aldosterone activity.[13,14,16-18,21-25]

Differential diagnosis: Various hyponatremic syndromes in head injured patients may be differentiated primarily on the clinical grounds.[2-7,12-15,25-30]

In low dietary intake, depletion of both ICF and ECF solute can lead to hyponatremia. In true sodium depletion due to nutritional neglect, hyponatremia is accompanied by an evidence of a contracted blood volume (low blood pressure, decreased skin turgor and elevated hematocrit). In dilutional hyponatremia due to excessive hypotonic fluid infusion, peripheral edema is a prominent feature and in addition, there may be an evidence of cerebral edema, congestive heart failure or hepatic disease. Urinary sodium concentration is less than 10 mmol/L in both aforementioned conditions: Chronic dietary salt depletion and dilutional hyponatremia due to hypotonic fluid therapy.

Pseudohyponatremia may result due to a decreased fractional water content of plasma in cases of hyperproteinemia (two times the normal values) and hyperlipidemia. An increase in positively charged paraproteins or a decrease in negatively charged albumin concentrations in plasma can displaces Na^+ from the plasma to the ICF compartment causing hyponatremia. Factitious hyponatremia therefore requires no special treatment.

Hyperosmolar hyponatremia: Hyperglycemia may also result in hyponatremia. When plasma solute concentrations (glucose) are increased, a shift of water from the ICF to the ECF causes dilutional hyponatremia. In addition, an increased serum osmolarity causes direct stimulation of osmoreceptors and ADH release leading to renal water retention that further worsens the hyponatremia. Moreover, such increase in ECF volume inhibits volume receptors controlling aldosterone secretion leading to renal loss of sodium (natriuresis). Following mannitol infusion (osmotic diuretic increases ECF volume and reduces ICF volume to treat cerebral edema), hyponatremia occurs due to the sum total effects of the aforementioned mechanisms.

The persistence of dilutional hyponatremia implies either SIADH or renal impairment (acute tubular necrosis). Dilutional hyponatremia (low serum proteins and low serum urea) indicates SIADH. In normal subjects, osmolarity of the maximally dilute urine is about 50 mmol/kg. In SIADH, osmolarity of urine is more than 50 mmol/kg, and peripheral edema is not a prominent feature whereas dilutional hyponatremia with a dilute urine with peripheral edema indicates renal impairment. Sodium depletion is seldom due to inadequate input (nutritional restriction) but more often due to excessive renal loss of sodium (CSWS or due to high ANP levels or urinary sodium loss in diuretic therapy). The clinical features of sodium depletion are primarily as a result of decrease in ECF volume. The plasma sodium will be normal if fluid is lost isotonically (bleeding) and increased if it is lost hypotonically (excessive sweating in hyperpyrexia, mechanical ventilation, or gastrointestinal hyperkinesia). Thus the plasma sodium concentration in sodium depletion may be variable (low, normal or high). Sodium loss never occurs alone but is always accompanied by some water loss. The fluid lost may be isotonic or hypotonic with respect to the plasma.

Hyponatremia is common after infusion of hypotonic fluids (5% dextrose or dextrose saline), when ability of the body to excrete water is depressed.

The common hyponatremic states in head injury patients—CSWS and SIADH: Initially, cerebral salt wasting syndrome (CSWS) was recognized in the early 1950's and later the syndrome of inappropriate (excess) antidiurctic harmone (SIADH) in 1957 by Schwartz.[5,31-33] Majority of head injury patients with hyponatremia present with CSWS or SIADH. In few cases, both conditions may coexist. CSWS and SIADH, both are characterized by hyponatremia, hyperosmolar urine and hypernatriuresis in patients with normal renal, suprarenal and thyroid functions. The major distinction among these conditions is the volume status of the patient. In CSWS, the ECF volume is contracted and the patient appears dehydrated; whereas in SIADH the ECF volume is expanded and a clinical picture of fluid overload is often seen. Patients with CSWS respond to fluid and sodium administration while those with SIADH respond to fluid restriction. In neurosurgical patients, CSWS is common than SIADH.

SYNDROME OF INAPPROPRIATE ADH SECRETION (SIADH)[1-15,22,33]

It usually begins in first or second week after head injury and with appropriate therapy, lasts no more than one to two weeks. In SIADH, there is a continuous secretion of ADH despite hyponatremia, hypo-osmolar serum and hypervolemia.

The typical clinical features of SIADH are hyponatremia, with concomitant hypervolemic hypo-osmolar ECF, relative hypernatriuresis with hyperosmolar urine and absence of clinical evidence of volume depletion (normal skin turgor, blood pressure). The clinical symptoms include anorexia, nausea, vomiting, irritability, personality changes and neurological signs (bulbar or pseudobulbar palsy, stupor, muscular weakness, loss of reflexes, positive **Babinski sign** and convulsions.

CEREBRAL SALT WASTING SYNDROME (CSWS)[1-5,16-19,22,30-32]

This syndrome is due to an unregulated release of atrial natriuretic peptite. It presents with hyponatremia, with concomitant hypovolemic hypo-osmolar ECF, hypernatriuresis with hyperosmolar urine and presence of clinical evidence of volume depletion. Persistence of high salt loss in the urine despite fluid restriction differentiates this condition from SIADH where salt loss depends on a liberal fluid intake. The estimation of intravascular volume (by CVP) and urinary sodium usually differentiates salt retaining states (SIADH) from salt losing states (CSWS). Peters et al[32] and Cort[31] described CSWS as a condition with hyponatremia with natriuresis and believed that the CNS normally influences the ability of the kidneys to reabsorb sodium in the proximal tubule and that a defect in this regulatory function can lead to natriuresis. Many workers have reported a reduction in the red cell mass in patients with CSWS. Vingerhoets and de Tribolet[34] distinguished between two clinical syndromes of hyponatremia and natriuresis, which differed in the interval between the neurological insult and the emergence of hyponatremia: The acute syndrome (<3 days) and the delayed syndrome (> 1 week). They found elevated serum ADH levels in patients with acute syndrome and depressed or normal in chronic syndrome. SIADH is commonly seen in acute and CSWS in chronic syndrome.

The main diagnostic criteria of SIADH and CSWS are outlined in Table 15.4.

Management

Hyponatremia is basically treated according to the underlying disease process, serum osmolality and clinical estimate of total body sodium. The cornerstone of therapy in SIADH is fluid restriction whereas in CSWS the volume replacement and correction of the hematocrit.[1-8,13-14,17,34-37]

SIADH:[1-6,9-14,16-18,34-37] The patients with SIADH are basically treated with fluid restriction usually below one liter/day until serum Na^+ returns to normal levels with some salt supplement or replacements. The free water restriction should be sufficient to decrease total body water by 0.5 to 1.0 L/day. The resultant reduction in glomerular filtration rate enhances proximal tubular reabsorption of salt and water and stimulates aldosterone secretion.

Mild cases (Na^+ > 125 mEq/L) are best treated with fluid restriction whereas moderate cases (Na^+<125 mEq/L to 120 mEq/L) with water restriction 600 to 800 ml 5 percent dextrose in 0.45 percent saline per 24 hr, with or without normal saline; diuresis usually occurs in 36 to 48 hours. Patients with severe hyponatremia (Na^+<120 mEq/L) or in coma or with seizures may require hypertonic saline, with furosemide; 20 to 40 mg.[19] The diuretic therapy is used with utmost caution and monitoring to promote water loss. When hypertonic saline therapy is considered then it should be given only to restore Na^+ concentration to levels that no longer represent a hazardous state. The end point of hypertonic saline therapy is generally a serum Na^+ of 120 mEq/L or absence of overt symptoms. Initially plasma Na^+ may be increased by 1 to 2 mEq/L /hr. Care should be taken to avoid hypernatremia by cautious correction so that the plasma Na^+ should not be increased more than 12 mEq/L in 24 hours or 25 mEq/L in 48 hours, or to a concentration greater than 130 mEq/L.[4,17,39] Demeclocycline (anti ADH synthetic hormone) antagonizes the action of ADH on the renal collecting ducts and therefore may be used (600 to 1200 mg/day) to induce nephrogenic resistance to ADH.[3-6,17,36] Phenytoin is used as an antiepileptic drug with an added benefit as an anti-ADH agent.[35] Fludrocortisone (0.3 to 3 mg daily) to inhibit action of ADH on aldosterone mechanism and helps in raising serum Na^+ levels.[40]

CSWS:[1-6,14,17,18,20,30,33,41] The principles of the management of hyponatremia associated with CSWS consists of the treatment of an underlying cause, restriction of intravascular volume, isotonic fluid (normal saline, plasma, blood) infusion and fludrocortisone in CSWS.[13,17,40,43] These measures are effective without jeopardizing ICP control in most cases.

The patients with CSWS are best managed with salt containing fluid orally, enterally or intravenously to maintain CVP around 10-12 mm Hg. Patient's hemoglobin and hematocrit levels are measured daily and if needed packed cell with isotonic fluid or whole blood is given as per requirement.

Rapid correction of chronic hyponatremia[8,13,14,39,42] has been associated with fatal central pontine and extrapontine myelinolysis; on the other hand, severe acute hyponatremia can cause fatal cerebral edema (tentorial herniation) and status epilepticus. Despite such concerns, the management of hyponatremia with diuretic therapy (furosemide) and saline (isotonic/hypertonic) is safe.

Rarely patient may develop malignant ventricular Tachycardia as a consequence of electrolyte imbalance (low magnesium and calcium concentration) resulting from head injury.[44]

MAINTENANCE OF VOLUME IN HYPERNATREMIC STATES

Hypernatremia (a high serum sodium concentration) is much less frequent in head injured patients than hyponatremia and is much more frequent of clinical significance. It is caused by either water loss or[2] sodium excess.

Etiopathogenesis:[1,7,12,17,25,27,44,45] In hypernatremic head injury patients, water depletion occurs due to increased water loss as in diabetes insipidus (lack of ADH), renal diabetes insipidus (ADH insensitivity), mannitol (osmotic diuresis), glycosuria (osmotic diuresis), prolonged hyperpyrexia (increased sweating); hyperventilation (increased insensible loss), antibiotics related diarrhea and due to decreased dietary water intake. The neurological causes include cerebral trauma, cerebral tumors (craniopharyngioma, secondary deposits, pituitary tumors), vascular disorders (Sheehan's syndrome, SAH or cerebral aneurysm), meningoencephalitis, surgery and idiopathic.

Despite the frequent pathological demonstration of pituitary and hypothalamic damage in head injury, the incidence of DI is relatively less. However, DI is a mortel sign in patients with massive brain injuries, uncontrollable intracranial hypertension.

In clinical practice, excessive water loss without much sodium loss is unusual except in diabetes insipidus. Pure water loss is borne by the total body water and not just the ECF, and therefore signs of a reduced ECF volume are not usually present. Severe water depletion causes cerebral dehydration that stimulates intracellular mechanisms for brain cells to synthesize osmotically active compounds and acute cerebral edema may then follow rapid fluid replacement with deleterious consequences. Severe water depletion is therefore corrected in cautious manner by 5 percent dextrose or hypotonic saline (2/3 deficits in the first 24 hours and 1/3 in next 24 hours).

Differential diagnosis:[1-5,12-15,21,29,44,45] The differential diagnosis of serum hyperosmolarity and polyuria following trauma in the region of hypothalamopituitary axis may be different due to the presence of variety of overlapping causes.

Polydipsia (thirst leading to increased intake) and polyuria are hallmark of DI. The differential diagnosis includes other conditions causing polyuria and polydipsia, i.e. renal diabetes insipidus, diabetes mellitus, chronic renal failure, hypercalcemia, hypokalemia and psychogenic polydipsia. Simple biochemical tests will easily eliminate many of these possibilities. Solute diuresis in hyperglycemia, uremia, osmotic or loop diuretics and aldosterone deficiency presents with a normal or slightly decreased serum sodium with only an occasional change in thirst mechanism. The urine specific gravity remains between 1.009 and 1.035 and urine osmolarity between 250 and 320 momol/kg whereas water diuresis (diabetes insipidus) presents with a normal or increased serum sodium levels and intense thirst and polyuria. The urine remains between 50 and 150 momol/kg. Whereas a normal (water deprived) individual will concentrate his urine with urine output of 0.5 ml/min and urine osmolarity of greater than 750 momol/kg. In diabetes insipidus decreased ADH secretion results in uncontrolled renal water loss (a dilute urine) with a dehydrational hypernatremia. Renal diabetes insipidus is due to renal insensitivity to ADH despite increased ADH levels in serum and urine, and psychogenic polydipsia-polyuria is due to a compulsive desire to drink. These conditions are differentiated with the help of either water deprivation tests or serum and urine ADH assays. Diabetes mellitus (hyperglycemia), hypercalcemia, chronic renal failure and hypokalemia may also cause polyuria and polydipsia but are easily differentiated from central diabetes insipidus by routine biochemical tests. If it is due to Demeclocycline (anti-ADH agent) this should be discontinued. If a random urine osmolality is greater than 750 mmol/kg, diabetes insipidus is basically excluded.

Diabetes insipidus:[1-8,13,15,16,21,29,44,45] Diabetes insipidus is a common phenomenon after craniofacial injury and basilar skull fractures, and can be permanent or transient disappearing in a few days or weeks. Trauma, hypoxia, hemorrhagic shock, surgery, fat embolism, drug overdose, etc. may cause diabetes insipidus. Hypothalamo-hypophyseal injury poses a particular risk of developing transient or permanent diabetes insipidus. It is transient in majority of patients lasting for 3-5 days, however, in one-fourth to one-third of cases it may be permanent.

Some patients show a triphasic response manifested by early diabetes insipidus, followed by return of normal urinary functions for 1-3 weeks and then relapse leading to permanent diabetes insipidus.

Clinical manifestations of diabetes insipidus:[3-5,8,29,44,45] Polyuria, (>2-3 L/ day), polydipsia, hypernatremia with hypovolemia, high serum osmolality (320-330 mOsm/kg), low urine osmolarity and a dilute urine (specific gravity less than 1005) and a urine to serum osmolarity ratio of less than one, implying a negative water balance are characteristic features of DI Diagnostic tests:[1-4,13,44,45] Serum and urine ADH assays and/or a water deprivation test are performed. A normal person on water deprivation for 8 hours will have urine output 0.5 ml/min and will concentrate urine to preserve water. Urine osmolarity will rise and become greater than 500 mOsm/kg. Patients with diabetes insipidus fail to concentrate their urine and the water loss continues as a dilute urine.

During the water deprivation testing, in diabetes insipidus, the urine does not become concentrated and the serum osmolarity rises during the eight hour test period, whereas a normal person will maintain serum osmolarity below 295 mmol/kg during this period. Serum osmolarity above 285 mmol/kg is a strong stimulus for ADH release to maintain serum osmolarity in normal range by retaining more water. On administration of desmopressin in patients suspected of DI, if the urine becomes concentrated and the serum osmolarity falls then the diagnosis of DI will be confirmed.

Measurement of ADH levels in urine and serum in relation to plasma osmolality is far more desirable than the water deprivation test in acute head injury patients as the latter may be highly inappropriate in many of these patients. If the ADH essays are not available then a therapeutic trial with desmopressin is highly indicated to resolve the diagnostic dilemma.

Management[1-8,13-16,18-21,29,44]

Daily measurements of body weight, fluid intake/output, hemoglobin, hematocrit, renal function tests (serum creatinine, BUN, sugar, electrolytes), serum osmolarity, urine specific gravity and urine osmolarity are performed. Treatment of hypernatremia by water loss basically consists of water replacement as well as repletion of associated deficits of sodium and other electrolytes. Hypernatremia is corrected slowly because of the risk of neurologic sequelae such as seizures and cerebral edema. The water deficit is corrected over 2~8 hours and plasma Na^+ is gradually reduced by 1-2 mEq/L/hr.

The aim of the fluid therapy is to replace hourly urine output with the usual estimate for the insensible loss with hypotonic fluids. The volume depletion leads to reduction in the mean systemic arterial pressure and subsequently a reduction in the cerebral perfusion pressure and therefore needs cautious correction.

Regardless of its cause, hypernatremia should initially be treated by administration of hypotonic fluids such as water (orally) or 5 percent dextrose (parenterally). The antidiuresis is enhanced by low sodium intake and diminished by high sodium. Urine output in DI may exceed 10 L/day although less than this is more usual. Adequate fluid replacement, desmopressin [Desmopressin (l-desamino-D-arginine-vasopressin) is a synthetic analog of ADH] for severe cases and chlorpropamide (oral hypoglycemic agent) 50 to 200 mg/day or carbamazepine (antiepileptic agent 600 mgs/day) for mild cases of DI may be used. Desmopressin is indicated if urine output exceeds 6 to 7 L/day, or urinary output remains more than 250 mL/hr for two to four consecutive hours or the patient is unable to maintain fluid balance and the normal intravascular volume. Treatment with vasopressin should not be withheld in verified cases of DI. There are many preparations of vasopressin which are highly effective:

a. Aqueous vasopressin (5-10 IU 1M/IV, 4 to 6 hourly)
b. Vasopressin Tannate-in-oil (5 IU IM/daily as initial therapy once in 2-3 days).
c. Lysine vasopressin nasal spray (21 IU/spray, 6-8 hourly).
d. DDA VP (1-deamino-8-D-arginine vasopressin) -10-20 mg intranasally on OD or BD basis.

Care must be exercised during the active treatment of DI/hypernatremia to prevent water intoxication (lethargy, confusion, seizures and coma) due to excessive desmopressin administration, hypoglycemia due to chlorpropamide therapy, and significant hypovolemia following diuretics therapy (by further contracting ECF volume). While controlling post-traumatic seizures, Carbamazepine stimulates ADH release in patients with diabetes insipidus. In patients with dangerously high serum sodium, the peritoneal dialysis/hemodialysis/hemofiltration to remove excess serum sodium may have to be considered. In terminal hypernatremia, the patient does not respond to any treatment and has the worst prognosis. Hemofiltration employs a filter containing a membrane with characteristics similar to those of capillary endothelial cells, in that water and smaller molecules (with a molecular weight <= 20,000) can pass freely across it. The filter is connected to arterial and venous lines and the hydrostatic pressure drives a solution similar to the ECF across the cell membrane. Hemofiltration in NICU has advantages over the conventional hemodialysis in fine control of fluid and electrolyte balance and removal of water soluble waste products and drugs.

CONCLUSION

Significant head injury results in marked hypermetabolism and hypercatabolism. Patients with injury to central neuraxis including the brainstem and hypothalamo-hypophyseal system causes the greatest response. Majority of the patients with head injury show no appreciable fluid and electrolyte abnormalities; however, a subset of significant head injury patients suffer from fluid and electrolyte disturbances. Neurological recovery in such patients occur rapidly if they are treated in time with adequate fluid and electrolyte therapy. To institute an appropriate therapy, a proper understanding of the etiopathological mechanisms, their diagnostic parameters and treatment protocols is necessary. Failure to execute such responsibility may lead to increased morbidity and mortality which may be avoidable in many of these critically ill head injury patients.

REFERENCES

1. Beck LH. Body fluid and electrolyte disorders. Medical Clinics of North Arne 1981;65:247-451.
2. Gill GV, Plear CTG. Hyponatraemia. Recent advances in clinical biochemistry 1985;3:149-59.
3. Marshall WJ. Water and sodium. In 'Clinical Chemistry'. WJ Marshall (ed) Und edition, Mosby Year Book, Europe Limited p. 1993;10-28.
4. Morgan DB (Ed). Electrolyte disorders. Clinics in Endocriology and Metabolism 1984;13:231-4.
5. Welt LG, Seldin DW, Nelson WP. Role of the central nervous system in metabolism of electrolytes and water. Am J Med 1952;90:355-78.
6. Young B, Ott L, Twyman D, et al. The effect of nutritional support outcomes from severe head injury. J Neurosurg 1987;67:668-76.
7. Bacic A, Gluncic I, Gluncic V. Disturbances in plasma sodium in patients with war head injuries. Mil Med 1999;164:214-7.
8. Darby JM, Nelson PB. Fluid electrolyte and acid base balance. In: Neurosurgical Intensive Care. Andrews BT (Ed). McGraw Hill Inc Baltimore 1993; p. 133-43.
9. Guggiari M, Georgrschu H. The injured brain. Basis for hydroelectrolyte and hemodynamic resuscitation. Ann Fr Anesth Reanim 1994;13:98-104.
10. Maclaurin RL, King LR. Recognition and treatment of metabolic disorders after head injuries. Clin Neurosurg 1972;19:281-95.
11. Orloff J, Handler JS. Cellular mode of action of antidiuretic hormone. Am J Med 1964;36:686-97.
12. Bakay RAE, Ward AA. Enzymatic changes in serum and cerebrospinal fluid in neurological injury. J Neurosurg 1983;58:27-37.

13. Lolin K, Jackowski A. Hyponatraemia in neurosurgical patients: Diagnosis using derived parameters of sodium and water homeostasis. Brit J Neurosurg 1992;6:457-66.
14. Crompton MR. Hypothalamic lesions following closed head injury. Brain 1971;94:165-9.
15. Griffin JM, Hartley JH, Crow RW, et al. Diabetes insipidus caused by craniofacial trauma. J Trauma 1976; 16:979-84.
16. Amer M, Hasse J, Holmegaard SN, Djurberg H. Cerebral salt wasting syndrome and syndrome of inappropriate antidiuretic hormone secretion in subarachnoid hemorrhage caused by ruptured berry aneurysms. Pan Arab Journal of Neurosurgery 2000;4(2):25-31.
17. Weinand ME, Boynick PL, Goetz KL. A study of serum antidiuretic hormone and atrial natriuretic peptide levels in a series of patients with intracranial disease and hyponatremia. Neurosurg 1990;25:781-5.
18. Decauy G, Waaterlot Y, Genette F, et al. Treatment of the syndrome of inappropriate secretion of anti-diuretic hormone with furosemide. N Eng J Med 1981;304:329-30.
19. lbarra-de-la-Rosa I, Perez Navero JL, Palocios Cordoba A, Montero Schiemann C, Montilla Lopez P, Ramanos Lezcano A. Inadequate secretion of atrial natriuretic peptide in children with acute brain injury. An Esp Pediatr 1999;51:27-32.
20. Brigham WF. The limits of cerebral dehydration in the treatment of head injury. Surg Neurol 1986;25:340-44.
21. Sivakumar V, Rajshekhar V, Chandy MJ. Management of Neurosurgical patients with hyponatraemia and natriuresis. Neurosurgery 1994;34:269-74.
22. Padilla G, Leake JA, Castro R, et al. Vasopressin levels and pediatric head trauma. Pediatrics 1989;97:62-70.
23. Steinbok P, Thompson GB. Metabolic disturbances after head injury. Abnormalities of sodium and water balance with special reference to the effects of alcohol intoxication. Neurosurgery 1978;3:9-16.
24. Becker RM, Daniel RK. Increased antidiuretic hormone production after trauma to the craniofacial complex. J Trauma 1973;13:112-5.
25. Simma B, Burger R, Falk M, Sacher P, Fanconi S. A prospective, randomized and controlled study of fluid management in children with severe head injury: Lactated Ringer's solution versus hypertonic saline. Crit Care Med 1998;26:1265-70.
26. Diringer M, Ladenson PW, Stern BJ, Schleimer J, Hanley DF. Plasma atrial natriuretic factor and subarachnoid haemorrhage. Stroke 1988;19:1119-24.
27. De Foer F, Mahler C, Dua G, et al. Post-traumatic diabetes insipidus. Acta Anesthesio! Belg 1987;38: 297-02.
28. Ganong CA, Kappy MS. Cerebral salt wasting in children. The need for recognition and treatment. Am J Dis Child 1993;147:167-9.
29. Cort JH. Cerebral salt wasting. Lancet 1954;1:752-4.
30. Peters JP, Welt LG, Sims EAH. A salt wasting syndrome associated with cerebral disease. Trans Assoc Am Physicians 1950;63:57-64.
31. Schwartz WB, Bennett W, Curelop S. A syndrome of renal sodium loss and hyponatraemia probably resulting from inappropriate secretion of antidiuretic hormone. Am J Med 1957;23:529-42.
32. Vingerhoets F, de Tribolet N. Hyponatraemia hypo-osmolarity in neurosurgical patients. Appropriate secretion of ADH and cerebral salt wasting syndrome. Acta Neurochir (Wien) 1988;91:50-54.
33. Fichman MP, Kleeman CR, Bethume JE. Inhibition of antidiuretic hormone secretion by diphenyl hydantoin. Arch Neurol 1970;22:45-53.
34. Forrest JN, Cox M, Hong C, et al. Superiority of demeclocycline over lithium in the treatment of chronic syndrome of inappropriate secretion of antidiuretic hormone. N Eng J Med 1978;298:173-7.
35. Fox JL, Falik JL, Shahoub RJ. Neurological hyponatraemia: The role of inappropriate antidiuresis. J Neurosurg 1971; 34:506-14.
36. Robertson CS, Narayan RK, Gokaslan ZL, et al. Cerebral arteriovenous oxygen difference as an estimate of cerebral blood flow in comatose patients. J Neurosurg 1989;70:222-30.
37. Cluitmans FAM, Meinders AE. Management of severe hyponatraemia: Rapid or slow correction? Am J Med 1990;88:161-6.
38. Ishikawa S, Saito T, Kaneko K, Okada K, Kuzuya T. Hyponatraemia response to fludrocortisone acetate in elderly patients after head injury. Am Intern Med 1987; 16:707-11.
39. Aviram A, Pfau A Czaczkes JW, et al. Hyperosmolality with hyponatraemia caused by inappropriate administration of mannitol. Am J Med 1967;42:648-50.
40. Swales JD. Dangers in treating hyponatraemia. BMJ 1987;294:261-2.
41. Yamakki T, Tano-oka A, Takahashi A, Imaizumi T, Suetake K, Hashi K. Cerebral salt wasting syndrome distinct from the syndrome of inappropriate secretion of antidiuretic hormone (SIADH). Acta Neurochir (Wien) 1992;115:156-62.
42. Norman DD, Mortek MA, Moses AM. Permanent diabetes insipidus following head trauma: Observations on ten patients and an approach to diagnosis. J Trauma 1980;20:599-602.
43. Sucart WA, Jackson I. Management of diabetes insipidus in neurosurgical patients. J Neurosurg 1976;44:65-71.
44. Khogali SS, Townsend JN, Marshal H. Ventricular tachycardia following head injury. Heart 2003;89(8):829.

16

Coagulopathy in Head Injury

Aditya Gupta, AK Mahapatra

SUMMARY

Coagulopathy following head injury may be a relatively common problem than is appreciated at present. Various alterations are hypothesized for the occurrence, but the basic abnormality remains the stimulation of the coagulation system owing to the brain tissue thromboplastins released as a result of brain injury. This may then lead to a brief period of fibrinolysis and the overall abnormality may flare into a full-fledged DIC syndrome. This requires timely evaluation of the coagulation status, and appropriate corrective measures when present. As the presence of coagulopathy is an independent predictor of high mortality and morbidity after head injury, all attempts should be made to detect and correct this dysfunctional state as early as possible. This is obviously paramount in patients with clinical evidence of DIC and those requiring urgent neurosurgical interventions. Even in the remaining, there may be a definite beneficial effect of treating the abnormal hemostasis. Prophylactic infusion of clotting factors is debatable at present, as is the beneficial impact of treating the coagulopathy following head injury. The pathogenesis and the management of this syndrome are discussed in relation to the currently available evidence for these aspects.

INTRODUCTION

Several reports have described coagulation abnormalities in patients with head trauma.[1-8]

Starting with preliminary reports in the 60s,[9-11] many reports have attempted to define the precise disturbances in the coagulation system. Similar reports have highlighted dysfunction of various coagulation components in other situations of brain injury as well as other neurological disorders.[1,9] Abnormalities consistent with a state of disseminated intravascular coagulation (DIC) have been shown to occur after acute head injury. The other abnormalities noted include alterations in platelet numbers[6] and function.[12] Additionally, "defibrination" has been reported in numerous reports and mainly refers to the consumption coagulopathy that follows severe DIC.

Patients with TBI develop platelet dysfunction which most likely contributes to bleeding complications. Thus dysfunction can be measured by thromboelastography, i.e. platelet mapping (TEG-PM) to identify the patients with high-risk of bleeding complication.[44]

It has been frequently suggested that the primary reason for development of DIC in head-injured patients is the release of brain thromboplastin. Additional factors as well as the evolving secondary events in these critically ill patients are certainly of much relevance in the development of fresh abnormalities and worsening of pre-existing ones. A good proportion of these patients require brain surgery mainly for decompressive purposes, especially when a lesion responsible for raised intracranial pressure (ICP) is evident. This adds the further confounding factor of general anesthesia and operative trauma and stress, all of which may very likely play a role. It is also recognized that coagulopathy can lead to delayed and progressive hematomas in patients with brain injury (Fig. 16.1). After surgery,

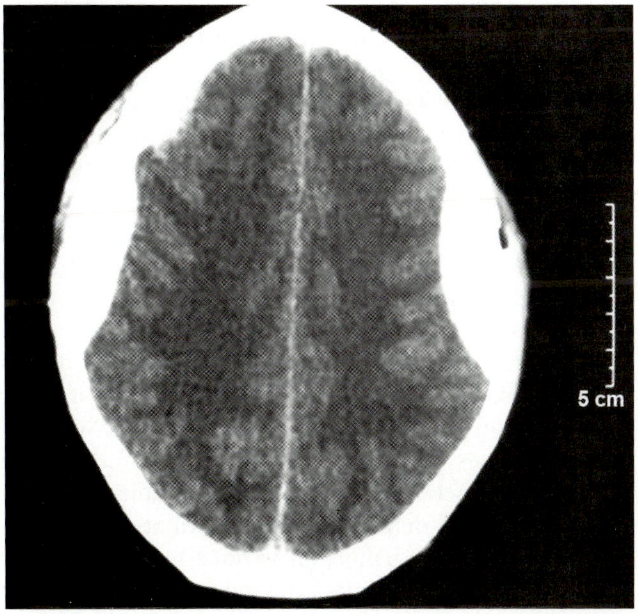

Fig. 16.1: CT showing bilateral frontoparietal extradural hematomas in a patient on anticoagulant drugs

these patients may develop recurrent hematomas that are extremely difficult to treat and carry a high morbidity and mortality.[13-15]

The mechanisms responsible for the spectrum of coagulation abnormalities following head trauma are varied and some continue to be controversial. There is similarly no consensus on the exact evaluation protocol for the detection of coagulation abnormalities in head-injured patients. There is also no agreement as to whether any prophylaxis for the impending coagulopathy is of any benefit to these patients. With the increasing trend of high velocity and missile injuries, it is possible that the neurosurgeon may encounter this kind of coagulopathy more frequently. Even otherwise, we feel that this kind of coagulation abnormality needs to be better recognized. We feel that this complication of head injury has been erroneously labeled as "rare" by numerous authors, without much more than anecdotal data. It is, therefore, of relevance to be aware of the various coagulation abnormalities, the mechanisms and the therapy in a neurosurgical setting. This review aims at discussing the above mentioned aspects with regard to the current state of knowledge. It is hoped that this brief overview would serve the purpose and provide some rational basis for management.

INCIDENCE OF COAGULOPATHY

An entire spectrum of coagulation abnormalities have been described, but the overall incidence of coagulopathy in head injury is difficult to estimate. Many reports cite the incidence as "rare" in passing, and very few reports exist detailing the incidence from large neurotrauma centers.

In the late 1960s, single case reports described this complication. From that time, many other reports are available. None of these systematically try to estimate the true magnitude of the problem.

There are two major approaches to address this issue: incidence based on laboratory test abnormalities, and based on autopsy studies.

Laboratory test abnormalities (later detailed) are a common feature in trauma patients.[13] These frequently are not associated with any clinical evidence of overt or occult bleeding. It should be realized that whereas normal values for these laboratory parameters are known, the exact cutoff values for the definition of DIC are still not well defined.[13] Further limitations include an inhomogeneous battery of various tests by various authors, in order to justify a diagnosis of DIC. It is also clear that only gross alterations (decline to 20–30% of normal) in coagulation factor levels lead to abnormal test results.[14,15] With these limitations in mind we can now place the available data in the correct perspective. It has been said that abnormal coagulation parameters are "common" in head-injured patients.[13-16] Several other reports cite the occurrence of abnormal coagulation parameters (suggestive of DIC) anywhere between 17 and 76 percent.[3-5,7,8,15,17,18] The most obvious reason for this vast range is primarily the varying criteria used for the diagnosis of DIC. Review of the larger series with some homogeneity as to the criteria for the diagnosis of DIC reveal that the actual range may lie somewhere between 20 and 50 percent.[5,7,15,17] The percentage of patients having a milder abnormality is much higher.

The percentage of clinically evident DIC has been estimated in only a few studies and probably lies between 1 to 24 percent.[3,14,15,17]

Few autopsy studies have also demonstrated clear evidence of fibrin deposition within the vasculature in many organs. The problem here is that this method is probably quite insensitive owing to the secondary fibrinolysis that may occur and not leave any fibrin deposits in tissues. It is also clear that routine autopsy surveys would markedly under report the microthrombi and special stains are required for this purpose. However, few available autopsy reports do give a clear indication of the existence of this syndrome, but are far too anecdotal to convey any idea about incidence of this complication.[1,19]

PATHOGENESIS

It is an often quoted fact that brain tissue has been frequently used as a rich source of tissue thromboplastin in performing the prothrombin time (PT) examination. Human brain tissue extract was used in the one stage method standardized by Quick as early as 1935. This leads us to probably the most important link in the pathogenesis of coagulopathy following head injury. It is now generally agreed that the most important factor leading to coagulopathy following head injury is the release of tissue thromboplastin from the brain tissue into the circulation, which then activates the coagulation cascade mainly through the extrinsic system.

The role of tissue thromboplastin was supported by the experiment of Cooper et al,[20] who produced DIC in dogs after infusing canine brain thromboplastin. This was implicated also in solitary case reports in 1970s[1,7] and later has been confirmed in several large studies.[3,6,8,17,19] In a report by Clark et al[21] the case reported developed florid DIC following head injury. The patient succumbed to the injuries, and autopsy revealed traumatized brain tissue within lacerated dural sinus. The authors implicated that thromboplastin may have reached the systemic circulation by this route. In another interesting study,[22] patient with a ventriculoatrial shunt sustained head injury and later developed DIC. The patient had traumatic intraventricular hemorrhage, and the authors postulate that the ventriculoatrial shunt may have drained the tissue thromboplastins into the general circulation. While we agree that the head injury and DIC in the above two cases were causally linked, we feel that the postulated route of entry of thromboplastins into the general circulation in both the above cases are over simplifications. It is clear that trauma leads to widespread blood-brain barrier alterations and these are then sufficient to allow leakage of tissue thromboplastin into the circulation. Other indications as to the truth of above statements come from various other clinical studies. It is worthwhile to highlight an important study by Goodnight et al.[3] They studied 13 patients each of head injury with and without obvious brain tissue destruction. The authors found highly significant differences between coagulation parameters in both the groups, with 9 of 13 patients with obvious brain tissue destruction having "defibrination". Other studies have also correlated the severity of the coagulopathy with the severity of head injury.[7,8,15,17,19] On the other hand, review of a report by Simmons and coworkers[23] reveals that among 240 combat casualties with extensive wounds but without head injuries, there were minor abnormalities of coagulation in a few cases.

While the role of tissue thromboplastin is important, the possible mechanisms of pathogenesis of DIC are mainly three:

- *Endothelial cell injury:* Leading to activation of the Hageman factor and then the intrinsic system.
- *Tissue injury:* Leading to thromboplastin release and activation of the extrinsic system.
- *Red cell or platelet injury* with release of procoagulant phospholipids.

The second pathway would seem to be the most important in our setting. So far, there is a general agreement as to the pathogenesis. There is controversy as to the exact triggering mechanism and few reports even deny the existence of coagulopathy following head injury. In two such reports, the first one[24] concluded that the authors could not identify any instance of DIC in 34 patients with moderate and severe head injury. These authors were able to identify a mild activation of the coagulation system. In the second report[25,40] trauma patients were studied, of which 15 had DIC. The authors stated that from their data, head injury did not significantly affect post-trauma coagulation or fibrinolysis. These authors feel that in general blood coagulation activity is enhanced and fibrinolytic activity is promoted on the day of trauma, but inhibited thereafter. This has found general acceptance, and most now believe that head injury initially induces a hypercoagulable state, which is then followed by fibrinolysis. A particular study demonstrated that the extent of fibrinolytic activity measured as early as 1 hour after injury correlates well with the extent of brain dranage.[26] Another recent study has attempted to address some of these controversies.[6] The authors studied 20 patients having isolated severe head injury with 4 patients having isolated bone fracture (control group). They performed sampling of both the central venous as well as jugular bulb blood samples. As in other reports, there was a significant difference in fibrinogen levels and platelet counts compared to the control group. Similarly, thrombin-antithrombin complex, prothrombin fragment and soluble fibrin concentrations were all higher in the head injury group. An important finding was that all but the latter concentrations were significantly higher in the cerebrovenous blood, thus indicating the source. On the other hand, as there was no difference in D-dimer and soluble fibrin levels between cerebral and central venous blood, it indicates the likely systemic source of these two coagulation factors. The authors therefore, state that there seems to be a marked activation of the systemic coagulation system following head injury, as a result of procoagulant influences from the brain tissue. This may "spark" DIC in some such head injury patients.

Apart from DIC, other coagulation abnormalities do exist. Platelet counts have been shown to be less in head trauma patients in numerous reports[3,5-8,14,15,17,19] The exact mechanism is not clear, but this finding may be also of equal importance from therapeutic aspect. Disturbances of platelet function have been reported in head injury patients.[12] In the study, authors studied ADP-induced platelet aggregation for 6 weeks in 34 head-injured patients. In all 8 patients dying within 24 hours of injury, the platelet aggregation was markedly reduced. In 17 patients that remained unconscious for four or more days, the platelet function was decreased and remained so for 9 days. Even the remaining 9 patients with mild decline in consciousness demonstrated subnormal function, which returned to normal by fourth day. This has important implications, as it implies the existence of neurohumoral factors that can directly influence platelet function. The authors postulate that serotonin or other catecholamine levels that rise after head injury may exert some influences on platelet functions through platelet β receptors. A recent study has attempted to define the differences between patients having symptomatic versus asymptomatic DIC after head injury.[27] The authors found that neutrophil elastase was significantly higher in the symptomatic DIC group. Neutrophil elastase is well known to mediate DIC after sepsis and causes tissue destruction and multiorgan failure. The authors suggest that monitoring neutrophil elastase early after head injury may help in identifying patients at risk for developing symptomatic DIC. Another valuable suggestion is that although laboratory parameters may reveal a DIC-like picture, the disorder may not truly be DIC as overall only very few patients become symptomatic, and neutrophil elastase elevation is present in only these patients.

LABORATORY EVALUATION

Reliable laboratory evaluation of coagulopathy is the cornerstone of diagnosing it, as it is the only available tool for identifying clinically silent abnormalities. However, the laboratory assessment has many limitations, which need to be understood. Firstly, the routine evaluation tests are quite insensitive to even substantial declines in coagulation factor levels. These become abnormal only when the levels decline to 20 to 30 percent of normal. This also means that abnormal parameters cannot be completely disregarded, even though the patient may not be symptomatic. The other problem is that head injury being a dynamic pathological state, one-time assessments may frequently be fallacious. The previous section has already told us the hypercoagulable state that exists in head-injured patients, with frequently coexistent fibrinolysis.

Prior to laboratory assessment, the following considerations merit attention:

- *Clinical status of the patient:* Time of injury; degree of blood loss and any replacement prior to sample collection; prior coagulation abnormality or history suggestive of it; intake of anti-inflammatory drugs or anticoagulants; existance of liver disease.
- *Careful collection of specimens:* Wrong dilutions or nonoptimal amount of reagent in collection tubes may all affect test results.
- Timely delivery of specimens to the laboratory.
- Assessment of test results by an experienced hematologist.

Six basic tests of coagulation function assessment are routinely recommended for any health care organization:

- Prothrombin time (PT)
- Activated partial thromboplastin time (APTT)
- Thrombin clotting time (TT)
- Platelet count
- Fibrinogen essay
- Fibrin degradation product essay (FDP).

In cases where hemodilution is suspected, concomitant performance of hematocrit should be done. This may be of importance in polytrauma patients, with significant blood loss. Taking into conjunction all these evaluations, different centers have devised their own grading systems for the diagnosis of DIC. There is yet no final consensus. In the absence of any underlying disease that could alter hemostasis, any abnormal result implies some coagulopathy. Abnormal PT mainly implies a derangement of the extrinsic system, and abnormal APTT implies a dysfunction of the intrinsic system. DIC usually causes prolongation of PT, APTT and TT accompanied by a low platelet count and elevation of FDP levels. The exact cutoff values are still controversial. For more details, a few grading scales are referred to.[28,29]

Certain specialized tests can be under some circumstances to better define the exact underlying mechanism,[6,12,13,19,25-29] and may provide some input of therapeutic significance:

- Fibrinopeptide A and B
- D-dimer
- Thrombin-antithrombin complex
- Protamine sulfate test
- Prothrombin fragment assay
- Platelet function tests, like platelet mapping (TEGPM).[44]

THERAPEUTIC CONSIDERATIONS

The therapy should be primarily based on clinical grounds and needs, and should not necessarily rely only on the biochemical evidence of a coagulopathy. The various parameters to be taken into consideration are:

- Active bleeding from skin, mucosae and other puncture sites
- Clinical and neurological state of the patient
- Severity of the intracranial injury and intracranial pressure
- Need for urgent operative decompression or repair
- Any underlying disease or drug intake predisposing to coagulopathy.

It is clear that patients having active bleed need urgent correction of the underlying coagulation abnormality. Any patient with clinically or biochemically evident coagulopathy needing urgent decompression should similarly undergo replacement of clotting factors prior to surgical intervention. This is of importance as operative stress, operative trauma including that to the brain tissue may further aggravate the existing coagulopathy. It has been clearly documented that these head-injured patients with coagulopathy are at risk for developing delayed and recurrent postoperative hematomas.[13,16,30-33] At the same time, it would be imprudent to make a patient with a large hematoma (especially an epidural hematoma) wait for decompression after obtaining a full report and correcting the abnormality as these patients can deteriorate rather rapidly. This can only be decided as per the merits of a particular case. However, in these patients we do perform simple bedside tests such as evaluations of bleeding and clotting times and start therapy as required by the urgency of the clinical situation. In such case, occasionally the replacement therapy and surgery may have to be done simultaneously. Surgically, in such a patient one should take care to minimize the time taken and further blood loss. The least extensive procedure should be planned in these patients. Adequate replacements of clotting factors should be available and transfusion of these should be continued throughout the procedure. In case of any doubt about adequacy of hemostasis, a drain should readily be left. Similarly, the same tube could be used to monitor the intracranial pressure after surgery. Postoperatively, check of the coagulation status should be carried out and replacement done to maintain adequate levels of coagulation function.

Coagulation disorders after head injury can contribute to progression of hemorrhage: In a small and highly individually selected series of patients with severe head injury, the administration of recombinant factor VIIa did not lead to adverse effect. The early use of recombinant factor VIIa without systematic coagulopathy may reduce the occurrence or enlargement of contusion, further need of operation and adverse outcome.[46]

The line of therapy for the actively bleeding patient and for the one requiring surgery is quite clear. Controversy exists regarding the optimal management of patients that are asymptomatic and do not require surgery. It has been previously stated that the biochemical coagulopathy only mimics DIC and is usually self-limiting. In this context, if only a minority of these patients is to develop full-blown DIC, it may not be cost-effective to treat all such patients with precious coagulation factors. It is also not clear whether in these patients therapy will be rewarded with improved outcome. It is possible that the DIC may only reflect the severity of the injury and thus appear to be associated with poor outcome without any benefit even if it is reversed. With all this in mind because DIC parallels outcome and it seems prudent to prevent further hemorrhagic complications in these critically ill patients we follow an aggressive approach. Some do not even agree to treat all abnormal coagulation parameteres,[34] but this remains a matter of debate. On the other hand, some recommend that the replacement therapy should be started on clinical grounds even before coagulation results are available.[3,13,35] May et al, in their patients have a greater mortality and hospital stay. Of their patients, 81 percent of those wih GCS of or below 6 were coagulopathies, compared to none with GCS above that. In such patients, the neurosurgical intervention was also delayed, which even included the placement of an ICP monitor. They recommend that empiric replacement therapy should be considered in patients with GCS of or below 6, as waiting for a full coagulation profile involves a delay of at least 1 to 1.5 hours. Our recommendations are to treat all abnormal coagulation tests and these abnormalities have also been shown to occur in patients with mild injuries and to affect outcomes even in these patients. We do not routinely infuse coagulation factors prior to obtain at least simple bedside estimates of hemostasis such as bleeding time and clotting time. If these indicate obvious abnormality and there is enough clinical evidence for coagulopathy or need for urgent correction, we do go ahead and replace clotting factors prior to obtain a full evaluation. We feel that these clotting factors are too valuable a resource to be wasted to patients who do not need them urgently and without firm justification.

The mainstay of the therapy is to replace the depleted coagulation factors, in adequate doses. Fresh frozen plasma (FFP) and platelet concentrates are the preparations of choice. If fresh frozen plasma is not available or fibrinogen level is extremely low, cryoprecipitate should be infused. It should be noted that fresh frozen plasma is a rich source of Factor V and cryoprecipitate of fibrinogen and Factor VIII. In their study, Goodnight et al replaced 12 bags of cryoprecipitate and two to four units of fresh frozen plasma while waiting for results of coagulation tests. The authors opinion was that the replacement was of benefit in the survival of at least two patients. Advice should certainly be sought from an experienced hematologist as to the replacement of these blood factors and should be titrated depending on the existing levels of these factors, with performance of repeat estimations. Platelets may not be required unless the count is below 75,000 per cubic mm. If the patient requires neurosurgical operation, the count should be kept at 100,000. As a general rule, the aim should be to administer the following doses:

- *Platelets*: One concentrate pack per 10 kg weight
- *Fibrinogen*: 50 mg/kg.

Most authors do not advise the administration of either procoagulant medications such as epsilon-aminocaproic acid (EACA) as it may cause unchecked thrombosis to occur, given the overall coagulation activation following head injury. Moreover, it may precipitate renal failure by preventing lysis of fibrin in glomerular capillaries.[36] The use of heparin is also to be avoided. In other situations, heparin is routinely' used in the management of DIC. In case of active bleed and in any patient with head injury heparin should probably not be used except as a last resort. No controlled studies are available in this regard. It is generally agreed that in head-injured patients some degree of disruption of the vascular tree can be assumed, and further intracranial hemorrhage has to be avoided.

Prognostic and Outcome Considerations

It has been shown in many studies that the presence of coagulopathy in head-injured patients is of definite prognostic value; coagulopathy has been shown to be linked to the extent of brain injury as well as the consciousness status of these adult and pediatric patients.[3,5,7,8,11,14-17,26,27,37,38] The problem therefore, is whether the presence of a coagulopathy is an independent prognostic factor or not. If not, then it may just appear to associate with prognosis and outcome as it is closely related to the severity of the injury. To address this issue, a few studies have used the statistical tool of multivariate analysis. In one such study,[37] the authors concluded that even a single abnormality in the PT or APTT within the first day of admission was significantly related to the mortality. Mortality was 80 percent in patients with coagulopathy and 7.4 percent in those without. The corresponding p value was less than 0.001 and odds ratio was 50. In the other study,[15] DIC was seen in 24 percent of patients overall and the highest incidence was in the acute subdural hematoma group. The mortality rate for patients with DIC was 58 percent. This study reveals two additional important points. Firstly, APTT value was the single most important predictor of survival in their study, even more than the GCS. This highlights the prognostic significance of DIC, if it is present in a head-injured patient. Other studies report that presence of coagulopathy was the second important predictive factor of survival, after GCS.[38,39] Secondly, in the patients in the DIC group, the fibrinogen level was the most important predictive factor for their survival. Another study has utilized logistic regression analysis to prove the independent predictive value of coagulopathy in survival of head-injured patients.[17] The authors noted that 38 percent of their patients had coagulation derangements, and for any particular value of GCS, the APTT, FDP and DIC scores had independent predictive value. In patients with GCS,[13-15] the FDP scores were significant predictors. In the GCS[6-12] subgroup, APTT and DIC scores were important predictors. Similarly, Van der Sande and coworkers[7] reported on 150 patients with head injury among whom 60 had deranged coagulation. They felt that FDP levels correlated most accurately with the extent of brain damage and outcome. In some cases, the FDP levels were better indicators of prognosis than the GCS. They cite example of two cases that were initially conscious but later deteriorated; both had deranged coagulation parameters. This finding bears striking similarity to that in the report quoted prior to this[17] and to the report by Olson et al.[29] The adverse prognostic impact of coagulopathy has also been studied in pediatric head injury,[38,40,41] pediatric abusive head trauma[42] and as a predictor of fetal mortality in trauma to pregnant patients.[43]

From the above discussion, it is clear that coagulopathy is an independent predictor of poor outcome in head injury patients. Coagulopathy following TBI is an important independent risk factor related to prognosis; hence a routine determination of coagulation status may be performed in all patients with TBI.[47]

The mortality, morbidity, hospital stay and poor outcome as assessed by the GOS are all much more in head-injured patients with coagulopathy. Another point to stress is the validity of this prognostic indicator even in alert and seemingly well patients. The mortality rate of patients once DIC is present is remarkably high, as mentioned and lies in the range of 40 to 60 percent.

Procoagulant microparticles are mainly platelet and endothelial in origin in CSF, their presence in CSF and plasma testify the activation of platelet and endothelial cells after severe TBI. A sustained generation of procoagulants in CSF could contribute to poor outcome.[45]

CONCLUSION

From the preceding review, it appears that coagulopathy after head injury is a common phenomenon than is routinely recognized. The mechanisms may vary, but the abundance of tissue thromboplastin in the brain is certainly of importance. This triggers the coagulation cascade and later fibrinolysis ensues. The coagulopathy itself is usually self-limiting and only few patients are symptomatic for this. Despite this, reliable evaluation of basic coagulation parameters should be performed as early as possible. The therapy should be urgently initiated and further decisions taken considering the presence of active bleeding or the need for a neurosurgical procedure. Even otherwise, any abnormal coagulation parameter should be treated, but there does not seem to be any clear role at present for prophylactic administration of clotting factors prior to establishing coagulopathy. There does not seem to be any indication for administration of other procoagulant or anticoagulant agents at present, such as EACA or heparin. Evaluation and therapy should be urgent because the presence of coagulopathy appears to have significant independent predictive value for the prognosis and survival of such patients and correcting it may have a beneficial effect on survival. The latter is more an expression of hope rather than a proven fact, and it is hoped that future studies would give us firmer indications and guidelines for management. At present, the mortality of DIC associated with head injury remains alarmingly high.

REFERENCES

1. Preston FE, Malia RG, Sworn MJ, Timperley WR, Blackburn EK. Disseminated intravascular coagulation as a consequence of cerebral damage. J Neurol Neurosurg Psychiatry 1974;37:241-8.
2. Vardi Y, Streifler M, Schujman E, Lowenthal M. Diffuse intravascular clotting associated with a primary brain tumor. J Neurol Neurosurg Psychiatry 1974;37:987-90.
3. Goodnight SH, Kenoyer G, Rapaport SI, Patch MJ, Lee JA, Kurze T. Defibrination after brain-tissue destruction: A serious complication of head injury. N Engl J Med 1974;(19):1043-7.
4. Pondaag W. Disseminated intravascular coagulation related to outcome in head injury. Acta Neurochir Suppl (Wien) 1979;28(1):98-102.
5. Khmer ME, Kaufman HH, Graham SH, Haar FH, Gildenberg PL. Disseminated intravascular coagulation fibrinolytic syndrome following head injury in children: Frequency and prognostic implications. J Pediatr 1982; 100:687-91.
6. Scherer RU, Spangenberg P. Procoagulant activity in patients with isolated severe head trauma. Crit Care Med 1998;26:149-56.
7. Van der Sande JJ, Veltkamp JJ, Boekhout Mussert RJ, Bouwhuis-Hoogerwerf ML. Head injury and coagulation disorders. J Neurosurg 1978;49:357-65.
8. Auer L. Disturbances of the coagulatory system in patients with severe cerebral trauma. I Acta Neurochir (Wien) 1978;43:51-9.
9. Bang NU, McDowell F. Cerebral infarction and blood clotting. Trans Am Neurol Assoc 1966;91:84-6.
10. Innes D, Sevitt S. Coagulation and fibrinolysis in injured patients. J Clin Path 1964;17:1-13.
11. Obrzut A, Jarzyna A, Skrzydiewski S. Thromboelastographical evaluation of the coagulative system of blood and fibrinolysis in craniocerebral injuries. Minerva Neurochir 1967;11:42-6.
12. Vecht CJ, Minderhoud JM, Sibinga CT. Platelet aggregability in relation to impaired consciousness after head injury. J Clin Pathol 1975;28:814-20.
13. Kaufman HH, Timberlake G, Voelker J, Pait TG. Medical complications of head injury. Med Clin North Am 1993; 77:43-60.
14. Kaufman HH, Moake JL, Olson JD, Miner ME, duCret RP, Pruessner JL, Gildenberg PL. Delayed and recurrent intracranial hematomas related to disseminated intravascular clotting and fibrinolysis in head injury. Neurosurgery 1980;7:445-9.
15. Kumura E, Sato M, Fukuda A, Takemoto Y, Tanaka S, Kohama A. Coagulation disorders following acute head injury. Acta Neurochir (Wien) 1987;85:23-8.
16. Mattson J, Hoots K, Contant C, et al. Influence of coagulopathy on prognosis in head-injured patients: A study of 2032 consecutive cases (abstract). Blood 1983; 62(suppl):276a.
17. Selladurai BM, Vickneswaran M, Duraisamy S, Atan M. Coagulopathy in acute head injury—a study of its role as a prognostic indicator. Br J Neurosurg 1997;11:398-404.
18. Anzil AP. Letter: Defibrination after head trauma. N Engl J Med 1974;291:632-3.
19. Kaufman HH, Hui KS, Mattson JC, Borit A, Childs TL, Hoots WK, Bernstein DP, Makela ME, Wagner KA, Kahan BD, et al. Clinicopathological correlations of disseminated intravascular coagulation in patients with head injury. Neurosurgery 1984;15:34-42.
20. Cooper HA, Bowie EJW, Owen CA. Chronic induced intravascular coagulation in dogs. Am J Physiol 1973; 225:1355-8.
21. Clark JA, Finelli RE, Netsky MG. Disseminated intravascular coagulation following cranial trauma. Case report. J Neurosurg 1980;52:266-9.
22. Tinnemans JG, Gerritsen SM. A fibrinogenemia and blunt head injury. Intensive Care Med 1980;6:211-3.
23. Simmons RL, Collins JA, Heistercamp CA III, et al. Coagulation disorders in combat casualties. I. Acute changes after wounding. II. Effects of massive transfusion. III. Post-resuscitative changes. Ann Surg 1969;169:455-82.
24. Vecht CJ, Sibinga CT, Minderhoud JM. Disseminated intravascular coagulation and head injury. J Neurol Neurosurg Psychiatry 1975;38:567-71.

25. Gando S, Tedo I, Kubota M. Post-trauma coagulation and fibrinolysis. Crit Care Med 1992;20:594-600.
26. Takahashi H, Urano T, Takada Y, Nagai N, Takada A. Fibrinolytic parameters as an admission prognostic marker of head injury in patients who talk and deteriorate. Neurosurgery 1997;86:768-72.
27. Takahashi H, Urano T, Nagai N, Takada Y, Takada A. Neutrophil elastase may play a key role in developing symptomatic disseminated intravascular coagulation and multiple organ failure in patients with head injury. J Trauma 2000;49(1):86-91.
28. Kaufman HH, Mattson JC. Coagulopathy in head injury. In Becker DP, Povlishock JT (Eds): Central Nervous System Trauma Status Report. Richmond, William Byrd Press 1985;187-206.
29. Olson JD, Kaufman HH, Moake I, O'Gorman TW, Hoots K, Wagner K, Brown CK, Gildenberg PL. The incidence and significance of hemostatic abnormalities in patients with head injuries. Neurosurgery 1989;24:825-32.
30. Kaufman HH. Delayed post-traumatic intracerebral hematoma. In Kaufman HH (Ed): Intracerebral hematomas. Etiology, Pathophysiology, Clinical presentation and Treatment. New York, Raven Press 1992;173-80.
31. Mellion BT, Narayan RK. Delayed traumatic intracerebral hematomas and coagulopathies. In Barrow DL (Ed): Complications and sequelae of head injury. Park Ridge, IL, American Association of Neurological Surgeons Publications Committee 1992;51-9.
32. Stein SC, Young GS, Talucci RC, Greenbaum BH, Ross SE. Delayed brain injury after head trauma: Significance of coagulopathy. Neurosurgery 1992;30:160-5.
33. Touho H, Hirakawa K, Hino A, Karasawa J, Ohno Y. Relationship between abnormalities of coagulation and fibrinolysis and postoperative intracranial hemorrhage in head injury. Neurosurgery 1986;19:523-31.
34. Winter JP, Plummer D, Bottini A, Rockswold GR, Ray D. Early fresh frozen plasma prophylaxis of abnormal coagulation parameters in the severely head-injured patient is not effective. Ann Emerg Med 1989;18:553-5.
35. May AK, Young JS, Butler K, Bassam D, Brady W. Coagulopathy in severe closed head injury: is empiric therapy warranted? Am Surg 1997;63:233-6; discussion 236-7.
36. McKay DC, Muller-Berghaus G. Therapeutic implications of disseminated intravascular coagulation. Am J Cardiol 1967;20:392-410.
37. Shaffrey ME, Polin RS, Phillips CD, et al. Classification of craniocerebral gunshot wounds: A multivariate analysis predictive of mortality. J Neurotrauma 1992;9(Suppl 1): S279-85.
38. Vavilala MS, Dunbar PJ, Rivara FP, Lam AM. Coagulopathy predicts poor outcome following head injury in children less than 16 years of age. J Neurosurg Anaesthesiol 2001;13:13-8.
39. Polin RS, Shaffrey ME, Phillips CD, Germanson T, Jane JA. Multivariate analysis and prediction of outcome following penetrating head injury. Neurosurg Clin N Am 1995;6:689-99.
40. Keller MS, Fendya DG, Weber TR. Glasgow coma scale predicts coagulopathy in pediatric trauma patients. Semin Pediatr Surg 2001;10:12-6.
41. Chiaretti A, Pezzotti P, Mestrovic J, Piastra M, Polidori G, Storti S, Velardi F, Di Rocco C. The influence of hemocoagulative disorders on the outcome of children with head injury. Pediatr Neurosurg 2001;34:131-7.
42. Hymel KP, Abshire TC, Luckey DW, Jenny C. Coagulopathy in pediatric abusive head trauma. Pediatrics 1997; 99:371-5.
43. Ali I, Yeo A, Gana TJ, McLellan BA. Predictors of fetal mortality in pregnant trauma patients. J Trauma 1997; 42:782-5.
44. Nekludov M, Bellender BM, Blombak M, Wallen HN. Platelet dysfunction in patients with severe TBI. J. Neurotrauma 2007;24(11)1:699-70.
45. Morel N, Morel O, Petit L, Hugil B, et al. Generation of procoagulant microparticles in CSF and blood after TBI. Trauma 2008;64(3):698-704.
46. Zaaroor M, Soustiel JF, Brenner B, et al. Administration of recombinant factor VIIa to the patients with blunt or penetrating brain injury without coagulopathy 2008; 150(7):663-8.
47. Harhangi BS, Kompanji EJ, Leebeek FW, Maas AI. Coagulation disorders after traumatic brain injury (TBI). Act a Neurochir (Wien) 2008;150(2):165-75.

17 Coagulopathy in Head Injury in Reference to Pediatric Patients

Raj Kumar, AK Mahapatra

INTRODUCTION

Trauma is the most frequent cause of death in children. While statistics in our country remain unknown, there are 6000 to 7000 deaths in the USA yearly among children below the age of 14. The leading cause of these is head injury. As in the USA, road traffic accidents contribute to a majority of these deaths.[1]

Broadly pediatric head injuries are divided into three categories, i.e. birth trauma, trauma below the age of 2 years and trauma in older children. As in adults coagulopathy is an important side-effect of head injury. But in children in addition undetected coagulation disorders may cause a relatively trivial trauma to have a grim prognosis a condition not seen as frequently in adults.[1]

OVERVIEW OF THE COAGULATION MECHANISM

Over the past decade it has become increasingly apparent that severe brain injury results in pathological changes in multiple organ systems. A number of reports noted that brain injuries can result in abnormalities of blood coagulation. These in turn can cause cerebral hemorrhage or infarction resulting in a self-perpetuating ever worsening vicious cycle resulting in a predictably poor outcome. Coagulopathy is one of the important causes of producing the so, called 'secondary insult' to the brain.[13] As neurosurgeons we must be aware of this complication, its early detection and strategies for successful treatment. To this end, the mechanisms of normal coagulation are briefly reviewed.

After a trauma that disrupts intimal continuity of a vessel, platelets aggregate at the site of hemorrhage and mechanically occlude the outflow of blood. This is followed by platelet activation a process that results in degranulation, release of vasoactive amines causing further vasoconstriction and recruitment of further platelets in the site. Then the clotting cascade comes into play. Two pathways are well-described extrinsic and intrinsic.[10]

Extrinsic pathway is initiated by tissue thromboplastin. It requires the action of Ca^{2+} ions and plasma factor VII. The brain has exceedingly high concentration of tissue thromboplastin. Intrinsic pathway on the other hand requires factor VIII, factor IX, Ca^{2+} ions and platelet phospholipid. Both pathways eventually generate activated factor X. This converts prothrombin to thrombin which in turn converts fibrinogen to fibrin monomers. These self-polymerize and yield a durable plug that finally seals the vessel.[4]

Intravascular coagulation is a process that occurs constantly in all organs. Similarly, fibrinolysis is a constantly occurring process. Plasminogen activator substance converts plasminogen to plasmin. This dissolves the fibrin clots by degrading the monomers into smaller molecules that are themselves antihemostatic by preventing further polymerization of monomers.[10]

PATHOPHYSIOLOGY OF COAGULOPATHY IN HEAD INJURY

Post-traumatic coagulopathy begins with the release of thromboplastin or plasmin or both from damaged brain cells. Widespread endothelial damage, pre-existing coagulopathy can exacerbate this process. This can result in discrete anomalies of, coagulation to systemic derangement's of the hemostatic process. This hypothesis is supported by high levels of specific markers like fibrinopeptide B 15/42, thrombin/antithrombin complexes and prothrombin fragments F 1+2.[2] The activation of monocytes and macrophages following injury can also contribute to thrombin generation through the release of cytokines like tumor necrosis factor.[6] The widespread, full blown picture of DIC may not be present in all cases of head injury. In fact a concept of local DIC has been propounded in milder degrees of head injury where fibrin degradation product (FDP) level anomalies may be the only detectable laboratory finding. Sometimes, altered coagulation profile in the jugular venous system is the only detectable abnormality, even when clotting studies on the peripheral blood disclose no anomalies.[13] The consequences of systemic DIC include vessel occlusion which causes ischemia to necrosis of the tissue supplied by the vessel or bleeding when there is lysis of clot and revascularization of infarcted tissue.

It has been realized that traumatic brain injury alone does not cause early coagulopathy, but must be coupled with hypoperfusion to lead to coagulation derangement, associated with activation of protein C pathway. It has an implication in treatment of coagulopathy associated TBI.[15]

Clinical Consequences of Altered Coagulation and Outcome

Kaufman et al noted that the CNS is the most common site of diffuse vascular thrombosis with coagulopathy. He also drew attention to the scattered petechial hemorrhages commonly found scattered in the brain and spinal cord of patients with altered coagulopathic profiles.[13]

The clinical consequences of coagulopathy are manifold. The dreaded full blown DIC results on one hand in runaway clot formation in small vessels (arteries and arterioles) leading to multisystem ischemia and on the other hand in a bleeding diathesis. In the CNS it can lead to delayed brain injury, infarction and venous thrombosis resulting in poor long-term recovery or even death. In the periphery poor renal perfusion can lead to renal shutdown, tubular necrosis and acute renal failure, hypoperfusion of the gastrointestinal tract can lead to bleeding, sloughing of the mucosa with increased risk of septicemia. ARDS, epiphyseal infarcts, retinal artery thrombosis, hepatic failure may also supervene. Bleeding diathesis is a result of uncontrolled fibrinolysis. It may manifest as delayed and recurrent intracerebral hematomas, delayed hematomas, difficulty in achieving hemostasis during surgery, hematomas related to ventriculostomies, etc. For these reasons DIC is also called consumptive coagulopathies.[5,9]

Use of serial CT imaging in patients with head injury yields a surprising number of new and progressive abnormalities with 37 to 60 percent of the follow-up studies showing worsening from the preadmission status and approximately 1/3rd of the scans showing fresh abnormalities. This delayed brain injury may take several forms: brain swelling, delayed intracerebral hematomas, ischemic and hemorrhagic lesions, enlargement of previously small hemorrhages and contusions.

In a seminal paper on the incidence and significance of hemostatic abnormalities in patients with head injury Olson and coworkers[13] grouped patients with trauma into four coma groups (depending upon their GCS) and calculated their DIC scores at admission. This score is an important concept in studying coagulopathy. Prothrombin time (PT), activated partial thromboplastin time (APTT), fibrinogen assay (FIB), fibrin degradation product (FDP), platelet count (PC), thrombin clotting time (TCT) are calculated. Points of 0-3 are given depending on severity. A patient may thus, have a minimum of 0 and a maximum of 18. The outcome of these patients was studied. They found severe or moderate thrombocytopenia was unusual and platelet count by itself was an unreliable predictor of outcome. APTT, fibrinogen level and thrombin clotting time had intermediate level of predictability. FDP was strong predictive of outcome and there was a good relationship between DIC score and outcome. APTT shortening was more strongly associated with death than prolongation.

With such a battery of tests being available, a stepwise logistic regression analysis was carried out to find the best possible combination of variables. The GCS at admission was found to have the highest predictive value singly but when clubbed with FDP (admission) and DIC score this combination was found to be the best possible one. The conclusion reached was that the hemostatic evaluation of all patients with head injury at time of admission is of value in determining the prognosis of the patient. Though GCS remains the most potent clinical indicator of outcome in acute head injury, patients within a specific GCS subgroup may have divergent outcomes. The predictive powers of hemostatic parameters were sharper when considered in specific GCS subsets.[11]

Stein et al[12] reviewed a series of 253 patients with head injury, 123 of whom required serial CT scans. In 45 percent of these they found evidence of delayed brain injury. In 55 percent of patients who had evidence of delayed brain injury as seen on serial scans, PT/APTT/platelet counts at admission were deranged as compared to only 9 percent in patients in whom follow-up scans were unchanged or improved. Again if coagulation studies at admission were normal, only 31 percent had a risk of developing delayed insult. The risk rose to 85 percent, if even a single parameter was altered. The mechanism of microvascular occlusion with secondary lysis and hemorrhage into damaged cerebral tissue has been hypothesized in the causation of delayed intracerebral hematomas, while diffuse brain edema is thought to result from the combination of initial damage to the endothelial walls and blood-brain barrier by the clot formation and subsequently reperfusion through the porous vessels.[7]

While Crone et al[3] reported coagulopathy in only 3 to 13 percent of patients with head injury their criteria was different. However, both they and Vander Sande et al[11] considered degree of coagulopathy to be an independent predictor of outcome. In fact, the latter authors after comparing CT scans, neurological status and clinical profile at admission hold that coagulation parameters are more sensitive than CT in picking up brain contusions. They hold that abnormal hemostatic parameters are more sensitive indicators of cerebral contusion than CT, especially in early stages of acute head injury. They also demonstrated that some patients who had laboratory evidence of DIC, had a poorer outcome despite not having developed delayed intracranial hematomas. Selladurai's study also highlights that there are patients who have a poorer outcome despite the absence of adverse predictors in CT and a significant majority of these had moderate to severe abnormalities in DIC scores.[11] Coagulopathy following TBI is an important independent risk factor related to prognosis; hence a protein determination of coagulation status may be performed in all patients with TBI.[16]

The scenario in children for long was assumed to be similar to that in adults. In a mark paper Concezio Di Rocco et al[2] studied prospectively the influence of hemocoagulative disorders on the outcome of head injury in 60 children. 45 percent of the patients had severe head injury, 21.7 percent had moderate head injury and 33.3 percent had mild head injury. 10 percent had DIC at the time of hospital admission all with a GCS of 4 and all of these patients died. PT was abnormal in 33.3 percent of children at the time of admission and 40 percent of these died, 10 percent had severe neurologic deficits at follow-up [GOS 1-3] and 50 percent were normal or near normal. Also a statistically significant association was shown between APTT, FDP, fibrinogen levels and platelet counts with neurological outcomes in traumatized children. The extent of this significance increases with variation of the parameters. They showed there is a direct correlation between the severity of head injury and the development of DIC. 22.2 percent of children with severe head injury and 100 percent of those who died developed DIC. However, surgical treatment of subdural hematoma with an, aggressive factor replacement in moderate hemophiliac infant may have good outcome.[14]

Chronic subdural hematomas in neonates may be rare (case report) but these may be secondary to an inherent coagulopathy.[17]

Tests of the Coagulation Pathway and their Significance in the Clinical Setting

Platelet count is important because platelet aggregation is the first step in the process of hemostasis. A count of less than 80,000/cumm is called thrombocytopenia. Prothrombin time screens abnormalities in the extrinsic pathway whereas activated partial thromboplastin time does the same for the intrinsic pathway. The latter two do not change till one or more factors fall to less than 20 to 30 percent of control values. Fibrinogen quantification gives an idea about the integrity of the final common pathway. A level less than 130 g/ml is considered by some authorities to be required to stamp a case as disseminated intravascular coagulation (DIC).[10]

The level of fibrin split products reflects the magnitude of fibrinolytic activity. This assay is highly sensitive but not very specific for DIC. Some workers require the presence of fibrin split products greater than 40 g/ml as a prerequisite for diagnosis of DIC.

Estimations of soluble fibrin, alpha 2-plasmin inhibitor, antithrombin 3 have been also considered to be sensitive indicators of early DIC.[4]

One question that is often raised particularly in centers with a heavy case burden is—"how much justification is there for using a wide variety of screening tests-to-test the integrity of clotting and fibrinolytic systems?"

Autopsy studies have shown the presence of microthrombi in various organs like lungs, kidneys and liver in patients with only brain injury.[8] Thus, anomalies of the hemostatic pathway may have profound effect on the outcome of patients with brain injury due to their propensity to cause multiple organ failure syndrome (MOFS). Studies show that derangement's in the extrinsic pathway is more common than in the intrinsic pathway. Though an abnormally low platelet count is rare, it is found in up to 5 percent of severely head injured patients (GCS < 7 postresuscitation). Patients with greater brain destruction (gunshot wounds and depressed skull fractures) have a greater incidence of coagulation abnormalities than those with closed head injury. However, the absence of demonstrable brain tissue loss does not rule out coagulopathy as it may occur from injury to other organ system; notably the liver in a poly trauma patient.

TREATMENT

A multidisciplinary team effort encompassing the neurosurgeon, intensivists, pediatricians, trauma specialists

Flow chart 17.1: Management of DIC

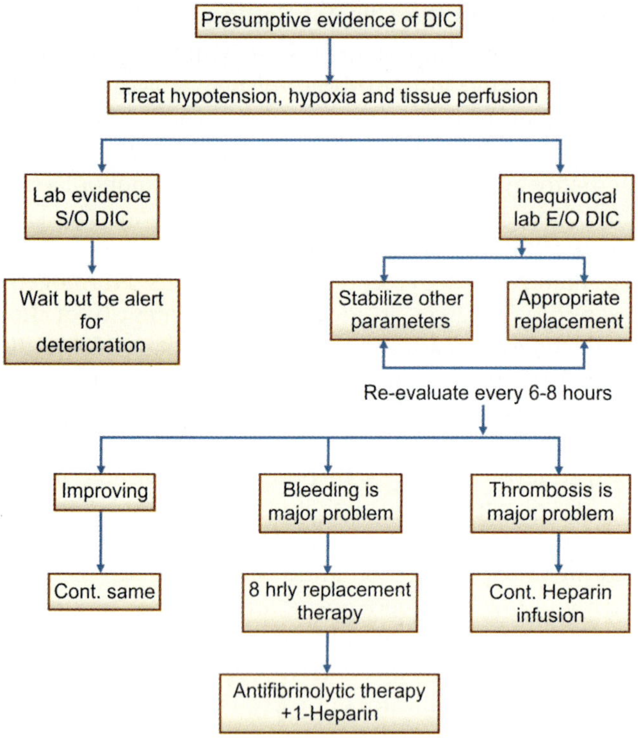

S/O = Suggestive of; E/O = Evidence of; Cont. = Continue

and hematologists is needed to salvage these patients (Flow chart 17.1). At admission, coagulation screening tests should be done for all patients with penetrating as well as diffuse brain injury. The broad principles of treatment are:[10]

1. Elimination of the precipitating factor if possible.
2. Replacement of coagulation factors and platelets.
3. Inhibitions of clotting process with heparin or other agents.

Fresh frozen plasma is used as the primary resuscitatory fluid once evidence of coagulopathy is present or if fibrinogen levels are less than 130 g/ dl. Platelets are transfused alongwith if counts are less than 1,00,000/ cumm. Whole blood transfusion preferably within 12 hours of collection is also beneficial though it may be inadequate to replenish some clotting factors. A non-emergent operation is to be delayed till coagulation studies normalize. But abnormal levels of fibrin split products are not regarded as a contraindication to surgery and patients can be taken up for emergency procedures under FFP cover. Heparin or enzyme inhibitors like aprotinin or Epsilon-aminocaproic acid (EACA) may be used with a careful watch being kept on bleeding parameters. The average requirement of heparin is 1000 IU/hr, but dose needs to be reduced in renal failure, hepatitis, circulatory failure, etc. Gabexate mesilate and nafamostat mesilate are two synthetic serine protease inhibitors used in clinical trials in Japan. 58 percent of patients were said to have improvement in coagulation parameters.[10]

A rise in serum fibrinogen within 12 hr is taken as a guide to successful treatment. All patients are to be rescanned on the 3-5th post-admission day. If recurrent or delayed intracerebral hematoma is found repeat coagulation profile is carried out. The general indications and principles of surgical intervention hold true bearing in mind that emergent lesions should not be delayed in an attempt to correct coagulation values.

ACKNOWLEDGMENT

The authors are greatful to Dr Prasad Krishnan, Senior Resident. Department of Neurosurgery, Sanjay Gandhi Postgraduate Institute of Medical Sciences, Lucknow, for his contribution in preparation of this chapter.

REFERENCES

1. Bruce DA. Pediatric head injury: Neurosurgery: Wilkins and Rengachary: McGraw-Hill; 2nd edn; 1996;266:2709-16.
2. Chiaretti A, Pezzotti P, Mestrovic J, et al. The influence of hemocoagulative disorders on the outcome of children with head injury. Pediatric Neurosurgery 2001;34:131-7.
3. Crone KR, Lee KS, Kelly DL Jr. Correlation of admission fibrin degradation products with outcome and respiratory failure in patients with severe head injury. Neurosurgery 1987;21:532-6.
4. de Gruchy. Clinical Hematology In Medical Practice: Firkin F, Chestern C, Remington D, Rust B (Eds). 5th edn. Chapter 15; Coagulation Disorders; 1994;406-54.
5. Enderson BL, Chen JP, et al. Fibrinolysis in multisystem trauma patients. The Journal of Trauma 1991;31(9): 1240-6.
6. Kearney TJ, Bennt L, et al. Coagulopathy and catecholamines in severe head injury. The Journal of Trauma 1992;32(5):608-12.
7. Miner ME. Delayed and recurrent intracranial hematomas and post-traumatic coagulopathies: Textbook of Neurosurgery: Wilkins and Rengachary: McGraw-Hill; 2nd edn 1996;277:2809-12.
8. Piek J, Chesnut RM, et al. Extracranial complications of severe head injury. Journal of Neurosurgery 1992; 77:901-7.
9. Rainhoff OD, Forbes CB. Disorders of hemostasis; 3rd edn; WB Saunders; Disseminated Intravascular Coagulation Rainhoff OD 1986;9:259-97.
10. Seligsohn U. Disseminated Intravascular Coagulation; Williams Hematology; 6th edn; McGraw Hill 1996; 126:1677-98.

11. Selladurai BM, Vickneswaran M, Duraisamy S, Atan M. Coagulopathy in acute head injury—a study of its role as a prognostic indicator. British Journal of Neurosurgery 1997;11(5):398-404.
12. Stein SC, Young GS, Talusci RC, Greenbaum BH, Ross SE. Delayed brain injury after head trauma-significance of coagulopathy. Neurosurgery 1992;30:160-5.
13. Olson JD, Kaufmann HH, Moake J, et al. Incidence and significance of hemostatic abnormalities in patients with head injury. Neurosurgery 1989;24:825-31.
14. Balak N, Silar G, Kilic Y, Timur C, et al. Successful surgical treatment of subdural hematoma with an aggressive factor replacement in moderate hemophilic infant with nontraumatic acute SDH, surg. Neurol 2007;68(5):537-40.
15. Cohen MJ, Brohi K, Ganter MT, Mantey GT, Mackersie RC, Pittet JF. Early coagulopathy after TBI, role of hypoperfusion and protein C pathway. J Trauma 2007; 63(6):1254-61.
16. Harhangi BS, Kompanji EJ, Leebeek FW, Maas AI. Coagulation disorders after traumatic brain injury (TBI). Act a Neurochir (Wien) 2008;150(2):165-75.
17. Powers CJ, Fuchs HE, George TM. Chronic subdural hematomas of neonates. Ped Neurol 2007;43(1):25-8.

18 Role of Surgery in Head Injury

AK Mahapatra, Raj Kumar

INTRODUCTION

Mortality and morbidity due to head injury is very high. It is also correct that the majority deaths are due to intracranial hematoma, leading to intracranial hypertension, hypoperfusion and ischemia. However, in significant number of cases, death is preventable,[1-6] if the diagnosis is made early and surgery is carried out timely. It is also right at this time to re-emphasize that head injury does not necessarily mean **hematoma nor intracranial hematoma means surgery and more importantly, surgery does not mean cure.** All these terminologies are not synonymous. Hence, there is a need for clear understanding, what is an intracranial hematoma? What are the indications for surgery? Having removed a hematoma, what is the expected outcome?

INDICATIONS FOR SURGERY IN HEAD INJURY

Basically, aims of the surgery in acute head injury are probably two: (a) first one is to remove a sizable intracranial hematoma producing mass effect, raised pressure and removal of hematoma is to reduce the intracranial pressure,[7-9] (b) the second aim is to operate open compound head injury to prevent CSF leak and meningitis.[6,10] Thus, the indications for definite surgery in acute head injuries are only two (Table 18.1). Surgery is also required for putting bolt or screw for the purpose of ICP monitoring or CSF drainage.[9]

A Surgery for Intracranial Hematomas

Large intracranial hematomas produce significant mass effect and raised ICP. The patients with severe intracranial hypertension are mostly comatose and do not show signs of clinical improvement.[10-13] Not infrequently, patients following initial coma improved and have a varying period of **lucid interval**.[3,14] During this period patients fully or partially improve in their conscious state and give a false impression that they are normal. These patients subsequently deteriorate in neurological status and may die if the hematoma is not evacuated timely and adequately. Thus, there are several situations: (a) Patients of head injury in coma from the time of injury and not showing signs of improvement, (b) Patients of head injury in coma from the time of injury but the level of coma is deteriorating, for example, motor scale 5 deteriorated to 3 or 4 (GCS from 6 or 7 deteriorated to scale 5, 4 or 3, (c) Patients with classical **lucid interval**, during which they are completely or partially lucid.[3,14,15] This means, patients following initial coma improved in conscious state, subsequently deteriorated again.

Table 18.1: Indications for surgery in head injury

A. In acute head injury

1. Large intracranial hematoma producing mass effect and raised ICP
   i. Patient is not improving
   ii. Patient is deteriorating
   iii. Patient having shown improvement then deteriorating.
2. Compound head injury
   i. Scalp laceration with compound comminuted fracture with CSF leak
      or CSF leak and oozing of brain tissue
   ii. Surgery for foreign body
      - Bullet, splinters
      - Knife, spear or sword
      - Penetrating woodpiece, etc.
      - Broken pencil or pen
   iii. Profuse CSF rhinorrhea or otorrhea not controlled on conservative management in 2-3 weeks time.
3. Surgery for putting bolt or screw
   For ICP monitoring indications are given elsewhere.

B. Surgery in chronic head injury

- Chronic SDH
- Subdural effusion
- Post-traumatic hydrocephalus
- CSF fistulae
- Cranial defect or growing skull fracture
- Hydrocephalus
- Osteomyelitis, brain abscess.

Table 18.2: Conservative management of intracranial hematoma

A. **Patients with good GCS (Mostly small children or elderly)**
   - Showing progressive improvement
   - Static with normal coma score

B. **Patients with hematoma with poor GCS**
   - ICP shows normal pressure

C. **Multiple small contusion or hematoma**
   - None of them individually producing mass effect

D. **Patients with hematoma in**
   - Brain death
   - Impending brain death

As an intracranial hematoma keeps on increasing in size, the conscious state goes on deteriorating. The deterioration is unpredictable, can be slow or rapid. These types of patients are the maximum priority group for surgery. Because, quick evacuation of hematoma is likely to result in good outcome. One must also remember that the surgery becomes futile if the evacuation of hematoma is significantly delayed,[14,15] during which patients may deteriorate to either GCS 3 or **brain death**. It indirectly **means severe deterioration might have resulted in irreversible brain damage (Table 18.2).**

On the other hand, some percentage of patients with intracranial hematomas are well, may be even conscious and oriented. This, happens more frequently in young children and elderly, in whom a large hematoma in brain can be accommodated without manifesting signs of raised ICP.[16,17] No doubt, these patients need close observation and may require ICP monitoring depending on the case. Close watch, repeat CT and clinical monitoring can avoid unnecessary surgery. **Recently, large number of papers have been published, reporting conservative treatment of intracranial hematomas.**[18-20]

Surgery in intracranial hematoma is aimed to reduce raised ICP. While, it is possible to totally remove an **extradural** hematoma and acute **subdural** hematoma, it may not be always possible to remove entire contusion or large intracerebral hematoma. Hence, the aim of surgery is to remove as much as possible, to achieve a significant lowering of ICP. At operation, **one can adjudge adequate removal by a lax and pulsating brain.** After the **evacuation** of hematoma in temporal lobe, one must incise the **tentorial edge** to relieve the **transtentorial herniation**.

Table 18.3: Indications for reoperation

A. **Operation for same hematoma**
   i. Recollection of hematoma
   ii. Inadequate evacuation and patient not showing improvement, CT showing significant clot
   iii. ICP remaining high postoperative

B. **Following removal of one hematoma**
   i. Patient may develop a new hematoma which is large
   ii. Smaller hematoma increased in size following evacuation of larger one

C. – Infected wound or bone flap
   – Postoperative abscess.

Indications for Reoperation or Second Surgery

Indications for **reoperation** are many (Table 18.3). Firstly, while removing contusion or intracerebral hematoma at the first operation, it is difficult to be sure about the amount of contusion/hematoma left. Surgeon stops when he feels adequate amount of pathological lesion is removed to provide significant reduction in raised ICP. However, **it is not unusual to see in repeat CT, the residual hematoma increased in size and producing significant mass effect**. In such a situation, if the ICP is high or patient not showing satisfactory improvement, a **reoperation** must be undertaken to remove the residual pathology to reduce raised ICP.

Secondly, reaccumulation of hematoma may be possible, which does not allow the patient to improve or ICP to normalize. There are two reasons for reaccumulation of **hematoma**. (a) **Inadequate or improper hemostasis during 1st surgery,** (b) **Bleeding abnormality resulting from severe head injury or due to excessive blood loss during first surgery.** Hence, in such a situation, before 2nd surgery, careful hematological evaluation is necessary, and if warranted **fresh blood, platelet or fresh frozen plasma** should be infused prior to second surgery and during surgery.

Thirdly, it is well known and repeatedly **reported** that a small hematoma elsewhere in the brain, may increase in size after removal of a large hematoma. It is also possible to have a fresh hematoma at a distant site to the first operation. The chance is more if the first operation is **performed** within 6 hours of injury, and CT scan is performed even earlier, when second hematoma was not formed.[21,22]

Surgery for Compound Head Injury

There are various types of compound head injuries:

1. *Open compound head injury:* It may be due to blunt injury or penetrating injury like bullet, splinter injury[23,24] or injury due to sharp weapons. Organic objects like sharp edge of a woodpiece or bamboo can enter the skull and damage brain. Rarely, injury can be due to pencil or pen, etc. The aim of surgery in such situations, is to convert an open injury to a close system by debriding the scalp, removing the bone fragments and damaged brain.[25] Sometimes, bone pieces are embedded in the damage brain tissue, which should also be removed. In bullet or splinter injury, the metallic foreign bodies should be removed. Adequate **debridement** and dura closure can prevent CSF leak and **meningitis**, to a great extent.[25] However, controversies exist when patients with compound injury come after 24 hours. Generally, it is believed that a wound is infected after 24 hours. When a patient comes after 24 hours he might already have wound infection or meningitis. Hence, antibiotics in antimeningitic dosage must be administered intravenously and observed.
2. *Closed compound injury:* These are the patients in whom there is no scalp laceration nor oozing brain tissue or CSF leak. The compound injury is because of CSF leak though paranasal sinuses or mastoid. The fracture of skull base also allow air entering into the cranial cavity, thus make it a closed compound head injury. When there is continuous CSF leak, there is chance of **meningitis.**[25] Frequently, CSF **rhinorrhea** or **otorrhea** stops in few days time, following injury. However, in small number of cases CSF leak may continue even after 2 weeks of conservative treatment. When CSF rhinorrhea or otorrhea persists, there is need for an operation to repair the dural defect in anterior cranial fossa floor, which is most frequent site for post-traumatic CSF rhinorrhea. In 90 to 95 percent cases CSF leak stops following surgery.
3. *Role of decompressive craniotomy/craniectomy:* Severe refractory intracranial hypertension in absence of focal intracranial pathology still remains a challenging situation. Craniectomy conducted in the past for severe brain swelling was proven to be useless. But in a series of 40 patients with intractable intracranial hypertension and at a very high-risk of brain death, decompressive craniectomy allowed 25 percent of patients to attain social rehabilitation at 1 year. The complications of meningitis and cerebral abscess need to be taken care of.[28]

However, with better understanding of CPP and availability of very good imaging facilities there is insurgence of interest in decompressive craniotomy.[26-28] It is generally believed that such type of surgery may save life but increase the number of vegetative or severely disable. Decompressive craniectomy led to sustained reduction in median ICP values [12.2 mm Hg (18.7: 24.2 mm Hg) preoperatively compared with 15.7 mm Hg (12.3: 19.2 mm Hg) postoperatively: P=0.01] in moderate to severely head injured patients with progressive brain edema. A similar improvement occurred in pressure volume compensatory reserve (RAP) index. A significant lower mean arterial pressure (MAP) was needed after decompressive craniotomy to maintain optimal cerebral perfusion pressure (CPP) level compared with preoperative period. The cerebral compliance is improved.[27] In patients, who otherwise will have poor functional outcome. Further studies are necessary in this subject.

CONCLUSION

Surgery in head injury is required in small percentage of patients. The aim of the surgery is to remove intracranial hematoma to reduce raised ICP or to operate open compound injury to prevent CSF leak and meningitis. Rarely, reoperation is also indicated if the residual hematoma is significant or a sizeable hematoma is encountered elsewhere. Prompt and adequate evacuation of hematoma are key points in surgery and overall outcome.

REFERENCES

1. Rose L, Valtonen S, Jennett B. Avoidable factors contributing to death after head injury. Br Med L 1977;2:615-18.
2. Kohi YM, Mendelow AD, Teasdale GM, et al. Extracranial insults and outcome in patients with acute head injury-relationship to GCS. Injury 1984;16:25-6.
3. Mahapatra AK. Lucid interval in fatal head injury. Ind J Surg, 1991.
4. Campbell S, Watkin G, Kreis D. Preventable death in a self-designated trauma system. Am Surg 1989;55:478-80.
5. Wilson D, Mcelligott, Fielding L. Identification of preventable trauma death. Confounded inquiries? J Trauma 1992;32:45-51.
6. Mahapatra AK. Management of head injury. Neurosciences Today 1997;1:197-204.
7. Miller JD, Becker DP, Ward JD, et al. Significance of intracranial hypertension in severe head injury. J Neurosurg, 1977;47:503-76.
8. Marshall LF, Gautille T, Klauber MR, et al. Outcome of severe closed head injury. J Neurosurg 1991;75:528-36.
9. Ghajar JB, Hariri RJ, Patterson RH. Improved outcome from traumatic coma using only venticular CSF drainage for ICP control (Class III) Adv Neurosurg 1993;21:173-7.

10. Mahapatra AK. Current management of head injury. Asian Arch Anae Rescu 1996;25:1-10.
11. Mahapatra AK, Tandon PN, Bhatia R, Banerji AK. Bilateral decerebration in head injury. Surg Neurol 1985;23:436-9.
12. Gentleman D, Nath F, MaCpherson P. Diagnosis and management of delayed traumatic intracerebral haematoma. Brit J Neurosurg 1989;3:367-72.
13. Jennett B, Teasdale G, Galbraith S, et al. Severe head injury in three countries. J Neurol Neurosurg Psychiat 1977;40:291-5.
14. Marshall LF, Toole B, Bower S. The National Traumatic Coma Data Bank. Part II. Patient who talk and deteriorate. Implication for treatment. J Neurosurg 1983;59:285.
15. Reilly PL, Adams JH, Graham Dr, Jennett B. Patients with head injury who talk and die. Lancet 1975;2:375-7.
16. Choux M, Grisoli F, Peragut JC. Extradural haematomas in children. Child's Brain 1075;1:337.
17. Choux M, Lena G, Geniton L. Intracranial haematoma. In Raimondi AJ (Ed): Head injury ill Newborn and Infants. Springer-Verlag, New York 1986, p. 203.
18. Bullock R, Smith RM, vanDellen JR. Nonoperative management of extradural haematoma. Neurosurgery, 1985;16:602-6.
19. Pozzati E, Togmetti F. Spontaneous healing of acute extradural haematomas: A study of twenty-two cases. Neurosurgery 1986;18:696-700.
20. Knuckey NW, Gelbard S, Epstein MH. The management of "asymptomatic epidural haematomas". A prospective study. J Neurosurg 1989;70:392-6.
21. Werner A. Diagnostic technique. In: NIMS. Basic and Clinical Approaches—Head injury Clinical Management and Research. E Frost (Ed) Vol AIREN, Geneva, Switzerland 1990;2(6):151-9.
22. Yague LG, et al. Contralateral extradural haematoma following craniotomy for traumatic intracranial lesion. Case report. J Neurosurg Sci 1991;35:107-9.
23. Carey ME, Young HF, Mathis JD. The neurosurgical treatment of craniocerebral missile wound in Vietnam. Surg Gynaecol Obstet 1972;13:386.
24. Carey ME, Sarna GG, Farrell JB, et al. Experimental missile wound to brain. J Neurosurg 1989;71:754.
25. Carey ME. Therapeutic Management. In: NINS Head Injury Clinical Management and Research. E Forst (Ed) AIREN, Geneva, Switzerland 1990;2:171-6.
26. Guerra WK, GM MR, Dietz H, et al. Surgical decompression for traumatic brain swelling, indications and results. J Neurosurg 1999;90:187-96.
27. Timofeev I, Czosnyka M, Nortje J, et al. Effect of decompressive craniectomy on intracranial pressure and CSF compensation following TBI. J Neurosurg 2008;108(1): 66-73.
28. Albanese J, Leone M, Alliez JR, et al. Decompressive craniectomy for sever TBI, evaluation of effect at 1 year. Crit Care Med 2003;31(10):2535-8.

19 The Role of Stereotactic Surgery in Head Injury

RR Sharma, Sanjay Pawar, RV Devadas, SD Lal

INTRODUCTION

Even in the current era of minimally invasive neurosurgery, majority of post-traumatic intracranial lesions are routinely managed with conventional neurosurgical procedures. Despite many limitations in conventional neurosurgical approaches, they remain preferred methods of managing acute post-traumatic intracranial mass lesions in many neurosurgical institutions around the globe.

Their familiarity and immediate availability overshadow their limitations. During such undertakings neurosurgeons are not infrequently faced with the task of attempting to reconstruct sequential two-dimensional CT or MR images into a three-dimensional 'mental image' of intracranial surgical targets. Not so in large post-traumatic lesions in the superficial intracranial sites; but determining the exact cranial site of entry, and cerebral trajectory to reach the deeper subcortical or basal ganglionic or brainstem lesions may be frustrating. In such situations, the neurosurgeons consider exploration when planning osteoplastic craniotomy flaps and can find themselves searching for the post-traumatic lesion during the brain surgery. More brain destruction/manipulation, though preventable by stereotactic neurosurgical procedures is largely inevitable in such circumstances. It is, therefore, increasingly realized that the intraparenchymal cerebral manipulations be minimized and be guided.[1,2]

GENERAL CONSIDERATIONS

In this modern era of microstereotactic neurosurgery, the precision of stereotactic localization removes the uncertainty commonly associated with conventional neurosurgical approaches in selected cases of acute and chronic post-traumatic intracranial lesions.[1-4]

Such stereotactic procedures provide an elegant solution by marking the chosen trajectory from the scalp to the desired intracranial target such as deep basal ganglionic hematoma. Therefore, the neuroimaging directed stereotactic neurosurgery is currently being increasingly employed in a selected subset of, post-traumatic intracranial lesions.[4,5]

Among neurosurgical centers, those who can obviously afford image guided stereotactic (frame-based or frameless) neurosurgery, the management of a selected subset of post-traumatic intracranial lesions should preferably be done with the aid of stereotaxy.[5-8] Free hand approaches and exploratory craniotomies are highly undesirable in the modern era of stereotactic precision.[1] **Stereotactic burr hole procedures** offer a safe, rapid, easily reproducible accurate **craniocortical** entry, transit and targeting whether it is a deep seated hematoma or a pinched cerebral ventricle. Whereas image guided precise **stereotactic minicraniotomy** is appropriate for conditions such as deep basal ganglionic hematoma and minimizes operative craniocerebral 'entry and transit' trauma in an already traumatized brain parenchyma. Those patients whose advanced age, associated medical illnesses or severe neurological disability pose unacceptable risks of conventional neurosurgical interventions under general anesthesia, will certainly be benefitted with a minimal interference by using image guided stereotactic burr hole procedures under local anesthesia. If a craniotomy is required then the **image guided stereotactic trephine craniotomy procedures** permits a small scalp incision, precise placement of a small bone flap, minimal dural opening and a controlled cerebral trauma. The neurosurgeon will have advantage of choosing the cranial site of entry, the operating cerebral trajectory and knowing the surgical target. In order to preserve functions, minimal surgical manipulations may then be performed using microsurgical techniques. Image guided stereotactic procedures achieve low morbidity and mortality, rapid convalescence and a short hospital stay when compared with the conventional neurosurgical procedures.[1-8] There are many stereotactic devices, all of which provide precise localization. The one used by an individual neurosurgeon is largely a matter of his training and experience.

The Spectrum of Post-traumatic Lesions: Conventional Neurosurgery vs Stereotaxy

Neurosurgical aspects in the management of significant head injury consist of dealing with a widespectrum of injuries of the scalp, skull and intracranial contents. According to the current practice, image guided stereotactic neurosurgery is superflush in the former two (scalp and skull) and useful in some subsets of the last group (intracranial contents).

A general outline of the current neurosurgical practice in a variety of post-traumatic intracranial lesions is as follows:

Acute Post-traumatic Intracranial Injuries

These are subdivided into two major groups: focal injuries and diffuse injuries.

Focal Injuries

a. Intracranial hemorrhage with and without significant cerebral contusion includes:
   i. Meningeal hemorrhage (EDH/SDH, SAH): EDH/SDH are best treated by the emergency conventional **neurosurgical** approaches and SAH by conservative surgical and medical therapy.
   ii. Cerebral hemorrhage [ICH/IVH]:
      - Superficial cortical and subcortical lesions are managed with emergency conventional neurosurgical techniques.
      - Deep subcortical, basal ganglionic, thalamic and brainstem hematomas are best approached by stereotactic procedures.
      - IVH is best treated with external ventricular drainage.
b. **Cerebral contusions/lacerations** are best managed by conventional **neurosurgical** approaches.
c. **Impairment injuries** are best treated by conventional neurosurgical approaches and only a select subset may need stereotactic surgery.
d. **Bullet injuries** are best treated by conventional neurosurgical approaches and only a select subset will need stereotactic surgery.

Diffuse Injuries

Concussion: Intensive neurosurgical observation (masterly inactivity and cat like observations).

Diffuse axonal injury: Intensive **neurosurgical** observations and **neurointensive** care.

Diffuse hypoxic encephalopathy: Intensive **neurosurgical** observations and **neurointensive** care.

Diffuse brain swelling: NICU care-stereotactic placement of intraventricular catheter for ICP monitoring and CSF diversion/drainage, care to protect brain.

Subacute and Chronic Post-traumatic Intracranial Injuries

Septate subdural hematoma: **Conventional** neurosurgery vs stereotactic surgery.
Intracerebral hematoma: Stereotactic burr hole aspiration.
Sinodural fistula with CSF leak: Stereotaxy guided endoscopic packing.

Sequalae of Head Injury

Post-traumatic movement disorders: Stereotactic thalamic/subthalamic lesions or stimulations.
Post-traumatic cerebellar syndrome: Stereotactic lesion/stimulations.
Post-traumatic intracerebral abscess: Stereotactic burr hole/minitrephine aspiration or removal of an abscess.
Post-traumatic spasticity: Antispasmodic drug therapy (dantrolene, baclofen, clonazepam, diazepam), Botox injection, intraspinal baclofen pump and spinal cord stimulation.

Definitive Indications of Stereotactic Neurosurgical Procedures in Significant Post-traumatic Intracranial Lesions/Disorders

Remarkable achievements have occurred in modern image guided stereotaxy during the past decade. Most importantly, the scientific concepts of this common modality are assimilated across the neurosurgical disciplines. The new facts and ideas developed in this arena of neurosurgery are having great impact on the concepts, important to other neurosurgical fields. The area of head injury also remained no exception to this important technique.

Currently, the image guided stereotactic procedures are indicated in the following post-traumatic intracranial lesions:

1. Stereotactic removal aspiration of **intracranial** hematomas:
   a. Acute post-traumatic space-occupying intracerebral contusion hematomas
      Basal ganglionic hematomas, thalamic hematomas and brainstem hematoma.
   b. Chronic septate subdural hematomas or chronic intracerebral hematoma.
2. Stereotactic ventriculostomy in severe generalized brain edema with small cerebral ventricle for ICP monitoring and CSF diversion/drainage.
3. Stereotactic removal of intracranial foreign body.
4. Stereotactic guided deep brain stimulation (DBS) or lesions for post-traumatic involuntary movements:
   a. Stereotactic thalamic lesions for post-traumatic resting tremors/Parkinson's syndrome.

   b. Stereotactic thalamic lesions for **post-traumatic** acute myoclonic syndrome.
   c. Stereotactic thalamotomy for **hemidystonia** due to focal post-traumatic basal ganglionic lesion.
   d. Stereotactic ventral intermediate **thalamotomy** for **post-traumatic** hemiballismus.
   e. Stereotaxic lesions for **post-traumatic** cerebellar syndrome.
5. Stereotactic guided surgical closure of post-traumatic craniosinus fistula in the sella turcica.
6. Stereotactic neurosurgery in post-traumatic intracerebral hematomas.

Traumatic intracerebral hemorrhage is a common neurosurgical emergency and an important cause of disability and death in head injured patient.[9-11] It may begin as a primary event at the time of impact but its effects manifest later on and therefore it is usually considered as a **secondary** complication of head injury. **Hematomas** manifesting in 24 hours following head injury are considered delayed. Traumatic **bleeding** may occur singly or in combination with **cerebral** contusion, laceration and hemorrhage in other areas (EDH/SDH/SAH/IVH).

Traumatic primary ICHs in their pure forms occur within the brain parenchyma and are not in contact with the surface of the brain. They occur in about 25 percent of severe head injury patients and are frequently multiple (20%). In about one-third to two-thirds of cases they are associated with EDH and in one-third to one-fourth of patients with SDH. They make up at least 30 to 40 percent of all intracranial hematomas being more common (80%) in the frontal and temporal regions and in the deep cerebral locations. Small deep ICH (usually less than 1 cm) are associated with diffuse axonal injuries. These can secondarily progress to large hematomas. Similarly secondary intracranial hematomas may result from damage to cerebral cortical vessels in the focus of cerebral contusions or lacerations in about 25 to 50 percent of cases. Multiple contusion hematomas occur in one-third of such patients and solitary ones in two-thirds. In the burst cerebral lobe (frontal and temporal polar regions) there is a coexisting cerebral contusion-laceration, intracerebral hematoma and subdural hematoma.

Deep ICHs arise due to rupture of intrinsic vessels deep in the brain at the time of injury and often penetrate ventricular systems. Post-traumatic basal ganglionic hematomas, thalamic hematomas and brainstem hematomas in head injury were thought to be uncommon entities in the past and their mechanisms have not been revealed clearly.

Traumatic deep basal ganglionic ICHs are probably secondary to the rupture of lenticulostriate or anterior choroidal branches. Thalamic hematomas due to posterior choroidal vessels and brainstem hematomas due to posterior perforating vessel, which are damaged by shearing forces in high velocity acceleration/deceleration injuries. The anterior and posterior perforating arteries are end arteries. Especially, the intermediate and lateral lenticulostriate arteries pursue a S-shaped course from their origin from the middle cerebral artery and enter the anterior perforated substance at an acute angle. The vessels are susceptible to damage where there is a transition from a fixed to a mobile segment; the perforators being more susceptible because of their redundant/S-shaped course and entry into the anterior perforated substance at an acute angle, during the *acceleration-deceleration* movements.[11]

Traumatic basal ganglia hematomas commonly occur as a part of the spectrum of lesions that may be seen in diffuse axonal injury (DAI) which is almost always related to the mechanisms of injury in which the rotational acceleration produces shear and tensile strains of high magnitude.[4,5] Most studies indicate that traumatic basal ganglia hematoma is a primary event and its identification in an early CT scan of the head suggests that the patient has sustained a severe diffuse brain damage at the time of impact. It would appear that the acceleration-deceleration forces are such that both the axons and the blood vessels in the brain are damaged simultaneously at the time of injury. Basal ganglia hematomas occurring in isolation are rare and occur especially in impacts along the long axis of the skull producing shear injury between the perforating vessels and the basal ganglias.

The prognosis differs markedly between the two entities.[12] Whereas the traumatic basal ganglia hematomas associated with DAI carries a very poor prognosis with mortality reaching 40 to 50 percent, the isolated hematomas in the basal ganglia usually carries a good prognosis, suggesting that the mortality is associated with the injuries produced in other parts of the brain.[12,13]

The CT scan is the method of choice to diagnose various characteristics of an acute ICH. It differentiates ICH from cerebral contusions, cerebral edema, cerebral infarction and diffuse axonal injuries.

The management of ICH depends on the clinical characteristics:[4,5,12-15]

- The patients with isolated ICH even though large but not causing raised ICP, brain shift, unconsciousness or progressive focal neurological deficits are managed on the expectant conservative lines with a close ICU monitoring and periodic CT brain scans. Multiple small ICHs involving hypothalamo-pituitary axis, basifrontal lobes and basal ganglia irrespective of the level of consciousness are best treated expectantly in majority of the cases.

- Patients with GCS of 10/15 and above, ICH of less than 4 cm and the absence of clinical as well as computed tomographic signs of brainstem compression are managed with nonoperative treatment.
- The lobar hematomas greater than 5 cm in diameter should be removed surgically if they are responsible for altered consciousness, focal neurological deficits and a shift of the midline structures.
- If removal of ICH is expected to make a significant reduction in the intractable raised ICP then it should be removed.

Various operative procedures are commonly used:[13-17]

Osteoplastic trephination and **encephalotomy** is the principle surgical method. Burr hole and needle aspiration may be resorted to if more than three-fourths of the volume of the hematoma can be aspirated. The stereotactic method is recommended for the removal of traumatic ICH situated in the region of basal ganglia, thalamus or brainstem with minimum risk and high accuracy. The potential usefulness of this surgery is positively suggested in the management of deep cerebral hematomas. Patients may show dramatic recovery with remarkable improvement in neurological deficits. Even in patients with disturbed level of consciousness in the absence of focal neurological deficits, the large basal ganglia hematomas are treated accordingly by CT guided stereotactic aspiration. Stereotactic removal of ICH is particularly useful in hematomas affecting several cerebral lobes simultaneously or in case of symmetrical hematomas.[14]

The stereotactically aimed treatment of ICH is an advance for the patient's benefit. The evacuation cannula is safely inserted to its target from a transcutaneous drill hole of the skull and thus the patient is spared the surgical trauma associated with a large craniotomy and further brain damage. If necessary, the focus of hemorrhage can be reached again by puncture via the channel in the bone, which navigates the cannula. The surgery under local anesthesia is rapid and the results are promising.[13] In a series of 37 traumatic ICH evacuated by a simplified stereotactic surgical procedure, the mortality was 80 percent in patients with Glasgow coma scale (GCS) scores of 3 to 5 and 25 percent in patients with scores of 6 to 7. There were no deaths in patients with GCS of 8 or more. The results were better than those achieved by wide craniotomy. The importance of reduced operative trauma in patients with ICHs which are often associated with multifocal or diffuse brain injuries[16] cannot be overemphasized. However, the stereotactic procedures are still rarely used. In Schneider et al series of 318 patients with severe head injury, 161 patients had cerebral contusion, and in about 90 percent of cases it was coexisting with other lesions (EDH 24 cases, SDH 29 cases, depressed skull fractures in 6 and traumatic SAH in 37 cases).[12] In their series, 10 patients underwent operative removal of their contusions-hematomas by trephination and only 2 others by stereotactic burr hole puncture aspiration.[12]

Chronic Septated SDH/ICH[18-20]

Chronic SDH are well delineated collections of fluid (blood) between duramater and the arachnoid membrane. Two forms of encapsulated chronic SDH can be distinguished: the non-septated and the septated form. The non-septated form can be treated easily using the burr hole drainage method, whereas treatment of septated chronic subdural hematoma remains a therapeutic problem. The main concern is about the division of the hematoma by neomembranes into compartments, which hinder the efflux of the hematoma fluid through one or two burr holes. In such situation a relatively large loculi can be well localized using the stereotaxy and then operated on using flexible steerable endoscopes through a burr hole approach. The flexible endoscopes may be fixed and guided as needed. For resection of neomembranes, small microscissors or microforceps may be used. This technique avoids blunt rupture of the membranes, which may cause bleeding. A closed drainage system is applied temporarily to guarantee the efflux of the remaining hematoma. Majorities of such patients have satisfactory evacuation of septated SDH.[19]

Stereotactic Ventriculostomy

In patients with severe head injury, the severe generalized brain swelling or edema and small cerebral ventricles are frequent CT findings. The raised intracranial pressure in these patients is invariably present. Therefore, ICP monitoring as well as CSF drainage form the diagnostic and therapeutic measures to treat these cases. In such pinched/small ventricles, stereotaxy is unquestionably beneficial to place the ventricular catheter in the lateral ventricles for ICP monitoring and CSF drainage.[1,2]

Stereotactic Removal of Foreign Body

Removal of a foreign body lodged in the deep brain tissue may need stereotactic approach without causing a significant brain injury. Using a stereotactic system any point in the intracranial compartment[21-27] and around the craniofacial skeleton[23-31] can be reached exactly with pre-calculated precision. Thus, a foreign body can be exposed and subsequently removed by a surgical approach that gives minimal discomfort and carries low risk. The target probe serves the surgeon as a guide bar whilst the tissue is dissected.[29] Kojima et al[23] reported an interesting case of a patient with air-gun bullets in the third ventricle associated with delayed ventricular hemorrhage. Through an anterior transcallosal approach they successfully removed the bullets without causing any significant permanent sequelae although they had to undertake a major craniotomy procedure. Hitchcock and Cowie reported the removal of air-gun pellet in the temporal lobe with the help of stereotaxy.[22]

Retained ventricular catheters are usually well tolerated but when infection is present then their removal becomes imperative because such catheters serve as a nidus for persistent infection. Minimally invasive methods for their removal are desirable. The removal of such catheters using stereotactic guided endoscopic surgery is a well proven minimally invasive technique.[21]

Stereotactic techniques certainly allow safe removal of a foreign body from a deep cerebral location with minimal traumal to the brain.[25]

Stereotactic Neurosurgery in Post-traumatic Movement Disorders

The sphere of stereotactic neurosurgery covers various post-traumatic intractable movement disorders, which are not controlled with maximal medicinal efforts.[32-34] The diagnosis is much more straightforward in these cases as compared to their idiopathic counterparts. The history of onset of movement disorder following head injury, progression during the convalescence period and the characteristics of the clinical features of the particular type of involuntary movement, provide reasonable clue for an accurate diagnosis of a specific post-traumatic movement disorder. Movement disorders commonly occur due to the injury to the extrapyramidal system, therefore the neurosurgical interventions are mainly directed at various portions of the extrapyramidal system.[32-35] However, indications of the stereotactic procedures with their implications (benefits, limitations and risks) must be carefully evaluated, expressed and discussed before these undertakings.

As widely recognized, extrapyramidal pathways concerning movement disorders are mainly two interlocking neuronal circuitry pathways involving the basal ganglia.[32-37] In the first pathway, the neurons of the corpus striatum (caudate and putamen) project to the globus pallidus, which gives two fiber bundles to the anterior nucleus of the thalamus. One fiber bundle (fasciculus) runs above the subthalamic nucleus of Luiz and other (ansa lenticularis) below the **subthalamic nucleus of Luiz**. Both bundles join above the subthalamic nucleus to form pallidothalamic bundle (thalamic fasciculus H1) in the **Forel's field- H** to reach to the ventral anterior thalamic nucleus. From here, the thalamic projections go to the supplementary motor cortex (which lies just anterior to the motor cortex) which in turn projects to the caudate nucleus to complete the pathways (caudate-putamen-globus pallidus-ventral anterior thalamus-supplementary motor cortex caudate). In the second pathway, the dentate nucleus of the cerebellum projects to the red nucleus then to ventrolateral thalamus from where the fiber projection goes to primary and secondary motor cortex. From these cortical areas **corticopontine** projection goes to pontine nuclei and then to cerebellar cortex which in turn projects to the dentate nuclei (**dentatorubro-thalamico-cortico-corticopontine-cerebellardentate pathways**).

Currently, in intractable movement disorders, stereotactic neurosurgical procedures are utilized to interup neuronal pathways in the **Forel's field** (compotory campus foreli),[35-37] ventrolateral nucleus of thalamus (thalamotomy)[35-37] or in the dentate nucleus for cerebellar syndrome (dentatotomy).[38]

Following intractable disabling post-traumatic movement disorders are treated with stereotactic procedures:

i. Hemiballism:[36,37] In an awake patient, constant irregular, hurling, frequently violent exhaustive **movements of the shoulder and proximal arm occur. Hemiballism is due to a partial lesion in the subthalamic nucleus** with a tendency to resolve spontaneously (1 to 3 months) in some patients. It may be effectively controlled with stereotactic surgery in up to two-thirds of cases by making a lesion in the ventrolateral thalamic nucleus thalamotomy or in the Forel's field (campotomy).

ii. Myoclonus:[39] It is characterized by **sudden unpredictable synchronous** severely **disabling** contractions of *the functionally synergestic muscles*. It causes a sudden jerk of a segment of the limb, head or part of the trunk. The movements involve mainly the proximal muscles and are usually bilateral and may be precipitated by any form of external stimuli but generally disappear during the sleep. Most of the time, *the dentate or olivary nuclei show abnormality*. *Serotoninergic* system may be involved. The stereotactic target is the *ventrolateral* *nucleus of the thalamus* (**thalamotomy**) or *Forel's field* (**campotomy**) *contralateral to the more severe movement disorder* with reasonably good results in majority of the cases.

iii. Post-traumatic resting tremors:[32-37] Resting tremors are commonly present in Parkinson's syndrome. Parkinson's syndrome is well known since 1817 and is characterized by tremor, rigidity, bradykinesia and disturbances of postural adjustment: pill-rolling tremor of the hand present at rest and usually stop at intention. Simultaneous contraction of the opposing muscles without hyperreflexia causes rigidity. However, bradykinesia is the most disabling and contributes to the characteristic gait. The characteristic posture is due to the changes in the postural reflexes. Mask like face with loss of autonomic facial statement occurs.

Parkinson's disease is usually an idiopathic disorder but Parkinson's syndrome may occur due to ischemic cerebral atherosclerotic disorder, postencephalitic syndrome or as a post-traumatic sequelae. At autopsy, commonly there is a loss of pigmented cells in the zona compacta of the substantia nigra and of the locus ceruleus. There is a deficiency of dopamine in basal ganglia, particularly in the substantia nigra. L-dopa (the precursor of dopamine) is administered orally which after absorption in the circulation crosses the blood-brain barrier to enter the brain where it is converted into dopamine to correct the deficiency. Carbidopa is given to avoid systemic and gastrointestinal side effects of the L-dopa. The disadvantages of the long-term medical treatment are well known, but many patients respond best to the medical therapy. However, for intractable cases, stereotactic surgery has been employed with some success. It relieves the tremor at best (after stereotactic campotomy or thalamotomy), rigidity next and bradykinesia least.

A combination of medical and surgical therapy may be optimal in many patients. Stereotactic pallidotomy is considered for severe bradykinesia.

Stereotactic surgery basically involves interruption of the extrapyramidal pathways in Forel's field (campotomy), in the ventrolateral or ventrointermediate nucleus of the thalamus (thalamotomy for tremors) or in the globus pallidus (pallidotomy for rigidity and bradykinesia). About 80 to 90 percent of the patients report relief in their tremors and 50 to 60 percent in rigidity and some in bradykinesia. Morbidity occurs in about 5 percent cases (changes in mentation, speech and equilibrium) and mortality in less than 1 percent cases.

iv. Post-traumatic intention tremors:[40-43] Among the variety of post-traumatic movement disorders especially following severe head injury, a moderate to severe intention tremor is often the major source of disability for the patients.[42]

Intention tremors occur in the distal part of the extremity as it approaches its target or when it performs fine distal movements. It is frequently due to cerebellar lesion. In Parkinson' s syndrome, tremors occur at rest and are suppressed by action, whereas action/postural tremors is an exaggeration of the physiological tremors (benign essential tremors) and occur when the muscles of a limb are contracted as and when the arms are outstretched (exaggerated by anxiety, thyrotoxicosis, alcohol withdrawal).

Intention tremors usually occur in Wilson's disease, multiple sclerosis, ischemic atherosclerotic cerebrovascular disorder, encephalitis or trauma. Beta-adrenergic receptors may be involved. Propanolol (if not contraindicated for the patient) helps. Stereotactic thalamotomy (ventrolateral nucleus or ventrointermediate nucleus) or campotomy usually results in relief in about 80 percent cases in non-progressive disorders.

Tremors following cerebellar trauma or stroke respond very well. However, the tremors should be severe enough to cause disability and show no response to medication.

The target for cerebellar tremor/essential tremor is same as for the Parkinson's tremor. Best results are obtained with a lesion in the ventrointermediate nucleus of the thalamus just in front of the sensory area for the hand as identified by intraoperative stimulation. Marks[42] reported the results of stereotactic ablation of the ventralis intermedius thalamic nucleus in seven patients with post-traumatic cerebellar syndrome, and found a good relief of their tremor in six patients and no appropriate benefit in one. For post-traumatic cerebellar syndrome, the conservative treatment is usually ineffective but in appropriately selected cases, stereotactic thalamotomy has a high degree of clinical success.

Thalamic targets in the treatment of involuntary movements usually include the lateral and the intermediate ventral nuclei. Destruction of their afferents in Forel's fields (campotomy) provides the same therapeutic results but the size of the lesion must then be very small due to the proximity of essential structures particularly corpus Luysii. Efficacy of treatment depends partly on the etiology of the involuntary movement; however, tremors of all types are usually improved or suppressed.

The CT stereotactic dentatotomy is well described by Weigel and Mundinger.[38] According to these authors, with modern CT imaging, ventriculography or pneumoencephalography is no longer needed to determine the target point.

In addition due to the direct representation of the anatomic structures in the CT, abnormal positions of the dentate nucleus may be taken into consideration in the determination of the target point and approach for the coagulation probe with reasonable good results.

v. Chorea:[32-37] Choreiform movement of an extremity progressively involves the other limbs. Despite medication if chorea is disabling, then stereotactic thalamotomy may offer some relief.

vi. Dystonia:[44-46] In dystonia, there is a sustained increase in the muscle tone without hyperreflexia. There is a limitation of voluntary activity. Asymmetrically increased tone in the opposing muscles gives a distorted posture. In **dystonia musculorum deformans,** it involves mainly the trunk and extremities, whereas spasmodic torticollis involves the neck muscles, and in **tardive dystonia** only extremities are involved. In most dystonias, the etiology remains unknown and it is rarely due to trauma. Dystonia musculorum deformans and tardive dystonia, however, respond to the stereotactic thalamotomy whereas spasmodic **torticollis** to the spinal cord stimulation. If there is a poor response to spinal cord stimulation then anterior **rhizotomy** or selective neurectomy may be tried.

Stereotactic Guided Surgical Closure of Post-traumatic Craniosinus CSF Fistula in the Sella Turcica[47-50]

Cerebrospinal fluid (CSF) leak may arise as a complication of trauma, trans-sphenoidal surgery, endoscopic sinus surgery or hydrocephalus, or may occur spontaneously without any identifiable cause. CSF leakage following head injury is a significant complication with a risk of meningitis and pneumocephalus especially in patients with fractures of the sella turcica or ethmoid bone. CT stereotaxy guided trans-sphenoidal/ethmoidal packing or injection of fibrin sealant through a 12-gauge needle or fibroendoscopic packing is a simple alternative to the conventional neurosurgical management of **CSF fistula**. This procedure avoids a large bifrontal craniotomy, preserves olfaction and avoids the risk of frontal lobe damage. Location and size of the leak, cause, technique and choice of the packing material used for the repair do not significantly affect the surgical outcome However, the presence of hydrocephalus influences the outcome utmost. Many patients with increased intraventricular pressure required a ventricular shunt in addition to a second endoscopic repair. Certainly the endoscopic repair of CSF rhinorrhea is a promising alternative to conventional surgical repair techniques. Since sphenoid/ethmoid sinuses have multiple septa and therefore, may behave like a maze. Stereotaxy may be used to localize precisely and identify a particular sinus compartment if needed.

The endoscopic repair of CSF rhinorrhea is a safe and effective approach that can be improved with stereotactic localization techniques. Proper graft placement is critical and lumbar drainage is an important adjunct in some cases. Following proper localization of the leak, repair is safely performed in most of the cases by endonasal route with the help of free mucoperiosteal flaps taken from the inferior or middle turbinates. CSF leakage bears high-risk of meningeal or intracranial infection and therefore should be repaired as soon as it is recognized that the conservative treatment has failed. The sphenoid sinus CSF fistula may be closed successfully using fascia, muscle and **gelfoam** or **fibrin glue** and gelfoam.

Where the skull base defect is accessible to the stereotactic-assisted endoscopic surgery, it should be considered as the preferred method. Its high success rate, low rate of morbidity and good long-term results recommend endonasal duroplasty as a primary treatment modality for frontobasal dural lesions. For extended traumatic frontobasal dural lesions, the conventional intracranial dural repair is preferred, however, the endonasal approach should then be reserved for the closure of the additional sphenoid sinus leaks in such cases. The excellent visualization and a traumatic surgical techniques of endoscopic sinus surgery combined with stereotactic localization results in successful outcome in majority of these complicated cases.

Pneumocephalus is a rare complication of stereotactic biopsy/surgery.[61]

Cortical and subcortical brain shift occurs during stereotactic surgery is a direct function of the volume of pneumocephalus, which probably reflects the volume of CSF that is lost, but clinically significant shift is uncommon.[60]

Advances in diffusion tensor imaging (DTI) is useful tool for visualization of white matter tracts, especially the corticospinal tract, which regulates motor function. In patients with intracranial hematoma by stereotactic aspiration, a clinical outcome can be predicted by preoperative DTI study.[59]

Implications of Stereotactic Surgery

The benefits of stereotactic surgery are enormous and the risk of morbidity and mortality is certainly low as compared to the conventional neurosurgical procedures ranging between 1 to 5 percent. However, postoperative hemorrhage, infection and neuronal damage may still occur.[1,2,51-53]

The postoperative artifacts should also be well recognized following stereotactic surgery if confusion is to be avoided.[54] The extent of resection bed usually does not change during the first week after operation and reduction of the size of artifact then began and continued up to 3 to 6 months. Mass effect and edema show no change during the first-four days; then they regress gradually. Pneumocephalus is found in about half of the cases in the first-three weeks. Benign surgically induced cerebral enhancement usually appears at the margins of the encephalotomy (and on the surface of the brain at the retractor site if used) at the end of the first postoperative week. It becomes more prominent during the following weeks and lasts up to 3 to 5 months. In many cases, such cerebral enhancement may prevent recognition of a residual lesion. Dural enhancement at the site of surgery is also noted in early postoperative period and may last for up to one year period.

CONCLUSION

The value of image guided stereotactic systems is directly dependant on the ease and speed of their use. In the past, most stereotactic techniques were complicated and time consuming to set up. They were exclusively used either for biopsing neoplasms[55-58] or for functional neurosurgery.[31-37] However, current systems equipped with advanced registration techniques are much simpler and faster to employ and indications for their use are rapidly increasing and certainly embrace head injury.[1,5,12-16,31-37,47-49]

REFERENCES

1. Sharma RR, Davis CHG, Lynch PG, Keogh AJ. Minimally invasive neurosurgery using CRW-3 Stereotaxy. Ann Saudi Med 1994;14(6):507-10.
2. Sharma RR, Lad SD, Pawar SJ, Sousa J, Mishra GP, Netalkar AS, Athale SD. The scope of image guided Leksell Stereotactic neurosurgery in Oman. Oman Medical Journal 1999;15(3):14-26.
3. Pawar SJ, Lad SD, Sharma RR, et al. CT guided stereotactic neurosurgery experience in Oman (Abstract). Pan Arab J Neurosurg 1999;3(2):73-4.
4. Delmendo A. Stereotaxy in head injuries and strokes in Oman. In Sharma RR, Pawar SJ, Mishra GP (Eds). Illustrated Synopsis: Helical CT guided microstereotactic neurosurgery in Oman. National Printers, Muscat, Oman June 1999;28.
5. Devadas RV, Mahapatra AK, Sharma RR, Lad SD. Traumatic primary Basal Ganglia Hematomas. In Sharma RR, Pawar SJ, Lad SD (Eds). Illustrated Synopsis: Management of Head Injury in Oman. AL Zahra Printers, Muscat, Oman, April 2000;97-8.
6. Brown AP, Dacey RG. New management techniques in neurosurgery. Curr Opin Neurol Neurosurgery 1992; 5:799-807.
7. Bucholz RD, Greco D. Image guided surgical techniques for infections and trauma of the central nervous system. Neurosurg Clin N Am 1996;7(2):187-200.
8. Ko K, Ghajar J, Hariri RJ. A method for monitoring intracranial temperature via tunneled ventricular catheter: Technical note. Neurosurgery 1994;34:927-30.
9. Broseta J, Gonzalez-Darder J, Barcia-Saloria JL. Stereotactic evacuation of intracerebral haematomas. Appl Neurophysiol 1982;45:443-8.
10. Hondo H, Matsumoto K. CT guided stereotactic evacuation of hypertensive and traumatic intracerebral haematomas experiences with 35 cases. No Shinkei Geka (Jap) 1983;1:35-48.
11. Jaykumar PN, Kolluri VR, Basavakumar DG, Arya BY, Das BS. Prognosis in traumatic basal ganglia haematoma. Acta Neurochir (Wien) 1989;3-4:114-6.
12. Schneider R, Mauer UM, Waldbaur H, Oldenkott P. Surgical indications in space occupying contusion haemorrhage. Unfallchirurg (German) 1993;96:191-200.
13. Fadrus P, Maca K, Smrcka V, Nadvornic P. Minimally invasive treatment of traumatic cerebral haematoma. Further experience with stereotactic evacuation. Rozhl Chir (Czech) 1998;77(10):441-4.
14. Chrastina J, Smrcka V, Nadvornik P, Zborilova E. Stereotactic therapy of post-traumatic cerebral haemorrhage. Rozhl Chir (Czech) 1996;75(7):330-33.
15. Yamamoto F, Eguchi G, Yoshimura K, Shigemori M, Kuramoto S. Massive traumatic haematoma localized in the basal ganglia: Treatment by CT-guided stereotactic aspiration surgery. No Shinkei Geka (Japanese) 1990; 18(6):563-5.
16. Coraddu M, Floris F, Nurchi G, Meleddu V, Lobina G, Marcucci M. Evacuation of traumatic intracerebral haematomas using a simplified stereotactic procedure. Acta Neurochir (Wien) 1994;129:6-10.
17. Potapov AA, Lantukh AV, Likhterman LB, Loshakov VA, Kravchuk AD, Melikian VG. The differentiated treatment of traumatic intracranial hematomas. Zh Vopr Neirokhir Im NN Burdenko (Russian) 1992;1:5-10.
18. Helling D, Kuhn TJ, Bauer BL, List-Hellwig E. Endoscopic treatment of septated chronic subdural haematoma. Surg Neurol 1996;45(3):272-7.
19. Hellwig D, Bauer BL. Minimally invasive neurosurgery by means of ultrathin endoscopes. Acta Neurochir Suppl (Wien) 1992;54:63-8.
20. Karakhan VB. Endof ibroscopic intracranial stereotopography and endof iberscopic neurosurgery. Acta Neurochir Suppl (Wien) 1992;54:11-25.

21. Blacklock JB, Maxwell RE. Stereotactic removal of a migrating ventricular catheter. Neurosurgery 1985; 16(2):230-31.
22. Hitchcock E, Cowie R. Stereotactic removal of intracranial foreign bodies: Review and case report. Injury 1983; 14(5):471-5.
23. Kojima T, Waga S, Kubo Y, Sbimazu T. Successful removal of air gun bullets from the third ventricle. Neurosurgery 1987;20:322-5.
24. Kosary IZ, Shacked Y, Ouaknine G. Removal of intracerebral foreign bodies with the aid of a stereotoxic procedure. Harefuah (Hebrew) 1971,80(5):243-4.
25. Muhammad AK, Maruno M, Maeda N, Kato A, Yoshimine T. Syringe needle located deep in the brain: Image guided removal. Surg Neurol 2000;54(6):458-63.
26. Schorf F. Stereotactic removal of foreign bodies form the visceral cranium. Fotschr Kiefer Gesichtschir (German) 1976;21:280-81.
27. Yoshijima S, Murayama Y, Matsumoto K. A case of successful removal of a deep-seated bullet in the brain by stereotactic approach. No Shinkei Geka (Jap) 1979;7(10): 989-94.
28. Eschler J, Scharf F, Rucker A. Localization and planned removal of foreign bodies in the maxillofacial region by means of a new stereotactic device. Disch Zahn Mund Kieferheilkd Zentralbl Gesamte (German) 1966;46:425-34.
29. Halling F, Merten HA, Dieckmann G, Luhr HG. Stereotactic removal of foreign bodies in the maxillo-facial area. Dentomaxillofac Radiol 1991;20(2):100-4.
30. Horton CE, McFadden JT. Stereotactic localization of a facial foreign body. Case report. Plast Reconstr Surg 1971;47:598-9.
31. McFadden JT, Horton CE. Stereotaxic localization of extracranial foreign bodies in the head. Am Surg 1971;37:353-6.
32. Bullard DE, Nashold BS. Stereotaxic thalamotomy for treatment of post-traumatic movement disorders. J Neurosurg 1984;61:316-21.
33. Derome PJ, Jedynak CP, Visot A, Delalande O. Treatment of abnormal movements by thalamic lesions. Rev Neurol (Paris) 1986;142(4):391-7.
34. Nizuma H, Kwak R, Ohyama H, Ikeda S, Ohtsuki T, Suzuki J, Sago S. Stereotactic thalamotomy for post-apoleptic and post-traumatic involuntary movements. Appl Neurophysiol 1982;45:295-8.
35. Tasker RR, Dostrovsky JO, Dolan EJ. Computerized Tomography (CT) is just as accurate as ventriculography for functional stereotactic thalamotomy. Stereotact Funct Neurosurg 1991;57(4):157-66.
36. Levesque MF, Markham CH. Ventral intermediate thalamotomy for post-traumatic hemiballismus. Stereotact Funct Neurosurg 1992;58:26-9.
37. Levesque MF, Markham CH, Makasato N. MR-guided ventral intermediate thalamotomy for post-traumatic hemilballismus. Stereotact Funct Neurosurg 1992; 58:88-9.
38. Weigel K, Mundinger F. Computerized tomography-guided stereotactic dentatotomy. Appl Neurophysiol 1986;49(6):301-6.
39. Eiras J, Garcia Cosamalon J. Post-traumatic myoclonic syndrome. Effectiveness of the thalamic lesions on the action of myoclonus. Arch Neurobiol (Madr) 1980;43:17-28.
40. Andrew J, Fowler CJ, Harrison MJ. Tremor after head injury and its treatment by stereotactic surgery. J Neurol Neurosurg Psychiatry 1982;45(9):815-9.
41. Fox JL, Kurtzke JF. Trauma Induced intention tremor relieved by stereotactic thalamotomy. Arch Neurol 1966;15(3):247-51.
42. Marks PV. Stereotactic surgery for post-traumatic cerebellar syndrome: An analysis of seven cases. Stereotact Funct Neurosurg 1993;60(4):157-67.
43. Van Manen J. Stereotaxic operations in cases of hereditary and intention tremor. Acta Neurochir (Wien) 1974; Suppl 21:49-55.
44. Andrew J, Fowler C, Harrison MJ. Hemidystonia due to focal basal ganglia lesion after head injury and improved by stereotactic thalamotomy. J Neurol Neurosurg Psychiatry 1982;45:276.
45. Andrew J, Fowler CJ, Harrison MJ. Stereotactic thalamotomy in 55 cases of dystonia. Brain 1983;106(pt 4).
46. Krauss JK, Mohadjer M, Braus DF, Wakhloo AK, Nobbe F, Mundinger F. Dystonia following head trauma: A report of nine patients and review of the literature. Mov Disord 1992;7(3):263-72.
47. Fraioli B, Pastore FS, Floris R, Vagnozzi R, Simonetti G, Liccardo G, Giuffre R. Computed tomography-guided trans-sphenoidal closure of post-surgical cerebrospinal fluid fistula: A transmucosal needle technique. Surg Neurol 1997;48(4):409-13.
48. Petr R. Surgical closure of a craniosinus fistula of iatrogenic origin in the area of the sella turcica. Rozhl Chir (Czech) 1966;45(11):731-4.
49. Zervas NT. Stereotaxic thermal pituitary ablation. Acta Neurochir (Wien) 1974;Suppl21:165-8.
50. Kurzeja A, Wenzel M, Korves B, Mosges R. Decompression of the optic nerve after fractures of the rhinobasal skull with computer assisted surgery. Laryngorhino-otologie (German) 1994;73:274-6.
51. Lafia DJ. Acute subdural haematoma as a complication of stereotaxic thalamotomy. Cof in Neurol 1965;26(3): 441-4.
52. Nashold BS. Operative complications due to stereotactic surgery. Coruin Neurol 1968;30(5):325-36.
53. Zarsi S, Sierpinski S, Mempel E, Pilipowska T. Intracranial haemorrhage as complications of stereotactic operations. Neurol Neurochir Pol 1971;5:29-35.
54. Herman M, Pozzi-Mucelli RS, Skrap M. CT and MRl findings after stereotactic resection of brain lesions. Eur J Radiol (Czech) 1996;75(7):330-3.

55. Pawar SJ, Lad SD, Sharma RR, et al. CT guided stereotactic neurosurgery experience in Oman (Abstract). Annual Meeting of the Egyptian Society of Neurological Surgeons, Cairo, Egypt 1999;8-12.
56. Sharma RR, Davis CHG. The impact of CT Stereotaxy on tumour surgery for the 90's. Paper presented at the 12th Annual Meeting of the British Neuro-Oncology Group, Bristol, UK (Abstract) 1992;8:25-6.
57. Sharma RR, Davis CHG, Lynch PG. Management of intra-third ventricular craniopharyngioma using Cosman-Roberts-Wells (CRW-III) Stereotaxy. Surgical Neurology 1994;42(6):551-2.
58. Sharma RR, Parekh HC, Davis CHG. The impact of CT Stereotaxy on tumour surgery for the 1990's Abstract of the 12th Annual Meeting of the British Neuro-Oncology Group. Br J Neurosurg 1993;7:105-6.
59. Hsieh CT, Chen CY, Chang CH, Chang CF. Role of diffusion tensor imaging in patients with spontaneous intracerebral hematoma created by stereotactic evaluation. Surg Neurol 2008;70(1):75-8.
60. Elias WJ, Fu KM, Frysinger RC. Carticle and subcartial brain shift during stereotactic procedures. J Neurosurg 2007;107(5):983-8.
61. Roth J, Avneri I, Nimrod A, Kanner AA. Stereotactic biopsy complicated by pneumocephalus and acute pulmonary edema. Surg Neurol 2007;68(5):573-6.

20 Endocrinal Abnormalities Following Head Injury

AK Mahapatra, Raj Kumar

INTRODUCTION

Despite of numerous case reports of patients with post-traumatic endocrinal disturbances,[1-5] prospective studies or even large retrospective studies are not available, dealing with trauma induced pituitary dysfunction. Moreover, pituitary function studies are infrequently considered in acute stage or even in long-term management of patients with traumatic brain injury, even though it is almost a well known fact that severe head injury offers considerable risk to pituitary function. Earlier autopsy studies had demonstrated anterior pituitary necrosis in as high as one-third fatal head injured patients.[6-8] However, in spite of development of neuroimaging and well established laboratory for neuroendocrinal assessment, the incidence, clinical significance and degree of risk due to endocrinal deficits, in head-injured patients are not well known. This chapter highlights many aspects of endocrinal abnormalities in patients with head injury and emphasizes the detail endocrinal evaluation and subsequent management which may improve the overall long-term outcome in these patients.

PATHOGENESIS OF ENDOCRINAL ABNORMALITIES

The exact incidence of pituitary dysfunction following head injury is not known. The endocrinal problem could result either due to pituitary or from hypothalamic damage following the head injury. No doubt, pituitary is highly vulnerable due to its location in sella turcica, and delicate infundibular hypothalamic structures. Autopsy studies in sixties had shown pituitary gland necrosis in one-third of fatal head injuries.[6,7] However, Daniel et al in 2000; had reported hypopituitarism in 40 percent of patients with moderate and severe head injury.

It is generally believed that the pituitary dysfunction following head injury is by and large due to diffuse swelling, hypotension or hypoxic insult.[10] However, primary pituitary damage is well described.[6-8] Prior to CT scans most of the evidences were autopsy based. In autopsy studies pituitary abnormality is recorded in almost 75 percent.[8] The significant primary abnormalities include capsular hemorrhage in over 50 percent, followed by posterior lobe and stalk hemorrhage in 30 and 20 percent cases approximately. Next to the hemorrhages, necrosis is another important finding. The common site of **necrosis** is anterior lobe followed by pituitary stalk (Table 20.1). In an autopsy study, Kornblum and Fisher in 1969,[8] had reported anterior pituitary necrosis in 35 percent patients of fatal head injuries those who had survived longer than 12 hours. Necrosis patterns always corresponds to the blood supply of the long **hypophyseal portal veins**. Long

Table 20.1: Pathology in pituitary gland following head injury

	Type of pathology	*Site*	%
Primary	Hemorrhage	– Capsular	50–55%
		– Posterior lobe	30%
		– Stalk	15%
	Necrosis	– Anterior pituitary	20%
		– Stalk	3%
Secondary	Hypoxia		–
	Edema		–
Direct stalk injury	Rupture of stalk		–
	Transection of stalk		–
	Stalk hemorrhage		–

portal veins pass through diaphragma sellae, where they are vulnerable to mechanical compression from swollen brain and swollen pituitary gland.[2,6,8] Long hypophyseal portal veins supply 70 percent blood to anterior pituitary. The somatotrophs and gonadotrophs are laterally placed, hence more frequently involved.[3] This anatomical arrangements very well explains the long-term hormonal insufficiency.

Direct stalk injury in form of stalk transection and stalk hemorrhage also lead to immediate and long-term hypopituitarism.[1,11-13] This can result due to fracture of the sella turcica.[1] With the advent of CT and MRI it is possible to demonstrate rupture of the pituitary stalk.[12,13]

Hypothalamic injury also can lead to hypopituitarism following severe head injury. By and large these patients do not survive to have long-term hypothalamic problems. Hypothalamic lesions in closed head injury. Recently, with improved imaging such lesions are more frequently diagnosed radiologically.[9,10,12] Traumatic SAH with or without vasospasm also contribute to hypothalamic and pituitary dysfunction.

Hypopituitarism is a common complication in TBI and aneurysmal subarachnoid hemorrhage, which might contribute to morbidity and poor outcome.[39]

CLINICAL PROBLEM

Clinical problem in head injury varies from acute stage to chronic problems. In acute stage there is likely have cortisol and ADH deficiency which can manifest persistent hypotension in absence of any obvious cause, as patients cannot withstand stress in presence of acute pituitary failure. Diabetes insipidus (DI) is not uncommon in severe head injury (Fig. 20.1). Failure of

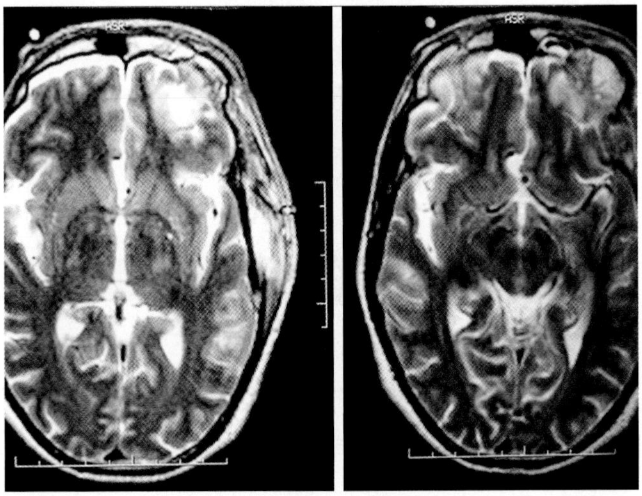

Fig. 20.1: MRI of a child showing bilateral basifrontal contusions, who developed diabetes insipidus after 5 days following trauma

posterior pituitary lead to fall of plasma ADH resulting in DI and easily diagnosed as patients pass large volume of urine which is of low specific gravity, serum osmolality is high and urinary osmolality is low.[13,14]

Syndrome of inappropriate ADH secretion in severe head injury is not rare and can be diagnosed on the biochemical parameters of serum and urine.

Pituitary dysfunctions are also reported in minor or moderate head injury. Ziaber et al[17] reported plasma cortisol and beta endorphin abnormality in minor head injury.

Diabetes insipidus is an important clinical problem in severe head injury.[13,14,18] In addition to DI, SIADH is not uncommon.[19] These clinical problems are also to be differentiated from patients with cerebral salt wasting (CSW). In these patients, serum sodium is low and 24 hours urinary sodium secretion is very high. For above reasons, only, a careful electrolyte balance should be monitored in severe head injury patients up to two weeks.[19] Electrolyte and plasma osmolality abnormalities are more frequent in patients with diabetes mellitus and chronic alcoholism. There remains high frequency of hypothalamic pituitary hormone deficiencies amongst the long-term survivors of TBI with approximately 25 percent having one or more pituitary hormonal deficiencies, marked changes are found in acute phase of TBI with 80 percent cases showing evidence of gonadotropin deficiency, 18 percent growth hormone deficiency and 16 percent corticotropin, 40 percent demonstrating vasopressin abnormalities resulting into diabetes insipidus or SIADH. Some of these are transient. Most of these cases remain undiagnosed.[15,40]

Clinically, significant **hypogonadism** is not uncommon in major head injury.[20-22] The hypogonadism could be transient[21] or long-term. Clark et al[20] in 1988 reported 33 male patients with major head injury in whom total free testosterone was significantly lower on third day. However, persistent hypogonadism was only reported in five of these 21 patients in whom the test were performed between 3 and 6 months after injury. They suggested repeated endocrinal assessment in patients with severe head injury. Woolf et al in 1986[21] reported transient hypogonadism following head injury. They included both severe and moderate head injury patients. They studied 31 male patients in whom testosterone and other hormonal assessments were performed shortly after injury and on the fourth day. They observed good correlation between severity of head injury and sex hormone abnormalities.

Table 20.2: Hormonal assessment			
	Test	*Method*	*Normal adult level*
GH	Insulin tolerance test (ITT)	RIA	–
ACTH	Insulin tolerance	RIA	9–50 ng/ml
TSH	TRH stimulation	Immunochemilluminescences assay	0.4–4.2 mu/l
Free thyroxin		RIA	5.5–11.51 J/dl
FSH (H)	GnRH stimulation test	Fluoroimmunometric assay	FHS 20–25 opg/dl
Serum testosterone	GnRH stimulation test	RIA	298-1043 ng/dl

Precocious puberty is another rare problem following severe head injury.[23] The precise mechanism is not still clear. Some authors have hypothesized extrahypothalamic involvement.

Neurobehavioral impact of hypopituitarism is significant. Chronic behavioral problems are recorded in significant number of patients with brain injury.[24-27] Both behavioral and cognitive defects are noticed even one year following injury.[2,26] Saatman et al,[27] in 1997 demonstrated cognitive abnormality in experimental brain injury. It is generally believed that the deficiency of growth hormone or insulin like growth factors[1] deficiency results in neurobehavioral and **cognitive** deficit.[27,28] Saatman et al[27] reported improvement in cognitive function by supplementing insulin like growth factor. Loss of memory, higher anxiety level, impaired motor skill and lower quality of life is also attributed to growth hormone deficiency.[9,31] Sex hormone deficiency also lead to mood disturbances and behavioral problems.

INVESTIGATIONS

Both anterior and posterior pituitary functions are tested (Table 20.2), when there is high degree suspicion of hypopituitarism.[16] (a) Insulin tolerance test is a simple test to find out corticotroph and somatotroph secretion by measuring GH and cortisole level. (b) A TRH stimulation test is important to assess the level of TSH and prolactin. (c) GnRH stimulation test is necessary to assess gonadotroph function. Blood is tested 30 minutes prior to record the baseline hormone level followed by stimulation. Blood samples are collected every 30 minutes for the next two hours. For stimulation insulin 0.14 units/kg is injected intravenously, while for thyrotrophs and gonadotroph 500 µg TRH and 100 µg GnRH are administered intravenously serum ACTH, TSH, thyroxine and cortisol are assessed. Serum level is assessed by using radioimmune assay (RIA).

Posterior pituitary function is not of less importance, realizing the problem of fluid electrolyte imbalance, problems of DI and SIADH. Hence, measurement of serum sodium, blood urea, nitrogen, creatinine and osmolality of plasma and urine are important (Table 20.3). In addition a regular check in urinary specific gravity and 24 hours urinary sodium excretion is also carried out to differentiate one from the other. Assessment of serum ADH level is also important.[9]

Overall growth hormone insufficiency is reported in 85 percent and **gonadotropin** in 95 percent. Approximately 30 percent patients developed DI during their illness. Isolated or combined somatotroph and gonadotroph dysfunction is most common as compared to corticotroph, thyrotroph and posterior pituitary dysfunctions.

Treatment of Hypopituitarism

No doubt endocrinal abnormality, be it in acute phase of head injury or chronic state require careful evaluation and replacement therapy. In acute stage patients with DI, or SIADH or cerebral salt wasting need treatment to correct the deficiency. The treatment may be long-term or short-term depending on the need, in an individual patient. DDA-VP nasal spray, arginine vasopressin and pitressin injections are widely used.[9,13,14] Several studies dealing with GH deficient patients showed beneficial role of GH replacement, which

Table 20.3: Biochemical test		
Serum	–	Na
	–	Creatinine
	–	Blood urea nitrogen
	–	Osmolality
Urine	–	Osmolality
	–	Specific gravity
	–	24 hours Na excretion

include improved memory, attention, comprehension and vocabulary. Improvement also included general well being of mood and reduction in depression and anxiety state.[28-31] GH also helps in increasing muscle mass. Some authors have used insulin like growth factor I and shown improvement in various cognitive functions.[27,28]

Other important replacement therapy include the deficiency of **testosterone**. **Testosterone** replacement in men helps in normalization of libido and sexual function helps in bone formation and increases the muscle mass.[32,33] Overall sex hormone replacement be it testosterone or **estrogen** therapy significantly improves the cognitive performance.[19,32] Sex hormone deficiency in women is adequately treated with estrogen therapy, which improves their neurobehavioral and cognitive functions.

Cerebral salt wasting (CSW) occurs due to **unregulated** release of **atrial natriuretic peptide.**[34-37] Patients present with persistent hyponatremia, hypernatriuresis with hyperosmolar urine. In CSW, volume is depleted, hence volume is replaced with Na containing fluid and hematocrit is to be restored. Infusion of saline, plasma and blood is necessary depending on the need. **Fludrocortisone acetate** is the specific treatment for CSW,[34,38] which helps in sodium retention with fluid and correct hyponatremia.

CONCLUSION

Endocrinal abnormality related problems in head injury is a neglected aspect. Overall, 40 percent of severe head injuries to develop either short-term or long-term endocrinal problems. Basic reasons may be hypothalamic or pituitary damage, may be primary or even secondary to hypoxia or hypotension. Both anterior or posterior pituitary get involved. Pituitary stalk necrosis or avulsion can also occur. Growth hormone deficiency, ADH secretion abnormalities and gonadotropin insufficiency are more common problems. GH and gonadotropin deficiency are also to some extent responsible for long-term behavioral and cognitive problems. Diabetes insipidus, inappropriate ADH secretion and CSW are quite frequent. All the endocrinal problems need proper evaluation and adequate short-term or long-term replacement to improve the overall outcome in patients with both severe and minor head injury.

REFERENCES

1. Bistritzer T, Theodor R, Inbar D, et al. Anterior hypopituitarism due to fracture sella turcica. Arne J Dis Child 1981;135:966-7.
2. Daniel PM, Prichard MML, Treip CS. Traumatic infarction of the anterior lobe of the pituitary gland. Lancet 1959; 2:927-30.
3. Edwards OM, Clark JDA. Post-traumatic hypopituitarism. Six cases and review of the literature. Medicine 1981; 65:281-90.
4. Halimi P, Sigal R, Doyon D, et al. Post-traumatic diabetes insipidus. MR demonstration of pituitary stalk rupture. J Comput Assist Tomogr 1988;12:135-7.
5. Miller WL, Kaplan SL, Grumbach MM. Child abuse as a cause of post-traumatic hypopituitarism. N Eng J Med 1980;302:724-8.
6. Ceballos R. Pituitary changes in head trauma (analysis of 102 consecutive cases of head injury). Albama J Med Sci 1966;3:185-98.
7. Daniel PM, Treip CS. The pathology of the pituitary gland in head injury. Mod Trends Endocrinol 1961;12:55-68.
8. Kornblum RN, Fisher RS. Pituitary lesions in craniocerebral injuries. Arch Patho 1969;188:242-8.
9. Kelly DF, Gonzalo ITG, Cohan P, et al. Hypopituitarism following traumatic brain injury and aneurysmal SAH: A preliminary report. J Neurosurg 2000;93:743-52.
10. Eisenberg HM, Gary HEJr, Aldrich EF, et al. Initial CT findings in 753 patients with severe head injury, a report from NIH traumatic coma Data Bank. J Neurosurg 1990; 73:686-98.
11. Adams JR, Daniel PM, Prichard MML. Transection of the pituitary stalk in man. Anatomical changes in pituitary glands of 21 patients. J Neurol Neurosurg Psychiat 1966; 29:545-55.
12. Hwang JL, Lieu AS, Howng SL, et al. Hypothalamic dysfunction in acute head injured patients with stress ulcer. Kaohsiung Journal of Medical Science 1998;14:554-60.
13. Halimi P, Sigal R, Doyon D, et al. Post-traumatic diabetes insipidus: MR demonstration of pituitary stalk rupture. J Comput Asst Tomogra 1988;12:135-7.
14. Massol J, Humbert P, Cattin F, et al. Post-traumatic diabetes insipidus and amenorrhoea-galactorrhoea syndrome after pituitary stalk rupture. Neuroradiol 1987;29:299-300.
15. Joete U, Endtz LJ. Traumatic disorders of pituitary hypothalamic function. Excretion of follicular stimulating hormone after closed head injury. A preliminary investigation. Applied Neurophysiol 1995;38:110-4.
16. NIH Consensus Development Panel on Rehabilitation of persons with Traumatic Brain Injury. JAMA 1999;282:974-83.
17. Ziaber J, Chmielewski H, Laskowski A, et al. Profile of daily secretion of ACTH, beta endorphin and cortisol in patients with minor craniocerebral trauma. Wiado Nosci Leakarskie 1995;48:36-9.
18. Trivedi HS, Nolph IC. Nephrogenic diabetes insipidus presenting after trauma. Arne J Nephrol 1994;14: 145-7.
19. Steinbok P, Thompson GB. Metabolic disturbances after head injury: Abnormalities of sodium and water

balance with specific reference to the effect of alcohol intoxication. Neurosurg 1978;3:9-15.
20. Clark JD, Raggatt PR, Edwards DM. Hypothalamic hypogonadism following major head injury. Clinical Endocrinol 1988;29:153-65.
21. Woolf PD, Hamill RW, McDonald N, Lee LA, et al. Transient hypogonadotropic hypogonadism after head trauma: Effect on steroid precursors and correlation with sympathetic nervous system activity. Clinical Endocrinol 1986;25:265-74.
22. Hackl JM. Metabolic disorders in severe head injuries. Fortschritte der Medizm 1981;99:1562-6.
23. Shaul PW, Towbin RB, Chernausek SD. Precocious puberty following severe head trauma. Arne J Dischild 1985;139:647-69.
24. Dikmen SS, Ross BL, Machamer JE, et al. One year psychological outcome in head injury. J Int Neuropsychol Soc 1995;1:67-77.
25. Hellawell DJ, Taylor RT, Pentland B. Cognitive and psychosocial outcome following moderate or severe traumatic brain injury. Brain Inj 1999;13:489-504.
26. Levin HS, Gary HE, Eisenberg HM, et al. Neurobehavioural outcome one year after severe head injury. Experience of the traumatic data bank. J Neurosurg 1990;73:699-709.
27. Saatman KE, Contreras PC, Smith DH, et al. Insulin like growth factor 1 (IGF1) improves both neurological motor and cognitive outcome following experimental brain injury. Exp Neurol 1997;1/147:418-27.
28. Rollero A, Munaldo G, Fonzi S, et al. Relationship between cognitive function, growth hormone and insulin like growth factor 1 plasma level in aged subjects. Neuropsychobiol 1998;38:73-9.
29. Burman P, Broman JE, Helta J, et al. Quality of life in adults with growth hormone deficiency response to treatment with recombinant human GH in a placebo controlled 21 months trial. J. Clin Endocrinol Metab 1995;80:3585-90.
30. Deijen JB, Vander Veen EA. The influence of growth hormone deficiency and GH replacement on quality of life in GH deficient patients. J Endocrinol Invest 1999;22 (Suppl. 5):127-36.
31. Bauma HBA, Katmelson L, Sherman JC, et al. The effect of physiological growth hormone on cognition and quality of life in patient with adult on set GH deficiency. J Clinical Endocrinol Metab 1993;76:309-17.
32. Wang C, Alexander G, Berman N, et al. Testosterone replacement therapy improve mood in hypogonadal mena clinical research center study. J Clin Endocrinol Metab 1996;81:3578-83.
33. Wang C, Eyre DR, Clark R, et al. Sublingual testosterone replacement improves muscle mass and strength, decreases bone resorption and increases bone formation markers in hypogonadal men-a clinical research center study. J Clin Endocrinol Metab 1996;81:3654-66.
34. Amor M, Hasse J, Holmegard SN, et al. Cerebral salt wasting syndrome and syndrome of inappropriate antidiuretic hormone secretion in SAH caused by ruptured berry aneurysm. Pan Arb J Neurosurg 2000; 4:25-31.
35. Weinand ME, Baynick PL, Goetz KL. A study of serum ADH and atrial natriuretic peptide level in a series of patients with intracranial disease and hyponatremia. Neurosurg 1990;25:781-5.
36. Ganong CA, Kappy MS. Cerebral salt wasting in children. The need for recognition and treatment. Ame J Dis Child 1993;147:167-9.
37. Simma B, Burger R, Falk M, et al. A prospective randomized and controlled study of fluid electrolyte management in children with severe head injury: Lactated Ringers solution vs hypertonic saline. Crit Care Med 1998;26:1265-70.
38. Ishikawa S, Saito T, Kaneko K, et al. Hyponatraemia response to fludrocortisone acetate in elderly patients with head trauma. Ann In Med 1987;16:707-11.
39. Schneider HJ, Kreistschmann-Andermahr I, et al. Hypothalamopituitary dysfunction following traumatic brain injury and aneurysmal subarachnoid hemorrhage: a systemic review. JAMA 2007;26,298(12):1429-38.
40. Behan LA, Phillips J, Thompson CJ, Agha A. Neuroendocrine disorders after TBI. J Neurol Neurosurg Psychiat 2008;79(7):753-9.

21 The Role of Hypothermia in Head Injury Management

Aditya Gupta, AK Mahapatra

SUMMARY

Outlook for patients with severe traumatic brain injury continues to be dismal despite of the dramatic advancements and improvements in diagnosis and management of most other neurological illness categories. Hypothermia is a recently proposed therapeutic modality for management of severe traumatic brain injury. A variety of proposed beneficial effects have been detailed in numerous reports. Currently available evidence does support a beneficial effect. Various protocols have been devised and used by numerous centers, active in this field. Complications are being recognized with the clinical use of hypothermia, and these merits familiarity by any clinician attempting to use this therapy. Despite of a spate of research activity evident in this field, it is clear that at present there does not exist evidence-based clear indications and contraindications for this novel modality of neuroprotection.

INTRODUCTION

The magnitude of head injury continues to pose a serious economic, social and health resource problem all over the world. A significantly high percentage of these patients have an extended stay in the hospital and are subject to a variety of neurological, behavioral, metabolic and infectious complications and sequelae. Not only this subgroup of severely head-injured patients have a sub-optimal outcome and a protracted recovery period, but also these, patients frequently use health resources and intensive care facilities that are extremely scarce in many areas of the world. The two main factors underlying the poor outcome in the patients with severe head injuries are injury to critical brain areas, and uncontrollable intracranial hypertension. In the remaining patients, the poor outcome could also relate to a variety of secondary insults, and a variety of other complications or a combination of many factors.

Various strategies have been evolving for the management of the patients with severe head injuries. This partly reflects the unsatisfactory outcome in many patients despite trying multiple approaches. Also, this is because the pathophysiology of traumatic brain injury (TBI) is complex and involves a multitude of both metabolic and hemodynamic factors.[1] In particular, the approach of using varying degrees of hypothermia has attracted, and continues to attract considerable attention and research effort. Understandably, there is also much controversy as to the indications for using this modality and the effect this has on the final outcome. The aim of this brief review is to highlight the different aspects, and the relevance of this approach to the treating neurosurgeon, as it appears from the current literature.

SYNOPSIS OF TBI PATHOPHYSIOLOGY

As it is readily appreciated, TBI leads to a complex cascade of interlinked, and at times contradictory hemodynamic and metabolic events simultaneously at micro- and macrolevels. Eventually, the final pathway is at the cell level when the results exceed the cellular capability for repair and compensation. From this point, a relatively well established chain of events results in irreversible cell damage and later cell death. At the macrolevel, the distribution of the cells that are already in the irreversibly damaged or dead state and the evolving metabolic events (such as continuing hypoxia or hypercarbia) and hemodynamic events (hypo- and hyperperfusion) together determine the future trend. Raised intracranial pressure, which may be due to a variety of causes, act at various levels to further depress the neurological function, and in effect speed up the vicious cycle where in the deterioration eventually becomes self-perpetuating.

Certain specific metabolic and hemodynamic events have been consistently recorded after TBI, and are thought to be at least partly modifiable with the use of hypothermia. Various teams studying the beneficial effects of hypothermia on head-injured patients have targeted these effects. The notable among these are listed below:

- Cerebral blood flow (CBF) changes following TBI have been well documented, and the more common initial response is mild to moderate reduction in CBF.[2] However, the major criticism of this being an important event is that these reductions still lie well above the conventionally accepted ischemic thresholds. CBF alterations may play a contributory role in conjunction with other unfavorable metabolic and hemodynamic alterations.

- Interestingly, some experimental studies have demonstrated post-traumatic elevations in local cerebral glucose consumption.[3,4] This phenomenon has been subsequently shown to be actually a marked region-specific uncoupling of local cerebral glucose metabolism and blood flow. Indeed, Ginsberg et al[5] have shown that there is a 2.5 fold elevation in local cerebral metabolic rate of glucose (LCMRglu)/local CBF ratio in experimentally lesioned zones. In this context, it now thought that in the setting of increased glucose demand, the relative local oligemia might lead to a bioenergetic stress contributing to the injury process.[5]
- Alterations in many neurochemical systems such as neurotransmitters, neuromodulators, endogenous antioxidants, nitric oxide system,[6,7] inflammatory mediators and adenosine[8,9] have been implicated in various reports. A comprehensive review is available by McIntosh et al. Adenosine has been demonstrated to cause a decline in cerebral metabolism, and yet induce local vasodilation by Al and A2 receptors, respectively.[8,9] This is thought to be a protective response, and the rise in CSF adenosine levels have been correlated with increased mortality.
- Blood-brain barrier alterations have been recognized to occur after TBI and have been shown to be beneficially altered by the use of hypothermia.[10]
- Traumatically induced axonal injury is a common feature of TBI in humans, and it has been shown in a study that the generation of traumatically induced axonal injury may be blunted by hypothermia,[11] This has been since validated by another study by Koizumi et al[12] who have used a better animal injury model as well as markers for axonal injury.
- Intracranial pressure (ICP) elevations follow severe TBI in a large proportion of cases, and clearly constitute an immediate detriment to the neurological function and meaningful survival. This is a very important target for hypothermia therapy as numerous reports have shown the beneficial effects of hypothermia in decreasing raising ICP that does not respond to other therapies.[13,17]

CLINICAL USE OF HYPOTHERMIA FOR TBI

In 1993, three clinical trials were published regarding the use of hypothermia for patients with severe TBI.[8,13,15] With these studies, which began in 1990, came the era of hypothermia as a therapeutic modality for TBI. All the studies have addressed the use of only mild hypothermia (Core temperature 32-34°C). Only patients with severe TBI have been evaluated for use of hypothermia, as any modality that alters the rather bleak prognosis would be welcome. The methods of induction of hypothermia have slightly differed between various groups working on this, and these have been subsequently adapted to suit their particular needs.

It is not entirely agreed upon at the present time at what juncture in the management of a patient with severe TBI, the hypothermia should be induced. Shiozaki et al[6,17] believe in hypothermia induction only when the conventional ICP control modalities—fail to control it below 20 mm Hg. Other centers and authors believe in hypothermia induction either in all patients with severe TBI or without any relation to patient ICP.[13,18] Experimental studies also remain divided over the issue of time of induction of hypothermia. The study by Marion and White[11] emphasizes that the hypothermia should be induced early to protect against emergence of axonal injury. The later study by Koizumi[12] demonstrated that even delayed hypothermia induction yielded a beneficial effect. Another study by Zhao et al[1] showed that in the early phase, the post-traumatic hypoperfusion is what may be deleterious, whereas the later induction of the same state of uncoupling of blood flow and metabolism is not. Extrapolated, it may be possible that in the acute phase, immediately following injury, hypothermia induced aggressively may be counterproductive.

Most groups have achieved mild hypothermia by surface cooling. This has been done by placing cool air or water circulating blankets above and below the patient. The circulation air or water temperature is titrated to the patient core temperature that is continuously monitored using a transducer. The intracranial temperature should be also monitored, and should lie in the same range. Shiozaki et al[16] recommend that the intracranial temperature be measured in the lateral ventricle (presumably where the catheter for concomitantly measuring the ICP would lie) and should be kept between 33.5 and 34.5°C. To maintain the hypothermia, it is imperative to simultaneously infuse barbiturates to suspend all corrective reflexes such as shivering. The barbiturate infusion is maintained at 6 to 8 mg/kg/hour.

Most centers continue hypothermia treatment for 48 to 72 hours and follow-up this with a gradual rewarming. On one hand, severe complications or ineffectiveness of this therapy may require cessation of therapy. On the other, a minority of patients may exhibit a rise of ICP during rewarming. In this, the cooling is again done and hypothermia continued for an additional period of time. It is extremely important for the rewarming to be gradual to avoid unwanted complications during this time. The recommended rate of rewarming is at 1 degree Celsius per day. At this time also the barbiturates need to be given at 2 mg/kg/hour to prevent shivering. With this protocol, by day 5, the patient usually becomes normothermic (intracranial temperature 37 degrees Celsius). After this, the barbiturates are tapered off and stopped.

At the present time, the debate still continues regarding the best time of initiation of therapy, the optimum temperature level, the duration and the precise indications for this mode of therapy.

CURRENT EVIDENCE FOR EFFICACY AND INDICATIONS

In an era of evidence-based medical therapeutics, it is always wise to critically analyze how robust is the evidence claiming the benefit of a new mode of therapy. At the present time, the various beneficial effects thought to be associated with hypothermia use have been listed in Table 21.1. Three initial clinical studies[13,15,18] led to a spate of clinical and experimental attempts to verify and further define the efficacy of hypothermia. In one of these studies by Shiozaki et al[15] there was convincing evidence for the efficacy of hypothermia treatment to lower the ICP, when it was refractory to other therapies. In their later studies[16,17] they regarded further the merits of this therapy. They found that mild hypothermia (as defined above) controlled the ICP rise in 35 (56.5%) of their 62 patients in whom it was more than 20 mm Hg despite "all therapies". The group in which the ICP was controlled had a much better functional outcome than the other group. In a study, of the 46 patients with an ICP higher than even 40 mm Hg, 12 (26.1%) had a functional recovery. This was in sharp contrast to the general experience and also the experience of Lobato et al[19] who did not find any survivor in their group of 26 patients with ICP higher than 40 without hypothermia. Patients those did not benefit from hypothermia treatment include with ICP more than 60 mm Hg prior to hypothermia, those with Glasgow coma scale (GCS) 3 or 4, midline shift of more than 13 mm on CT and those with diffuse brain swelling. The patients with ICP more than 60, GCS of 3 or 4 or midline shift more than 13 millimeters probably indicate the therapeutic limit for hypothermia beyond which it becomes ineffective. These limits probably indicate the irreversible point for decline of brain function beyond which all therapies cease to benefit. Patients with diffuse brain swelling may have direct severe injury to the whole of the brain, including critical areas such as the brainstem. The major criticism for all the studies by this group of Shiozaki et al[15,16] is that the authors neither use mannitol for any of their patients, nor they use optimized hyperventilation therapy. They only used moderate hyperventilation therapy. This fact does cast a doubt on the actual margin of benefit attained with use of hypothermia. In their recent paper, the same group also documented the lack of benefit of hypothermia therapy in patients[16] with severe TBI, but with low ICP. The two groups of patients, one of which received and the other which did not receive hypothermia therapy did not differ in relation to either the clinical outcome or CSF concentrations of cytokines, etc. Following a meta-analysis of previous data, the Brain Trauma Foundation and American Association of Neurological Surgeons (BTF & AANS) have issued a level III recommendation for optional and cautious use of hypothermia for adults with TBI.[28]

The other major point of focus has been on the experimental demonstration of prevention against emergence of axonal injury by the use of hypothermia. This beneficial effect, if it stands the test of time and is substantive, certainly constitutes an exciting development in the field of neuroprotection. Two studies are noteworthy in this regard. The initial study by Marion and White[11] in 1996 showed the protective effect of early hypothermia following experimentally induced brain injury in rodents by a cortical impact. The above authors used antibodies against cytoskeletal markers to determine the extent of axonal damage. However, the rewarming induced was rather abrupt and is in contrast to the gradual rewarming recommended for patients after hypothermia. Another finding was that delayed hypothermia did not confer the

Table 21.1: Proposed beneficial effects of hypothermia used for severe TBI

- Decline in brain metabolism and oxygen consumption
- Lowering of ICP
- Protective effect on blood-brain barrier
- Protection against emergence of axonal injury
- Beneficial alteration in EAAS
- Alteration in neuromodulators
- Alteration in antioxidants and nitric oxide system
- Decline in release of cytokines and other inflammatory mediators

protective effect. The more recent study by Koizumi et al[12] used an experimental injury model based on impact acceleration. The induced hypothermia and subsequent rewarming were as per the human protocols being followed. Antibodies against amyloid precursor proteins (APPs) were used to reflect densities of axonal profiles that appeared injured. The authors' results showed a distinct beneficial effect of not only early but also delayed hypothermia. The authors postulate that hypothermia could act on some or many of the pathogenic processes that result in the progression of swollen axonal end bulbs to disconnection. The axolemma appears to be stabilized as also the organelles and cytoskeletal components. The major limitation was that the assessment was made only at 24 hours post-trauma. Later study may well have shown emergence of injured axons. However, these results certainly give scope for some of this beneficial effect taking place in humans. Obviously, one cannot obtain pathological proof in human subjects (especially in those who fare well) but it is likely that this effect may constitute a portion of the overall beneficial effect that has been documented in numerous studies. Treating any patient with severe TBI on the grounds of this early evidence cannot be said to be on firm scientific grounds.

The beneficial effects of hypothermia on the release of cytokines, excitatory amino acids (EAAs) and other mediators have also been reported in some series.[14,20,21] The role of glutamate and aspartate has been realized in TBI in humans.[14,20] A study by Busto et al[21] showed that mild hypothermia (but not normothermia) in the area of ischemia inhibited extracellular glutamate concentrations. These findings may not have reflected in the study by Shiozaki et al[16] because the concentrations in severe TBI patients with low ICP may have been low. This fact has previously been reported by Bullock et al.[22] They used a microdialysis technique to show the relationship between sustained high ICP and glutamate levels. Similarly, several types of cytokines have been shown to be increased in CSF following TBI. These may be the factors responsible for secondary brain injury. It has again been claimed that apart of the beneficial effect of hypothermia on TBI may relate to this effect.[11,13]

Other effects have been claimed with the use of hypothermia, such as stabilization of blood-brain barrier. Newer aspects and insights are hoped to emerge with the use of clinically applicable intracerebral microdialysis systems for use in severe TBI patients.

In short the indications for the clinical use of hypothermia in severe TBI are not scientifically well defined at present. Although the weight of evidence does suggest beneficial effects exact indications are unclear with the possible exception of refractory raised ICP.

COMPLICATIONS OF HYPOTHERMIA TREATMENT

The use of hypothermia seem to be associated with a definite risk of complications, as outlined in Table 21.2. In fact, the use of hypothermia remains partly controversial because of occasionally encountered severe complications.

Cardiac tachyarrhythmias reported after hypothermia, but the risk of developing these substantial is only when the temperature is lowered below 30 degrees Celsius.[23] Therefore, during clinical use mild hypothermia for severe TBI, the risk of cardiac tachyarrhythmias is relatively small.

There is probably an increase in the incidence of pneumonia in the hypothermic patients.[16] This fact correlates well with the earlier demonstration by Kurz and colleagues[24] that perioperative hypothermia predisposed operated patients to culture-positive surgical infections. It has further been shown that WBC count and activity both decline during hypothermia, which can very well explain the increased infection rate. This fact should be carefully considered in the context of patients with severe TBI as many other unfavorable factors are clustered. Stress, prolonged insertion of a variety of catheters and tubes, surgical procedures further aggravate the risk of infection in these patients. Though, there is likely a definite predisposition towards infection, the magnitude cannot be judged accurately as other reports do not experience,[11,13,17] this.

Hypernatremia may result due to diabetes insipidus (DI). This is largely the result of cold induced diuresis, which is usually mild and self-limiting. It is important to realize that these patients with severe TBI may already be predisposed to developing DI as a direct consequence of the trauma.[25] Additionally;

Table 21.2: Possible complications of hypothermia therapy

- Cardiac (tachy) arrhythmias
- Coagulopathy
- Increased infections
- Pneumonitis
- Hypernatremia (cold diuresis)
- Hypokalemia
- Hypomagnesemia
- Hypophosphatemia
- Acidosis

these patients are routinely administered mannitol and other diuretics, which may also result in polyuria and hypernatremia.

Excessive diuresis owing to the aforementioned reasons can also lead to the losses of various electrolytes including Mg, K and phosphate. This may lead to serious clinical implications for the patient. Hypokalemia may cause cardiac arrhythmias, especially in patients with ischemic cardiac disease or ventricular hypertrophy. Whereas potassium is important for the Na-K pump, magnesium deficiency may lead to cardiac arrhythmias, neuromuscular irritability, hypertension and vasoconstriction.[26] It has been shown that hypomagnesemia is an independent risk factor for increased mortality in the ICU.[27] Hypophosphatemia leads to low intracellular levels of adenosine triphosphate (ATP), and results in muscle weakness, respiratory failure, and a decrease in cardiac output.[26] When more than one of the above electrolyte abnormalities are present, the result may be cumulative.

Hypothermia causes vasoconstriction, and usually some acidosis. One particular group reported that on an average, the pH decreased from 7.37 to 7.31 in their patients.[26] This could also then be responsible for other electrolyte abnormalities as a consequence of intracellular shifts.

Coagulopathy has also been recognized to occur following hypothermia[23,25] but the available data is rather scanty, and no firm conclusions can be arrived at. In children with sever TBI, hypothermia that is initiated within 8 hours of injury and continued for 24 hours does not improve outcome and may increase mortality.[29]

Increasing and recent evidences suggest that induction of mild hypothermia (32-35°C) in first hour after an ischemic event can prevent or mitigate permanent injuries; it applies more for postanoxic brain injuries. However, the rate of rewarming seems to be an important factor in establishing successful use of hypothermia in treatment of neurological injuries.[30]

CONCLUSION

The use of hypothermia for patients with severe TBI is presently an object of active ongoing research efforts, and early evidence does seem to support a somewhat neuroprotective effect. This has been attributed to a host of suspected and extrapolated beneficial effects. However, owing to the differences in clinical situations in which it has been studied and the varying protocols used, no clear indications exist at the present time, various centers continue to further evaluate and use this therapy with varying results. It is evident from reports of beneficial results of this novel approach that very soon we would have modality, and what results to expect. Similarly, it is already becoming clear that hypothermia is hardly a panacea for all patients, and some patients would not derive any benefit whatsoever. A definite risk of complications should be always kept in mind prior to instituting this therapy. It is also hoped that other ongoing comprehensive armamentarium of therapies for use in these unrewarding conditions.

REFERENCES

1. Zhao W, Alonso OF, Loar JY, Busto R, Ginsberg MD. Influence of early post-traumatic hypothermia therapy on local cerebral blood flow and glucose metabolism after fluid-percussion brain injury. J Neurosurg 1999;90:510-19.
2. Hossman KA. Peri-infarct depolarization. Cerebrovasc Br Metab Rev 1996;8:195-208.
3. Kawamura T, Katayama Y, Hovda DA, et al. Administration of excitatory amino acid antagonists via microdialysis attenuates the increase in glucose utilization seen following concussive brain injury. J Cereb Blood Flow Metab 1992;12:12-24.
4. Yoshino A, Hovda DA, Katayama Y, et al. Hippocampal CA 3 lesion prevents postconcussive metabolic dysfunction in CA 1. J Cereb Blood Flow Metab 1992;12:996-1006.
5. Ginsberg MD, Zhao D, Alonso OF, et al. Uncoupling of local cerebral glucose metabolism and blood flow after acute fluid-percussion injury in rats. Am J Physiol 1997;272:H2859-H2868.
6. DeWitt DS, Smith TG, Deyo DJ, et al. L-arginine and superoxide dismutase prevent or reverse cerebral hypoperfusion after fluid-percussion traumatic brain injury. J Neurotrauma 1997;14:223-33.
7. McIntosh TK. Neurochemical sequelae of traumatic brain injury: therapeutic implications. Cerebrovasc Br Metab Rev 1994;6:109-163.
8. Headrich JP, Bendall R, Faden AI, et al. Dissociation of adenosine levels from bioenergetic state in experimental brain trauma: potential role in secondary injury. J Cereb Blood Flow Metab 1994;14:853-61.
9. Phillis JW, Kostopoulos GK, Limacher JJ. A potent depressant action of adenosine derivatives on cerebral cortical neurones. Eur J Pharmacol 1975;30:125-9.
10. Smith SL, Hall Ed. Mild pre and post-traumatic hypothermia attenuates blood-brain barrier damage following controlled corticald impact injury in the rat. J Neurotrauma 1996;13:1-9.
11. Marion DW, White MJ. Treatment of experimental brain injury with moderate hypothermia and 21-aminosteroids. J Neurotrauma 1996;13:139-47.
12. Koizumi H, Povlishock JT. Post-traumatic hypothermia in the treatment of axonal damage in an animal model of traumatic axonal injury. J Neurosurg 1998;89:303-09.

13. Marion DW, Obrist WD, Carlier PM, et al. The use of moderate therapeutic hypothermia for patients with severe head injuries: a preliminary report. J Neurosurg 1993;79:354-62.
14. Metz C, Holzschuh M, Bein T, et al. Moderate hypothermia in patients with severe head injury: cerebral and extracerebral effects. J Neurosurg 1996;85:533-41.
15. Shiozaki T, Sugimoto H, Taneda M, et al. Effect of mild hypothermia on uncontrollable intracranial hypertension after severe head injury. J Neurosurg 1993;79:363-8.
16. Shiozaki T, Kato A, Taneda M, et al. Little benefit from mild hypothermia therapy for severely head injured patients with low intracranial pressure. J Neurosurg 1999;91:185-91.
17. Shiozaki T, Sugimoto H, Taneda M, et al. Selection of severely head injured patients for mild hypothermia therapy. J Neurosurg 1998;89:206-11.
18. Clifton GL, Allen S, Barrodale P, et al. A phase II study of moderate hypothermia in severe brain injury. J Neurotrauma 1993;10:263-73.
19. Lobato RD, Sarabia R, Cordobes F, et al. Post-traumatic cerebral hemispheric swelling. Analysis of 55 cases studied with computerized tomography. J Neurosurg 1988;68:417-23.
20. Baker AJ, Moulton RJ, MacMillan VH, et al. Excitatory amino acids in cerebrospinal fluid following traumatic brain injury in humans. J Neurosurg 1993;79:369-72.
21. Busto R, Globus MYT, Dietrich WD, et al. Effect of mild hypothermia on ischemia-induced release of neurotransmitters and free fatty acids in rat brain. Stroke 1989;20:904-10.
22. Bullock R, Zauner A, Woodward JJ, et al. Factors affecting excitatory amino acid release following severe human head injury. J Neurosurg 1998;89:507-18.
23. Weinberg AD. Hypothermia. Ann Emerg Med 1993; 22:370-77.
24. Kurz A, Sessler Dr, Lenhardt R, et al. Perioperative normothermia to reduce the incidence of surgical-wound infection and shorten hospitalization. N Engl J Med 1996;334:1209-15.
25. Kaufman HH, Timberlake G, Voelker J, et al. Medical complications of head injury. Med Clin North Am 1993;77:43-60.
26. Polderman KH, Peerdeman SM, Girbes ARJ. Hypophosphatemia and hypomagnesemia induced by cooling in patients with severe head injury. J Neurosurg 2001;94:697-705.
27. Chernow B, Bamberger S, Stoiko M, et al. Hypomagnesemia in patients in postoperative intensive care. Chest 1989;95:391-7.
28. Peterson K, Larson S, Carney N. Hypothermia treatment for TBI: A systemic review and meta-analysis. J Neurotrauma 2008;25(1):62-71.
29. Hutchison JS, Ward RE and Lacroix J, et al. Hypothermia therapy after TBI in children. N Eng J Med 2008; 5:358(23):2447-56.
30. Polderman KH. Induced hypothermia and fever control for prevention of treatment of neurological injuries. Lancet 2008;371(9628):1893-5.

22 Prognosis and Outcome in Head Injury

AK Mahapatra, Raj Kumar

INTRODUCTION

Patient's early clinical condition defines the severity of head injury but the most important measure of severity of trauma is the impact that the injury has on the patient's final functional outcome. Early determination of severity, prognosis determination and outcome assessment are interconnected and they need to be discussed simultaneously. High cost of treatment of head injury patients has focussed attention on cost-effectiveness, with increasing reliance on prognosis for allocation of resources. Assessment of outcome in relation to initial clinical and nonclinical features of head-injured patients provide insight into pathophysiology of head injury and better understanding of complex variables determining outcome. Prognostication for head injury has changed dramatically over past decades and is presently based on collective experience based on systemic research into factors contributing to outcome. This also has helped in focussing attention of physicians on neuropsychiatric and psychosocial disabilities of survivors of head injury. Standardized methods of assessment of severity and outcome (especially **Glasgow coma scale** (GCS), and **Glasgow outcome scale** (GOS)[1,2] have provided practical framework for detailed studies of prognosis. Multicenter efforts to integrate data in a systemic way (e.g. **International Data Bank: IDB and Traumatic Coma Data Bank: TCDB**)[2a,2b] to determine predictive factors in head injury and contributed to better understanding of head injury (Table 22.1).

CLINICAL FACTORS INFLUENCING OUTCOME IN HEAD INJURY PATIENTS

Mechanism of injury has been correlated with outcome but not as an independent variable. TCDB study[3] showed that pedestrians had worse outcome and high (48%) mortality. But in IDB[4] study gunshot wound was the only significant mechanism correlating with worse outcome. In a study by Luerssen et al,[5] falls were more common in children (<16 years) and elderly (>60 years), whereas RTA was more common in 16 to 59 years old. Incidence of surgically treatable hematomas increases with age.[6] Leurssen et al[5] also showed that at same GCS adults had worse outcome than children (Table 22.2).

In children, mortality is highest at 1 to 2 years[5a,5b] and decreases till adolescence, being minimum at 12 years.

Table 22.1: Factors affecting outcome

I. A. Clinical
– Mechanism of injury
– Age
– Motor response
– Pupillary reflex
– Eye movement
– Systemic factors
– Duration of coma
– Associated injury
B. Physiological
– Intracranial pressure (ICP)
– Evoked potentials, EEG
– Cerebral blood flow (CBF)
– Coagulation defect
C. Radiological
– CT
Midline shift, intracranial hematoma (intra/extra-axial)
– MRI
Diffuse axonal injury
D. Biochemical
– CSF
– Blood-catecholamines, sugar levels
II. Assessment of head injury Severity/outcome
– GCS
– GLS
– GOS
III. Sequalae of head injury
– Physical
– Neurological
– Neuropsychological
IV. Timing of outcome assessment

Table 22.2: Outcome according to age in head injury[5]

GCS	*Children*	*Adults (Mortality)*
3–8	28.4%	47.7%
9–12	1.4%	6.8%
13–15	0.0%	0.9%

Multiple medical problems, e.g. DM, HT, myocardial infraction, COAD add to the increased mortality. Although several authors have contested this old belief and age may not have an effect in all types of head injury, e.g. Alberico[7] showed same mortality for children and adults with raised ICP but better outcome in children with low/normal ICP. Children do better in case of diffuse injury (16% vs 35%). Similarly, mortality for EDH was significantly greater in adults (4.3% in children and 21.5% in adults).[5] GCS has been widely used in assessing severity and predicting outcome. Motor component alone has been used as single important predictor. Placidity has worse outcome (~100%) mortality. Becker et al,[8] found that 68 percent patients had worse outcome with M1-2 response, whereas patients with normal motor response had less mortality 19 percent. The difference was greater when diffuse axonal injury was taken (76% mortality with M2 response and 8 percent mortality with normal movements).

In the IDB, 91 percent patients with nonreactive pupils died or were vegetative (Fig. 22.1) compared to 39% with reacting pupils. Braakman et al[9] reported patients with only one reactive pupil had 50 percent mortality compared to 90 percent in bilateral nonreactive pupils. Similar results were obtained from a study at AIIMS.[13,13a] Brainstem centers for ocular movements are usually injured in association with other significant injuries. Becker et al[8] and Levati et al[10] reported 73 percent mortality in patients with impaired/absent oculocephalic response. Braak-man et al[9] showed absent oculovestibular reflexes associate with 95 percent mortality. Alexandar et al[11] showed that patients with normal oculovestibular reflex were generally free of significant deficit 2 years after the injury.

Hypoxia (PO_2 <60) and **hypotension** (BP < 90), when associated with head injury leads to worse outcome by causing secondary brain insults.[9a,9b] Stocchetti et al, role of hypoxia and hypotension recorded at accident site and outcome. No doubt early or delayed resuscitation of hypotension alter the outcome. Jennett et al,[4] defined coma as being unable to obey commands, utter words or open eyes. Thus, patients with GCS ≤ 8 are comatose and those ≥9 are not. **Post-traumatic amnesia** is defined

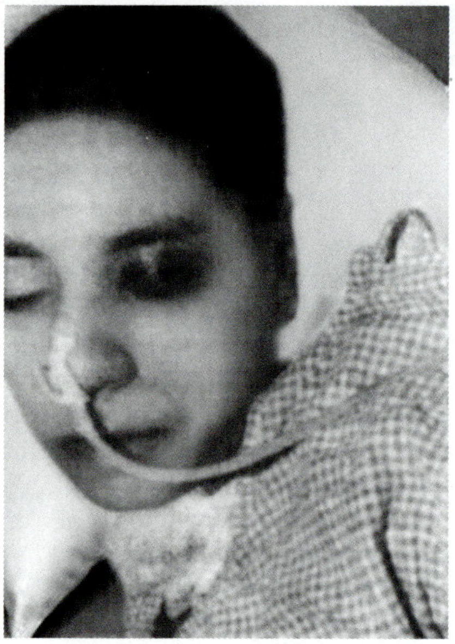

Fig. 22.1: A severe head injured patient who was still vegetative at 3 months

as time interval from the moment of impact to the time from where continuous **registration of facts starts. Jennett** et al[2] found 90 percent patient with PTA < 7 days had good outcomes. Groswasser et al,[12] identified 6 features predictive of failure to regain consciousness fever of central origin, diffuse sweating, disturbance of ADH secretion, abnormal motor reactivity, respiratory disturbance, diffuse non-neurological injury.

Associated injuries like rib fracture, abdominal injuries, spinal injuries may require surgical intervention in their own merit. These also interfere with postoperative nursing care leading to more postoperative complications, like chest infection, DVT, etc. Delay in operating and surgical lesion has been correlated with worse outcome.[15] Deep vein thrombosis and pulmonary embolisms are frequent complications in head injured patients and incidence can be as high as 50 to 55 percent.[15a] Routine heparin therapy may not be considered safe in early postinjury period, however, after few days low molecular heparin may help.[15b,15c]

PHYSIOLOGICAL FACTORS

Miller et al[16] demonstrated poor outcome in patients with raised ICP. Mortality was 18 percent in patients with normal ICP and was considerably high in patients with raised ICP, (26%) in patient with raised ICP-treatable and 92 percent in unresponsive raised (ICP). A study at AIIMS in 1995 showed that patients with raised ICP had significantly raised mortality than with normal ICP.[14] Also higher values of ICP

Table 22.3: Outcome related to ICP[14] result of study carried out at AIIMS

ICP Values	*GR*	*MD*	*SD*	*PVS*	*Death (%)*
Normal	11	11	45	11	22
Raised	12	3	33	0	52
Peak ICP Value	*GR*	*MD*	*SD*	*PVS*	*Death (% outcome)*
<15 (n = 18)	11	11	45	11	22
16–30 (n = 21)	19	5	38	0	38
31–50 (n = 10)	0	0	30	0	70
>50 (n = 2)	0	0	0	0	100

were associated with higher mortality rate (Table 22.3). Marmarow et al[17] showed that raised ICP was among first four significant variables affecting outcome and ICP was superior to CPP in predicting outcome. Secondary size in ICP is reported to have worse outcome.[18] It has been shown that SSEP and VEP and BERA correlate well with GCS and other clinical indicators of severity,[19,20] but they did not help in the outcome prediction. Evaluation of CBF in head injury is affected by various variables. It has been shown that decreased CBF is associated with poor outcome.[21]

RADIOLOGICAL FACTORS

Computed tomography (CT) provides a rapid and reliable method of detecting intracranial pathology and therefore, CT findings do have a significant role in predicting the outcome. Also, it is important to repeat the scan within 72 hours of injury as hematomas may enlarge, have more mass effect because of surrounding edema, new lesions may appear. In a study at AIIMS we found that as many as 36 percent patients in which second scan was done within 72 hours showed new hematomas or change in the size of previous hematomas. Appearance of new lesion is highly predictive. Cooper et al[22] showed that 25 (83.3%) of 30 patients with new lesion had poor outcome, but 8 (28.6%) of 28 patients without new hematomas had poor outcome. Genarellic et al[23] showed that patients with acute SDH with GCS 3 to 5 had mortality rate of 74 percent whereas patients with diffuse injury in same GCS had 51 percent mortality and EDH had 21 percent deaths. Lobato et al[24] on a different classification system of lesions on CT scan came to similar conclusions. In a study at AIIMS 1991-92, 158 patients with severe head injury were studied. Patients with normal CT had best survival (72.7%). Patients with single lesion on CT had better outcome (60.6% survival) than

Table 22.4: Correlation of CT findings with survival (Results of a study at AIIMS)

CT Finding	*No. of Cases*	*Survived (%)*
Normal	44	32 (72.7%)
Single Lesion		
- GCS <5	16	05 (31.25%)
- GCS 5-8	17	1/15 (88.23%)
Multiple Lesions		
- GCS <5	21	7 (33%)
- GCS 6-8	24	12 (50%)
Midline Shift		
Nil	97	63 (64.9%) P< .001
<3 mm	16	08 (50%)
>3 mm	09	00 (0%)

those with multiple lesion (42.2% survival). Different types of lesion leads to different neuropsychological sequelae.[25] Midline shift had also been correlated with survival. We found that 64 percent patients without midline shift survived,[13] whereas 50 percent survival was noted with shift ≤ 3 mm. None of the patients with midlines shift ≥ 3 mm survived (P < 0.001) (Table 22.4). Late CT scan findings have been correlated with outcome and patients with wider IIIrd ventricle (related to **diencephalic atrophy**) had poorer cognitive status.[26]

Magnetic resonance imaging (MRI) in acute head injury has limited role because of increased scan time, cost, incompatibility with life support system. CT and MRI have similar sensitivity for acute hemorrhage but old hemorrhage and hemosiderin is better demonstrated on MRI.[27] MRI is most useful when clinical status do not correlate with CT scan finding, especially when diffuse axonal injury is suspected. Also the chronic effects of head injury like demyelination, hemorrhage, hemosiderin and old parenchymal injuries are better revealed with MRI.[27] MRI findings have been correlated with outcome by Wilson et al[29] and Levin et al.[28]

BIOCHEMICAL PARAMETERS

CSF levels of creatinine kinase-BB,[30,31] Lactic dehydrogenase and lactate[32,33] have been shown to correlate with outcome. Niedeggen et al,[31] showed that all patients with CK-BB > 50 ng/ml died whereas <25 ng/ml was associated with minimal deficits. Serum catecholamines have shown to correlate well with GCS score and they also have independent predictive value.[34] Levels of serum glucose rise in response to stress. High glucose levels with poor GCS scores have been shown to have very poor outcome.[35] Similarly deranged coagulation parameters (especially raised FDP levels) have been shown to be associated with poor outcome.[36]

Alteration of sodium levels critical and may occur in as high as 50 percent comatose patients.[36a-36c] Both hyponatremia and syndrome of inappropriate ADH secretion and cerebral salt wasting results in increased sodium loss. Elevated sodium level may indicate dehydration or DI.

CEREBRAL PERFUSION AND CEREBRAL BLOOD FLOW

In children with severe head injury, an initial ICP and CPP measurement were useful prognostic factors. Children with initial CPP between 40 and 70 mm Hg were found to have better neurological prognosis than those with CPP either higher or lower than that range.[46]

A low cerebral blood flow (CBF) and cerebral perfusion pressure (CPP) is associated with poor outcome in TBI. It is less clear whether altering CBF/CPP will lead to clinical improvement. A targeted CPP at 70 mm Hg (1996 guideline of trauma foundation) showed no demonstrable effect but had increase in complication rates. More recently, evidence that autoregulation may be disrupted after TBI has led some authors to propose an individualized approach to CPP management. A close neuromonitoring techniques can monitor the effects of hemodynamic manipulations on cerebral metabolism.[47]

STANDARDIZED ASSESSMENT

It is essential to follow a standardized protocol for trauma assessment so that results of studies can be compared. GCS is the most widely used scale. There are eight different types of coma scales available of which GCS is most accepted. It has low inter observer variability[37,38] and the scores have been shown to correlate with outcome.[39] GLS incorporates brainstem reflexes into GCS.[40] Glasgow outcome scale was introduced in 1975 by Jennett and Bond to provide a standardized method of assessment. It divides outcome into five categories—dead (D), persistent vegetative state (PVS), severe disability (SD), moderate disability (MD), good recovery. Timing of outcome assessment is an important aspect of outcome determination. Jennett and others[41] have demonstrated that the distribution of outcome for a group of head-injured patients changes significantly over first year. Therefore, premature outcome assessment may under estimate recovery and affect decision adversely regarding rehabilitation. Jennett et al[4] found that patients classified on MD or GR at 1 year—60 percent of them had reached this status by 3 months and 90 percent by 6 months.

Table 22.5: Recovery time of cognitive deficits after mild to moderate head injury

Function	*Recovery time (months)*
Motor skill and speed	0–3
Language skills	3–6
Attention/concentration	6–12
Memory/learning	6–12
Complex problem-solving	6–24
Mental stamina	6–24

Heider et al[42] reported that while SD was most common outcome at 1 month, 68 percent of these improved to MD and GR at 6 months and 72 percent reached (MD or GR) this status at 1 year. Bricolo et al[43] states that the diagnosis of PVS should not be made till 1 year post-head injury. Most of the cognitive function recovers in first 6 months.[44] However, different functions recover at different rates (Table 22.5).

CONCLUSION

The concept of primary and secondary brain damage has greatly changed the treatment of head injury, while primary brain injury can only be prevented. Hypotension and hypoxia are the worst events that can happen after head injury and injured brain tolerates them poorly. Maintenance of good cerebral blood flow, and CPP above 70 mm Hg is the key factor in good outcome. Almost any improvement in management, like timely resuscitation, better transportation and prehospital care, management of associated injuries, rapid imaging and surgery may prevent secondary damage and affect final outcome.

REFERENCES

1. Teasdale G, Jennett B. Assessment of coma and impaired consciousness—a practical scale. Lancet 1974;2:81-4.
2. Jennett B, Bond MR. Assessment of outcome after severe brain damage—a practical scale. Lancet 1975;1:480-4.

2a. Eisenberg HM, Frankowski RF, Contant CF, et al. Initial CT findings in 753 patients with severe head injury. A report from NIH Traumatic Coma Data Bank. J Neurosurg 1990;73:688-98.

2b. Foulkes MA, Eisenberg HM, Jane JA, et al. The Traumatic Coma Data Bank: Design, Method and Baseline Characteristics. J Neurosurg 1991;78:S8-S13.

3. Marshall LF, Gantille T, Klauber MR. The outcome of severe closed head injury. J Neurosurg 1991;75 (Suppl.): 28-36.
4. Jennett B, Teasdale G, Galbraith S, et al. Severe head injuries in three countries. J Neurol Neurosurg Psychiat, 1977;40:291-8.

5. Luerssen TG, Klauber MR, Marshall LF. Outcome from head injury related to patient's age. J Neurosurg 1988;68:409-16.
5a. White JR, Farukhiz, Bull C, et al. Predictions of outcome in severely-head injured children. Crit Care Med. 2001; 29:534-40.
5b. Pervin RG, Rutka JT, Drake JM, et al. Management and Outcome of Posterior Fossa subdural haematomas in neonates. Neurosurg 1997;40:1190-1220.
6. Vollmer DG, Tomer JC, Jane JA, et al. Age and outcome following traumatic coma: Why do older patients fare worse? J Neurosurg 1991;75 (Suppl.):37-49.
7. Alberico AM, Ward JD, Choi SC, et al. Outcome after severe head injury. Relationship to mass lesions, diffuse injury, and ICP course in paediatric and adult patients. J Neurosurg 1987;67:648-56.
7a. Lannoo E, Van Rietvalde F, Colardyn F, et al. Early predictor of mortality and morbidity after severe closed head injury. J Neurotrauma 2000;17:403-14.
8. Becker D, Miller JD, Ward JD, et al. The outcome from severe head injury with early diagnosis and intensive management. J Neurosurg 1977;47:491-502.
9. Braakman R, Glepke GJ, Habbema JDF, et al. Systematic selection of prognosis features in patients with severe head injury. Neurosurgery 1980;6:362-70.
9a. Chesnut RM. Avoidance of hypotension: Condition sine 949 non of successful head injury management. J Trauma 1997;42:54-9.
9b. Guidelines for cerebral perfusion pressure. J Neurotrauma 2000;17:507-11.
9c. Stocchetti N, Furlan A, Volta F. Hypoxemia and arterial hypotension at the accident scene in head injury. J Trauma 1996;40:764-7.
10. Levati A, Farina ML, Vecchi G, et al. Prognosis of severe head injuries. J Neurosurg 1982;57:779-83.
11. Alexandre A, Colombo F, Nertempi P, Benedetti A. Cognitive outcome and early indices of severity of head injury. J Neurosurg 1983;59:751-61.
12. Groswasser Z, Sazbon L. Outcome in 134 patients with prolonged post-traumatic unawareness. Part 2: Functional outcome of 72 patients recovering consciousness. J Neurosurg 1990;72:81-4.
13. Mahapatra AK. Some evidence based management of head injury at AIIMS. Neurosciences Today 2002;6:97-102.
13a. Sousa J, Sharma RR, Power SJ, Mahapatra AK, Lad SD. Bilateral dilated unveiling pupils in pediatric patients following severe head injury. Pan Arob J Neurosurg 2002;6:39-46.
14. Bansal S. A study of 51 patients of head injury—relation of ICP to outcome of patients. Thesis submitted to AIIMS in 1995.
15. Seelig JN, Becker DP, Miller JD, et al. Traumatic acute subdural haematoma. Major mortality reduction in comatose patients treated within four hours. N Engl J Med 1981;304:1511-8.
15a. Geerts WH, Code KI, Jay RM, et al. Prospective study of venous thromboembolism after major trauma. N Engl J Med 1994;331:1601-6.
15b. Knudson MM, Morabito D, Paiemen GD, et al. Use of low molecular heparin in preventing thromboembolism in trauma patients. J Trauma 1996;41:446-59.
15c. Spain DA, Richardson JD, Polk He, et al. Venous thromboembolism in the high-risk trauma patients: Do risks justify aggressive screening and prophylaxis. T Trauma 1997;42:463-9.
16. Miller JD, Becker DP, Ward JD, et al. Significance of intracranial hypertension in severe head injury. J Neurosurg 1977;47:503-16.
17. Marmarou A, Anderson RL, Ward JD, et al. Impact of ICP instability and hypotension on outcome in patients with severe head trauma. J Neurosurg 1991;75 (Suppl): 59-66.
18. Unterberg A, Kiening K, Schmiedek P, Lanksch W. Long-term observation of intracranial pressure after severe head injury. The phenomenon of secondary rise of intracranial pressure. Neurosurgery 1993;32:17-23.
19. Greenburg RP, Becker DP, Miller JD, et al. Evaluation of brain function in severe human head trauma with multimodality evoked potentials. Part 2: Localization of brain dysfunction and correlation with post-traumatic neurological conditions. J Neurosurg 1977;47:163-77.
20. Lindsay KW, Carlin J, Kennedy I, et al. Evoked potentials in severe head injury—analysis and relation to outcome. J Neurol Neurosurg Psychiat 1981;44:796-802.
21. Robertson CS, Contant CF, Narayan RK, Grossman RG. Cerebral blood flow, $AVDO_2$ and neurologic outcome in head injured patients. J Neurotrauma 1992;9 (Suppl): 349-58.
22. Cooper PR, Maravilla K, Moodly S, et al. Serial computerized tomographic scanning and the prognosis of severe head injury. Neurosurg 1979;5:566-9.
23. Gennarelli TA, Spielman GM, Langfitt TW, et al. Influence of the type of intracranial lesion on outcome from severe head injury. A multicenter study using a new classification system. J Neurosurg 1982;56:26-32.
24. Lobato RD, Cordobes F, Rival JJ, et al. Outcome from severe head injury related to the type of intracranial lesion. A computed tomographic study. J Neurosurg 1983;59:762-74.
25. Uzzell BP, Dolinskas CA, Wiser RF, Langfitt TW. Influence of lesions detected by computed tomography on outcome and neuropsychological recovery after severe head injury. Neurosurgery 1987;20:396-402.
26. Reider-Groswasser I, Cohen M, et al. Late CT findings in brain trauma: Relationship to cognitive and behavioural sequelae and to vocational outcome. AJR 1993;160:142-52.
27. Zimmerman RA, Bilaniuk LT, et al. Head injury early results of comparing CT and high-field MR. AJR 1986;147:1215-22.

28. Levin HS, Williams D, Crofford MJ, et al. Relationship of depth of brain lesions to consciousness and outcome after closed head injury. J Neurosurg 1988;69:861.
29. Wilson JTL, Wiedmann KD, Hadley DM, et al. Early and late magnetic resonance imaging and neuropsychological outcome after head injury. J Neurol Neurosurg Psychiat 1988;51:391-6.
30. Bakay RAE, Ward AA Jr. Enzymatic changes in serum and cerebrospinal fluid in neurological injury. J Neurosurg 1983;58:27-37.
31. Niedeggen A, Adelt D, Berndt R, et al. Creatine-kinase-BB after severe head injury as an index of prognosis in relation to nature of trauma and patient's age. Acta Neurochir (Wien) 1989;101:117-20.
32. DeSalles AAF, et al. Prognostic significance of ventricular CSF lactic acidosis in severe head injury. J Neurosurg 1986;65:615-24.
33. Rabow L, DeSalles AF, Becker DP, et al. CSF brain creatine kinase levels and lactic acidosis in severe head injury. J Neurosurgery 1986;65:625-29.
34. Woolf PD, Hamill RW, Lee LA, et al. The predictive value of catecholamines in assessing outcome in traumatic brain injury. J Neurosurg 1987;66:875-82.
35. Lam AM, Winn HR, Cullen BF, et al. Hyperglycemia and neurological outcome in patients with head injury. J Neurosurg 1991;75:545-51.
36. Crone KR, Lee KS, Kelly DL J. Correlation of admission of fibrin degradation products with outcome and respiratory failure in patients with severe head injury. Neurosurgery 1987;21:532-6.
36a. Harrigan MR. Cerebral Salt Wasting. Crit Care Clin 2001;17:125-138.
36b. Zafonte RD, Mann NR. Cerebral Salt Wasting Syndrome in brain injury patients: A potential cause of hyponatremia. Arch Phys Med Rehabil 1997;78:540.
36c. Peterson B, Khanna S, Fisher B, et al. Prolonged hypernatremia controls elevated pressure in head injured pediatric patients. Crit Cave Med 2000;28:1136-43.
37. Braakman R, Avezaat CJJ, Maas AIR, et al. Interobserver agreement in the assessment of the motor response of the Glasgow coma scale. Clin Neurol Neurosurg 1977;80:100-6.
38. Teasdale G, Knill-Jones R, Van der Sande J. Observer variability in assessing impaired consciousness and coma. J Neurol Neurosurg Psychiat 1978;41:603-10.
39. Jane JA, Rimel RW. Prognosis in head injury. Coo Neurosurg 1982;29:346.
40. Born JD, Albert A, Hans P, et al. Relative prognostic value of best motor response and brainstem reflexes in patients with severe head injury. Neurosurgery 1985;16:595-601.
41. Jennett B, Snoek J, Bond MR, et al. Disability after severe head injury observations on the use of the Glasgow outcome scale. J Neurol Neurosurg Psychiat 1981;44:285-93.
42. Heiden JS, Small R, Caton W, et al. Severe Head Injury. Clinical assessment and outcome. Phys Ther 1983;63: 1946-51.
43. Bricolo A, Turazzi S, Feriotti G. Prolonged post-traumatic unconsciousness. Therapeutic assets and liabilities. J Neurosurg 1980;52:625-34.
44. Bond MR. Assessment of the psychosocial outcome of severe head injury. Acta Neurochir (Wien) 1976;34:57-70.
45. Wagner AK, Sassor He, Hammond FM, et al. Internal traumatic brain injury: Epidemiology, risk factors and association of injury severity and outcome. J Trauma 2000;49:404-10.
46. Catala-Temprano A, Claret Teruel G, Cambralasaosa FJ, et al. ICP and CPP as risk factors in children with TBI. J Neurosurg 2007;106(6 Suppl):463-6.
47. White H, Venkalesh B. Cerebral perfusion pressure in neurotrauma: a review. Anesth Analog 2008;107(3):979-88.

23 Improving Outcome after Traumatic Brain Injury

P Sarat Chandra

INTRODUCTION

In the past, the outcome from serious head injury was often dismal. There has been however research and development in the last 25 years that has significantly changed the management and outcome of head injuries. These include a better understanding in the anatomy, physiology, pathology and biochemical changes at the cellular level. Each aspect is briefly discussed.

Anatomy of Injury-Imaging the Injured Brain

By far the most important single advance was the introduction of cross-sectional imaging of the head in the 1970s (computed axial tomography). This led the clinician to see into the brain, identify normal and abnormal structures, and plan treatment with confidence.[1,2] Magnetic resonance imaging (MRI) has so far had less impact in the management of head injury because of the practical difficulties of getting MR images in an acutely injured patient. However, it can provide more detail about structural brain damage.[3,4] This may become useful for predicting specific residual deficits on which rehabilitative efforts can be targeted.

Physiology of Injury-Measuring Neurological Disturbance

Clinicians need a reliable method to quantify disturbed neurological function after head injury, and to monitor its progress. The Glasgow coma scale (GCS)[5] is simple and practical. Its worldwide adoption over the last 30 years underlines its usefulness with some limitations in clinical practice.[6-8]

Pathology of Injury Understanding Events in the Injured Brain

Concepts of 'secondary' brain damage is the end result of biochemical and pharmacological cascades which begin in the brain at the moment of injury.[9-12] The anatomical basis of primary brain damage is mechanical disruption of neurons and the cerebral microcirculation at the time of injury, varying from contusions to diffuse axonal injury.[13] Neuropathological study of fatal head injury cases has shown that often, traumatic brain damage is the result of events which occur after the time of injury and which may therefore, be preventable.[13] Secondary brain damage the 'second insult' has commanded much attention over the last 25 years. Jennett's group described head-injured patients who 'talked and died', whose death was due to causes other than overwhelming primary brain damage.[14] They turned the spotlight on to raised intracranial pressure (ICP) from hematoma or brain swelling and identified 'avoidable factors' which had caused or contributed to the death of these patients: delay in evacuating hematomas; uncontrolled intracranial infection or epilepsy; and failure to correct systemic hypoxia, hypercarbia, and shock.[15-17]

The aim is to define what should and should not be done, in the early hours and days after injury, in order to optimize the outcome. It is now well known that inadequate oxygen supply to the injured brain is often associated with reduced cerebral blood flow and a rise in ICP.[18] Mechanically injured neurons are highly susceptible to hypoxic-ischemic damage. The depth and duration of the insult determine the extent and reversibility of this damage.[19]

Biochemistry of Injury-Analyzing the Chemical Environment

The last decade had seen an explosion in our understanding of the biochemical cascades, which follow brain injury. Injured neurons can be further compromised by the action of metabolites and ions in their immediate environment. Depolarization by excitotoxic neurotransmitters, degradation of phospholipid membranes, inflammatory tissue changes, and disruption of the regulatory mechanisms for transmembrane sodium and calcium ion transport can further damage the injured neurons and worsen clinical outcome.[9-13] Brain is especially prone to tissue damage induced by free radicals. The lipid membranes, rich in cholesterol and polysaturated fatty acids are the primary targets for such damage. Iron, which is abundant in brain, is the most likely initiator of free radicals in brain injury. Superoxide anion, hydrogen peroxide and hydroxyl radicals are the most destructive of the free radicals known. A number of compounds like mannitol, ascorbic acid, vitamin E, glutathione peroxidase, barbiturates, dimethyl-sulfoxide deferoxamine and catalase have been shown to act as free radical scavengers and have neuroprotective properties.[9-13,20-25] The search for better neuroprotective agents is still on.

RESUSCITATION AND TRANSFER

Initial resuscitation plays the most important role in the final outcome of head injuries. Hypoxemia, hypercarbia, and hypovolemic shock are potent causes of avoidable death and disability after injury independent of the patient's conscious level and the CT scan findings.[18-21] Some complications of head injury carry a high-risk of hypoxemia and hypercarbia: uncontrolled seizures, inadequate breathing, and obstruction of the airway by vomitous, blood or dentures.[17] Victims of high velocity injuries such as road accidents and falls from a height often suffer serious blood loss from major extracranial injuries.[26,27] To miss or underestimate these injuries puts the patient at substantial risk of hypovolemic shock and secondary brain damage.[28]

The risk to the airway is closely related to the patient's conscious level, and it is now widely accepted that the only effective way to protect the airways of a patient who is unconscious (or nearly so) is by the endotracheal intubation and ventilation. Optimal ventilation of the patient is thus very essential. The pCO_2 should be maintained at 30 to 35 mm Hg. Hyperventilation has not been found to be very useful because it causes vasoconstriction and can exacerbate ischemia. In patients with a seriously altered conscious level, the airway can become obstructed at any time accident scene, ambulance, emergency department, ward, intensive care or neurosurgical unit. Oxygenation must be guaranteed at every stage. Bringing the doctor or paramedic to the scene of the accident can secure the airway early on, but it is now generally accepted that a severely injured patient cannot be fully stabilized in the field, so quick shifting of the patient to the nearest hospital or airlifting is advocated to reduce time of transportation. Seriously head injured patients remain liable to develop airway obstruction and hypoxemia even after arrival at the hospital, especially when moved between the departments or taken to another hospital for the CT scanning or specialist treatment.[23] Complications often follow suboptimal management of the airway before and during transfer to the neurosurgical unit, and recognition of this had led to improved airway care and arrangements for quick transfer, and improved outcome. Overall the ABC (airways, breathing, and circulation) must be given the top priority while resuscitating the patient.[24,25] In patients who do not require surgery, i.e. with diffuse axonal injuries, diffuse contusions or small contusions or hematomas, intracranial pressure monitoring may be performed using a subarachnoid bolt or an intraparenchymal pressure monitoring device. If the pressures are continuously high (> 20 mm Hg) various maneuvers like brain decongestants (mannitol, frusemide), thiopentol infusion (barbiturate coma), and ventricular drainage may be performed. Some surgeons have advocated decompressive craniotomies but its usefulness is still to be documented.[24-28]

Post-traumatic transtentorial herniation and intractable intracranial hypertension are ominous signs. Aggressive procedure such as lobectomies may help few of these patients. Among the study of different risk factors other than age, gender, mechanism, hypotensions, initial GCS score and other injuries, it was the blunt trauma which had significantly higher mortality in lobectomy group also. A logistic regression analysis identified blunt, trauma low GCS score and frontal lobectomy as independent risk factors for poor outcome. The servival and functional outcome after lobectomy in sever head injury group are acceptable.[42]

Concepts of Rehabilitation

This process involves the disabled person and his/her family and has to go beyond the confines of physical disease and must deal with the psychological consequences of physical disability and with the social milieu in which the disabled person has to operate. Modern rehabilitation practice is based around the concepts of impairment, disability and handicap as outlined by the World Health Organization (WHO) in 1980 (Table 23.1).

Against the above background it can be seen that the *rehabilitation is an active and dynamic process*, which assists the disabled person to acquire the necessary knowledge and skills, in order to maximize, their own physical, psychological, and social function. Rehabilitation uses three basic approaches: (i) approaches to reduce disability; (ii) approaches designed to acquire new skills and strategies that will reduce the impact of disability; and (iii) approaches that help to alter the environment, both physical and social, so that a given disability carries as little handicap as possible.[29-32]

Table 23.1: WHO's international definition classification of impairment, disability and handicap, Geneva 1980

a. *Impairment:* Any loss or abnormality of psychological, physiological or anatomical structure of function.
b. *Disability:* Any restriction or lack of activity resulting from an impairment to perform an activity in the range considered normal for people of the same age, sex and culture.
c. *Handicap:* A disadvantage for a given individual resulting from impairment or disability that limits or prevents the fulfillment of a role that would otherwise be normal for that individual.

Goal Setting

Some disabled individuals will wish to take a major leading role in developing their own rehabilitation goals, while others will wish to take a more passive role and reply on the expertise of the team. Whichever approach is adopted, realistic goal setting is the key to a good quality rehabilitation prograrm.[29-32]

Setting of Rehabilitation

Rehabilitation should start as early as possible. Regrettably, muscle contractures, pressure sores and unnecessary aggressive behavior are not unusual. If the rehabilitation team can be involved in the early stage, even on the intensive care unit, then it is more likely that such complications can be avoided. The recovery curve is steepest in the first-three months or so after injury and it is important to capitalize as much as possible on this phase of rapid improvement. Outpatient or day care center rehabilitation should continue at least until physical recovery has plateaued. Thus, long-term support, or at least the ability to contact the head injury team, should be maintained for sometimes after discharge and probably at least for two years.

SEVERE PHYSICAL DISABILITY

The long-term problems of traumatic brain injury will tend to be cognitive intellectual, behavior and emotional difficulties rather than the physical problems. This has been confirmed by a number of studies.[33,34] Spasticity can be particularly troublesome after traumatic brain injury and, if not treated aggressively, can often lead to muscle contracture and a functionally useless limb. Passive stretching in the acute phase is important as may be the use of orthoses or even serial splinting and casts in order to prevent such contracture. Botulinum toxin injection has been also found useful.[35,36] *Heterotopic ossification* is fortunately unusual but, nevertheless, a troublesome and irritating complication which remains rather difficult to treat effectively.[37] The onset is usually 1 to 4 months after injury and sings will include a decreased range of movement.[3] *Nutrition* is a particular problem. The reasons are two-fold an increased catabolic rate immediately after brain trauma compounded by the common occurrence of swallowing difficulties. If maintenance of good nutritional status is difficult, then fine bore percutaneous endoscopic gastrostomy (PEG) tube should inserted. This is a relatively simple and straight forward procedure with few complications.[23] *Pressure sores* themselves remain unfortunately rather common and are nearly always avoidable. Rigid adherence to regular turning regimens, as well as the use of appropriate pressure relieving mattresses, and to appropriate lifting and handling techniques should avoid the occurrence of pressure sores.[38]

Fecal and urinary incontinence can also be troublesome after head injury. Whilst in the short-term indwelling catheterization is useful, in the long-term, this is a most undesirable solution. If there remains impairment of bladder emptying then the technique of clean intermittent self-catheterization can be invaluable either performed by the patient or sometimes by an appropriate caretaker.[39] Language problems can be troublesome after brain injury. Thus, an assessment by a speech therapist is important and various speech and language interventions can obviously be of benefit, particularly for dysarthria and dysphagia.[40]

Cognitive and Intellectual Problems

These are a whole variety of important cognitive impairments that can follow a head injury.[40,41] The most common are those associated with attention deficits, problems with concentration, memory, perception, and information processing speed and problem solving. Natural recovery of neuropsychological difficulties can take place over a prolonged period of time and certainly up to two years post-injury.

Persistent Coma and Vegetative State

Fortunately there are very few individuals who remain in prolonged coma or vegetative state following brain injury. One study[41] found that 0.6 percent of all brain injured individuals admitted to a neurosurgical unit remained in prolonged coma (of more than 2 weeks duration). Care certainly needs to be taken in the early diagnosis of coma or vegetative state as later recovery has clearly been documented. Prolonged reassessment is necessary in order to ensure that some form of cognitive recovery is not taking place. Obviously, the best long-term outcome, in those of working age, is to return to the pre-accident employment situation.

CHALLENGES IN MANAGEMENT OF HEAD INJURIES

Despite many advances, prevention of head injuries still remains the best solution. There are still many gross limitations in management of head injuries. The challenges are many: *miles to go before we sleep*.

There are still no clear-cut insights into the pathophysiological basis of head injuries. Despite several advances, the pathology still remains complex and difficult to understand. Various aspects of pathology like the 'diffuse brain swelling' are still not understood completely. All the present advances have been structured to prevent or minimize the secondary injury. It is still not possible to treat or reverse the primary injury, as the brain has little or no capacity to regenerate. A lot of basic research is emerging the usefulness of functional imaging for head injuries, the introduction of various neuroprotective agents, and the use of fetal transplants for neuroregeneration. It remains to be seen that how much of this basic research can be effectively and practically translated into clinical practice. There still remain a lot of lacunae in management in terms of mobilization of adequate task force, quick transport facilities, and optimal rehabilitation, all of which add to long-term favorable recovery.

REFERENCES

1. Ambrose J, Gooding M, Uttley D. EMI scan on the management of head injuries. Lancet I 1976;847-8.
2. French BN, Dublin AB. The value of computerized tomography in the management of 1000 consecutive head injuries. Surg Neurol 1977;7:171-83.
3. Hadely DM, Teasdale GM, Jenkin A, et al. Magnetic resonance imaging in acute head injury. Clin Radiol 1988;39:131-9.
4. Mittl RL, Grossman RI, Hiehle JF, et al. Prevalence of MR evidence of diffuse axonal injury in patients with mild head injury and normal head CT findings. Am J Neurol Rad 1994;15:1583-9.
5. Teasdale GM, Jennett B. Assessment of coma and impaired consciousness. Lancet ii 1974;81-4.
6. Teasdale G, Knill-Jones R, Vander Sande J. Observer variability in assessing impaired consciousness and coma. J Neurol Neurosurg Psychiatry 1978;41:603-10.
7. Bardt TF, Unterberg AW, Kiening KL, Schneider GH, Lanksch WR. Multimodal cerebral monitoring in comatose head-injury patients. Acta Neurochir (Wien) 1998;140:357-65.
8. Prasad K. The Glasgow Coma Scale: A critical appraisal of its clinimetric properties. J Clin Epidemiol 1996; 24:362-72.
9. Povlishock JA, Christman CW. The pathobiology of traumatically induced axonal injury in animals and humans: a review of current thoughts. J Neurotrauma 1995;12:555-64.
10. Mexwell WL, Povlishock JT, Graham DI. A mechanistic analysis of non-disruptive axonal injury: a review. J Neurotrauma 1997;14:419-40.
11. Katayama Y, Becker DP, Tamura T, Hovda DA. Massive increases in extracellular potassium and the indiscriminate release of glutamate following concussive brain injury. J Neurosurg 1990;73:889-900.
12. Faden AI, Demediuk P, Panter SS, et al. The role of excitatory amino acids and NMDA receptors in traumatic brain injury. Science 1989;244:798-800.
13. Adams JH. The neuropathology of head injuries. In: Vinken PJ, Bruyn G (Eds). Handbook of Clinical Neurology, Vol 23. Amsterdam: North Holland 1975;35.
14. Reilly PL, Asams JH, Graham KL, Jennett B. Patient with head injury. Who talk and die. Lancet ii 1975;375-7.
15. Rose J, Valtonen S, Jennett B. Avoidable factors contributing to death after head injury. BMJ ii 1977;615.
16. Jennett B, Carlin J. Preventable mortality and morbidity after head injury. Injury 1978;10:1-39.
17. Gentleman D, Jennett B. Hazards of inter-hospital transfer of comatose head injured patients. Lancet ii 1981;853-5.
18. Miller JD, Sweet RC, Narayan RK, Becker DP. Early insults to the injured brain. JAMA 1978;240:439-42.
19. Ishige N, Pitts LH, Hashimoto T, Nishimura MC, Bartkowski HM. Effect of hypoxia on traumatic brain injury in rats. Neurosurgery 1987;20:848-53.
20. McIntosh TK. Novel pharmacologic therapies in the treatment of experimental traumatic brain injury: a review. J Neurotrauma 1993;10:215-61.
21. Harders A, Kakarieka A, Braakman R, and the German. Subarachnoid Hemorrhage Study Group. Traumatic subarachnoid hemorrhage and its treatment with nimodipine. J Neurosurg 1996;85:82-9.
22. Gorio A. Gangliosides as a possible treatment affecting neuronal repair processes. Adv Neurol 1998;47:523-30.
23. Andrews PJD, Piper IR, Dearden NM, et al. Secondary insults during intrahospital transport of head-injured patients. Lancet 1990;335:327-30.
24. Vyvyan HAL, Kee S, Bristow A. A survey of secondary transfers of head injured patients in the south of England. Anaesthesia 1991;46:395-7.
25. Lambert SM, Willett K. Transfer of multiple injured patients for neurosurgical opinion: a study of the adequacy of assessment and resuscitation. Injury 1993;24: 333-6.
26. McLaren CAN, Robertson C, Little K. Missed orthopaedic injuries in the resuscitation room. JR Coll Surg Edinb 1983;28:399-401.

27. Gentleman D, Teasdale G, Murray L. Cause of severe head injury and risk of complications. BMJ 1996;292: 449.
28. Piek J, Chesnut RM, Marshall LF, et al. Extracranial complications of severe head injury. J Neurosurg 1992;77:901-7.
29. Wade DT, Collin C. The Barthel ADL index: a standard measure of physical disability? Int Dis Studies 1988;10: 64-7.
30. Granger CV, Hamilton BB, Sherwin FS. Guide for the Use of the Uniform Data set for Medical Rehabilitation. New York: Buffalo General Hospital 1986.
31. Turner-Stokes K, et al. The Northwick Park Dependence scale—a measure of nursing dependency, which translates into care, needs in the community. Clin Rehabil 1998;12:304-18.
32. Semlyen JK, Summers SJ, Barnes MP. The predictive validity of the Newcastle Independence Assessment form Research (NIAF-R): Further development of an alternative measure. J Neurol Rehabil 1997;11:213-8.
33. Mckinlay WW, Brooks DN, Bond LR, et al. The short-term outcome of severe blunt head injury as reported by relatives of the injured persons. J Neurol Neurosurg Psychiatry 1981;44:527-33.
34. Oddy M, Humphrey M, Uttley D. Stresses upon the relatives of head injured patients. Br J Psychiatry 1978;133:507-13.
35. Simpson DM, Alexander DN, O'Brien CF, et al. Botulinum toxin type A in the treatment of upper extremity spasticity: a randomized, double-blind, placebo controlled trial. Neurology 1996;46:1306-10.
36. Yablon SA, Agana BT, Ivanhoe CB, et al. Botulinum toxin in severe upper extremity spasticity among patients with traumatic brain injury: an open labelled trial. Neurology 1996;47:939-44.
37. Rogers RC. Heterotopic ossification in severe head injury: a preventive program. Brain Inj 1988;2:163-73.
38. Bader DL (Ed). Pressure Sores-Clinical Practice and Scientific Approach. London: MacMillan 1990.
39. Lipides J, Diokno AC, Lowe BS, et al. Follow-up on sterile, intermittent self-catheterisation. J Urol 1974;111:184-7.
40. Brooks DN. Closed Head Injury: Psychological, Social and Family Consequences. Oxford: Oxford University Press 1984.
41. Briccolo A, Turazzi S, Feriotti G. Prolonged post-traumatic unconsciousness. J Neurosurg 1980;52:625-34.
42. Oncel D, Demetriades D, Gruen P, Salim A, et al. Brain lobectomy for severe head injury is not hopeless procedure. J trauma 2007;63(5):1010-3.

24 Extradural Hematoma

AK Mahapatra, Raj Kumar

INTRODUCTION

Extradural hematoma (EDH) is a collection of blood between the dura and the skull bone. Incidence of extradural hematoma inpatients admitted to the hospital for head injury ranges between one to three percent.[1,2] In patients with GCS scores of 8 or less at admission the frequency of extradural hematoma can be as high as 9 percent.[3]

Extradural hematomas commonly occur between the ages of 10 to 40 years.[4] EDH are rare over the age 60 years because of close adherence of the dura to the inner table of the skull. It is commonly found in males (M:F ratio is 4:1).

The usual sites of occurrence for epidural hematomas are temporal (62–80%) and frontal (7–18%).[5] The other sites for EDH are middle fossa, parieto-occipital region, parasagittal region, and the posterior fossa.

The type of trauma that cause EDH are the same as those that cause other types of head injuries, i.e. falls, vehicular accidents, and assault.[6,7]

PATHOGENESIS

Following impact, the skull bends which can result in stripping of dura from the inner table of the skull. This bending of skull can also result in fracture of the skull. Skull bending, dural stripping and fractured skull are sufficient to cause vascular tears. The vascular tears cause bleeding into areas created by stripping of dura from the inner table of skull and the dura is further stripped by collecting extradural hematoma. Extradural hematomas are associated with **skull fractures** in more than 90 percent of patients.[5,8,8a] In children the incidence of associated fracture is lower owing to increased deformability of the skull in children.

The middle meningeal artery or vein is the most common source of bleeding in patients with extradural hematoma, responsible in over 80 percent of patients, followed by torn dural venous sinuses or **diploic veins** (Figs 24.1A and B). The hematomas are generally unilateral, and most are found in the temporal region.

Bilateral extradural hematomas have been reported, chiefly after assault injuries (Fig. 24.2).[8]

Associated Injuries

Extradural hematomas are associated with other intracranial injuries in 10 to 15 percent of cases.[5,9] In presence of associated intracranial injuries the mortality increases.

Clinical Manifestations

The clinical course of presentation of a patient with an extradural hematoma can take one of five patterns:[2-5]

1. Conscious throughout (8–24%).
2. Unconscious throughout (23–24%).
3. Initially unconscious and subsequently recovered (20–28%).
4. Initially conscious, followed by loss of consciousness (14–21%).[2a,2b]
5. Initially unconscious followed by recovery followed by a second loss of consciousness (2–34%).

Pattern 5 represents the classic lucid interval which occurs in one-third or fewer patients with extradural hematomas and is not pathognomonic.[8] The most important single sign of a developing extradural hematoma is clouding of consciousness or progressive depression of the level of consciousness.

There are no definite symptoms of extradural hematomas. The triad of head injury with lucid interval, mydriasis on the side of a hematoma and contralateral paresis occurs only in 18 percent of cases and mainly in temporoparietal region.

The dilated and nonreactive pupil can be associated with ipsilateral hemiplegia. This is due to indentation of the contralateral cerebral peduncle by the edge of the tentorium cerebelli (Kernohan's notch).

Initially pupil on the side of extradural hematoma contracts due to irritation of the oculomotor nerve, the opposite pupil remains normal in size. In the next stage the ipsilateral pupil dilates due to paralysis of oculomotor nerve. Finally the pupils of both sides become dilated and fixed (Hutchinson's pupil). Paralysis of extraocular muscles supplied by oculomotor nerve occurs little after pupillary changes as pupillary fibers are more sensitive to pressure because of their peripheral arrangement in the oculomotor nerve.

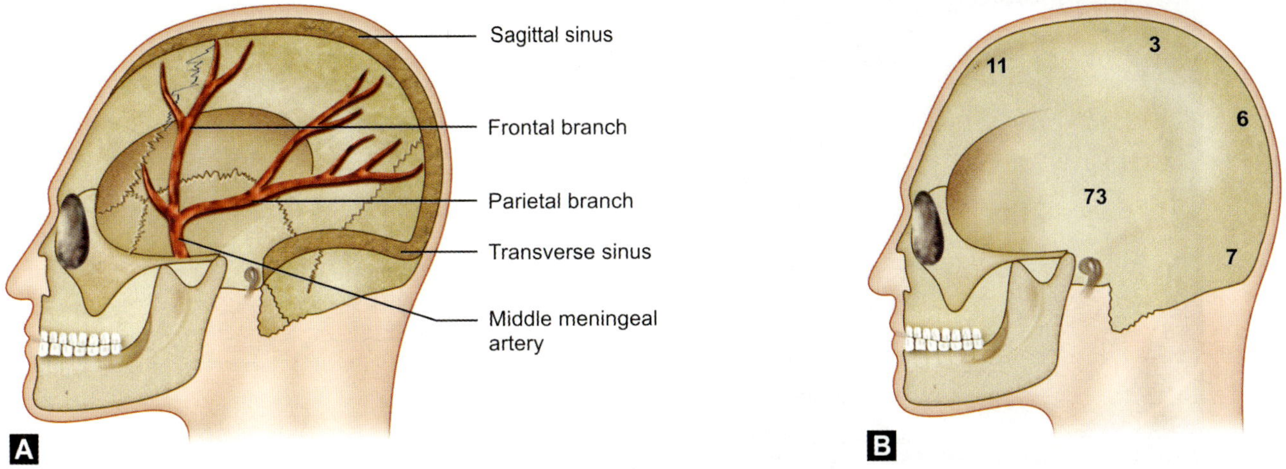

Figs 24.1A and B: (A) Distribution of vessels from which epidural hematomas may arise; (B) Percentage distribution of site of epidural hematoma

DIAGNOSIS OF ACUTE POST-TRAUMATIC EXTRADURAL HEMATOMA

The operative mortality for EDH is directly related to the **level of consciousness** at the time of surgery.[11,13] Hooper had analyzed the mortality from epidural hematoma in patients who had optimal management with rapid diagnosis and early surgery and had concluded that a mortality of less then 10 percent should be reasonable. The mortality of EDH removal in awake, neurologically intact individual should be essentially zero regardless of hematoma size or location, but mortality dramatically increases to 40 percent if the patient is allowed to deteriorate to coma.[3]

EDH deserves a high index of suspicion in every patient with head injury of any type. Any patient with history of head injury and altered sensorium should undergo CT evaluation. Any patient with an abnormal neurological examination, clouding of consciousness by alcohol or drugs, or who may be lost to follow-up examination should undergo CT scan of head (Fig. 24.3).

A CT head can safely and quickly rule out an EDH and identify associated intracranial lesions (Fig. 24.4).

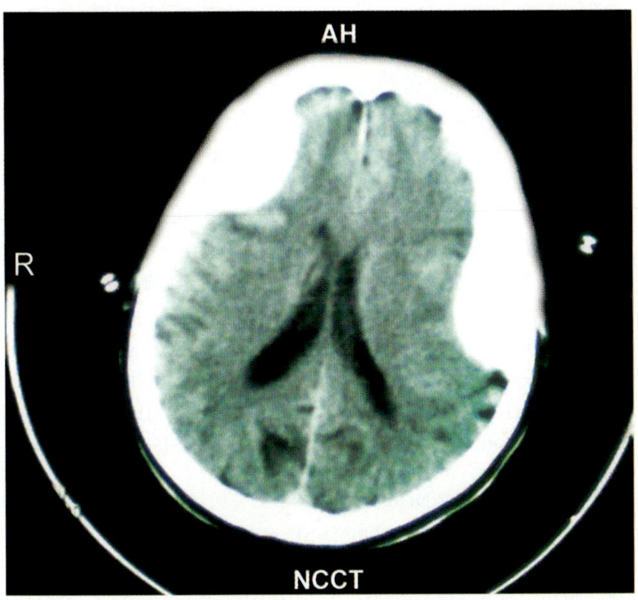

Fig. 24.2: Plain CT head depicting bifrontal extradural acute hematomas

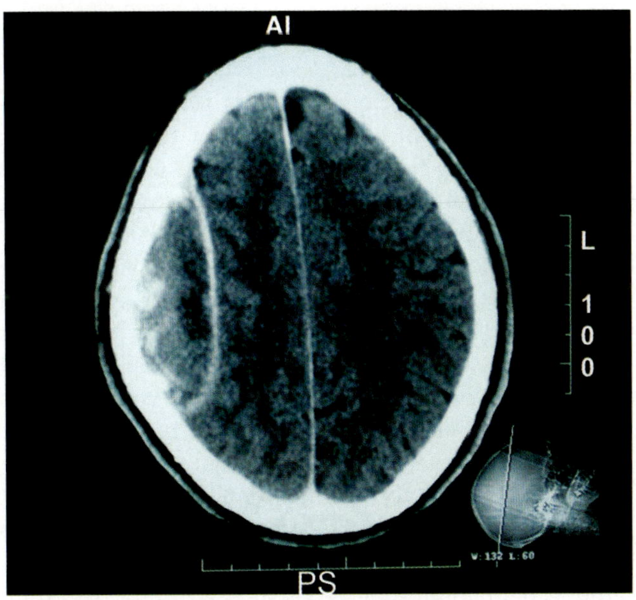

Fig. 24.3: CT showing extradural hematoma with fluid level in a patient with bleeding diasthesis

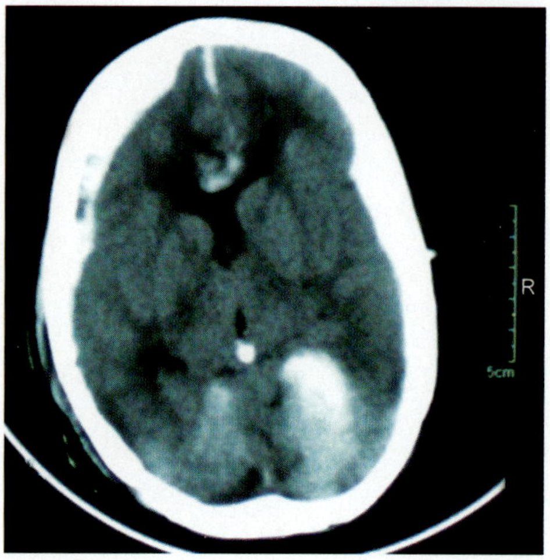

Fig. 24.4: CT showing right extradural hematoma, anterior corpus callosum bleed and large tentorial bleed, was better seen in lower cuts

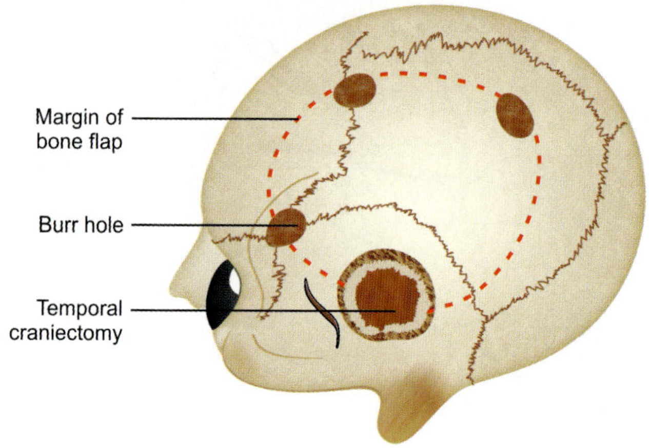

Fig. 24.5: Temporal craniectomy or bone flap

If a patient is admitted to a hospital without neurosurgeon or CT scanner then he should be immediately shifted to a hospital with these facilities.

Skull X-ray should be done in conscious patient, since the presence of skull fracture, increases the risk of an intracranial hematoma. Mendelow et al,[12] estimated that, for an alert patient without a skull fracture, the risk of developing an intracranial hematoma is about 1:6000, compared to 1:4 risk in a patient with an altered level of consciousness and a skull fracture. A fracture seen on skull X-ray is an indication of CT scan.

CT APPEARANCE

The acute extradural hematoma is a relatively stereotyped lesion. Because the dura mater tends to adhere to the skull, the hematoma is seen on CT sections as a dense area immediately beneath the skull vault, convex towards both the brain and the vault.

Conventionally acute extradural hematomas are described as biconvex lens-shaped hyperdense lesion on CT scan. The temporoparietal convexity is the most common site, in which the lesions are easily detected on axial sections (Fig. 24.5). Additional, coronal views may be necessary to identify the rare hematoma over the vertex. Large extradural hematoma may show significant mass effect with evidence of herniation.

A severe temporal lobe contusion may also obscure the EDH, although the temporal contusion or intracerebral hematoma may be of such size that operation would be performed regardless of the evidence of EDH.

TREATMENT OF ACUTE EXTRADURAL HEMATOMA

If a significant extradural hematoma is diagnosed on CT scanning with evidence of herniation or rapid neurological deterioration, then the patient should be directly taken to operation theater for immediate removal of hematoma. With strong clinical diagnosis of extradural hematoma urgent exploratory burr hole exploration is mandatory when CT scan is not available or will be delayed significantly and the patient is deteriorating fast neurologically with evidence of **transtentorial herniation.** For the patient who can be scanned rapidly and taken directly to the operating room, CT scanning is preferred to the placement of burr holes.

Patients who are conscious with no neurological deficit and who is discovered to have an extradural hematoma the necessity of surgical decompression can be questioned. Epidural hematoma may resolve on conservative treatment provided patient is under constant supervision with early detection of deterioration and operation. But this will result in prolonged stay in hospital. Such **conservative approach** should be avoided unless the hematoma is very small.

Epidural hematomas in newborn are rare, which occur more frequently in newborns that experienced difficult delivery from nulliparous mothers. Few of these can be managed conservatively also.[22]

Operative Technique

The classical epidural hematoma is due to the arterial bleeding from the middle meningeal artery and its branches. The patient should be placed on the operating table with the head positioned with the hematoma uppermost, and a skin and bone flap should

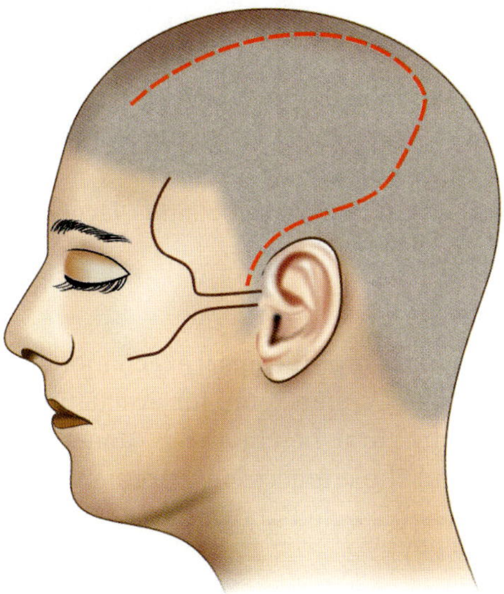

Fig. 24.6: Skin incision for removal of extradural hematoma

be fashioned that encloses the area of hematoma as much as possible.

The vertical incision is placed one inch anterior to the external acoustic meatus, is about 7 cm long, and reaches down to the zygomatic process. The incision should not go below the zygomatic process in order to prevent cutting the branches of the facial nerve which innervates the frontalis and orbicularis oculi muscles. The temporalis muscle and fascia are incised along their fibers and retracted by a self-retaining retractor. **A burr hole is made and enlarged with a rongeur (Figs 24.6 and 24.7).** The craniectomy is carried down to the floor of the temporal fossa and the hematoma is evacuated by suction. The burr

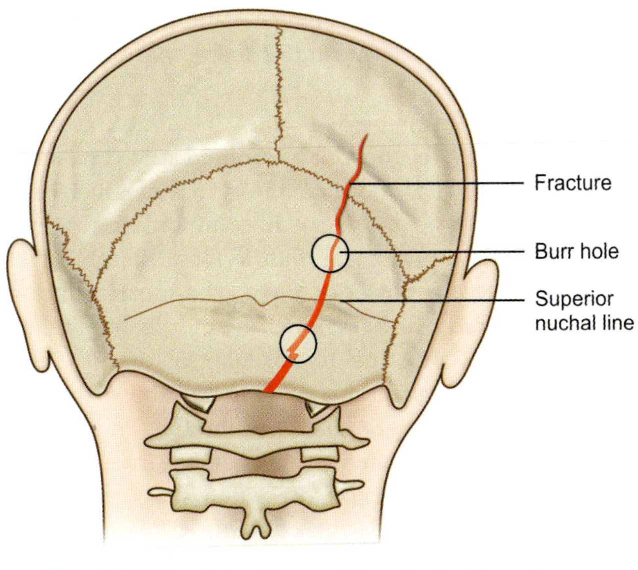

Fig. 24.7: Burr hole placement in extradural hematoma over occipital and suboccipital area

hole should be made as quickly as possible so that extradural hematoma is decompressed rapidly. This reduces ICP quickly, hence improves the outcome.

The single burr hole can be converted into a craniotomy flap with craniotome or by making a trephine.

If the **middle meningeal artery** lies just over the fracture site, it may be coagulated at this point or it may be necessary to coagulate it at the **foramen spinosum.** In some patients, the bleeding may originate directly from the foramen spinosum, with no visible artery available to coagulate. In these cases, foramen spinosum is plugged with bone wax for controlling the hemorrhage. Bleeding from fracture site will stop with application of bone wax.

After evacuation of clot and adequate hemostasis, a small incision in dura should be made to look acute subdural hematoma. The dura must be tacked securely around the perimeter of craniotomy or craniectomy **(Hitch stitches)**. One dural stitch can be placed near the middle of exposed dura which passes through the corresponding holes near the center of craniotomy flap.

A pilot study demonstrated that a thrombolytic evacuation of a post craniotomy EDH using closed suction drain is feasible without complication. 6 urokinase instillations lasting 12 hours or 12 urokinase instillations in 24 hours can be used depending on the thickness of EDH.[20]

OUTCOME OF PATIENTS WITH EXTRADURAL HEMATOMA

The mortality from epidural hematomas should be less than 10 percent.[12] However, in large series, the overall mortality for epidural hematomas ranges from 20 to 30 percent.[15-17] Mortality is higher in patients over 40 years of age. The outcome is directly related to the level of consciousness at the time of operation.

Patients who were conscious at the time of surgery had a mortality of 6.2 percent whereas in unconscious patients mortality may as high as 39 percent. Some authors have reported zero mortality rate in noncomatosed patients. Mortality also varies significantly with modes of presentation as studied by McKissock et al (Table 24.1).[5]

Table 24.1: Mode of presentation and mortality

Mode of presentation	*Mortality %*
1. Conscious throughout	0%
2. Unconscious throughout	57%
3. Initially unconscious and recovered	8%
4. Initially conscious, followed by loss of consciousness	29%
5. Initially unconscious followed by recovery followed by second loss of consciousness	27%

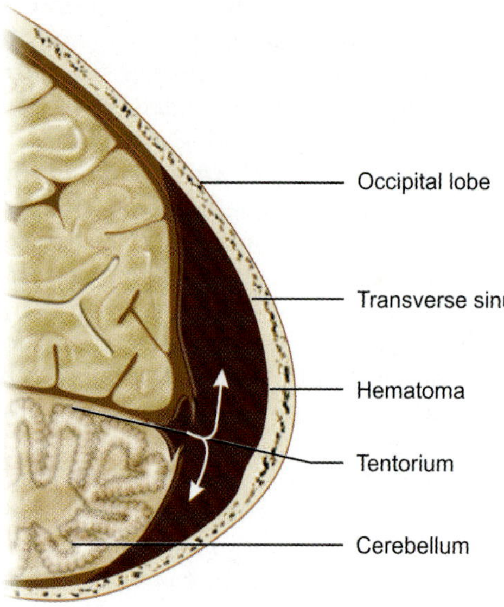

Fig. 24.8: Extradural hematoma over occipital and suboccipital area due to laceration of transverse sinus

Extradural hematomas in elderly patients have been known for poor prognosis. The elderly are less likely to manifest with clinical features of increased intracranial pressure due to cerebral atrophy, hematomas were seen in parietal region in one study. The postoperative results are found to be satisfactory with one death out of 14 operated elderly patients (with mean age 74 years).[21]

Posterior Fossa Extradural Hematoma

Extradural hematoma in the posterior fossa is the most frequently encountered traumatic mass lesion in the posterior fossa.[15,16] It occurs in 3 to 13 percent of all post-traumatic extradural hematomas. It is common in young adults. Extradural hematoma of posterior fossa is almost always associated with a **fracture of occipital bone** which extends towards foramen magnum, and usually crosses the **transverse sinus** (Fig. 24.8).

Clinically, deterioration may be rapid, with respiratory depression occurring without any pupillary change or motor signs. Headache, nausea, vomiting and stiffness are the most common signs.[16,17] The clue to the diagnosis is an occipital injury, such as occipital bone fracture, scalp laceration in the occipital region.[8a,19]

Superior Nuchal Line

Patient may present with classic lucid interval, but in acute cases, patients more commonly present with signs of brainstem compression of rapid onset.[17a]

Extradural clots in the posterior fossa may be recognized only when appropriate cuts are taken. Typical CT findings are those of a characteristic biconvex or lenticular area of increased density. These hematomas can extend above tentorium.

In these cases, a transverse sinus laceration has to be considered.

Management

Prompt diagnosis, rapid surgical evacuation is essential.

A suboccipital craniectomy for evacuation of posterior fossa extradural hematoma is done, but it may need to extend the craniectomy supratentorially if the hematoma has dissected above the level of transverse sinus (Fig. 24.8).

Operative Technique

The patient is placed in the prone position. The length of the skin incision is shown in Figure 24.8. The trapezium muscle is cut 1 cm below its insertion and parallel to the superior nuchal line and scraped off the occipital bone with periosteal elevator. Two burr holes are made above and below the superior nuchal line. (The superior nuchal line corresponds to the transverse sinus). The burr holes are enlarged by a rongeur. The extradural hematoma is removed by suction and irrigation. Bleeding from sinus is usually controlled by placing surgicel and gelfoam. Dural sagging sutures are placed.

CONCLUSION

Early diagnosis and surgical intervention have reduced the mortality rate from posterior fossa epidural hematoma.[17,18]

Extradural hematoma occurs in about one to three percent of the hospital admitted cases of acute head injury. EDH is more common in males between the ages of 10 and 40 years. It commonly occurs in temporal, frontal and basal middle fossa. Rarely EDH may be present in posterior fossa. The most common source of extradural hematoma is middle meningeal artery. EDH occurs due to vascular tear and dural stripping following trauma. EDH should be suspected in patients with progressive deterioration in level of consciousness and patients with lucid interval. CT scan is the investigation of choice and shows biconvex lenticular hyperdense lesion on plain CT head. Early diagnosis and quick surgical evacuation is key to good

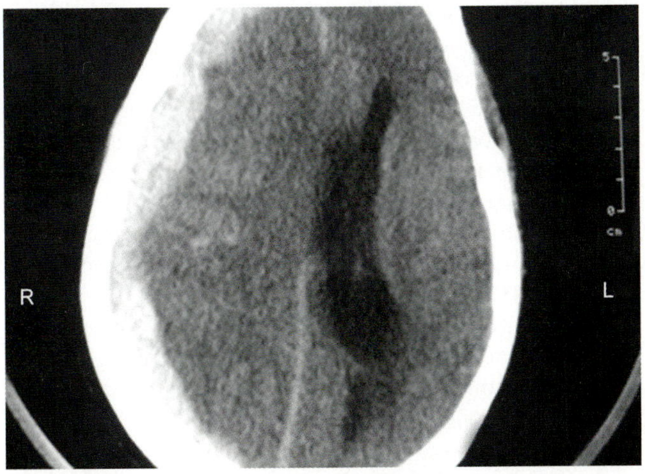

Fig. 24.9: CT showing acute subdural hematoma

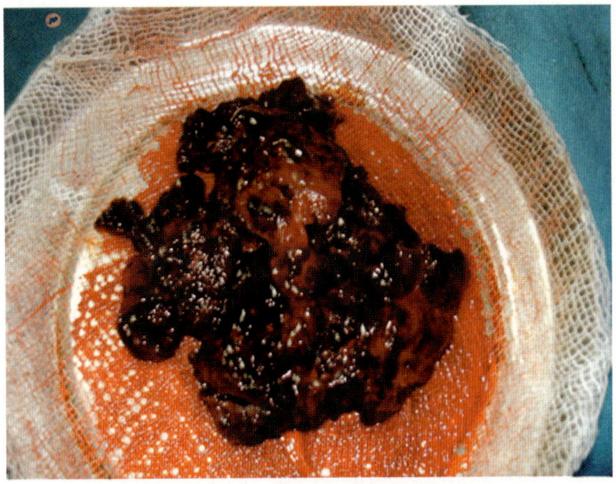

Fig. 24.11: Acute subdural hematoma evacuated

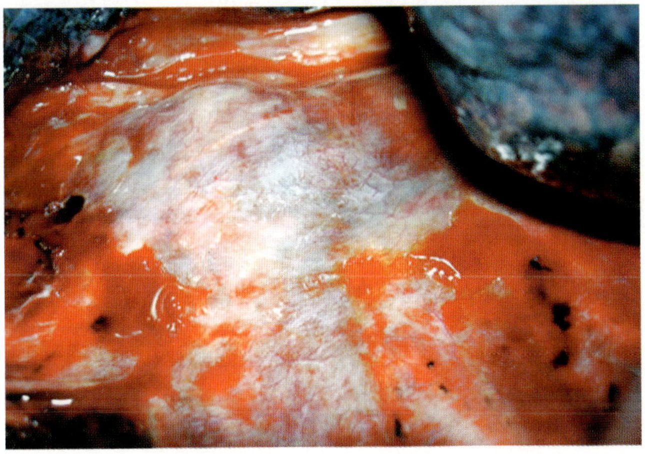

Fig. 24.10: Dura tense on exploration of acute subdural hematoma

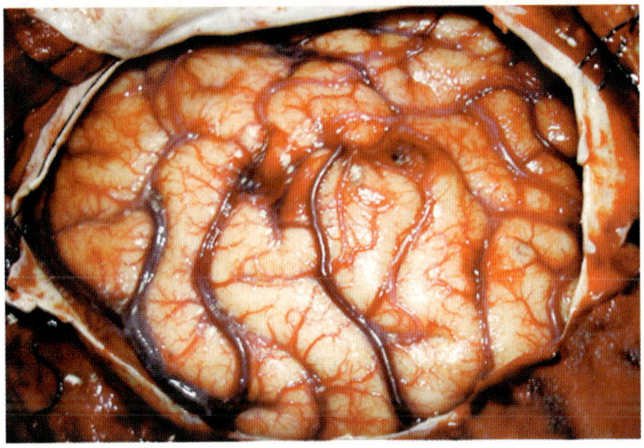

Fig. 24.12: Brain lax following removal of acute subdural hematoma

result. Outcome depends on the level of consciousness at the time of operation, and associated brain and systemic injuries.

REFERENCES

1. Cordobes F, Lobata RD, et al. Observation on 82 patients with extradural hematoma. J Neurosurg 1981;54:179-86.
2. Jamieson KG, Yelland JDN. Extradural hematoma. Report of 167 cases. J Neurosurg 1968;28:13-23.

2a. Eisenberg HM, Gary HE Jr, Aldrich EF, et al. Initial CT Finding in 753 patients with severe head injury. A report from NIH Traumatic Coma Bank. J Neurosurg 1990;73:88-98.

2b. Gusmao SN, Pittella JE. Extradural hematoma and DA, in victims of fatal road traffic accidents. Br J Neurosurg 1998;12:123-26.

3. Seelig JM, Marshall LF, et al. Traumatic acute epidural-haematoma: Unrecognized high lethality in comatose patients. Neurosurg 1984;15:617-20.
4. Heiskanen O. Epidural haematoma. Surg Neurol 1975; 4:23-6.
5. Mc Kissock W, Taylor JC, Bloom WH, et al. Extradural haematoma. Observations on 125 cases. Lancet 1960;1:167-72.
6. Cook RJ, Dorsch NWC, et al. Outcome prediction in extradural hematomas. Acta Neurochir (Wien) 1988; 95:90-94.
7. Gutman MB, Moulton RJ, Sullivan I, et al. Risk factors predicting operable intracranial haematomas in head injury. J Neurosurg 1992;77:9-14.
8. Samudrala S, Cooper P. Traumatic intracranial haematomas In: Wilkins R, Rengachary S Neurosurgery, New York: McGraw Hill 1997:2797-807.

8a. Gupta PK, Mahapatra AK, Lad SD. Posterior fossa extradural haematoma. The Oman experience. Pan Arab J Neurosurg 2001;5:1-7.

9. Subramaniam MV, Rajendra Prasad G, Dibbala Rao B. Bilateral extradural haematoma. Br J Surg 1975;62:5.

10. Jaya Kumar PN, Sastry KVR, et al. Prognosis in centre coup intracranial haematomas a clinical and radiological study of 63 patients. Acta Neurodrir (Wien) 1991;108:30-3.
11. Gallaghar JP, Browder EJ. Extradural haematoma. Experience with 167 patients. J Neurosurg 1968;29:1.
12. Mendelow AD, Teasdale G, Jennett B, et al. Risks of intracranial haematoma in head injured adults. Br Med J 1983;287:1173-6.
13. Kvarnes T, Trumpy JH. Extradural haematoma. Report of 132 cases. Acta Neurochir (Wien), 1978;41:223-31.
14. Hooper RS. Observations on extradural hemorrhage. Br J Surg 1959;47:71-87.
15. Hooper RS. Extradural hemorrhages of the posterior fossa. Br J Surg 1954;42:19-26.
16. Tsai FY, Teal JS, et al. Computed tomography of posterior fossa trauma. J Compute Assistant Tomogr 1980;4:291-305.
17. Stone JL, Schaffer L, et al. Epidural haematomas of the posterior fossa. Surg Neurol 1979;11:419-24.
17a. Gupta PK, Mahapatra AK, Lad SD. Limitation in management of extradural haematoma and their remedy. Oman Medical Journal 2001;18:28-32.
18. Reigh EE, O' Connell TJ. Extradural haematoma of the posterior fossa with concomitant supratentorial subdural haematoma. Report of a case and review of literature. J Neurosurg 1962;19:359-64.
19. Mahapatra AK, Bhatia R, Banerji AK. Posterior fossa extradural haematoma. A report of 5 cases. Neurology India 1982;30:239-44.
20. Park J, Kim GJ, Hwang SK. Thrombolytic evacuation of postcraniotomy epidural hematomas using closed suction drain: a pilot study: Acta Neurochir (wien) 2008;150(4):359-66.
21. Hemlat A, Mazzon A, And M, et al. Intracranial epidural hematoma in elderly patients observation in 14 patients. Acta Neurochir 2005;147(10):1055-60.
22. Heyman R, Heckly A, Magagi J, Pladys P, Hamlet A. Intracranial epidural hematoma in newborn infants: Clinical study of 15 cases: Neurosurg 2005;57(5):924-9.

25 Posterior Fossa Extradural Hematoma

PK Gupta, AK Mahapatra

INTRODUCTION AND EPIDEMIOLOGY

Traumatic space occupying lesions of the posterior fossa are uncommon, however, extradural hematoma is probably the most common amongst them. It is seen in 0.1 to 0.3 percent of all head injury patients and 1.1 to 5.8 percent of all head injury patients requiring surgery.[1-4] It accounts for up to 10 percent of extradural hematoma in our experience.[5] Males are affected in almost 90 percent of the cases and this is primarily due to protected lifestyle of females. Mostly younger individuals are affected in their most productive life and it is rare in extremes of age, less than 2 years and more than 60 years, due to the dense adherence of the dura to the overlying bone. Two-thirds of our patients were in pediatric age group, less than 16 years of age.[6]

MODE OF INJURY

RTA and fall from height are the usual modes of injuries causing posterior fossa extradural hematoma (PFEDH). Though extradural hematomas (EDHs) are caused by trivial/minor injuries, slow traffic usually causes supratentorial EDH and PFEDH is less frequent due to protected location, smaller area and excessive bony reinforcement by stresses. High-speed traffic and severe impact is more often associated with PFEDH. Assault is yet another but uncommon mode of injury causing PFEDH.

PATHOGENESIS

Hematoma usually evolves slowly and takes 18 hours to few days to manifest. Hyperacute EDH in the posterior fossa is unusual as the bleeding is not arterial in most of the cases.

Usual source of bleeding is venous, i.e. dural sinuses or one of the draining veins and fracture hematoma. At some stage, bleeding stop due to the tamponade effect of the cerebellum. Hence, the patients take sometime to accumulate enough PFEDH to become symptomatic. Exceptionally, the source of bleeding is arterial. The occipital branch of the vertebral artery and distal branches of middle meningeal artery are usual blood vessel involved.[7-9] Source of bleeding is, identifiable in 60 to 65 percent of the patients only.[10,11] Once a significant volume gets accumulated, then the clinical course is rapid and catastrophic in most of the cases. Almost 50 to 60 percent of the cases presents within 18 to 24 hours (acute) following trauma. Remaining patients may present as subacute or even chronic (after 7 days). Hematoma may be confined to posterior fossa unilaterally or may extend to both the sides or may sometimes even extend into supratentorial compartments.[5] Bilateral separate PFEDH has been very infrequently reported.[12] Pediatric PFEDH is more often confined to posterior fossa whereas the PFEDH in adults tend to extend supratentorial.[13] Up to 40 percent of cases have associated intracranial pathology.[1,5,14]

CLINICAL PROFILE

Early symptoms and signs of PFEDH are uncertain and unpredictable. Patient can remain unconscious or conscious throughout, may have single or double lucid interval[15] or may remain conscious initially to lapse into unconsciousness later. A conscious patient may complain of persistent and severe occipital pain and persistent vomiting. Large numbers of patients have external evidence of occipital trauma. Battles sign may also indicate presence of ongoing PFEDH collection but it is not a common sign and has been reported in less than five percent of the cases.[5] Neurological examination of these patients may reveal papilledema as early as 6 to 8 hours due to acute hydrocephalus that may be missed in an unconscious patient unless specifically looked for. In chronic cases, the patient may present with classical symptoms and signs of cerebellar mass lesion. Rarely a patient may present with torticollis. In subacute cases, the clinical picture will be indistinct and only a thoughtful/fastidious clinician will be able to pick up the subtle signs and reach the diagnosis. Initial assessment has no bearing on the diagnosis, hence it is important to closely and continuously observe such patients. Evolution of localizing signs, failure to improve completely, persistent altered state of consciousness and persistent headache and vomiting are indications to further investigate such patients. Clinical deterioration once sets in, is usually rapid and even an asymptomatic significant PFEDH will not give time to act. Only prompt decompression can save the life and limit of the morbidity. However, small and insignificant PFEDH with no mass effect can still be treated conservatively and expectantly under close observation. High index of suspicion is essential to identify such cases in time.

In extradural posterior fossa hematomas, the vomiting may be a risk factor of acute clinical deterioration in occipital head trauma cases. The patients with occipital fracture and vomiting must be observed closely. An initial normal CT can miss the diagnosis.[21,22]

INVESTIGATIONS

In centers, where CT scanning is not a routine norm in the initial evaluation of head injury patients, X-ray of the skull (including the Towne's view) is a good screening investigation for radiological evaluation of such patient. Occipital fracture is noted in 55 to 100 percent of the cases when Towne's view is also included in the initial radiological assessment of the patient in best center.[1] A CT scan should evaluate a patient with occipital fracture, even though only 6 to 8 percent of occipital fractures are associated with PFEDH, irrespective of clinical status of the patient. CT scan is the most valuable investigation. CT scan helps in early diagnosis, as it is reliable and predictive and also shows associated intracranial pathologies in almost one-third of the cases. CT scan shows biconvex hyper/iso- or mixed density lesion besides compression of the cerebellum, shift of the IVth ventricle, compression of the brainstem and obstructive hydrocephalus involving both lateral and IIIrd ventricle and fracture of the occipital bone in bone windows. Compared to supratentorial EDH, PFEDH are usually less dense on CT scanning, more so in younger age group.[13] CT scan done soon after injury (within 6 hours of trauma), small EDH and a fracture overlying a vascular marking stands high chances of delayed deterioration due to hematoma enlargement and even if asymptomatic, CT scan should be repeated in them before expiry of 24 hours.[16] Rapidly evolving hydrocephalus and direct compression over the brainstem are the usual causes of mortality whereas associated intra- and extracranial lesions are primarily responsible for morbidity.[17]

TREATMENT/SURGERY

Posterior fossa extradural hemotoma (PFEDH) more than 15 mm in thickness, compressing and obliterating IVth ventricle causing obstructive hydrocephalus, poor visualization of the posterior fossa cisterns and compression of brainstem irrespective of GCS/ neurological status should be promptly evacuated to achieve good result.[18] Hematoma less than 15 mm in thickness, less than 10 ml in volume with a maximum of 5 mm shift of midline structures and no associated intracranial pathologies can still be observed but even mild deterioration in such situation warrants immediate evacuation of PFEDH.[19] Posterior fossa craniectomy with or without supratentorial craniotomy is necessary to evacuate a solid acute or subacute clot, however, a chronic PFEDH with liquid blood requites only a burr hole to drain out the fluid hematoma.

OUTCOME

Outcome is good provided the condition, is identified and treated in time, before any catastrophic deterioration occurs. Poor outcome is associated with delayed or missed diagnosis, poor primary neurological status, associated intra- and extracranial injuries and unstable cardiopulmonary functions.[5,17,20] Compared to supratentorial EDH, PFEDH has a poorer outcome. Noninvasive imaging techniques like CT and MR scanning has tremendously changed the prognosis in such patients, as they are identified well in time and treated, to an extent that now zero mortality has been obtained in these patients[5] at the cost of increasing morbidity due to associated lesions or poor primary neurological status.

Traumatic epidural hematoma of posterior cranial fossa (TEH PCF) are rare but have higher mortality than supratentorial hematomas. An early diagnosis and prompt surgical evacuation provides on excellent recovery. Active use of CT Scan in suspicious cases plays a major role in diagnosis.[23]

CONCLUSION

Posterior fossa EDH is a rare condition and constitutes less than 10 percent of cranial EDH. Clinical presentation is varied, however, diagnosis must be kept in mind in patients having impact over occipital or suboccipital region or in patients having radiological evidence of occipital fracture. A patient with an acute PFEDH is an acute neurosurgical emergency and if treated in time, can result in good outcome. CT scan has significantly facilitated early, prompt and appropriate diagnosis. Associated brain pathology, presence of an acute hematoma and acute hydrocephalus are few prognosticating factors. High index of suspicion, early diagnosis and prompt evacuation are the essential components of good outcome.

REFERENCES

1. Mahajan RK, Sharma BS, Khosla VK, Tewari MK, Mathuriya SN, Pathak A, Kak VK. Posterior fossa extradural haematoma. Annals Academy of Medicine 1993; 22:410-3.
2. Mahapatra AK, Bhatia R, Banerji AK. Posterior fossa extradural haematoma. Report of 5 cases. Neurology India 1982;30:239-44.
3. Sadik AR, Epstein FJ, Ransohoff J. Epidural haematoma of posterior fossa. NY State J Med 1978;78:801-3.
4. Thomas LM, Gurdjian ES. Intracranial haematomas of traumatic origin. In: Youmans JR (Ed), Neurological Surgery vol 2 Philadelphia: WB Saunders 1973;960-8.
5. Gupta PK, Mahapatra AK, Lad SD. Posterior fossa extradural hematoma an Oman experience. Pan Arab J Neurosurg 2001;5:1-7.
6. Gupta PK, Mahapatra AK, Lad SD. Pediatric posterior fossa extradural hematoma. Ind J pediatrics. In press.
7. Garza-Mercado R. Extradural haematomas of the posterior cranial fossa. J Neurosurg 1983;59:664-72.
8. Jamieson KG. Angiographic demonstration of bleeding points in posterior fossa extradural haematoma. J Neurosurg 1972;36:644-5.
9. Perot P, Ethier R, Wong A. An arterial posterior fossa extradural haematoma demonstrated by vertebral angiography. J Neurosurg 1967;26:255-60.
10. Koc RK, Pasaoglu A, Menku A, Oktem S, Meral M. Extradural haematomas of the posterior fossa. Neurosurg Rev 1998;21:52-7.
11. Holzschuh M, Schuknecht B. Traumatic epidural haematomas of the posterior fossa: 20 new cases and a review of the literature since 1961. Br J Neurosurg 1989;3:171-80.
12. Gelabert M, Prieto A, Allut AG. Acute bilateral extradural haematomas of the posterior cranial fossa. Br J Neurosurg 1997;11:573-5.
13. Suyama Y, Kajikawa H, Yamamura K, Sumioka S, Kajikawa M. Acute epidural haematoma of posterior fossa: comparative analysis between 20 cases in adults and 10 cases in children. No Shinkei Geka 1996;24:621-4.
14. Roda JM, Gimenez D, Perez-Higueras A, Blazquez MG, Perez-Alvarez M. Posterior fossa epidural haematomas: a review and synthesis. Surg Neurol 1983;19:419-24.
15. Parkinson D, Hunt B, Shields C. Double lucid interval in patients with extradural haematoma of the posterior fossa. J Neurosurg 1971;34:534-6.
16. Knuckey NW, Gelbard S, Epstein MH. The management of asymptomatic epidural haematomas. A prospective study 1989;70:392-6.
17. Kawakami Y, Tamiya T, Tanimoto, Shimamura Y, Hattori S, Veda T, Ishida T. Non-surgical treatment of posterior fossa epidural haematoma. Pediatr Neurol 1990;6:112-8.
18. Otsuka S, Nakatsu S, Matsumoto S, Sato S, Motozaki T, Ban S, Yamamoto T. Study on cases with posterior fossa epidural haematoma clinical features and indications for operation. Neurol Med Chir (Tokyo) 1990;30:24-8.
19. Wong CW. The CT criterion for conservative treatment but under close clinical observation of posterior fossa epidural haematoma. Acta Neurochir (Wien) 1994;126:124-7.
20. Pozzati E, Tognetti F, Cavallo M, Acciarri N. Extradural haematomas of the posterior cranial fossa. Surg Neurol 1989;32:300-3.
21. Faiz AU, Mahapatra AK. Intraoperative development of posterior fossa extradural hematoma during evacuation of frontal contusion Neurol. India 2006;54(2):219-20.
22. Hayashi T, Kameyama M, Imaizumi S, et al. Acute epidural hematoma of posterior fossa, case of acute clinical deterioration. Am J Emerg Med 2007;25(9):989-95.
23. Karasu A, Sabanchi PA, Izki N, Imer M, et al. Traumatic epidural hematoma of posterior fossa. Surg. Neurol 2008;69(3):247-51.

26 Acute Subdural Hematomas

Raj Kamal

INTRODUCTION

Subdural hematomas (SDHs) can be classified into:

1. Acute subdural hematoma presents within 48 to 72 hours of injury.
2. Subacute subdural hematoma between 3 and 20 days.
3. Chronic subdural hematoma presents from three weeks to several months.

Acute subdural hematoma: An acute subdural hematoma is a collection of fresh blood under the dura, which may compress the brain.

The source of acute subdural blood is bridging cortical vein near sagittal sinus, veins from sylvian fissure to sphenoparietal sinus, the inferior cerebral veins draining into the transverse and the superior petrosal sinuses.

EPIDEMIOLOGY

Acute SDH occurs in approximately 10 to 30 percent of patients with severe head injury.[1,1a] Males are much more likely to present with acute subdural hematomas than females. In 80 of acute SDH it is the extent of the underlying brain injury which determines the outcome.[2a] The reported male to female ratio varies from 3:1 to 6:1.[1] Falls and assaults are the most frequent mechanisms of injury associated with acute subdural hematomas. Older people have a greater risk of developing acute SDH, and the average age of patient with acute subdural hematoma is greater than other types of head injury.[3]

PATHOGENESIS

Acute subdural hematomas are caused by rupture of parasagittal or sylvian bridging veins draining into dural venous sinuses. Acute SDH result entirely from inertial forces. The parasagittal veins are susceptible to damage during short duration angular acceleration of the head as they are superficially located.[4] Rarely, acute SDH can be due to rupture of cortical artery.[4a] Matsumaya et al[4a] in 1997 reported a series of 19 cases of SDH due to arterial rupture.

When the head strikes a broad, hard surface (as in fall), the impact energy causes brain to accelerate within the skull. The strain that occurs during these conditions is confined to the surface, if the acceleration is present for a brief period of time. The types of injury that can be produced in these circumstances are those at the brain surface and those to vascular tissue (bridging veins). If the duration of acceleration is prolonged, the strains penetrate deeper into brain and cause *diffuse axonal injury (DAI)*. Hence, acute SDHs and DAI often coexist. This diffuse brain injury can have a greater influence on the patients outcome and prognosis than the presence of a hematoma in the subdural spaces.

Another source of bleeding that can result in subdural hematoma is laceration or rupture of small cortical arteries and veins associated with cerebral contusion or injury. Subdural hematomas are usually located over cerebral convexities. The most common site of cerebral contusion associated with a subdural hematoma is the temporal pole, followed by frontal pole and cerebral convexity. Subdural hematoma extends to nearest dural reflection. It may extend along the tentorium.

Subdural hematomas may occur medially between falx and medial surface of cerebral hemisphere. Acute SDHs at this site occur due to rupture of veins bridging the medial aspect of the hemisphere and superior sagittal sinus. This is commonly called as parafalcine subdural hematoma, which is clinically characterized by contralateral hemiparesis in which the lower extremity is weaker than the upper extremity (*Falx syndrome*).

INJURIES ASSOCIATED WITH ACUTE SUBDURAL HEMATOMA

Acute subdural hematomas are commonly associated with **conter coup** injuries, including contusions and lacerations of frontal and temporal poles (Fig. 26.1). If an acute SDH is associated with an extensive area of lobar contusion and intracerebral hemorrhage this combination is often referred to as **burst lobe**.

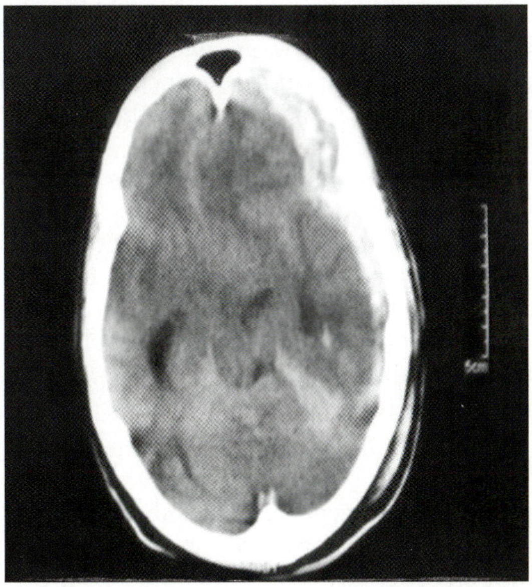

Fig. 26.1: CT head shows left frontotemporal acute to subacute subdural hematoma with midline shift

The contusions frontal poles and temporal poles are common because brain sustains an impact against irregular bony prominences at the time of injury. Other associated injuries are epidural hematomas, posterior fossa lesions, and contralateral subdural hematomas.[1]

As already stated, diffuse axonal injuries of the brain are commonly associated with acute SDH. This finding may explain the high morbidity and mortality rates in patients with acute SDHs, despite appropriate management of these hematomas.

Clinical Findings (Table 26.1)

The clinical finding in patients with acute subdural hematoma are related to an acute raised intracranial pressure and the severity of diffuse injury to the brain. The evolution of symptoms may be rapid and thus simulate the picture of an acute extradural hemorrhage.[6]

It is too early for papilledema to develop in a patient with an acute subdural hematoma, though an occasional case is seen where severe papilledema with or without retinal hemorrhages may be seen within a day or two of the injury.[7,8] Patients who sustain severe injuries, become unconscious with decerebrating posture since the time of injury or decerebrate rapidly may be assumed to have sustained diffuse cerebral injury.

In patients with less severe injuries, the deteriorating level of consciousness is determined by the severity of brain injury at the time of impact and the rate of growth of hematoma. Transtentorial herniation is indicated by the bradycardia associated with hypertension **(Cushing's response)**.

Table 26.1: Clinical symptoms and signs in patient with acute supratentorial subdural hematoma

Symptoms and signs	*Mckissock et al*[10]	*Jamieson*[1]
Pupillary abnormalities	57	43
Hemiparesis	44	40
Seizures	6	11
Aphasia	6.1	7.5
Decerebrate posturing	–	16

Table 26.2: True and false localizing signs

True localizing signs

1. Ipsilateral pupillary dilatation with nonreaction.
2. Contralateral motor weakness.

False localizing signs

1. Contralateral pupillary dilatation (cause—optic or oculomotor nerve injury)
2. Ipsilateral motor weakness (Kernohan's notch)

Patients with minor head injuries may lose consciousness initially because of concussion and later on become unconscious due to collecting hematoma **(lucid interval)**.

Lateralizing findings (Localizing signs): It includes ipsilateral pupillary dilatation with impaired reaction and motor deficit. Usually the pupillary dilatation will be ipsilateral and motor deficit (hemiparesis or hemiplegia) will be contralateral to the site of subdural hematoma (Table 26.2).

False localizing signs may also occur such as contralateral pupillary dilatation due to opposite optic nerve injury or oculomotor nerve injury. Another false localizing sign would be motor weakness of same side due to compression of the contralateral cerebral peduncle against tentorial edge (Kernohan's notch).[9]

Diagnosis

In the presence of lateralizing signs the diagnosis between epidural and subdural hematoma is usually impossible. Early onset disturbances of consciousness are indicative of SDH.

The role of skull X-ray in evaluating patient of an intracranial mass lesion is controversial. The skull X-ray provides little information that will help the neurosurgeons to make therapeutic decisions. However, the risk of an intracranial hematoma is increased 50 times when a skull fracture is present.[11] Therefore, CT scanning is essential in any patient with an abnormal skull film.

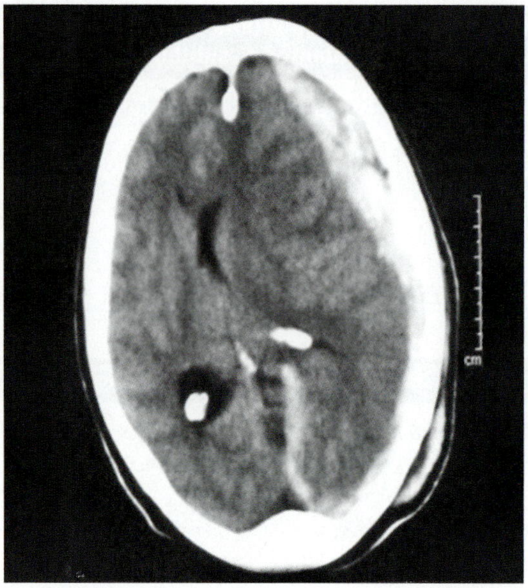

Fig. 26.2: CT head of same patient shows posterior parenchymal extension of same hematoma

On CT scan (Fig. 26.2) an acute subdural hematoma appears as a hyperdense extra-axial collection which are usually crescent shaped.[12]

The concavity of the crescent follows the brain surface. The inner surface of the hematoma outline the contours of the brain and therefore, a characteristic saw tooth appearance in the region of sylvian fissure.

The subdural hematomas as do not cross the falx or tentorium. Rarely, acute SDH can be present in interhemispheric fissure. There may be mass effect on brain in the form of compression of ipsilateral ventricle, midline shift and obliteration of basal cisterns.

A typical CT findings include mixed density subdural hematomas with varying degree of hypodensity within the high density clot due to CSF within the subdural space or due to clot retraction.

MAGNETIC RESONANCE IMAGING

Magnetic resonance imaging (MRI) is superior at identifying subacute or chronic traumatic lesions, including intracerebral or extra-axial hematomas, particularly in the posterior fossa or brainstem. However, MRI is not as sensitive as CT scan in diagnosing acute hemorrhage because fresh blood is not well delineated; MRI takes longer time. In sick patients on monitors/ventilators MRI scanning is often not possible.

BURR HOLES AS DIAGNOSTIC AIDS

When the symptoms are developing rapidly and there is no time for investigations, it is best to make exploratory burr holes in the frontal, parietal and temporal region on both sides of the skull. Acute subdural hematoma can be diagnosed by presence of fresh blood or blood clot beneath the dura after incising the dura in a cruciate manner. The advantage of this procedure is that it combines treatment also.[12]

Transcranial high resolution grey scale (TGS) sonography allows diagnosis and monitoring of subdural hematoma and extracerebral fluid collection in infants. TGS is able to detect subdural hematomas in 88 percent adults, the extant of SDH measured by TGS and CT sean also correlates. Hence, TGS may be a possible monitoring method in cases of SDH. But it is not suitable for diagnosis of SDH currently in adult cases.[25]

TREATMENT

The initial management of acute subdural hematoma includes maintenance of airway, maintenance of blood pressure and measures to lower intracranial pressure (ICP). The aim of decreasing ICP and maintaining BP is to maintain cerebral perfusion pressure (CPP).

The treatment for a subdural hematoma causing increased intracranial pressure, significant midline shift and signs of brainstem compression is surgical evacuation. In general, all SDHs that are more than 5 mm thick with midline shift are considered for surgical evacuation.

At the other extreme, patients with absent brainstem reflexes after resuscitation will almost certainly have a poor result and are rarely operative candidates.[13,14]

Patients with good Glasgow coma scale (GCS) with small subdural hematoma may not need surgery.

An acute subdural hematoma should be removed by wide craniotomy centered over maximum width of hematoma. Adequate exposure will allow to remove complete removal of subdural clot with visualization and control of the source of hemorrhage. Removal and debridement of underlying contusion or intracerebral hemorrhage may be accomplished at the time of evacuation of the subdural hematoma.

SURGICAL TECHNIQUE

The mechanism of injury responsible for producing acute SDH also leads to high incidence of temporal and frontal contusions and tearing of midline **bridging veins**. To achieve all the surgical objectives, the operative exposure must provide access to the frontal and temporal lobes.

Skin incision: A large **frontotemporoparietal** skin flap is made by using a question mark incision. The incision starts 1 cm anterior to the tragus at the level of the zygomatic arch and turns posterosuperiorly and then curved anteriorly towards frontal region as shown in Figure 26.3.

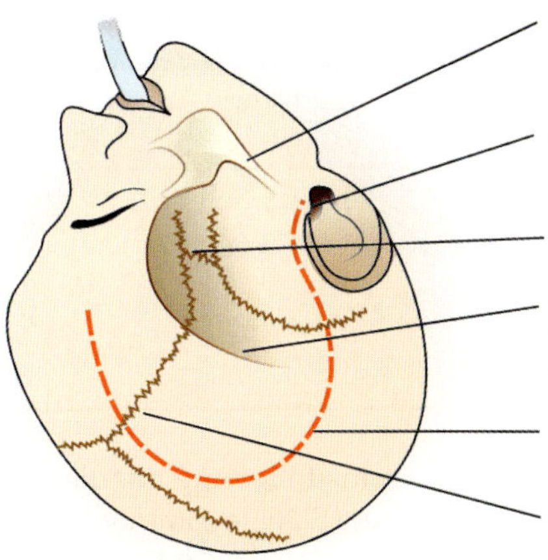

Fig. 26.3: Dotted line indicates skin incision

Incision over the temporal region should be made first, because in patients who are deteriorating rapidly quick decompression can be achieved by making a burr hole craniectomy followed by cruciate dural incision. This cruciate dural incision allows rapid surgical decompression and may be crucial for the patient.

Bone flap is made as shown in Figure 26.4.

Dural opening and evacuation of hematoma: Dura is opened in C shaped manner. The dura is opened by gently curving the incision anteriorly. Care should be taken not to injure the cortical vessels particularly in sylvian fissure.

After dura is opened, the clot is removed gently from the cortical surface with the help of suction catheter and irrigation. Frontal lobe or temporal lobe contusions, if present, are evacuated. Hemostasis should be meticulously done with bipolar.

Closure: Dura should be closed in all cases with or without dural graft. Bone flap is replaced and fixed.

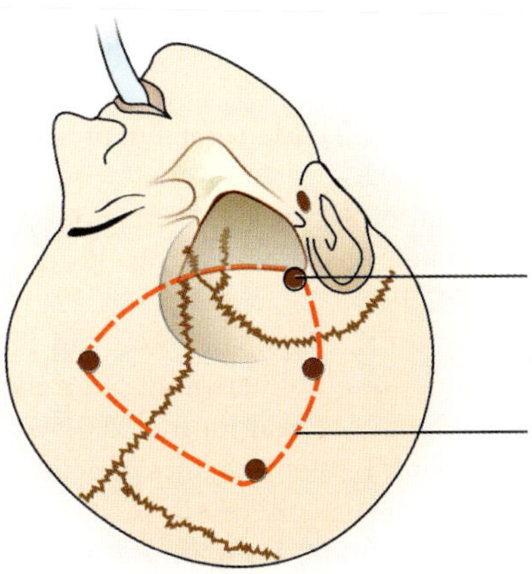

Fig. 26.4: Position of burr holes. Burr holes are connected with gigli wires (dotted line). Bone is nibbled out in hatched area

Multiple tack-up sutures (Hitch sutures) should be used to prevent postoperative extradural hematoma. If possible, intracranial pressure (ICP) monitoring should be done in all cases postoperatively.

Following problems are frequently encountered during evacuation of acute post-traumatic subdural hematoma.

1. Intraoperative brain swelling.
2. Intraoperative bleeding.

Intraoperative Brain Swelling

This is not an uncommon problem. Immediately after opening the dura and evacuation of SDH, the brain starts swelling up into the incision. If this happens, the endotracheal tube and position of patient should be checked.

Causes of intraoperative swelling can be:

1. Cerebral vascular engorgement.
2. Epidural hematoma on opposite side.
3. Intracerebral contusion hematoma.
4. Residual hematoma.

Intraoperatively mannitol should be administered or a bolus of phenobarbitone (10 mg/kg) may be beneficial, provided patient is not hypotensive.

Brain swelling can result from cerebral vascular engorgement following failure of cerebral autoregulation. Practical problem of massive brain swelling is closure of dura and whether to replace bone flap or not. It is recommended that dural should be closed with dural grafts. Some authors advocates that the dura should not be closed and the bone flap should be left out. However, this will usually lead to infarction of herniated brain. Aldrich and Eisenberg[15] strongly recommend replacement of bone flap.

Intraoperative Bleeding

Venous hemorrhage is an important cause of acute subdural hematoma.

Important veins from which bleeding can occur:

1. Bridging veins along the sagittal and transverse sinus.
2. Vein at the anterior aspect of the sylvian fissure.
3. Inferior cerebral veins and dural sinuses.

These veins may continue to bleed as the subdural hematoma is removed because of release of tamponade effect. Sinus bleeding can be controlled by packing with surgical or gelfoam.

Bleeding from cortical arteries are not uncommon.

In few cases of acute SDH, surgery may not be necessary, because of the reason that SDH is thin and not producing mass effect, patient may be in good GCS or patients may be unfit for surgery. Thus, conservative management can be used in selected cases.[22] Rarely, acute SDH can disappear rapidly in 12 to 24 hours.

Conservative Treatment

A study of conservative treatment of acute subdural hematomas shows that patients with GCS score greater than 8 had functionally independent outcome in 78 percent of the cases. Patients with thickness of hematoma < or 10 mm and midline shift < or = 5 mm showed functionally independent outcome in 82 percent cases. Hence, conservative management may be a viable option in certain cases.[23]

Outcome of Patients with Acute Post-traumatic Subdural Hematomas

Acute subdural hematomas are associated with high mortality ranging from 36 to 90 percent (Table 26.3).

Of various factors attributing to mortality, the level of consciousness at the time of presentation and at the time of operation is highly predictive of outcome. In the series of Gennarelli et al mortality correlated directly with Glasgow coma scale (GCS) score; patients with a GCS score of 3 to 5 and an acute subdural hematoma had a mortality of 76 percent, while patients with a GCS score of 6 to 8 had a mortality rate of 36 percent.[5]

Mortality and morbidity are lower in patients who are conscious when the decision to operate is made compared with those who have lucid intervals with subsequent deterioration to unconsciousness or who are unconscious throughout.

Patients who present with pupillary dilatation is strongly predictive of high mortality and morbidity.[1,20] Unilateral pupillary abnormality have mortality of ranging from 41 to 74 percent, while bilateral pupillary abnormalities ranges from 82 to 98 percent.

Younger patients have better outcome than older patients with acute subdural hematoma.[21]

In one series, mortality increased from 39 percent in patients at or under 40 years of age to 70 percent in those older than 40 years.

Poor prognostic factors

1. Patients older than 40 years.
2. Glasgow coma scale <8.
3. Pupillary abnormalities.
4. Postoperatively raised intracranial pressure.
5. Delay in diagnosis and operation.[24]

CONCLUSION

Acute subdural hematoma is a collection of blood under dura which results from rupture of parasagittal and Sylvian bridging veins following angular acceleration injuries to brain. Acute SDH is commonly associated *contrecoup injuries* and DAI. The clinical presentation in patients with acute subdural hematoma are related to increased ICP and the severity of diffuse injury to the brain. In severe injuries patient may become unconscious since the time of injury. CT scan is the investigation of choice. Acute SDH appears as a hyperdense, crescentic extra-axial collection with or without mass effect. Surgical intervention is required in patients with thick subdural hematomas with midline shift. Intraoperative brain swelling is a common problem, which results due to vascular engorgement, EDH on opposite side and increase in intracerebral contusion/hematoma. Acute subdural hematomas have high mortality rate ranging from 36 to 90 percent. In selected cases patients can be managed conservatively.

Table 26.3: Outcomes from acute subdural hematoma

Source	*Mortality (%)*	*Severe disability (%)*
Gennarelli et al[16]	74 (GCS 3-5) 36 (GCS 6-7)	16%
Stone et al[17]	59	14%
Wilberger et al[18]	66	15%
Marshall et al[19]	50	36%

REFERENCES

1. Jamieson KG, Yelland JDN. Surgically treated traumatic subdural haematomas. J Neurosurg 1972;37:137-49.

1a. Sosin DM, Sniezek JE, Waxweiler RJ. Trends in death associated with traumatic brain injury, 1979 through 1992: Success and failure. JAMA 1995;273:1778-80.

2. Seelig JM, Becker DP, et al. Traumatic acute subdural haematoma: Major mortality reduction in comatose patients treated within four hours. N Eng J Med 1981; 304;1511-18.

2a. Paul ME, Joseph V, Todd T. Management of head trauma. Chest 2002;122:699-711.

3. Gutman MB, Moulton RJ, et al. Risk factors predicting operable intracranial haematomas in head injury. J Neurosurg 1992;77:9-14.

3a. AL Hani Q, Gupta PK, Mahapatra AK, Lad SD. Development of chronic subdural hematoma. A reminder for its pathogenes. Oman Medical Journal 2001;17:20-24.

4. Gennarelli T, Jhibault L. Biomechanics of acute subdural haematoma. J Trauma 1982;22:680-6.

4a. Matsuyama T, Shimomura T, Okumura Y, et al. Acute subdural haematoma due to rupture of cortical arteries: A study of the points of rupture in 19 cases. Surg Neurol 1997;47:423-7.

5. Marshall LF, Gautile T, et al. The outcome of severe head injury. J Neurosurg 1991;75(Suppl):28-36.
6. Balasubramaniam V, Ramamurthi B. Subdural hematoma. J Ind Med Assn 1961;36:1.
7. Kalyanraman S, Ramamurthi B, et al. Subdural hematoma. Neurol (India) 1970;18:18.
8. Kalyanraman S. Traumatic intracranial hemorrhage. In: Ramamurthi B, Tandon PN (Eds). Textbook of Neurosurgery, Second edn, BJ. Churchill Livingstone 1996;307-14.
9. Kernohan JW, Woltman HW. Incisura of the cinus due to contralateral brain tumour. Arch Neurol Psychi 1929; 27:274-87.
10. McKissock W, Richardson A, et al. Subdural haematoma. A review of 389 cases. Lancet 1960;1:1365-9.
11. Mendelow AD, Teasdale G, Jennett B, et al. Risks of intracranial haematoma in head injured adults. BMJ 1983;287:1173-6.
12. Samudrala S, Cooper PR. Traumatic intracranial hematomas. In Wilkin RH, Rengachary SS (Eds): Neurosurgery McGraw Hill 1996;2797-2807.
13. Obana WG, Pitts LH. Extracerebral Lesions. Neurosurg Clin N Am 1991;2,351-72.
14. Meyer SH, Chesnut RM. Post-traumatic extra-axial mass lesions: Subdural and extradural haematoma. In Tindall GT, Cooper PR, Barrow DL (Eds): The Practice of Neurosurgery, Williams and Wilkins 1996;1461-72.
15. Aldrich EF, Eisenberg HW. Acute subdural haematoma. In Apuzzo MLZ (Ed). Brain Surgery complication Avoidance and Management. Churchill Livingstone 1993;1283-98.
16. Gennarelli TA, Spielman GM, Langfitt TW. Influence of the type of intracranial lesion on outcome from severe head injury. J Neurosurg 1982;56:26-36.
17. Stone JL, Lowe RJ, et al. Acute subdural haematoma: Direct admission to a trauma centre yields improved results. J Trauma 1986;26:445-50.
18. Wilberger JJ, Harris M, et al. Acute subdural haematoma: Morbidity, mortality, and operative timing. J Neurosurg 1991;74:212-18.
19. Marshall LF, Toole B, et al. The National Traumatic Coma Data Bank Part 2: Patients who talk and deteriorate: implications for treatment. J Neurosurg 1983;59:285-8.
20. Mc Laurin RL, Tutor FT. Acute subdural haematoma. Review of ninety cases. J Neurosurg 1961;18:61-7.
21. Jennett B, Bond M. Assessment of outcome after severe brain damage: a practical scale. Lancet 1975;1:480-4.
22. Croce MA, Dent DL, Menke PG, et al. Acute subdural haematoma: nonsurgical management of selected patients. J Trauma 1994;36:820-6.
23. Feliciano CC, De Jesus O. Conservative management outcomes of traumatic acute subdural hematomas. PR Health Sci J 2008;27(3):220-3.
24. Tian HL, Chen SW, Xu T, Hu J, et al. Risk factors related to hospital mortality in patients with isolated traumatic acute SDH analysis of 308 patients undergone surgery. Clin Med J (Eng) 2008;121(12):1080-4.
25. Niesen WD, Burkhardt D, Hoeltje J, et al. Transcranial grey scale of sonography of subdural hematoma in adults. Ultrasound Med 2006;27(3):251-5.

27 Cerebral Contusion and Intracerebral Hematoma

Raj Kamal

INTRODUCTION

A cortical contusion is a bruise of the brain's parenchyma. It consists of heterogeneous areas of hemorrhage, brain necrosis and infarction.[1] A cerebral contusion is distinctive of mechanical injury. Contusions formed at the site of cranial impact are coup contusions and those opposite the cranial impact are contrecoup contusions. Herniation contusions occur in the margins of brain hernias located most frequently along the margin of the falx cerebri, tentorium or foramen magnum.[2] In several series of head-injured patients studied by CT scan, the occurrence of cerebral contusion has varied from 30 to 40 percent.[3-5]

Traumatic parenchymal hematoma may result from the coalescene of the hemorrhages within contusion. The pathogenesis of production of intracerebral hematomas are similar to pathogenesis of contusions.

PATHOLOGY AND PATHOGENESIS

Coup contusions due to direct injury to the brain tissue and its surface vessels by fracture fragments.

The direct injury causes highly localized compressive strains. Coup contusions also result from high negative pressure that develop when an area of inbent skull rapidly snaps back are into place (see chapter on biomechanics of head injury). This results in high tensile strains causing rupture of pial vessels, cortical vessels and brain tissue.[6]

Contrecoup contusions result from translational or angular head motion. Angular head motion produces high tensile strains throughout the brain. According to Gennarelli,[6] if these tensile strains exceeds the vascular tolerance in a given region, contusion results. These tensile strains are concentrated in certain regions of the brain due to geometric effects. These areas are adjacent to the bony structures with considerable irregularity to the surface of the frontal lobe and the temporal lobes. In clinical practice, contusions of frontal and temporal lobe are very common.[7,8] Contusion of the occipital lobe is rare because it is surrounded by the falx cerebri and the tentorium on two sides and on the third side by the smooth, curving skull adjacent to the occipital lobe.

Contusions involve gyral crests, are wedge shaped extending through the cortex to the white matter. According to definition if the pia is torn then the injury becomes cerebral laceration.

Lindenberg and Freytag[9] described gliding contusion as areas of focal hemorrhages along superior medial margins of cerebral hemispheres. These are deep parenchymal injuries that may or may not be comparable to surface contusion.[2,9]

Pathogenesis of intracerebral hematoma is similar to cerebral contusion. The mechanisms of coup and contrecoup injury described for cerebral contusion also apply for intracerebral hematoma.[10] Intracerebral hematomas frequently occur in frontal and/or temporal lobes. Hematomas can be adjacent to contusion. Traumatic intracerebral hematoma can be present without cerebral contusion. In 20 percent case hematomas are multiple and in 30 to 60 percent are associated with extracerebral hematomas.[11,13,13a]

Certain factors such as loss of autoregulation and post-traumatic coagulopathies can lead to delayed formation and increase in size of intracerebral hematoma.[14,16] Delayed post-traumatic hematoma have been noted following surgical removal of cerebral contusions. This most probably occurs because of loss of initial tamponade effects of mass lesion.[17]

CLINICAL FEATURES

There is no specific clinical picture that suggests cortical contusion. It is progressive neurological deterioration following head injury that makes contusions and intracerebral hematoma likely especially if there has been progressive deterioration of consciousness with localizing signs.[11] Signs of brainstem compression and transtentorial herniation are more common in temporal contusion and hematoma. Traumatic temporal contusion and hematomas produce brainstem compression because of their location in the middle fossa with bone on their inferior, lateral, and anterior side. The path of least resistance would appear to be towards the brainstem.[11,18]

Bifrontal contusions can produce delayed neurological deterioration in the patient. The shift in bifrontal contusion may be more in anteroposterior direction than in lateral direction.[10,18] Temporal contusions and hematomas can be dangerous because they can produce brainstem compression in presence of normal or slightly raised ICP.

Delayed intracerebral hematoma is diagnosed by serial CT scans. The indication for repeat CT scan are:

i. Development of focal neurological deficit.
ii. Failure to improve.
iii. Neurological deterioration.

Gudeman et al[16] found the incidence of delayed intracerebral hematoma to be eight percent among 162 consecutive severe closed head injuries. In 90 percent cases the diagnosis of delayed traumatic intracerebral hematoma by CT was within 48 hours.

Cerebellar hematoma following head injury are uncommon and results from coup injury. They are associated with occipital bone fracture and cerebellar contusion. They can cause brainstem compression and obstructive hydrocephalus.[20-22]

A study aiming to see the frequency of tentorial hematomas revealed traumatic subarachnoid hemorrhage and cerebral contusion in 60 percent patients, subdural hematomas in 45 percent, intracerebral hematoma in 31 percent pathology in posterior fossa in 12 percent and epidural hematomas in 8 percent.[28]

Neurogenic stunned myocardium (NSM) is known to occur with subarachnoid hemorrhage, but a case of NSM is reported with hemorrhagic brain contusion

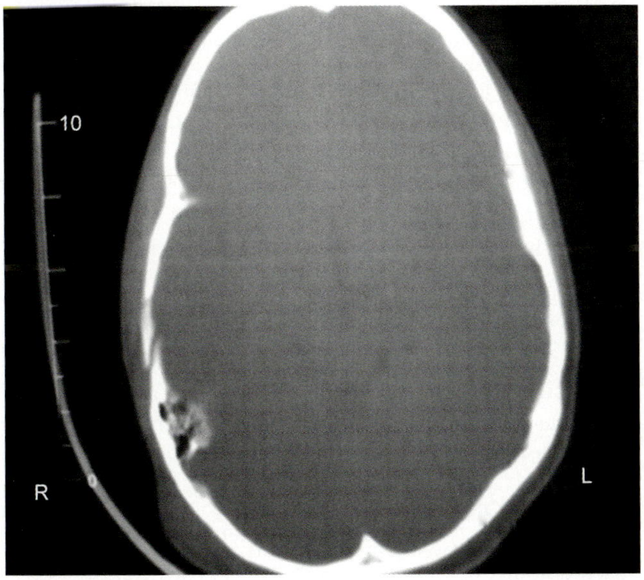

Fig. 27.1: CT of a child showing temporal bone fracture

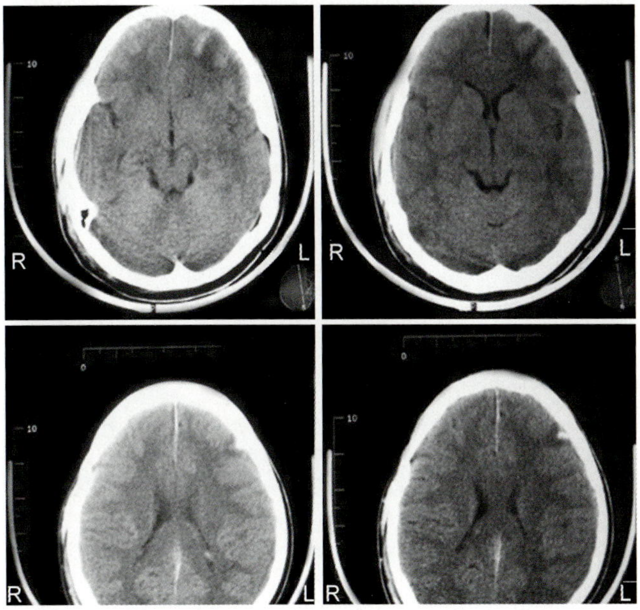

Fig. 27.2: CT of a child shows left frontal contusion

associated with cerebral edema. The role of intracranial pressure triggering a sympathetic outflow might be responsible for NSM.[29]

CT SCAN FINDINGS

On CT scan, contusions appear as lesions of mixed density, with areas of high density blood surrounded by low density areas of edema and tissue necrosis with or without mass effect (Figs 27.1 and 27.2) They may be entirely of low density after 24 to 48 hours due to resorption of blood.[24,27]

On CT scan, traumatic intracerebral hematoma is visualized as a focal, well defined rounded areas of abnormal density in the brain. Traumatic parenchymal hematomas may result from the coalescence of the hemorrhages within contusion. Normal, fresh whole blood is hyperdense (50 to 60 Hounsfield units [HU) relative to normal brain (20 to 35 HU) (Figs 27.3 and 27.5). This density is accounted for almost entirely by the globin (protein) moiety of hemoglobin. CT scan may fail to show nonhemorrhagic contusion or small contusion in brainstem, which can be well visualized by MR scan.

MANAGEMENT

The optimal management of cerebral contusion and hematoma is variable. Management depends upon clinical condition of the patient, size of contusion and intracranial pressure. Patients with small, deep, lesions are managed conservatively.[27] Patients with large intracerebral hematoma and/or contusion with mass effect, altered sensorium should be surgically evacuated.

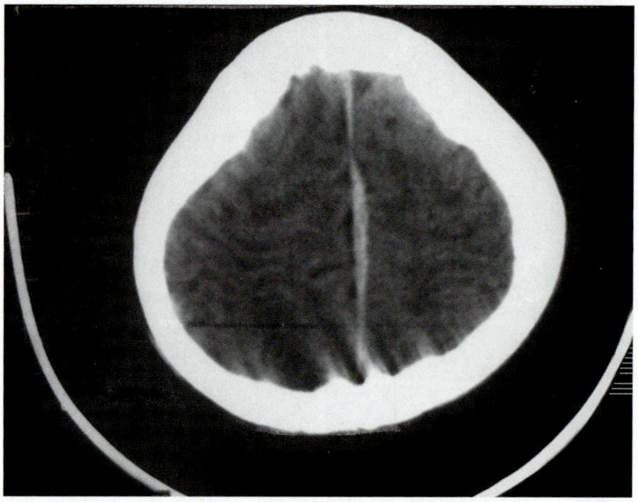

Fig. 27.3: CT of child showing blood along the falx following head injury

Patients whose hematomas are small (irrespective of neurological deficit) and patients with hemorrhages involving the deep white matter, basal ganglia or in brainstem usually do not require surgery.[1] Intracranial pressure monitoring should be done in all severe head injury patients with intracerebral hematoma and/or contusion. Intracranial hypertensive unresponsive to medical treatment, midline shift on CT on deteriorating neurological condition are indications for surgical removal of contusion/hematoma.

Intracranial pressure of over 20 mm Hg sustained for more than 5 minutes should be treated. In patients

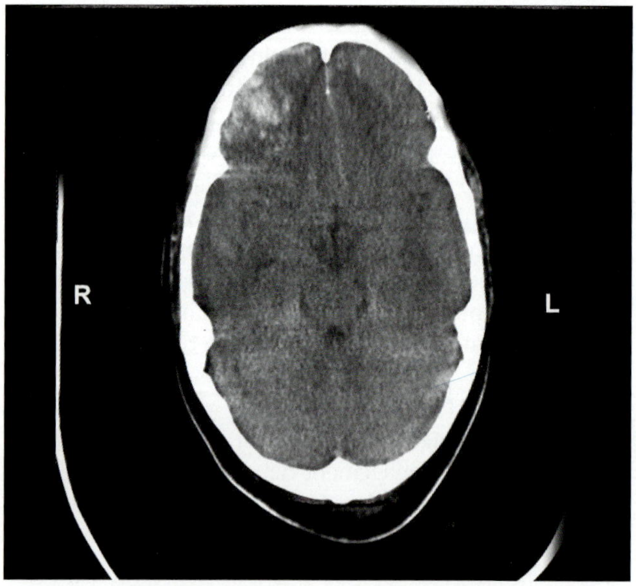

Fig. 27.4: CT showing multiple basifrontal contusions and diffuse clot on right side without mass significant mass effect

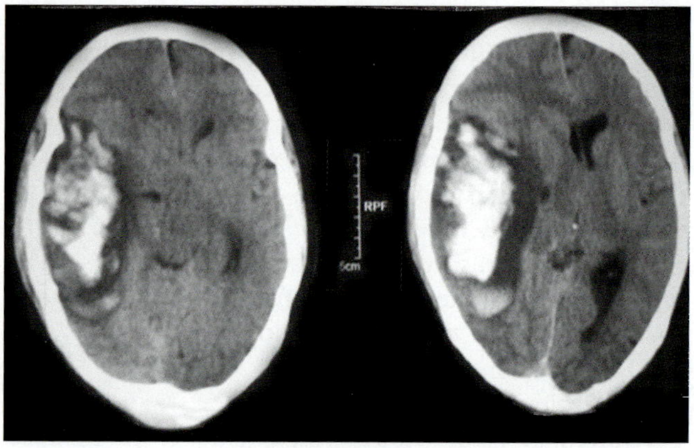

Fig. 27.5: Plain CT showing a large temporal hematoma, edema and midline shift hospitalized late to require ventilator

with temporal lobe or deep frontal lobe lesions in whom the risk of uncal herniation is greater, and ICP of over 15 mm Hg should be treated.[19,20]

Measures to control intracranial hypertension includes normothermia, head elevation, sedation, hyperventilation, ventricular drainage, mannitol and barbiturate coma. These measures are described in detail elsewhere in this book.

If the ICP is not controlled by above means then repeat CT scan should be done to rule out new or increasing intracerebral hematoma. Phenytoin should be given postoperatively for prophylaxis against post-traumatic seizures.

Post-traumatic cerebellar hematoma larger than 30 cc and/or greater than 3 cm should be evacuated through suboccipital craniectomy. Cerebellar hematomas cause direct brainstem compression and needs urgent attention.

OUTCOME

Outcome in intracerebral hematomas and cerebral contusions vary widely (Figs 27.4 and 27.5). Mortality and morbidity depends on the neurological status at the time of operation.

Associated intracranial lesions, as well as the severity of the primary brain injury itself markedly influences the prognosis.

Intracerebral hematomas: Mortality rate varies from 25 to 72 percent.[23,25]

Contusion: Mortality rate varies from 25 to 60 percent. For delayed intracerebral hematomas mortality is more than 50 percent.[14]

CONCLUSION

Contusion and post-traumatic intracerebral hematomas are relatively frequent in head injury. The pathogenesis of traumatic intracerebral hematoma is similar to cerebral contusion. Cerebral contusion and traumatic intracerebral hematoma occur due to coup and contrecoup injuries. These frequently occur in frontal and temporal lobes because of bony irregularities and high tensile strains in these areas of brain. Clinical symptoms and signs vary with location and size of the intracerebral hematoma. Larger contusions produce significant neurological deterioration in the patient. Temporal lobe contusion and hematoma can present with deteriorating level of consciousness, oculomotor nerve palsy or an uncal herniation syndrome. Large bifrontal contusions result in delayed, abrupt clinical deterioration. Traumatic intracerebral hematoma and contusions can be diagnosed easily by CT scan. Contusions and hematomas producing mass effect should be evacuated surgically. Small contusion with no mass effect should be managed conservatively.

REFERENCES

1. Samudrala S, Cooper PR. Traumatic intracranial haematomas. In: Wilkins RH, Rengachary SS (Eds), Neurosurgery, Second edn. McGraw Hill 1996;2797-2807.
2. Hardman JM. Cerebrospinal trauma. In: Davis RL, Robertson DM (Eds). Textbook of Neuropathology, 3rd edn. Williams and Wilkins 1997;1179-1232.
3. Dublin AB, French BN, Rennick JM. Computed tomography in head trauma. Radiol 1977;122:365-9.
4. French BN, Dublin AB. The value of computed tomography in the management of 1000 consecutive head injuries. Surg Neurol 1977;7:171-83.
5. MacPherson BCM, MacPherson P, Jennett B. CT evidence of intracranial contusion and haematoma in relation to the presence, site and type of skull fracture. Clin Radiol 1990;42:321-6.
6. Gennarelli TA, Meaney DF. Cranial trauma. In: Wilkins RH, Rengachary SS (Eds). Neurosurgery, Second edn. McGraw Hill 1996;2611-21.
7. Hirsh LF. Delayed traumatic intracerebral hematomas after surgical decompression. Neurosurg 1979;5(6):653-5.
8. Stender A, Schulze A. The surgical treatment of space occupying contusions and intracerebral haematoma after blunt cerebral trauma. Excepta Med-Intern Congress Series 1966;110:231-5.
9. Lindenberg R, Freytag E. A mechanism of cerebral contusions: A pathologic-anatomic study. Arch Pathol 1960;69:440-69.
10. Rockswod GL. Post-traumatic intra-axial mass lesions: haematomas, Contusions, Edema. In: Tindall GT, Cooper PR, Barrow DL (Eds). The practice of Neurogery, 1st edn. Williams and Wilkins 1995;1461-72.
11. Browder J, Turney MF. Intracerebral hemorrhage of traumatic origin: Its surgical treatment. NY state J Med 1942;42:2230-5.
12. Dublin AB, French BN, Rennick JM. Computed tomography in head trauma. Radiol 1977;122:365-9.
13. Solonick D, Pitts LH, et al. Traumatic intracerebral haematomas: Timing of appearance and indications for operative removal. J Trauma 1986;26:787-94. Rockswold GL. Post-traumatic Intra-axial Mass Lesions.

13a. Fukamachi A, Kohnok, Nagaseki Y, et al. The incidence of delayed traumatic intracerebral haematoma with extradural hemorrhage. J Trauma 1985;25:145-9.

14. Diaz FG, Yock DH, Larson D, et al. Early diagnosis of delayed post-traumatic intracerebral haematomas. J Neurosurg 1979;50:217-23.
15. Evans JP, Scheinker IM. Histological studies of the brain following head trauma II. Post-traumatic petechial and massive intracerebral hemorrhage. J Neurosurg 1946;3:101-13.
16. Gudeman SK, Kishore PRS, et al. The genesis and significance of delayed traumatic intracerebral haematoma. Neurosurg 1979;5:309-13.

16a. Gupta PK, Mahapatra AK, Lad SD. Delayed hematoma in head injury. Pan Arab J Neurosurg 2003;7:40-5.

17. Hirsh LF. Delayed traumatic intracerebral hematomas after surgical decompression. Neurosurg 1979;5(6):653-5.
18. Statham PF, Johnston RA, MacPherson P. Delayed deterioration in patients with traumatic frontal contusions. J Neurol Neurosurg Psychi 1989;52:351-4.
19. Chestnut RM, Marshall LF, Marshall SB. Medical management of intracranial pressure, in Cooper PR (Ed): Head Injury, 3rd edn. Baltimore, Williams and Wilkins 1993; 225-46.
20. Kelly DF, Mebride DQ, Becker DP. Surgical management of severe closed head Injury in Adults. In: Schmidek HH, Sweet WH (Eds). Operative Neurosurgical Techniques. Indications, Methods, and Results, 3rd edn. WB Saunders Company 1995;47-67.
21. Firsching R, Frowein R, Thun F. Intracerebellar hematoma: Eleven traumatic and non-traumatic cases and a review of literature. Neurochirurgia 1989;30:182-5.
22. Nagata K, Ishikawa T, et al. Delayed traumatic intracerebellar haematoma: Correlation between the location of the haematoma and the pre-existing cerebellar contusion. Neurol Med Chir (Tokyo) 1991;31:792-6.
23. Bullock R, Golek J, Blake G. Traumatic intracerebral haematoma—which patient should undergo surgical evacuation? CT scan features and ICP monitoring as a basis for decision-making. Surg Neurol 1989;32:181-7.
24. Jamieson KG, Yelland JDNR. Traumatic intracerebral haematoma: report of 63 surgically treated cases. J Neurosurg 1972;37:528-32.
25. Jaya Kumar PN, Sastry KVR, et al. Prognosis in contrecoup intracranial haematoma a clinical and radiological study of 63 patients. Acta Neurochir (Wien) 1991;108:30-33.

26. Lane B, Stevens JM, Moseley IF. Cranial and intracranial pathology.[3] In Grainger RG, Allison DJ (Eds), Grainger and Allison's Diagnostic Radiology, A Textbook of Medical Imaging, Churchill Livingstone 1997:2127-48.
27. Soloniuk D, Pitts LH, Lovely M, et al. Traumatic intracerebral haematomas: Timing of appearance and indications for operative removal. J Trauma 1986;26:787-94.
28. Moskala M, Polak J, Moskala A, et al. Hematoma in tentorium cerebeli, new pathology or new prognostic factor in neurotraumatology. A preliminary report. Neurol Neurochir Pol 2007;41(3):234-40.
29. Deleu D, Kettern MA, Hanssens Y, et al. Neurogenic stunned myocardium following hemorrhagic cerebral contusion. Saudi Med J 2007;28(2):283-5.

28 Penetrating Head Injuries

Raj Kamal

INTRODUCTION

Penetrating head injuries are commonly encountered in both military and civilian practice. It is a leading cause of mortality or morbidity in both civilians and military combatants. The aim of management of penetrating head injury should be to prevent or decrease the secondary brain damage, control intracranial hypertension and prevent infection.

Penetrating head injuries are of two types: (i) Penetrating missile injuries caused by bullet or shrapnel, (ii) Penetrating stab injuries caused by knife, nails, screwdrivers, etc.

EPIDEMIOLOGY

Penetrating head injuries are the cause of mortality in about 50 percent cases.[1,2] The annual incidence of deaths related to head injury due to gunshot injury in the US has been estimated at 2.4 per 100,000.[3] Overall incidence is higher in males as compared to females and occurs most frequently in young adults.

BALLISTICS AND PATHOPHYSIOLOGY

The energy dissipated in the brain by a bullet is proportional to the impact velocity of the bullet.[4]

Military rifles typically have muzzle velocities that exceed 2500 feet/s (750 m/s) while most civilian injuries are caused by handguns with muzzle velocities between 800 and 1400 feet/sec.[5]

The most severe wounds are produced by rifles whose bullets have an initial velocity exceeding 2000-3000 feet/s (750 m/s). Shell fragments and bullets from handgun produce much less destructive wounds. The speed of sound (320 m/s) is taken as an arbitrary velocity which separates high velocity missiles from low velocity missiles.

The energy transferred from moving missile depends on the velocity of entry and velocity of exit of the bullet and can be expressed as ½ M x (Velocity of entry – Velocity of exit).[2] M = Mass of bullet, V = Velocity of bullet. Hence, higher the velocity of entry higher will be energy transfer and brain damage.[6]

Missile causes brain parenchymal damage through three mechanisms.[6,7]

a. Direct crushing and laceration along the tract of missile.
b. Cavitation.
c. Shock waves.

Crushing and laceration along the tract of missile is caused by the direct penetration of both low velocity and higher velocity missile injuries. Direct crushing and laceration of brain can also be caused by indriven bone fragments.

At low velocities the missile tends simply to lacerate the tissue it passes through. As the velocity increases, it moves tissue away from the track. At high velocities (> 320 m/sec) the tissue may be displaced several centimeters from the wound track, this phenomenon is known as cavitation.[8] The size of resulting cavitation is much larger than the diameter of missile.

High speed shock waves cause structural and functional disruption well beyond the course of missile. Shock waves can explain brainstem dysfunction when the path of the missile has been distant from it.[7]

'Yaw' of missile is defined as the deviation of the long axis of the projectile from its line of flight. Increasing degree of yaw will cause increasing severity of damage. For example, a stabilized round from a high velocity rifle may pass straight causing less damage with only a small entry and exit wound. If, on the other hand, the round yaws more than 10° from its flight path, it will tumble rapidly in tissue giving up much of its energy and will, thereby, cause severe damage.[5]

Missile injuries to the cranium has been studied in certain experimental studies. Following penetrating missile injury there is immediate and steep rise in the intracranial pressure (ICP) secondary to the cavitation.[9] This initial rise in ICP is followed by moderate rise in ICP due to intracranial contusion, hematoma and swelling. Increased ICP is associated with bradycardia with hypertension. Following penetrating missile injuries cerebral autoregulation may fail. All the factors lead to decreased cerebral perfusion pressure.

As already mentioned shock waves and cavitation cause indirect brainstem injury which may be distant from the injury site. Resulting brainstem injury may explain the post-injury apnea and hypotension which are found frequently following missile injuries.[9-11]

MANAGEMENT OF PENETRATING INJURIES

The initial evaluation, neurological examination and resuscitation are similar to closed head injury. Entire body must be examined for entry and exit wound as the gunshot wounds are often multiple. The initial evaluation and management can be done in a quick stepwise manner:

1. Systemic examination.
2. Resuscitation.
3. Neurological examination.
4. Radiological investigations.
5. Definitive management.

Systemic Examination

Thorough systemic examination should be done to assess pulse rate, BP, respiration and associated injuries such as thoracic or abdominal injuries. Severity of thoracic and abdominal injury should be assessed by appropriate investigation as treatment of an associated injury such as thoracoabdominal injury will take precedence.

Resuscitation

Resuscitation should be initiated at the site of injury. The airway, breathing and circulation (ABC) should be checked and an attempt is made to maintain them during transport to specialized center. Endotracheal intubation may be needed to maintain airway. The use of helicopters in the transport of severely injured patients may aid in reducing the transit time in certain situations.

Aggressive resuscitative measures have known to improve the outcome of patients with penetrating head injury.[12,13] Significant bleeding from the scalp should be controlled. In suspected associated cervical injury, adequate immobilization of the spine should be done while shifting the patient.

Neurological Examination

A rapid neurological examination should be done which includes Glasgow coma scale (GCS) score, pupillary response, and brainstem reflexes. Severity of penetrating injury can be classified depending upon GCS score. A brief description of detailed neurological examination can be found elsewhere in this book.

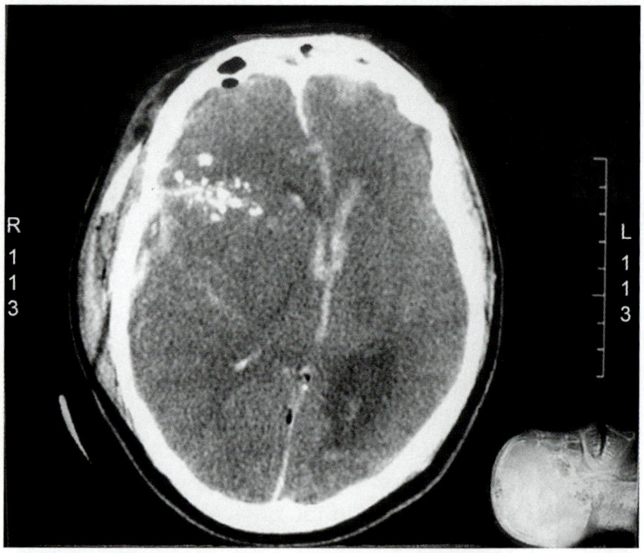

Fig. 28.1: CT showing bullet injury track (clots) and severe midline shift, caused from point blank distance at temporal region, patient died within 6 hours[2]

Focal deficit may or may not be present. Focal deficits may be absent if the missile traverses only through non-eloquent area of brain. An enlarging intracranial mass lesion should be suspected when there is deteriorating level of consciousness with pupillary changes.

Complete shaving of the head should be done to demonstrate entry or exit wounds. Open wounds caused by missile or stab injury should be bandaged properly.

Radiological Investigations

Plain X-rays of the skull identifies the presence, size and location of bullet, metallic fragments and bone fragment (Fig. 28.1). Plain X-rays can demonstrate penetrating stab injuries caused by knife. From X-ray of skull one can assess the trajectory of the missile.

CT scan head is the investigation of choice. All patients with penetrating head injuries should undergo an immediate CT scan with the exception of those who present brain dead and remain so after resuscitation. CT scan demonstrates the missile track, as well as missile fragments and fractured in driven bone fragments.

Contusions, hematomas and brain edema are also clearly demonstrated on CT scan.[14,15]

Cerebral angiogram is required when there is suspected major vascular injury. Suspicion of major intracranial vessel is based on track of bullet or path of penetrating stab injury by knife or any other similar sharp object.

Table 28.1: Prognostic factors in penetrating craniocerebral trauma

Favorable factors	*Poor prognostic factors*
Good GCS score	Poor GCS score
Normal BP	Suicidal attempts
Normal CT scan	Through and through perforating wounds
Young age	Elevated ICP and hypotension
	CT findings
	Transventricular injury
	Subarachnoid
	Intraventricular
	Hemorrhage
	Compression of basal cisterns
	Bihemispheric injury and midline shift

Definitive Management

After initial evaluation resuscitation and investigation, surgeon should decide operability of the particular case. The favorable and unfavorable prognostic factors for penetrating injuries are given in Table 28.1.

Grahm et al[12] proposed that all patients (who are not brain dead) should be aggressively resuscitated. Surgery is reserved for following group of patients:

1. A GCS score of 3 to 5 and large extra-axial hematoma.
2. A GCS score of 6 to 8 without transventricular or bihemispheric injury.
3. A GCS score of 9 to 15.

No treatment is given to those patients with a GCS score of 3 to 5 without hematoma or a GCS score of 6 to 8 with intraventricular, bihemispheric, or multilobar dominant hemisphere injury.[12-16]

The selection of patients appropriate for surgical intervention continues to require judgment and experience on the part of neurosurgeon as no universally accepted formula or protocol is available. The decision to withhold operative treatment appears to be justified for most severely injured patients. However, great care must be exercised, lest potentially salvageable patients be missed.[17]

Taha et al[18] in their prospective study on patients with penetrating invisible injuries of the brain were treated with wound debridement and closure only in patients with stable neurological examinations and GCS scores greater than 10. Additionally, the patients had to be evaluated within 6 hours of being wounded, have entry wound less than 2 cm in diameter, and have no exit wound or missile trajectory that traversed proximal Sylvian fissure. These patients were treated with simple wound debridement and closure with intravenous antibiotics for two weeks.

OPERATIVE TECHNIQUE

The goals of surgical intervention in the management of penetrating craniocerebral trauma should be accomplished by:[17]

1. Debridement: Removal of debris, bone and missile fragments along the trajectory.
2. Evacuation of any significant intracranial hematoma.
3. Hemostasis.
4. Meticulous dural and scalp closure.

Missile Injuries

Preoperative treatment with:

1. Antibiotics-penicillin + Chloramphenicol or any broad spectrum antistaphylococcal antibiotics.
2. IV mannitol (1 gm/kg).
3. Phenytoin-loading dose 15 mg/kg IV @50 mg/min.

Complete head should be shaved and cleaned so that access to both entry and exit wound must be provided. Thigh should also be prepared for fascia lata graft.

A curvilinear incision with broad based scalp flap with adequate blood supply should be made. The entry or exit wound of missile should be placed at the center of the flap and for stab injury with knife *in situ*, it should be planned accordingly.

Circumferential craniectomy is performed. The craniectomy method is applied to limited injuries without large mass or any suspicion of vascular or dural sinus injury. The craniectomy should be large enough to remove all comminuted bone fragments, contused and necrotic brain. The size of craniectomy is usually 5 × 5 cm. Aggressive debridement of brain is not recommended. Secondary operation can be done to remove retained debris. The aim should be to preserve as much as neural tissue.[18-20]

After removal of debris, hematoma, good hemostasis should be obtained. The dura should be closed meticulously and frequently requiring a patch graft. The graft may be obtained from local tissues (pericranium, temporalis fascia) or, in more extensive dural defect fascia lata may be employed.

Nonmissile Injuries

The surgical management of nonmissile injuries is similar to that for missile injuries. Weapons such as knife still in place at the time of presentation should not be removed.[1] These patients should undergo preoperative carotid angiogram to rule out any possible major vascular injury. The weapon should be removed only in operation theater after making craniectomy or craniotomy. If there is any vascular injury it should be dealt accordingly. Wound and track debridement and dural repair are similar to that of missile penetrating injury.

Postoperative Care

Postoperative intensive care management of penetrating injury is similar to the closed head injury. Following measures to be taken and monitoring to be done during postoperative course (details can be found elsewhere in this book).

1. **Intracranial pressure monitoring:** ICP should be kept below 20 mm Hg. Bolus infusion of osmotic diuretics, sedatives and neuromuscular blocking agents should be given as and when required.
2. **Hyperventilation:** Hyperventilation to keep $PaCO_2$ between 30 to 35 mm Hg also reduces ICP. However, ischemic damage may occur if the $PaCO_2$ becomes less than 25 mm Hg.
3. **Antibiotics:** Broad spectrum antibiotics should be used during postoperative course. A combination of vancomycin, ceftazidime and metrogyl for 10 days is recommended.[17]
4. **Anticonvulsant:** Prophylactic anticonvulsant such as phenytoin should be used in postoperative period.

Special Surgical Considerations

Vascular injuries: Following penetrating missile injuries of head, various vascular injuries are reported, e.g. post-traumatic aneurysms, vascular occlusion, dural sinus injuries, anterovenous fistula.[21] Traumatic intracranial aneurysm following penetrating injuries are usually false aneurysms that develop after disruption of the arterial wall followed by periarterial hematoma formation and cavitation. They tend to occur more distally and are multiple in 20 percent of cases. They have more malignant course than congenital aneurysms. The risk of repeat hemorrhage and mortality is higher.[22,23] Hence, surgical or endovascular treatment should be considered whenever such post-traumatic pseudoaneurysms are diagnosed on any angiogram.

Dural venous sinus injuries must be anticipated and diagnosed. Small rents can be easily controlled by packing with gelfoam.

Injury to anterior 1/3rd of sagittal sinus can be treated by packing or by ligating the anterior one-third of superior sagittal sinus. Injury to dominant transverse sinus or posterior sagittal sinus may require microsurgical repair which can be extremely difficult in given situation, hence any depressed bony fragments involving dural sinuses should not be removed.[19]

Tangential Wounds

Tangential wounds are caused by glancing blows from the missile injury. There is no penetration of calvarium. Underlying brain contusion and hematoma can be diagnosed by CT scan and treated accordingly.

Migratory projectiles: Bullets are known to migrate intracranially. The cause for migration of bullet is related to its site of impaction. Migratory bullets can be found in within the ventricular system, within a cavity of pus or hematoma. The mobile bullet may damage important tracts and hence should be removed whenever possible.[16]

Complications of Penetrating Head Injuries

1. CSF fistulae.
2. Infection: Wound infection, meningitis, ventriculitis and intracranial abscess.
3. Post-traumatic epilepsy.

The management of CSF fistula is described in detail elsewhere in this book. CSF fistula is seen frequently following transbasal or transfacial gunshot wounds. Postoperative CSF leak indicates improper closure of dura at operation. CSF fistulae is an important risk factor in the development of meningitis and brain abscess. Any postoperative CSF leak beyond two weeks should be repaired surgically. Metrizamide cisternography can be done before taking up for second surgery.

Infection rate is higher in patient in whom the bone fragment is retained, i.e. inadequate debridement. Hagan[24] reported on patients evacuated from Vietnam war that a retained bone fragment to be the evidence of incomplete brain debridement.

If the primary operation is performed within 2 hours then the risk of infection becomes considerably less even in the presence of retained bone fragment. Since reoperation for retained bone fragment is not without risk, hence it may be desirable to accept the possibility of late infection rather than undertaking repeated operations of the brain.[25,26]

Cognitive Recovery

The patients with penetrating head injury demonstrated a greater degree of cognitive decline overall during the years following recovery from head injury compared with uninjured controlled group of Vietnam Veterans. This became increasingly significant in later life. Preinjury intelligence was the most consistent predictor of cognitive outcome across all phases of recovery and decline after penetrating injuries.[27]

CONCLUSION

Penetrating craniocerebral injuries are classified as penetrating missile injuries (bullet, shrapnel) and penetrating stab injuries (knife, nails, screwdrivers). Penetrating injuries occur during war and in civilian practice. Penetrating missile injuries are either high velocity or low velocity missile wounds. Missile wound causes structural and functional cerebral injury by direct injury, cavitation and shock waves. These factors cause intracranial hypertension and decreased cerebral perfusion. Indirect brainstem injury is caused by shock waves and cavitation. Aggressive resuscitative measures should be taken for all patients and operability in individual case should be decided. Surgery is indicated in patients: (i) GCS score of 9 to 15, (ii) GCS score of 6 to 8 without bihemisphere injury, (iii) GCS score of 3 to 5 and large extra-axial hematoma. The aim of surgery in missile injuries are debridement, evacuation of any significant intracranial mass lesion, meticulous dural and scalp closure.

Nonmissile injuries should undergo preoperative angiogram to rule out any vascular injury. Complications of penetrating head injuries are CSF fistula, infection and seizures.

REFERENCES

1. Ameen A. Penetrating craniocerebral injuries: Observations in the Iraqi-Iranian war. Mil Med 1987;152:76-9.
2. Rish B, Dillon J, Weiss G. Mortality following penetrating craniocerebral injuries. J Neurosurg 1983;59:775-80.
3. Sosin D, Sacks J, Smith S. Head injury—associated deaths in the United States from 1979-86. JAMA 1989;262: 2251-5.
4. Crockard HA, Brown FD, et al. An experimental cerebral missile injury model in primates. J Neurosurg 1977; 46:776.
5. Dagi T. Emergency management of missile injuries to the brain: Resuscitation, treatment and preoperative stabilization. Am J Emerg Med 1987;5:140-8.
6. Hopkinson D, Marshall T. Firearm injuries. Br J Surg 1967;54:344-53.
7. Kirk Patrick J, Di Maio V. Civilian gunshot wounds of the brain. J Neurosurg 1978;49:185-98.
8. Mellor SG. Modern war wounds. In Mason JK (Eds), The Pathology of Trauma, 2nd edn. Hodder and Stoughton Ltd 1993;86-96.
9. Crockard A, Brown F, Calica A, et al. Physiological consequences of experimental cerebral missile injury and use of data analysis to predict survival. J Neurosurg 1977;46:784-94.
10. Allen I, Scott R, Tannel J. Experimental high velocity head injury. Injury 1982;14:183-93.
11. Carey M, Gurcharan S, et al. Experimental missile wounds to brain. J Neurosurg 1989;71:754-64.
12. Graham TW, Williams FC Jr, et al. Civilian gunshot wounds to the head: a prospective study. Neurosurg 1990;27:696-700.
13. Siccardi D, Cavaliere R, et al. Penetrating craniocerebral missile injuries in civilians: A retrospective analysis of 314 cases. Surg Neurol 1991;35:455-60.
14. Cooper P, Maravilla K, Cone J. Computerized tomographic scan and gunshot wounds of the head: Indications and radiographic findings. Neurosurg 1979;22:373-80.
15. Clark W, Mulbaner M, et al. Analysis of 76 civilian craniocerebral gunshot wounds. J Neurosurg 1986;65: 9-14.
16. Rosenberg WS, Harsh GR. Penetrating Wounds of the head. In Wilkins RH, Rengachary SS (Eds). Neurosurgery. 2nd edn. McGraw Hill 1996;2813-20.
17. Trask T, Narayan RK. Management of Penetrating Head Injuries. In Tindall GT, Cooper PR, Barrow DL, The practice of Neurosurgery, Williams and Wilkins 1995; 1517-33.
18. Taha JM, Saba MI, Brown JA. Missile injuries to the brain treated by simple wound closure: Results of a protocol during the Lebanese conflict. Neurosurg 1991;29:380-4.
19. Benzel EC, Day WT, et al. Civilian craniocerebral gunshot wounds. Neurosurg 1991;29:67-72.
20. Nagib MG, Rockswold GL, Sherman RS, et al. Civilian gunshot wounds to the brain: Prognosis and management. Neurosurg 1986;18:533-7.
21. Jinkins J, Dadsefan M, et al. Value of acute-phase angiography in the detection of vascular injuries caused by gunshot wounds to the head: Analysis of 12 cases. AJR 1992;159:365-8.
22. Aarabi B. Traumatic aneurysms of the brain due to high velocity missile head wounds. Neurosurg 1988;22:1056-63.
23. Haddad F, Haddad G, Taha J. Traumatic intracranial aneurysms caused by missiles: Their presentation and management. Neurosurg 1991;28:1-7.
24. Hagan RE. Early complications following penetrating wounds of the brain. J Neurosurg 1971;34:132-41.
25. Carey ME, Young H, et al. A bacteriological study of craniocerebral missile wounds from Vietnam. J Neurosurg 1971;34:145-54.
26. Meirowsky AM, Harsh GR. The surgical management of cerebritis complicating penetrating wounds of the brain. J. Neurosurg 1953;10:373-9.
27. Raymount V, Great house A, Reding K, et al. Demographic, structural and genetic prediction of late cognitive decline after penetrating head injury. Brain 2008;131(pt2):543-58.

29 Traumatic Diffuse Axonal Injury

Raj Kamal, Raj Kumar, AK Mahapatra

INTRODUCTION

Diffuse brain injury is defined as the pathology of comatose patients who are unconscious from the moment of impact and do not experience a lucid interval without evidence of space occupying intracranial lesions on computed tomography (CT) scan or magnetic resonance imaging (MRI). The two subgroups of diffuse brain injury are traumatic diffuse axonal injury (TDAI) and diffuse brain swelling.

Traumatic diffuse axonal injury (TDAI) was first described by Strich as "diffuse degeneration of white matter following severe head injury".[1] Since then, a number of terms have been used to describe TDAI and include "shearing injury," "diffuse white matter shearing injury" and "inner cerebral trauma".

The new definition includes severely head-injured patients with normal scans (Figs 29.1A and B), tissue tear hemorrhages, traumatic subarachnoid and intraventricular hemorrhages, diffuse brain swelling, and unilateral swelling with midline shifts.

In diffuse axonal injury case, the brain may appear surprisingly normal when viewed with the naked eye. However, distinctive gross and microscopic features characterize severe TDAI. Axonal swelling ("retraction balls") are the microscopic hallmark of TDAI. Widely distributed lesions contain reactive axonal swellings in the cerebral white matter, corpus callosum, and upper brainstem.

PATHOGENESIS

It is caused by angular or rotational acceleration and deceleration inertial effects and not by contact phenomena. The severity of axonal damage is related to the magnitude, duration, and onset rate of the angular acceleration.[2]

The direction of impact plays an important role. Sagittal movement is the best tolerated by the brain whereas lateral and horizontal movements are not well tolerated. The angular acceleration results in shearing and tensile strains on axons, typically at the gray, white matter interphases.[2] In response to a lateral head motion, small centers of rotation occurs in temporal and superior frontal lobes. Xiao-Sheng et al,[2a] had demonstrated diffuse axonal injury in rats due to lateral head rotation. The regions shown in the figure indicate the areas where the brain is the most prone to axonal damage due to high level of strain at the site.

By only using angular acceleration in monkeys, Gennarelli et al,[2] produced injury patterns seen in

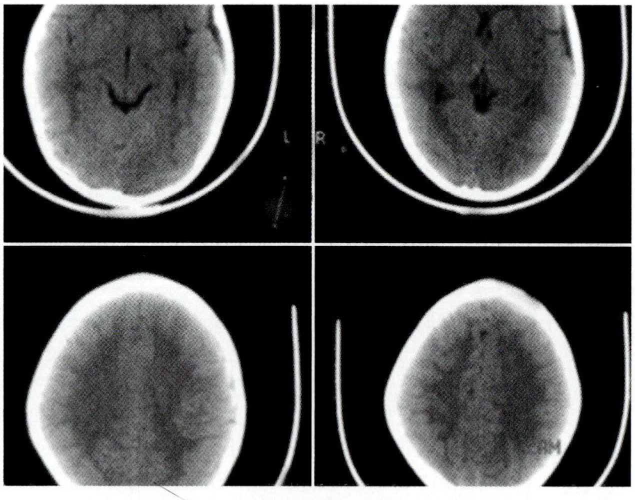

Fig. 29.1A: Child with DAI shows nearly normal CT 4 days following head trauma

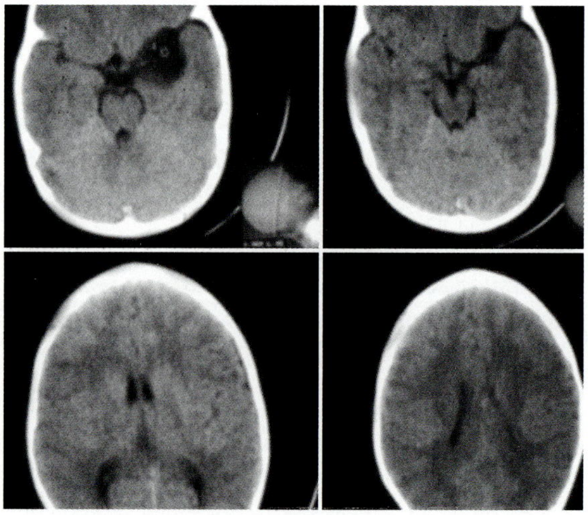

Fig. 29.1B: Child with diffuse axonal injury showing incidental left Sylvian arachnoid cyst, otherwise nearly normal CT

humans. Such injuries result from shear and/or tensile strains on axons in the cerebral white matter, corpus callosum, and brainstem. The severity of axonal injury was proportional to the rapidity of angular acceleration of head. These findings suggest that minute injuries sometimes found after concussion may also be the result of angular acceleration.

Remaining surviving axons may be vulnerable because of secondary events leading to hypoxia, ischemia and subsequent release of excitatory amino acids and free radicals. The ultimate event in the neuronal death appears to be the influx of calcium ions.[3] Buki et al[3a,3b] had demonstrated calpain mediated sped in proteolysis in pathogenesis of traumatically induced axonal injury. In another study they reported Cytochrome C release and caspase activation in DAI.

PATHOLOGY

Three "Classic" lesions, characterize severe TDAI:[4]

I. Reactive axonal "retraction" balls.
II. Hemorrhagic necrosis in the dorsolateral quadrant of the rostral brainstem.
III. Hemorrhagic necrosis in the corpus callosum.

The axonal swellings are the microscopic hallmark of TDAI. They become apparent within hours after injury and may persist for a year or more. Microglial stars develop in these damaged sites and may eventually replace the swollen axons. Degeneration of long tracts will evolve and ventricular dilation will follow.[5]

The lesion in the dorsolateral quadrant of the rostral brainstem are usually hemorrhagic and involve dorsolateral-lateral part of midbrain and the rostral pons, almost always involving the superior cerebellar peduncle.

The lesions in corpus callosum usually lie lateral to the midline, affect the inferior and posterior part of corpus callosum. These lesion may extend over several centimeters. The callosal injury may be focal, may be segmental, or may extend from the genu to the splenium.

Traumatic diffuse axonal injury (TDAI) appears to be a distinct entity which may develop after mild concussion up to and including persistant coma. The finding of occasional clusters of microglia in patients dying soon after head injury suggested that axonal injury has occurred. More recently antibody against β-amyloid precursor protein has been demonstrated in patients who died from unrelated causes after sustaining a minor head injury.[6,7]

Recently evidence from animal experiments[8] and observations in humans[9] have shown that the initial axonal injury is in continuity. The disruption of axon occurs only later, as a result of a so called secondary or delayed axotomy.

Accumulation of precursor protein of amyloid within 2 or 3 hours of injury indicates beginning of delayed axotomy. This process may continue for 24 hours or more.[9-11] The exact mechanisms causing secondary axotomy are not yet known. But proposed mechanisms include increased permeability to Ca^{2+} in the region of Ranvier's node or, alternatively, within the internal cytoskeleton itself.[12] This leads to disorganization of microtubules and neurofilaments hence block in axonal transport resulting in axonal focal swelling. Later on classical axonal bulb appears. Any measure which prevents or minimize secondary axotomy can improve clinical outcome. Till now no such specific measure is available for use in human beings.

INCIDENCE

The incidence of TDAI will be higher at autopsy than would be obvious on radiographic (CT, MRI) examination.

Adams et al[13,14] found TDAI in 28 percent of non-missile head injuries histologically at autopsy. In 20 percent of these cases, the diagnosis of TDAI could not have been made without microscopic examination. The CT incidence of TDAI in various series varies from 2.4 to 15.5 percent.[15,16]

CLINICAL PRESENTATION

TDAI occurs most commonly in patient injured in high velocity traffic accidents. The hallmarks of severe diffuse brain injury are coma from the onset of trauma, with the majority of severely injured patients showing a combination of generalized extensor posture or flexion. Classically these patients become unconscious immediately upon impact. About one-third of TDAI patients may recover sufficiently from the initial head injury to talk before lapsing into coma.

DIAGNOSTIC STUDIES

Computed Tomography

The classic CT appearance of TDAI is small focal punctate tissue tear hemorrhages in the cerebral white matter, basal ganglia, corpus callosum or dorsal part of the brainstem. The three most common locations for the hemorrhages are the lobar white matter, corpus

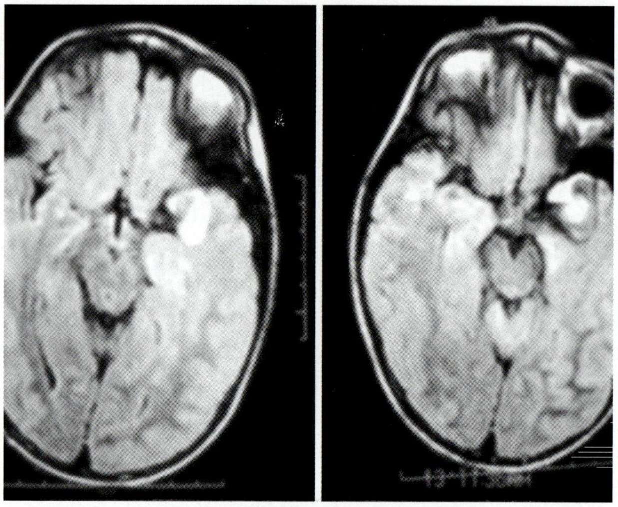

Fig. 29.2: MRI of same child with DAI showing multiple parenchymal hyperintensities

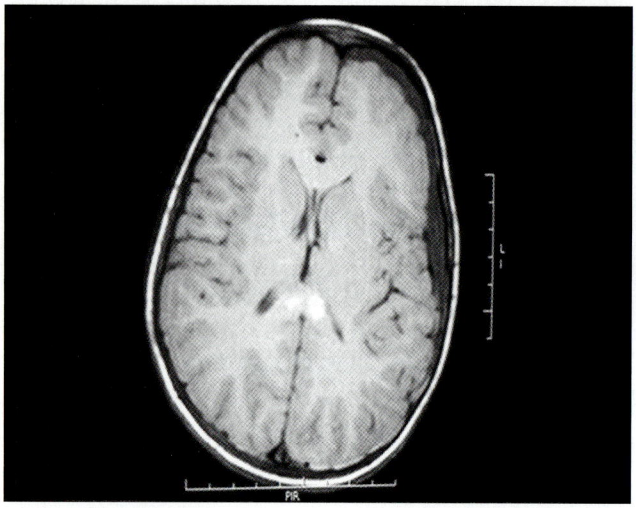

Fig. 29.3: MRI of same child shows hyperintensities in the region of posterior corpus callosum

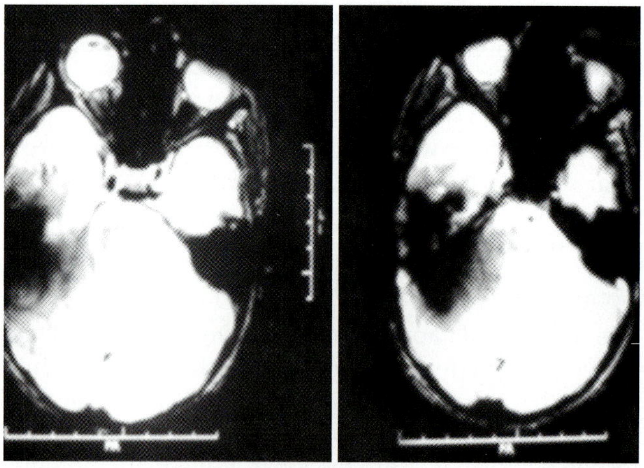

Fig. 29.4: Child with DAI difffusion restriction is seen in right temporal lobe on DWI MR imaging

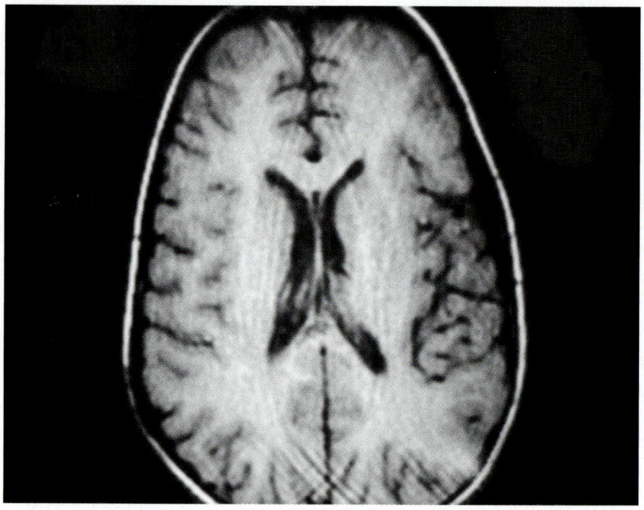

Fig. 29.5: MRI of same child showing significant improvement at 3 months follow-up

callosum and the dorsolateral quadrant of rostral brainstem in the region of superior cerebral peduncle (Figs 29.2 to 29.5).

Tissue tear hemorrhages characteristically appear as small, discreet areas without mass effect or other associated abnormalities. The size of these lesions vary from 0.5 to 2.5 cm. They may not be evident in early CT scans. Normal CT scan have been reported in about 10 to 12 percent of cases.

MRI

Magnetic resonance imaging (MRI) is superior to CT in depicting nonhemorrhagic contusions, which appear as high intensity areas on T2-weighted images and as isointense or hypointense areas on T-weighted images.

Magnetic resonance imaging (MRI) is more sensitive than CT scan in detecting tissue tear hemorrhages. A comparison between T2-weighted MRI and CT scanning showed that non-hemorrhagic lesions were identified in 90 percent of the cases diagnosed with MRI, but in only 20 percent on CT scan. However, small hemorrhagic lesions were seen with approximately the same frequency on both CT scans and MRI studies.

Using high resolution structural MRI evaluation of volume loss in TBI showed widespread effect in white matter volume and sulcal/subdural CSF. Most reliable effects were observed in frontal, temporal and cingulated regions. Although the effects were observed to varying degree in nearly every brain region. Focal lesions were associated with greater volume loss in frontal and temporal region. The pattern of parenchymal volumetric changes can differentiate among the level of traumatic injury severely.[19]

In diffuse axonal injury, diffusion tensor (imaging) tactography-based quantitative analysis at the acute stage of injury has the potential to serve as a valuable biomarker of diffuse axonal injury and predict long-term outcome.[21]

The role of magnetic resonance imaging, specifically magnetic resonance spectroscopy MRS and susceptibility-weighted imaging (SWI) has emerged in evaluation of cases with TBI for better predictability. Specifically the number and volume of hemorrhagic Diffuse axonal injury (DAI) lesious as well as changes in spectral metabolites such as reduced N-acetyl aspartate or elevation in choline related compounds correlate with neurological disability and impairment of global intelligence, memory and attention.[20]

Treatment of Traumatic Diffuse Axonal Injury

Following basic principles are applicable for managing patients with diffuse axonal injuries:

1. Immediate establishment of ventilation and circulation at the accident site.
2. Aggressive monitoring and control of intracranial pressure.
3. Intensive care to achieve neuronal recovery.

The patency of the respiratory tract must be maintained or established and restoration of an adequate ventilation should have top priority. Endotracheal intubation is often necessary to protect the airway and maintain ventilation.

Cerebral perfusion pressure (CPP) is defined as mean arterial pressure (MAP) minus intracranial pressure. CPP = MAP – ICP. The initial approach to maintain MAP (hence CPP) is to establishment and maintenance of circulatory volume by administering adequate volumes of crystalloids, colloid, or blood products, as appropriate.

It is important to identify the patient who are at risk of developing increased intracranial pressure. Risk factors, which can predict intracranial hypertension are:

1. Subarachnoid hemorrhage
2. Midline shift
3. Abnormal mesencephalic cistern.

Patients with subarachnoid hemorrhage are twice likely to develop increased ICP and presence of abnormal mesencephalic cistern are almost three times prone to develop increased ICP. More the midline shift more is the chance of developing raised ICP.

Severe head-injured patients with a normal CT scan have 10 to 15 percent chance of developing intracranial hypertension after 72 hours, hence serial follow-up CT scans are necessary. Most investigators report improved outcome with treatment at levels from 15 to 20 mm Hg. ICP may be measured from intraventricular, intraparenchymal, subdural and extradural sites. At our center, we are using subdural bolt for measuring ICP. A bolt utilizes the technology of fluid filled systems with an external transducer that is consistently referred to a point on the patients head as the zero level (external auditory meatus).

Various medical methods for controlling an increased intracranial pressure are:

1. *Hyperventilation:* Hyperventilation induces hypocapnia which rapidly lowers the ICP by the mechanism of metabolic autoregulation. There is vasoconstriction which decreases the cerebral blood volume. $PaCO_2$ is usually kept around 30 to 33 mm Hg using sedation, analgesia and full neuromuscular blockage.
2. *Position of the patient's head:* Elevating the head of the bed in the range of 15 to 30° from horizontal decreases ICP by improving venous outflow.
3. *Osmotherapy and diuretics:* Mannitol is the drug of choice to reduce ICP. It increases osmotic gradient across the blood-brain barrier (BBB) leading to water movement from area of edema across area of BBB. Mannitol also increases erythrocyte membrane flexibility, which decreases blood viscosity and results in reflex vasoconstriction and decreased cerebrovascular volume. These effects are pronounced if mannitol is administered in bolus.

Barbiturates: It effectively reduces increased ICP by sedation, vasoconstriction, reducing $CMRO_2$ and by inhibiting free radical-induced lipid peroxidation. Important side effects of barbiturate are hypotension and myocardial depression.

Dosage: Loading dose (10 mg/kg) of thiopental given during 30 min.

Maintenance: 1 mg/kg /hr infusion loading dose should be given in well equipped ICU under supervision.

Treatment of barbiturate induced hypotension.

Intravascular volume should be increased and dopamine/dobutamine to be started.

Cerebrospinal fluid drainage: It is an effective means of reducing ICP. Complications are infection and hemorrhage.

Prognosis: In diffuse axonal injuries little can be done about the primary axonal injury. Measures to reduce intracranial pressure and measures to prevent or reverse the secondary insults (such as edema, ischemia and secondary neuronal death) should be taken aggressively as it may improve the mortality and morbidity in diffuse axonal injuries.

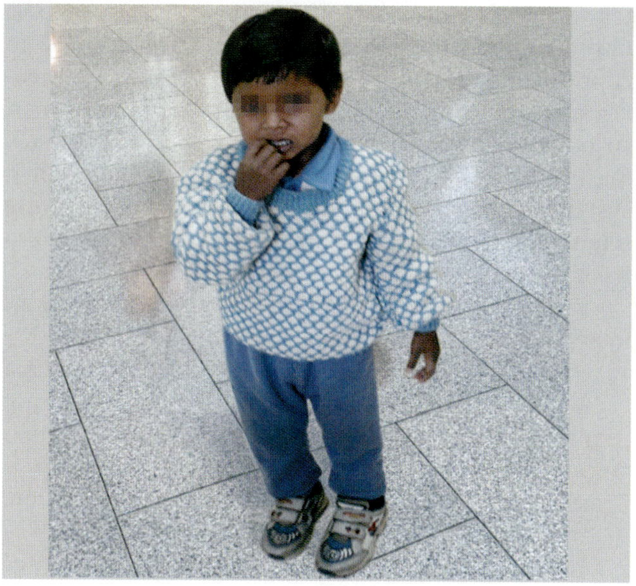

Fig. 29.6: Child recovered from diffuse axonal injury, follow-up at 6 months

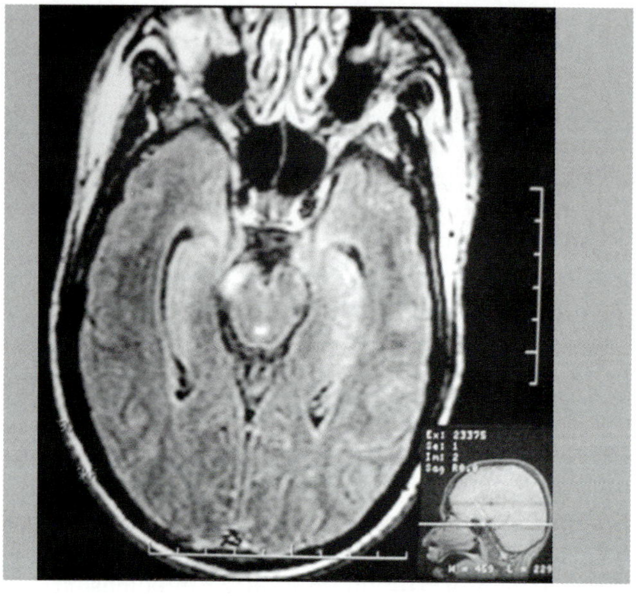

Fig. 29.7: MRI of a patient with DAI showing hyperintensity changes in right cerebral peduncle

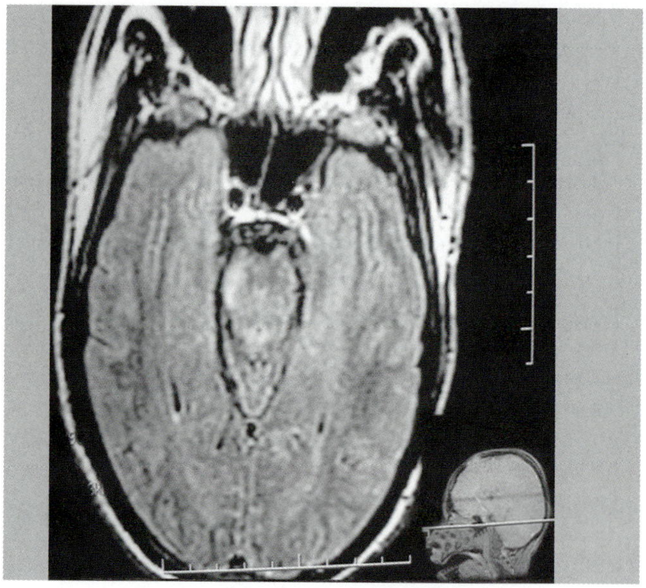

Fig. 29.8: Same patient of DAI showing hyperintensities in right lateral pons

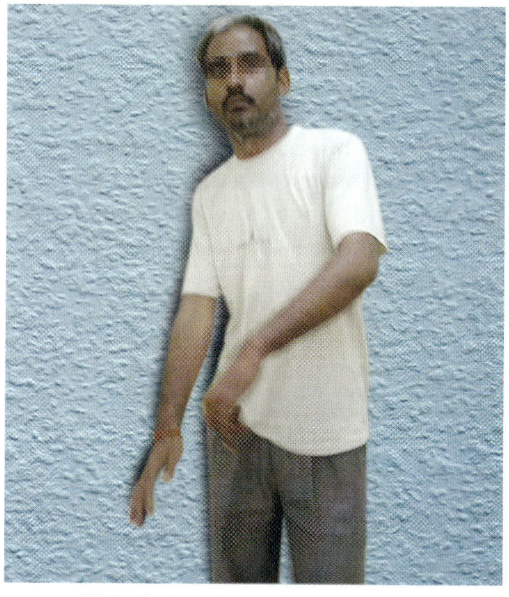

Fig. 29.9: Clinical print of same a patient recovering from DAI having residual weakness in left upper limb

Wilberger et al[16] found a correlation between the admission GCS scores and the eventual outcomes of patient with diffuse axonal injury.

In severe head injury 42 percent of the patients either died or were severely disabled or vegetative at discharge. Mild and moderate head injuries did well; no patient was severely disabled or vegetative at discharge, and no patient died. In patients with brainstem or corpus callosum tissue tear hemorrhages, the outcome were especially poor.[16] Patenkis et al,[17] in 2000 had reported outcome in patients of TDAI and highlighted prognostic role of MRI (See Figs 29.1 to 29.6).

An increase in ventricular CSF total tau (microtubular binding protein) probably reflects the axonal damage, known to be central pathological mechanism in TBI. This increase may be an important neuromarker for predicting long-term outcome in severe TBI.[18]

CONCLUSION

Traumatic diffuse axonal injury is characterized by reactive axonal 'retraction' balls, hemorrhagic necrosis in dorsolateral quadrant of brainstem (Figs 29.7 to 29.9), hemorrhagic necrosis in the corpus callosum. Diffuse axonal injury is caused by angular acceleration or rotational acceleration, the extent of axonal damage depends upon magnitude, duration and rate of angular acceleration. Classically these patients become unconscious immediately upon impact. CT shows small focal punctate hemorrhages in the cerebral white matter, basal ganglia, corpus callosum or dorsal part of the brainstem. MRI is superior to CT scan in demonstrating nonhemorrhagic contusions. Maintenance of cerebral perfusion pressure and aggressive monitoring and control of intracranial pressure are mainstay of medical management.

REFERENCES

1. Strich SJ. Diffuse degeneration of the cerebral white matter in severe dementia following head injury. 3 Neurol Neurosurg Psychiatry 1956;19:163-85.
2. Gennarelli TA, Thibault LE, Adam JH, et al. Diffuse axonal injury and traumatic coma in the primate. Ann Neurol 1982;12:564-74.
2a. Xiao-Sheng H, Sheng YuY, Xiang Z, et al. Diffuse axonal injury due to lateral head rotation in rat model. J. Neurosurg 2000;93:626-33.
3. Aldrich EF, Eisenberg HM. Diffuse Brain Injury. In Tindal GT, Cooper PR, Barrow DL (Eds). The Practice of Neurosurgery, Williams and Wilkins 1996;1490-1501.
3a. Buki A, Povlishock JT. Evidence for Calpain mediated spectin proteolysis in the pathogenesis of traumatically induced axonal injury. J Neuropathol Exp Neurol 1999; 58:365-75.
3b. Buki A, Okonkwo DO, Wang KKW, et al. Cytochrome C release and caspase activation in traumatic axonal injury. J Neurosci 2000;20:2825-34.
4. Mc Cormick WF. Pathology of closed Head Injury. In Wilkins RH, Rengachary SS (Eds). Neurosurgery McGraw Hill 1997;2639-66.
5. Hardman JM. Cerebrospinal trauma. In Davis RL, Robertson DM (Eds). Textbook of neuropathology. Williams and Wilkins 1997;1179-232.
6. Blumbergs PC, Scott G, et al. Staining of amyloid precursor protein to study axonal damage in mild head injury. Lancet 1994;344:1055.
7. Grady MS, Mc Laughin MR, et al. The use of antibodies targetted against the neurofilament subunits for the detection of diffuse axonal injuries in humans. J Neuropathol Exp Neurol 1993;52:143.
8. Povlishock JT, Jenkins LW. Are the pathobiological changes evoked by traumatic brain injury immediate and irreversible? Brain Pathol 1995;5:415-26.
9. Mc Kenzie KJ, Mc Lellan DR, Gentleman SM, et al. Is β-APP, a marker of axonal damage in short surviving head injury? Acta Neuropathol (Berl) 1996;92:608-13.
10. Sherriff FE, Bridges LR, et al. Markers of axonal injury in postmortem human brain. Acta Neuropathol (Berl) 1994;88:433-9.
11. Gentleman SM, Roberts GW, Gennarelli TA, et al. Axonal Injury: A universal consequence of fatal closed head injury. Acta Neuropathol (Berl) 1995;89:537-43.
12. Teasdale GM, Graham GI. Craniocerebral Trauma: Protection and retrieval of neuronal population after injury. Neurosurgery 1998;43:723-38.
13. Adam JH, Doyle D, et al. Diffuse Axonal Injury definition, diagnosis and grading. Histopathology 1989;15:49-59.
14. Adam JH, Dajle D, et al. Microscopic diffuse axonal injury in cases of head injury. Med Sci Law 1985;25:265-9.
15. Lindenberg R, Fisher R, et al. Lesions of corpus callosum following blunt mechanical trauma to the head. Am J Pathol 1955;31:297-317.
16. Wilberger JE, Rothfus WE, et al. Acute tissue tear hemorrhages of the brain: Computed tomography and clinicopathological correlations. Neurosurgery 1990;27:208-13.
17. Paterakis K, Karantanas AH, Komnos A, et al. Outcome of patients with diffuse axonal injury: the significance and prognostic value of MRI in the acute phase. J Trauma 2000;49:1071-5.
18. Ost M, Mylen K, Csajbok L, et al. Initial CSF total Tau correlates with 1 year outcome in patient with TBI. Neurol 2006;67(9):1600-4.
19. Levine D, Kovacevic N, Nica EI, et al. The Toronto traumatic brain injury study. Injury severity and quantified. MRI Neurology 2008;70(10):771-8.
20. Ashwal S, babikian T, Gardener-Nichols J, et al. Susceptibility Wt Imaging and proton magnetic resonance spectroscopy in assessment of outcome in pediatric TBI, Arch Phys Med Rehabl 2006;87(12 suppl 2):550-8.
21. Wang JY, Bakhadirov K, Devons MD Sr, et al. Diffusion tensor tractography of traumatic diffuse axonal injury. Arch Neurol 2008;65(5):619-26.

30 Pediatric Head Injury

Raj Kumar, AK Mahapatra

INTRODUCTION

It is almost 30 years Professor McLaurin, a famous Pediatric Neurosurgeon said, "Child is not a small adult". When he said that, he tried to emphasize that the management protocol being used in adult cannot be applicable to children, especially so, if the children are less than 5 years of age. In India over 40 percent population is under 15 years of age and belongs to pediatric age group. A questionnaire circulated by me in 1995, gave an impression that 30 percent of head injury subjects are in fact, children under 15 years. Considering that the total number of head injuries in a year in India is over 600,000 pediatric population approximately contribute to around 200,000. The magnitude of the problem is therefore, immense. The mechanism of injury, type of pathology, mode of management and specific problems, in the pediatric age group makes these an entirely different management problem compared to that the adult population. The above points justify the need for a special consideration of pediatric head trauma.

MECHANISM OF INJURY

The pediatric population can be distinctly subdivided into four groups: (a) Patient below 1 year, which also include, neonates, (b) Between 1 and 5 years, (c) Above 5 years and less than 10 years and (d) Above 10 years. The frequent mode of head injury in neonates, is birth trauma which is not uncommon. The causes are prolonged labor, cephalopelvic disproportion and difficult labor (Table 30.1). Injury can also be due to the use of forceps or vacuum. The above mentioned causes lead to injury during engagement. During the moulding of fetal head, there is overriding of parietal bones over each other and of the frontal and occipital bones over the parietal bones. These normal processes get exaggerated during an obstructed labor leading to various intracranial hemorrhages and brain edema. The above situation can be made worse due to the application of forceps and vacuum extractors. All the above complications in the neonates are partly avoidable by the use of cesarean section.

Table 30.1: Neonatal head injury

Causes	*Types of labors*
a. Prolonged labor	a. Intracranial hemorrhage
b. Cephalopelvic disproportion	– Subarachnoid
c. Difficult labor	– Intracerebral hematoma
d. Use of forceps and vacuum extractors	– Intraventricular hemorrhage
	– Posterior fossa hematoma
	b. Brain edema

Brain Edema

Injury in toddlers below 5 years are more frequently due to falls, from a height, or object falling on the head of child. Falls constitute over 80 percent of injury in this group, however, when all pediatric age groups are put together falls contribute to injury in over 55 percent cases. Sambasivan had reported occasional head injury in children due to coconut falls. This is common in coastal areas where children play under the coconut trees. Older children more often get injured in road accidents. Recently school accidents have significantly contributed to pediatric head injury. Rarely head injury can occur in children during recreational activities (Tables 30.2A and B).

Table 30.2A: Mode of injury in children—AIIMS observation in 183 patients

Mode	*Number*
a. Fall from a height	101
b. Road traffic accidents	71
c. Assault	9
d. Sports injury	2

Table 30.2B: Other causes or head injury in children

i. Birth injuries
ii. Objects falling over the head (Coconut injury)
iii. Industrial injury
iv. Battered children (Repeated infliction of head injury)

PATHOLOGY

Pathology of head injury in children is similar to those in adults. However, larger number of factors modify the ultimate changes in the brain. The factors are thickness of the skull, presence of open fontanelle type of sutures and developing brain. Pathological changes in brain are: (a) Primary or (b) Secondary. Primary injury includes all types of hematomas, cerebral contusion and laceration, while secondary changes are mainly cerebral edema, hypoxic and ischemic injury (Table 30.3). Hyponatremia is also a known complication of traumatic cerebral injury, often related to SIADH, and also to the elaboration of atrial natriuretic peptide, which can be a cause of seizures after brain injury.[44]

Specific Injuries, Scalp Hematoma and Skull Fracture

Newborns and neonates: Some degree of birth trauma occurs to each newborn during moulding leading to edema of the scalp. Scalp hematoma may occur. However, these conditions often be treated by the pediatricians and usually not referred to neurosurgeon. This condition is called caput succedaneum, which is nothing but scalp edema. Occasionally a larger cephalohematoma can give rise to hypovolemic shock, needing blood transfusion. Fractures in neonate are rare. However, due to elasticity of bone a typical fracture called "Ping Pong fracture" can develop. The fracture could be fissured fracture or even depressed fracture. The linear fracture is the most common type. As the dura is densely adherent to the bone, the dura gets torn and can frequently lead to growing skull fractures. This occurs in children less than 5 years. Due to nonpneumatized paranasal sinuses, the fracture through anterior cranial fossa is also common in children which can lead to CSF leak through the nose.

Table 30.3: Common lesions in children

A. Neonates	– Cephalohematoma
	– Ping-Pong skull fracture
	– Acute subdural hematology
	– Intracerebral hematology
	– Brain swelling
B. Toddlers	– Depressed and common fracture
	– Concussion
	– Extradural and subdural hematoma
	– Contusion
	– Laceration
	– Brain swelling
	– Combinations
C. Older children	– Extradural hematology
	– Subdural hematology
	– Cerebral contusion/laceration
	– Intracerebral hematology
	– Ischemic hypoxic injury
	– Brain swelling

Intracranial Hemorrhage

An exaggerated moulding of skull bones during labor or rough use of forceps can lead to intracranial hemorrhage in neonates. Extradural hematomas are rare in neonates, as in infants the dura is densely adherent to the skull bone. Rupture of delicate surface veins lead to acute subdural hematoma, which is not rare in newborns. Sometimes, subdural hematoma may occur in the posterior fossa. Rarely these hematomas can be large enough to cause herniation and death. Hematoma can be formed even without fracture of the skull.[4,5] About 20 to 25 percent of neonatal deaths are due to intracranial hemorrhage.[10]

Toddlers and Older Children

Children between 5 to 15 years fall from roof tops due to a lack of parent supervision, or during kite-flying. Another cause of injury can also be due to automobile accident, described as "Baby Dashboard syndrome". When small babies are allowed to travel standing or sitting unharnessed on the seat, and the car is suddenly brought to a halt by a head on collision, the head of the baby is squashed between mother and the dashboard.

Fracture of the Skull

The fractures are usually linear and parietal in location. Fractures can cross suture lines and vascular grooves. In younger children, skull is pliable and depressed fracture may look like a dimple on a gutta-percha doll's head. Children falling from greater heights can have comminuted fractures. These fractures lead to dural tears and laceration of brain, and are more often compound in nature. Over 50 to 80 percent children with fracture have associated brain injury. Fractures can also involve anterior or middle fossa giving rise to CSF rhinorrhea or otorrhea. Fracture of anterior fossa may involve orbit and give rise to orbital hematoma and black eyes known as 'Raccoon' eyes. Fracture going through orbit rarely can give rise to blindness. When fracture line involves the petrous bone, the skin overlying the mastoid process is discolored and is popularly known as "Battle's sign".

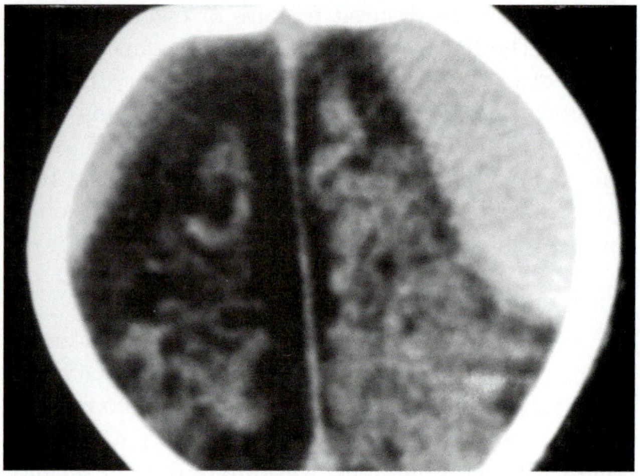

Fig. 30.1: CT of a child showing bifrontal acute subdural hematomas left more than right with cortical atrophy secondary to birth hypoxia

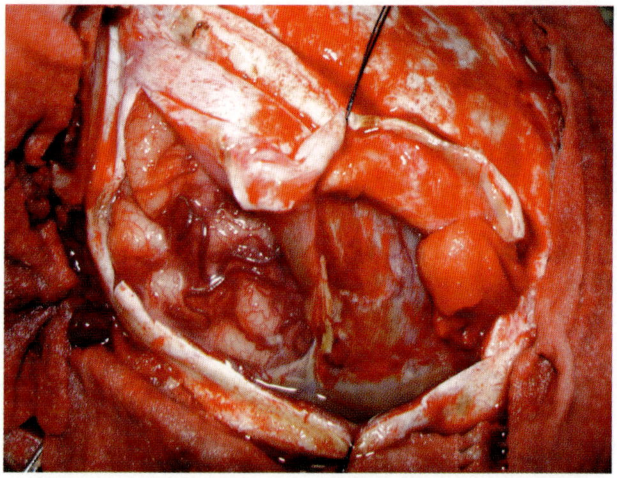

Fig. 30.2: The child of acute subdural hematoma shows organized clot, when operated a week after CT

In shaken baby syndrome, a diffuse axonal injury can be verified by autopsy findings. These children may demonstrate multilayered retinal hemorrhages and acute subdural hematomas along with the changes suggestive of DAI. These findings may be present in older and heavior children.[44]

Concussion of the Brain

Concussion generally means a reversible neurologic dysfunction. This can follow trivial injuries, with transient loss of consciousness. Memory loss is a part of concussion leading to both retrograde and post-traumatic amnesia (PTA). Small children may be "stunned" for a short time do not give classical history of unconsciousness. The etiology of concussion is the injury in the occipital area and shearing strain at brainstem level. Loss of consciousness may also be due to kinking of posterior cerebral arteries. The children recover faster than adults. CT scan usually does not show any abnormalities. However, in experimental animals concussion has shown diffuse damage to axons, both in cerebral cortex and brainstem.

Extradural Hematoma

In younger children extradural hematomas are rare. Hematomas may be of arterial or venous in origin, depending on the type of fracture and type of vessel involved by the fracture. The hematoma can also collect as a result of bleeding from fracture line, and this usually is a thin layer of clot. Most hematomas are temporal or frontal in location. Rarely, posterior fossa extradural hematomas are also observed.[11,12] Ammarati and Tomita[12] reviewed 36 cases of posterior fossa extradural hematomas in children till 1985. These

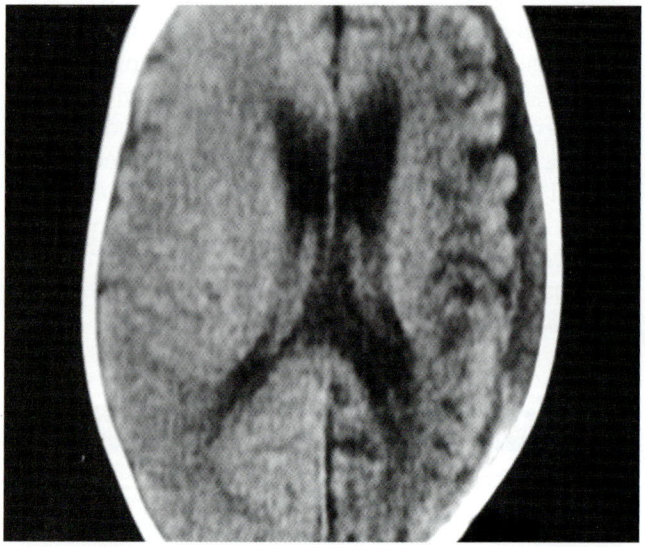

Fig. 30.3: CT of child with tentorial bleed having pre-existing left MCA infarct and atrophy of hemisphere along with subdural effusion

hematomas can also extend above the tentorium in significant number of cases.[11]

Acute Subdural Hematoma

Acute subdural hematomas are common in children. There are two peaks, one in infancy and the another being in older children. Acute SDH is usually a result of severe injury, only rarely it may be due to minor injury in children with bleeding disorders. Frequent falls and injury to the head accounts for a higher incidence of SDH. When the sutures are not fused, the hematoma can grow slowly and is termed as subdural hematoma. The hematoma may remain silent for sometime, as the cranium can expand to accommodate the SDH. When the fontanelle is open, the raised ICP is indicated by tense anterior fontanelle and may be wrongly diagnosed as hydrocephalus by the treating doctor. Rarely acute subdural hematoma can be located in the posterior fossa.

Chronic Subdural Hygroma/Effusion

Subdural fluid collections in neonates and children have varying etiologies; birth trauma is one of them. Majority are seen in infants, predominantly male, with 93 percent under 3 years of age.[38] Other causes of subdural effusion are meningitis, head injury, unknown etiology, postoperative, child abuse, hemorrhagic diathesis and ruptured arachnoid cyst.

The symptoms and signs of extracerebral fluid collection are as follows:

- Seizure
- Macrocrania
- Bulging fontanelle
- Irritability anemia
- Psychomotor retardation
- Cranial nerve palsies
- Hemiparesis.

Different modalities of treatment have been instituted in dealing with these including burr hole drainage, repeated tapping, membranectomy and superior sagittal sinus reconstruction. The most accepted modality of treatment presently is subduroperitoneal shunting. Of course all complications of shunt surgery follow: obstruction, migration, infection, unilateral drainage, skin necrosis, bowel perforation and ileus.[38]

Brain Edema

There are certain differences the way child's brain responds to injury, as compared to that of an adult. In adults the edema is more often due to increased water content, otherwise called vasogenic edema. In children the swelling is intractable and the brain volume increases rapidly, and the condition is termed as malignant brain edema.[13,14] This is by and large due to venous congestion or stasis. Brain injuries lead to release of excitatory neurotransmitters.[15,17,18,33] These substances disturb the autoregulation, leading to breakdown in blood-brain barrier (BBB)[17] and there is leakage of fluid into the extravascular spaces giving rise to brain edema (Table 30.4). Edema could be focal around a contusion or generalized as seen in CT scan.

Table 30.4: Mechanism of edema formation

Head trauma
↓
Disturbance of autoregulation
↓
Deranged microcirculation

(a)	*(b)*
– Opening of tight junction	– Release of vasoactive neurotransmitters
– Breakdown of BBB	– Release of free radicals
– Exudation of fluid	– Opening of calcium channel
– Edema	– Development of edema

Brain Swelling

Recently brain swelling is more and more recognized. This is basically due to vascular congestion. In the past, a term called "luxury perfusion" was described in angiography, which means increased circulation in an infarcted area. Similar findings are occasionally seen in angiogram of the head injured patients. Sometimes children may die rapidly due to generalized brain swelling. Labato et al[18,19] described acute hemispheric brain swelling. Pathophysiological mechanism of brain swelling is, however, not clear. Postmortem usually reveals venous congestion. Control of cerebral circulation following trauma is poorly understood. In contusion or intracerebral hematoma, the focal brain swelling can be well conceived, because of the release of neurotransmitters.

However, formation of diffuse edema or swelling in absence of focal brain lesion is difficult to understand. The only mechanism possible is due to hypoxia occurring during concussion, when a patient is unconscious and the airway may get obstructed due to variety of causes. It is sometimes difficult to understand, whether the vasocongestion is a neurogenic vasoparalysis or is caused by hypoxic autoregulation failure leading to vasodilatation and increased blood flow. Recently transcranial Doppler studies have shown significant flow velocity and pulsatility index abnormalities.

Traumatic Ischemic Damage

Over the last 2 decades, it has been clearly established that the ischemic brain damage is an important pathological finding in the brain, following the head injury. The studies conducted by Graham et al[21,23] have shown that the incidence of ischemic damage is 85 percent, 90 percent in cases of fatal head injuries. Ischemia may be focal or diffuse due to microcirculatory failure. The hypoxic ischemic damage is probably the most frequent mechanism of secondary brain injury. Ischemic damage is not uncommon in children. The fine vasculature in

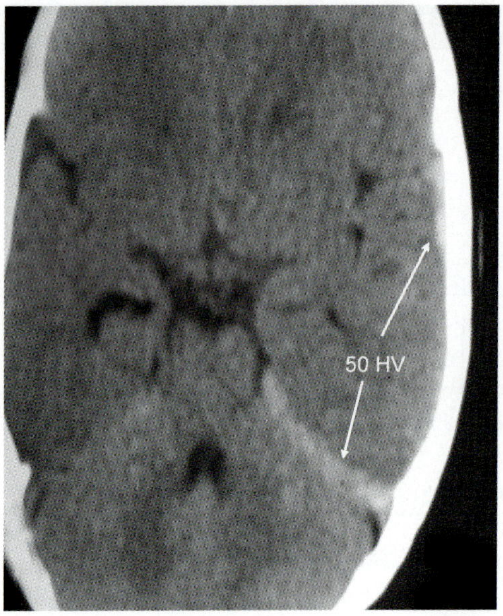

Fig. 30.4: CT of child showing post-traumatic tentorial bleed with cortical atrophy on contralateral side

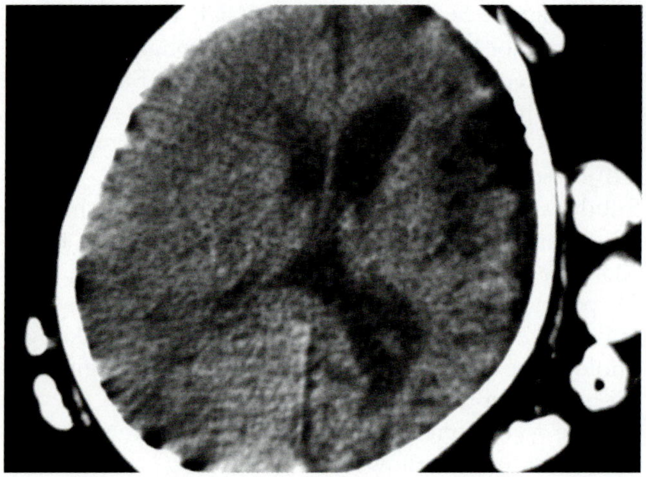

Fig. 30.5: CT of same child following evacuation of subdural effusion showed significant clinical improvement at follow-up

children and the sludging effect of blood in capillaries due to increased viscosity may lead to microcirculatory failure. The potent cause of ischemia is hypotension and raised ICP. Fall in cerebral perfusion pressure below 60 to 70 mm Hg can lead to hypoperfusion and ischemia leading to anaerobic glucose metabolism, and accumulation of lactic acid and glutamate, production of oxygen free radicals, opening of calcium channels and damage to the cells. The ischemic damage is more common in the hippocampus and basal ganglia.[22,23]

Occlusion of major vessels does occur in head injury. Size of ischemia depends upon the size of the vessel occluded. Recently after the availability of CT scan radiological diagnosis of ischemic damage secondary to occlusion of a vessel is possible. In a study on pediatric head injury from our institute, Walia reported large infarcts on CT scans in 8 children.

CLINICAL ASSESSMENT

Breathing

Quick clinical assessment is a key point in management. Evaluation of breathing is most important aspect. This is particularly so in children, and hypoxia is poorly tolerated by the children. Respiratory obstruction for few minutes can lead to irreversible brain damage and is the most potent and preventable cause of death. On the other hand, children do have a high oxygen demand, as compared to adults and consume oxygen, which is double that of the adults. In children air passage is narrower, and the tonsils and adenoids are larger than in adults; thus the probability of respiratory obstruction is higher. The tracheal rings are soft hence flexion of neck can easily obstruct the trachea. (a) Presence of blood, saliva and foreign bodies are likely to obstruct the airway, (b) flexion, extension of neck is likely to compress the larynx and trachea, and (c) the delicate vocal cords and larynx can easily get damaged by repeated suction and repeated attempt to intubate a child. In whom intubation is rather much more difficult as compared to that of adults. The simplest method of evaluation of breathing is to look at the chest movement. One should also observe whether

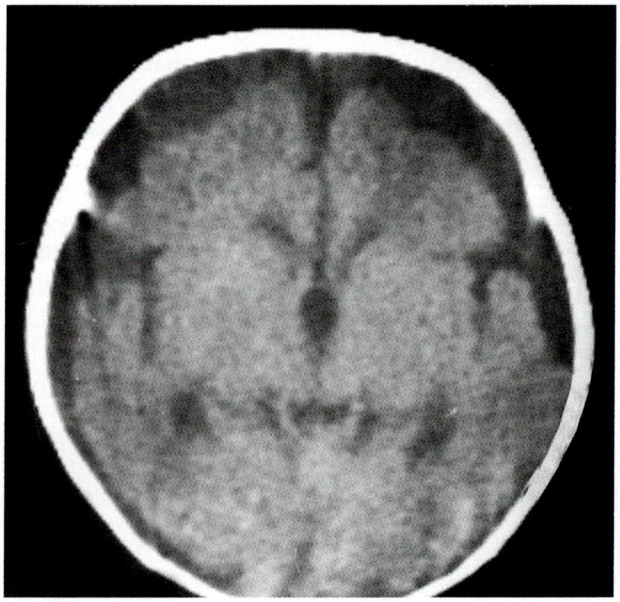

Fig. 30.6: CT of an infant showing post-traumatic subdural effusion

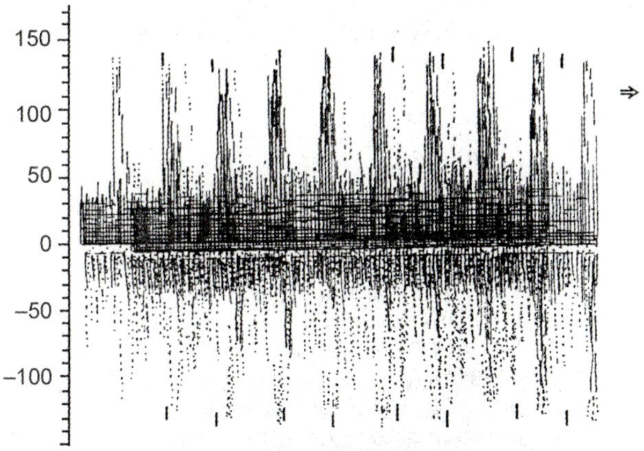

Fig. 30.7: TCD from MCA shows increased PI value in a child with head injury

the breathing is noisy or quite. Noisy bring indirectly means partial construction to air passage.

Fractured ribs make the respiration painful and even in the absence of obstructed breathing respiration can be inadequate, leading to hypoxia. Hence, a careful evaluation of chest injury is mandatory in children, who have poor tolerance to pain. Children have a tendency to swallow air, and develop gastric distention which can further worsen the breathing as diaphragm is pushed upwards.

Assessment of Blood Pressure

Generally head injury does not produce shock. However, neonates and children can develop shock due to scalp hematoma or bleeding from lacerated wound. Children have an increased blood volume of 20 to 25 percent by weight. A simple long bone fracture may lead to 70 to 100 ml blood loss and can result in shock in a child with 10 kg weight. The children also have a poor response to blood loss. Only 10 to 15 percent blood loss is tolerated in children, as compared to adults, who can stand blood loss up to 30 to 40 percent.

Systemic Examination

Thorough examination of limbs for fracture, and of the abdomen for an occult abdominal, pelvic or retroperitoneal injury is also important. Distention of urinary bladder results in an irritable state. Evacuation of urinary bladder reduces abdominal distention and normalizes the respiration.

Neurological Assessment

Neurological assessment helps in determining the extent of the damage to the min. However, assessment

Table 30.5: Pediatric rapid score

A	–	Alert on fully conscious
V	–	Responds to verbal command
P	–	Responds to pain
U	–	Unresponsive

in children under 2 years of age is much more difficult, while children above 10 years of age do not pose difficulty in examination. Neurological examination is undertaken in similar headings as in adults. The examination of the level of consciousness and the presence of focal neurological deficit are the two most important aspects:

a. *Level of consciousness:* Since the time Teasdale and Jennett designed the Glasgow coma score (GSS) it has been universally accepted to evaluate the condition of patients, especially, the level of consciousness. However, over the years its limitations have been realized in assessing the pediatric patients. Hence, pediatric coma score has been developed considering six important factors: (1) Size, (2) Respiratory status, (3) Systolic blood pressure, (4) CNS status, (5) Open wound and (6) Fractures.

   The abnormalities classified into three grades: (a) +2 score for minor abnormality or no abnormality, (b) +1 score for major abnormality and (c) –1 is for severe and life-threatening abnormality. Thus, the total scores ranges from –6 to +12, –6 score signifies 100 percent mortality, while +12 score indicates an excellent outcome.

   For rapid evaluation some pediatric neurosurgeons have modified Glasgow coma score and called AVPU. A for Alert and conscious. V signifies-responses to verbal command, P denotes that the patients response to pain, while U-symbolizes unresponsiveness (Table 30.5). The above assessment system is simple and rapid, however, does not include the systemic factors. Overall 25 percent children are admitted with history of loss of consciousness, and another 25 percent may be drowsy and irritable. Drowsy or lethargic state in a child should be taken seriously as a large number of these children can have intracranial hematoma and can deteriorate rapidly. A typical lucid interval is uncommon in children.

b. *Focal neurological deficit:* Presence of hemiparesis, monoparesis or hemiplegia is indicative of focal brain damage. Examination of cranial nerves is important. Third nerve palsy is considered to be the most significant finding in head injury. Presence of unilateral or bilateral dilated fixed pupils are not uncommon, depending on severity of injury and transtentorial herniation.[27] Bilateral fixed dilated pupils usually indicate a severe injury and signifies, a poor outcome. Rarely a child can be conscious and have a fixed dilated pupil, with a positive consensual light reflex. This is indicative of an optic nerve injury. Mahapatra and Tandon in 1994 reported 50 children with optic nerve injury.[27] Seventh nerve involvement may be of upper motor type as a part of hemiparesis. Lower motor facial palsy can occur due to petrous temporal bone fracture. In such cases Battle's sign and bleeding through the ipsilateral ear may be associated. Hearing loss and CSF otorrhea, may also be associated with facial palsy. Cerebellar signs are rarely observed in head injured children. When present, are always indicative of posterior fossa lesions, such as extradural or subdural hematomas and cerebellar contusion.[11,12,28] Rarely acute subdural hematomas can occur in neonates due to birth trauma and till 1997 less than 100 cases have been reported in the world literature.[28] Irritability, hypotonia, lethargy, tense fontanelle and rarely opisthotonic posture are the characteristic findings in these neonates. In cases of extradural hematoma, patients may remain drowsy and a fine horizontal nystagmus is a significant finding.[11,12]

INVESTIGATIONS

X-ray Skull

Role of X-ray skull, following the availability of CT scan has been a subject of controversy. There is little doubt about the medicolegal significance of X-ray skull. Presence of fracture in a minor head injury warns of the possibility of intracranial hematoma. It is difficult to get a good quality X-ray skull in children, as the quality of X-ray deteriorates due to movement. In unconscious patients and patients with compound head injury, with brain herniation, CT scan is the investigation of choice. In minor head injury, when CT scan is not indicated, X-ray skull must be considered as a mandatory investigation. X-ray skull can reveal various types of skull fractures, PNS opacity, and more importantly, foreign bodies such as metallic fragments or bullet. In a comminuted fracture, X-ray skull may give an indication of displaced bone fragment. However, the use of skull X-ray, to decide whether or not a CT scan is needed is not warranted, as significant intracranial pathology can exist without evidence of skull fracture.[32]

Carotid Angiogram

Carotid angiogram considered as the investigation of choice in adults in the past is no longer used today. Even when CT was not available, carotid anglo was not considered in children because of its invasiveness and the inherent difficulty in obtaining good quality angiogram in children.

CT Scan

CT scan is now considered as the investigation of choice in evaluating brain injury. It is rapidly obtained, more informative, and can be easily repeated.[31] It delineates the intracranial pathology including edema and infarction. Evaluation of posterior fossa is also an important point in favor of CT scan, and shows hematoma distinctly. CT scans are also used to evaluate long-term sequele of head injury.

We at the institute regularly performed CT scan in pediatric head injury (Table 30.6). It is only after the availability of CT scan that it was possible to diagnose brainstem hematoma.

MRI

Magnetic resonance imaging (MRI) although prohibitive in cost and has limitations with excess motion (which can be overcome with latest generation fast scanners), however, can be used for the diagnosis of all pathologies in head injury except skull fractures and subarachnoid hemorrhage. It gives a better resolution of parenchymal injury and posterior fossa. MRI is more sensitive to the presence of intraparenchymal injury, edema, diffuse axonal injury, small contusions and hematomas. The most sensitive neuroimaging study available for brain injury is MRI scan. The ability to measure cerebral

Table 30.6: CT scan finding in pediatric head injury, experience at AIIMS

Type of lesion	*Number of patients*
Extradural hematoma	15
Subdural hematoma	29
Cerebral contusion/cerebral hematoma	85
Brain edema	37
CMUSE axonal injury	14
Intraventricular hemorrhage	5
Brainstem hematoma	6
Cerebral infarction	8
Normal scan	31

blood flow (CBF), cerebral blood volume (CBV) and to identify location, of edema fluid, inn or extracellularly is now possible with MRI.

MRI spectroscopy will allow the clinicians to subdivide further types of head trauma, and to define certain aspects of pathology in better fashion. These will be the location of ongoing ischemia if it exist, frequency of vasogenic edema, and contribution to raised ICP, and the presence and distribution of intracellular edema as well as its role in elevated JCP, can be determined.[31]

The role of magnetic resonance imaging, specifically magnetic resonance spectroscopy (MRS) and susceptibility-weighted imaging (SWI) has emerged in evaluation of cases with TBI for better predictability. Specifically the number and volume of hemorrhagic Diffuse axonal injury (DAI) lesions as well as changes in spectral metabolites such as reduced N-acetyl aspartate or elevation in choline related compounds correlate with neurological disability and impairment of global intelligence, memory and attention.[45]

MANAGEMENT

Management of head injury should ideally start from the site of accidents, however, in the best of the situation it may not be possible. Hence, the real treatment starts from the casualty. There is no doubt that the 1st golden hour following trauma is important for both adult and pediatric patients. Events happening within 1 to 2 hours almost always indicate the long-term outcome.

As it is generally accepted and by and large is correct that respiratory obstruction and hypotension are the two most important killers, followed by intracranial hematomas. Intracranial hematoma takes time and requires CT scan to establish the diagnosis contrary to respiratory obstruction which kills the patient rapidly and do not require investigation for its management. Hence, adequate oxygenation is the most important step in the patients management. Frequently, patients need endotracheal intubation and elective ventilation (Tables 30.7 and 30.8). Starting of proper intravenous fluid therapy and adequate replacement of fresh blood is the 2nd most important treatment in patients with shock. Concept of dehydrating the patient is wrong and specially so in children, as children tolerate dehydration poorly and likely to develop renal problems. Patients with raised ICP or intracranial hematoma need mannitol 0.5 to 1 gm per kg of body weight. Ringer's lactate is considered as the fluid of choice. However, to avoid hypoglycemia one must add glucose containing fluid. If necessary an indwelling catheter is placed to prevent the bladder distention and also for exact measurement of urine output.

Table 30.7: Intensive care criteria for imaging after head Injury[34]

A. Criteria for imaging after head injury
• Loss of consciousness or amnesia suspected at any time
• Neurological symptoms, e.g. headache, vomiting, irritability on handling, inappropriate behavior
• CSF or blood from the nose or ear
• Suspected penetrating injury
• Scalp bruising or swelling laceration down to the bone
• Under fives when the mechanism of injury is not deemed to be trivial
• Suspected non-accidental injury.
Note: Skull X-ray is not necessary if CT scan is to be performed; clinical judgment is necessary particularly with regard to the force of injury.
B. Indications for admission to hospital
• All children with altered level of consciousness
• In an oriented child:
– Skull fracture
– Persisting neurological signs and symptoms
– Difficulty in assessment
• Other medical conditions
• Lack of responsible adult to supervise child if discharged.
C. Indications for consultation with the head injury center (when admitted in non-neurosurgical unit)
• Decreased level of consciousness after resuscitation
• Deteriorating consciousness or progressive neurological signs
• Skull fracture with: Irritability, inappropriate behavior, seizures, or neurological signs

Anticonvulsants are important.[37] Children are prone for hypoxia and hypoglycemia and both are potent causes of post-traumatic fits. During the fit the intracranial pressure is increased significantly. Hence, phenytoin must be administered. In an unconscious patient proper antibiotics are likely to reduce chest and urinary infection. Infection significantly increases the risk of death and morbidity. Prevention of bed sore and nutrition requirements must be managed judiciously.

Role of Surgery

As in adults the surgery must be offered to: (a) Compound injury with brain herniation, (b) Large hematoma with significantly raised ICP. Removal of clot is a quick method of reducing the raised ICP.

Table 30.8: Intensive care

A. Nursing
- Nurse head-up tilt 20°
- Ensure optimal mid
- Line head and neck position so that neck veins are not obstructed
- Keep head in the midline when turning the patient.

B. Glasgow Coma Score
- Oral enacheal intubation using rapid sequence induction
- Mechanical ventilation with, 100% oxygen
- Intravenous access at two sites
- Place on cardiac monitor
- Blood test: Full blood count, blood type, glucose.

Note: Indications for intubation include hypoxia, chest and facial fractures, deteriorating neurology, multiple repeated seizures, or if moderate/severe case needing transfer. If in shock give 20 ml/kg of intravenous isotonic crystalloid colloid or blood product as and when indicated.

C. Intubated Patient
- Ensure uptimal analgesia, sedation and neuromuscular blockade
- Optimize blood gases
- Seizure activity: Use loading dose of phenytoin 20 mg/kg following intravenous guidelines
- Protect the eyes
- Aim to keep temperature normal using paracetamol; counsider cooling if >38°C
- Give mannitol 0.25–0.5 g/kg over 15 minutes for acute rise in ICP or pupillary changes.

D. Fluids after Resuscitation
- Normal saline with appropriate potassium chloride at the rate of 75% maintenance
- Add glucose when serum glucose in the normal range
- Hypoglycemia: Treat with 2–4 ml/kg 25% dextrose in water.

A significant percentage of children do have compound head injury. A study reported from AIIMS showed that compound head injury was the largest group in operated cases (Table 30.9). Amongst 84 operated, 38 had (36%) compound head injury. Hematoma was removed in 15 patients and craniotomy and lobectomy or removal of contusion was carried out in 22 patients. The aim of the surgery in compound injury is to debride the wound and to perform a water tight dural closure, after excising the damaged brain.

In general, experienced anesthetist, quick surgery and adequate replacement of fresh blood are the three most important points. As far as possible, narcotics must be avoided as they produce respiratory depression and also interfere with postoperative evaluation. Care must be taken to ventilate the children postoperatively till the time they have good respiration.[6,7,34] If a patient needs long-term ventilation an elective tracheostomy is necessary which helps in reducing the dead space and easy aspiration of tracheobronchial secretions.

Table 30.9: Indications for surgery in pediatric head injury, experience at AIIMS

Surgical procedure	*Number of patient*
Evacuation of EDH	9
Evacuation of SOH	15
Removal of contusion	22
Debridement and duraplasty	38
Tracheostomy	20

Children have a very little glycogen or fat reserve. Hence in severe head injury, a nasogastric feeding should be started as soon as possible. Nasogastric feeding also helps in administering drugs. In compound head injury, intravenous antibiotics are given to prevent wound infection and meningitis. Antibiotics must be prescribed as the protocol of the unit considering the common pathogens and their antibiotic sensitivity.

Predictors of the Severity of Injury

In addition to well established clinical parameters such as infant coma score at time of presentation and the history of loss of consciousness, a bulging fontanelle, bilateral 3rd nerve palsy, irregular respiration and unresponsiveness, other parameters also are known to have a positive correlation with the severity of brain injury even in the presence of an apparently normal neurological examination. Hemocoagulative abnormalities deranged activated partial thromboplastin time (APTT), fibrinogen level, fibrin-degradation products (FDP) and platelet counts have a positive correlation with the severity of injury and Glasgow outcome score.[39,43] Also the development of early post-traumatic seizures correlates with the severity of injury.[37]

Age under one year has a strong correlation with high mortality.[36] Patients with a less than 6 hours post-trauma low GCS score or less than 135 mm systolic BP correlate with a poor prognosis for survival. Children as a group have a better prognosis. Very young and pre-school children have a worse outcomes and long-term disability. Aggressive management to prevent secondary injury will improve outcome.[41,42]

Table 30.10: Factors influencing outcome
a. Coma score
b. Associated injury
c. Age of the patient
d. Hypotension
e. Fixed dilated pupils
f. Decerebrate rigidity or decortication
g. Cold caloric response

OUTCOME

The overall mortality in severe head injury is high, can range 20 to 60 percent.[6-8,29,30] The mortality is multifactorial and depends upon large number of factors.[6,7,30] The factor influencing the outcome listed in Table 30.10. Age below 2 years has been reported as a poor prognostic factor.[6,7]

The study reported by Walias observed a 97 percent mortality when the GCS was three to four. Zuccarello et al[8] reported 85 percent mortality in patients with GCS three to four. The study reported from AIIMS reported an overall mortality of 22 percent and good recovery in 57 percent children.

The predictive critical score of GCS should be set at 5 for pediatric TBI. Because it strongly correlates with outcome in this age group. Subarachnoid hemorrhage with brain swelling and edema, subdural, intracerebral hemorrhage and basal ganglion lesions are associated with severe injury and poor outcome ($P<0.05$). However, cortical lesions do not effect severity and outcome.[43]

Although the mortality rates for children with severe TBI remains high, but decompressive craniectomy is effective in reducing ICP is associated with good outcomes in surviving patients.[48]

CONCLUSION

Head injury is frequent in pediatric age group. Pediatric head injury constitutes 25 to 30 percent of all head injuries in India. Wide range of etiologies are encountered depending on the age group. Birth trauma is a more frequent cause in neonate, while falls are causative in toddlers. Extradural hematomas are rare in young children. However, young children are prone for malignant brain swelling and ischemic brain damage. Children withstand blood loss and hypoxia poorly. Surgery in children require experienced anesthetist and surgeon. Infants and younger children have poorer prognosis than older children. Overall mortalities in children ranges from 20 to 50 percent.

REFERENCES

1. Mahapatra AK. Monitoring in paediatric head injury patients. Neurology India (Suppl) 1995;43:67-70.
2. King DR. Trauma in infancy and childhood: Initial evaluation and management. Paediatric Clinic of North America 1995;32:1299-1303.
3. Moront ML. The injured child. An approach to care. Paediatric Clinic of North America 1994;41:1201-26.
4. Sambasivan M. Epidemiology-Paediatric Head Injuries. Neurology India (Supple) 1995;43:57-58.
5. Chidambaram B. Head injuries. Special problems in children. Neurology India (Supple) 1995;43:68-73.
6. Walia severe paediatric head injury. An analysis of 138 patients. M Ch. Thesis submitted to AIIMS, 2010.
7. Bruce DA, Scheet C, Ware JD, Sutton LN. Outcome following severe head injury in children. J Neurosurg 1978;48:679-88.
8. Zuccarello M, Facco E, Zampieri P, Zanardi I, Andrioli GC. Severe head injury in children. Early diagnosis and outcome. Child's Nervous System 1985;1:158-62.
9. Baker DP, Flower C, Li G, Laine M. Head injuries incurred by children and young adults during informal recreation. Ame J Publ Health 1994;84:649-52.
10. Bagchi AK. Head Injury in neonates. In an introduction to head injury. Chapter 11, AK Bagchi (Ed), Oxford University Press, 1980;77-80.
11. Mahapatra AK. Posterior fossa extradural haematoma. Indian Paediatrics 1990;27:989-92.
12. Ammarati M, Tomita T. Posterior fossa. Extradural haematoma in children. Neurosurgery 1985;14:541-4.
13. Bruce DA, Alavi A, Bilanink L, et al. Diffuse cerebral swelling following head injuries in children. The syndrome of "malignant brain oedema". J Neurosurg 1981;54:170 8.
14. Lang DA, Teasdale GM, et al. Diffuse brain swelling after head injury, more often malignant in children than adults. J Neurosurg 1991;80:875-80.
15. Mohanty S, Dey PK, Ray AK. Role of serotonin in cerebral edema. Ind J Med Res 1979;69:1001-7.
16. Mohanty S, Dey PK, et al. Role of histamine in traumatic brain oedema. An experimental study in rats. J Neurol Sciences 1989;90:87-97.
17. Long DM. Traumatic brain edema. Clinical Neurosurg 1982;29:174-202.
18. Lobato RD, Savania R, Cordabes F, Civas JJ. Post-traumatic cerebral hemispheric swelling. Analysis of 55 cases studied with CT. J Neurosurg 1988;68:417-23.
19. Lobato RD. Post-traumatic brain swelling. In Advances and technical standarders in neurosurgery. Symon L (Ed) 1993, Springer Verlag (Wine) New York vol. 21, 3-38.
20. Yang BO, Feng Z, Zhang Z. Sun H. A transcranial Doppler study of drainage of cerebrospinal fluid and intracranial haematoma. In: Modern Trends in Management of Neurotrauma. Ramani PS, and Sharma A (Eds), Lavanya Print Pvt. Ltd. Bombay, 1994, 36.

21. Graham DI. Pathology of hypoxic damage in brain, hopoxia and ischaemia. J Clin Path 30 (Supplement) 1977;11:170-80.
22. Dharker SR, Mittal RS, Bhargav N. Ischaemic lesion in basal ganglia in children after minor head injury. In: Neurology India Supplement 1995;43:61-3.
23. Graham DI, Adama JH, Doyle O. Ischaemic brain damage in brain in fatal nonmissile head injuries. J Neurol Sciences 1976;39:213-34.
24. Miller JD. Relevance of primary and secondary brain damage for outcome of head injury. In Mechanism of secondary brain damage. Brethmann A, Go KC, Unterberg A (Eds). New York, Plenum Press, 1986;323-8.
25. Bakshi A, Mahapatra AK. TCD change in basilar artery in severe head injury (Abstract) Neuro Euro and Critical Care Conf 1998 Feb Brussel.
26. Moront ML, et al. The injured child. An approach to care, Paediatric Clinic of North America 1984;41:1201-29.
27. Mahapatra AK, Tandon DA. Traumatic optic neuropathy in children. A prospective study of 50 patients. Paediatric Neurosurgery 1993;19:34-39.
28. Pervin RG, Rutka JT, Drake JM, et al. Management and outcome of posterior fossa subdural haematoma in neonates. Neurosurg 1997;40:1190-1200.
29. Hendrick EB. The use of hypothermia in severe head injury in children. Arch Surg 1985;79:362-4.
30. Pazzoglia P, Frank G, Frank F, Gaist G. Clinical Course and Prognosis of acute post-traumatic coma. N Neurol Neurosur, Psychiat 1992;38:149-54.
31. Bruce DA. Imaging after head trauma: Why, when and which. Child Nervous System 2000;16:755-9.
32. Murgio A, Patrick PD, Andrade FA, Boetto S, Leung KM, Sanchez MAM. International study of emergency depart-ment care for paediatric traumatic brain injury and the role of CT scanning. Child Nervous System 2001;17:257-62.
33. Glass TE (Ed). The Journal of Paediatrics 2001;138(1):1-3.
34. Tasker RC. Symposium: Intensive care-I, Neurocritical care and traumatic brain injury. Indian Journal of Paedia-trics 2001;68(3):257.
35. Tomia T. Management of acute-stage head trauma in childhood. No To Hattatsu 2000;32(2):132-4.
36. Tilford JM, Simpson PM, Yeh TS, Lensing S, Aitken ME, Green JW, Harr J, Fiser DH. Variation in therapy and outcome for paediatric head trauma: patients. Crit Care Med 2001;29:1056-61.
37. Chiaretti At, De Benedictis R, Polidori G, Piastre M, Iannelli A, Di Rocco C. Early post-traumatic seizures in children with head injury. Child Nervous System 2001; 16:862-6.
38. Ersahin V, Tabur E, Kocaman S, Mutluer S. Complications of it sub-duroperitoneal shunting. Child Nervous System 2000;16:433-6.
39. Chiaretti A, Pezzotti P, Mestrovic J, et al. The influence of Hemocoagulative disorders on the outcome of children with head injury. Paediatric Neurosurgery 2001;34:131-7.
40. White JR, Farukhi Z, Bull C, Christensen J, et al. Predictors of outcome in severely head-injured children. Crit Care Med 2001;29:534-40.
41. Adelson PD. Paediatric trauma made simple. Clin Neurosurg 2000;47:319-35.
42. Abbate B, Donati P, Cagnoni G. Head Injuries in children, consideration on 3,715 consecutive cases. Minerva Pediatr 2000;52:623-8.
43. Keller MS, Fendya DG, Weber TR. Glasgow coma scale predicts coagulopathy in pediatric trauma patients. Semin Pediatr Surg 2001;10:12-6.
44. Donati-Genet PC, Dubuis JM, Girardin E, Rimensberger PC. Acute symptomatic hyponatremia and cerebral salt wasting after head injury: An important clinical entity. J Pediatr Surg 2001;36(7):1094-7.
45. Chung CY, Chen CL, Chang PT, See LG, et al. Critical score of GCS for pediatric traumatic brain injury. Pediatr Neurol 2006;34(5):379-87.
46. Salehi- Had H, Brandt JD, Rosas AJ, Rogers KK. Findings in older children with abusive head injury: does shaken child syndrome exist: Pediatrics 2006;117(5):e1039-44.
47. Ashwal S, Babikian T, Gardener-Nichols J, et al. Sus-ceptibility Wt Imaging and proton magnetic resonance spectroscopy in assessment of outcome in pediatric TBI. Arch Phys Med Rehab. L 2006;87(12 suppl 2):550-8.
48. Ost M, Mylen K, Csajbok L, et al. Initial CSF total Tau correlates with 1 year outcome in patient with TBI. Neurol 2006;67(9):1600-4.
49. Imataka G, Miyamoto K, Fujiyama Y, et al. Acute purulent meningitis associated with chrome subdural hematoma and subdural hygroma. Turk J Pediatr 2007;49(4):437-40.
50. Jagannathan J, Okankavo DO, Dumont AS, Ahmed H, et al. Outcome following decompressive craniectomy in children with severe traumatic brain injury. 10 years single center experience with long-term follow-up. J Neurosurg 2007;106(4):268-75.

31 Head Injury in Elderly

AK Mahapatra, Raj Kumar

INTRODUCTION

Outcome of head injury is multifactorial and amongst those the age is an important prognostic factor. The outcome in extreme age groups is unfavorable. Mortality and morbidity due to moderate and severe head injury in elderly is twice as high as younger patients.[1-4] The term elderly is also confusing. With increased longevity today, a large section of population in the society is surviving over 60 years. According to well accepted terminology, people above 60 years of age are termed as elderly. Surprisingly, there is very little literature on this topic.[1,4-7] I feel, with increasing incidence of head injury and enhanced life-expectancy, the number of people suffering from head injury above 60 years of age is going to increase. Hence, there is need for special awareness of management of head injury in elderly patients.

INCIDENCE

The exact incidence of head injury in elderly is not known. However, several studies have reported the incidence ranging from 2.7 to 15 percent.[4-6] As early as 1969, Jain and Kankanady[6] reported 6 percent incidence of head injury above the age of 50 years, in a study analysing 1500 head injury, in Delhi. A multicentric study on head injury[3] comparing head injury outcome at Delhi and Charlottesville, USA, showed incidence of head injury in elderly above the age of 60 years is 2.7 percent at Delhi as compared to 15 percent at Charlottesville, Virginia. This is quite expected as larger section of US population is above 60 years of age as compared to India. In a retrospective study dealing with 2476 patients from AIIMS, Sinha et al[7] reported 4.4 percent incidence of head injury above 60 years (110 out of 2476 patients).

Mode of Injury

The most common cause of head injury is the road traffic accidents, which account for 75 to 80 percent of head injuries.[2,3] However, the situation is slightly different for elderly patients. The most frequent cause of head injury in elderly is fail.[3,5,6,8] Galbraith in 1989,[5] Goodman and Englander[8] (1990) had reported fall as a frequent cause of head injury in elderly, as compared to the road traffic accident in younger age group. In another report, Jain and Kankanady[6] observed, fall contributing to head injury around 52 percent of patients above 50 years of age. Surprisingly, report from AIIMS[7] quoted 63 percent of all head injury in elderly due to road traffic accidents and 32 percent due to fall. The remaining 5 percent were due to assaults. The usual history is fall in the bathroom or during climbing the stairs. There are several factors which contribute to the fall in an elderly individual.[8] Few important factors are, visual and auditory impairment, high blood pressure, osteoarthritis, parkinsonism and rarely dementia. Sometimes, it is difficult to determine the cause of head injury in a patient and could be likely due to one of the above medical problem.

Pathological Lesions in the Brain

Pathological nature of lesions, in general, are similar in all age groups. However, the incidence of various pathology vary significantly in patients with different age groups. This is basically because of several factors, such as thickness of the skull bone, adhesion of dura to the innertable of skull, associated cerebral atrophy and status of intracranial and cerebral blood vessel. Associated conditions like diabetes, high blood pressure and long-term use of drugs such as aspirin and other anticoagulants do influence the clot formation in the brain following the head injury. Hence, these conditions must be carefully enquired in patients with head injury. It is also important to remember that the consumption of alcohol does play an important role in outcome of traumatic brain lesions.

It is correct that extradural hematoma is rare in elderly. Cortical atrophy due to aging brain, helps in tearing of the bridging veins due to shearing movement, even following minor injury. Hence, there is a high possibility of formation of acute subdural hematoma (SDH). As there is a lot of space due to cortical atrophy, there is less of tamponade effect to stop bleeding, which lead to a large amount of blood collection. However, development of raised pressure is prevented due to availability of space to accommodate a large hematoma. Hence, patient's clinical condition may not deteriorate for a longer time as compared to young patients. Extradural hematomas in elderly patients have been known for poor prognosis. The elderly are less likely to manifest with clinical features of increased intracranial pressure due to cerebral atrophy, hematomas were seen in parietal region in one study. The postoperative results are found to be satisfactory with one death out of 14 operated elderly patients (with mean age 74 years).[17]

Patients with ischemic heart disease or hypertension, are likely to develop large intracerebral hematoma. Klashee et al[9] in 1980 reported 4 times higher incidence of intracranial hematomas in patients above 45 years, in whom there was associated hypertension. In a study from AIIMS, Sinha et al[7] had observed higher incidence of cerebral contusion or intracerebral hematomas (ICHs) (40/97) and only 3 patients had extradural hematoma (Table 31.1). In his study, 34 (35%) patients showed normal CT scan. A thin layer acute subdural hematoma may be formed in old people following a very minor head trauma, patients are usually asymptomatic or have mild headache. Over the period of 2 to 3 weeks, a large amount of liquid blood get collected in subdural space giving rise to clinical problem. This condition is termed as chronic subdural hematoma, with an outer and an inner membrane. The chronic SDH is a common condition in elderly. Troller in 1914[10] was the first to describe the traumatic SDH. Due to cortical atrophy, bilateral SDH is common in elderly.

Therapeutic anticoagulation with warfarin, rather than warfarin use itself is associated with adverse outcome in elderly patients with TBI.[18]

Table 31.1: Nature of pathology diagnosed in CT scan

CT scan findings	*No.*	*Number operated*
Extradural hematoma (EDH)	3	1
Subdural hematoma (SDH)	14	9
Cerebral contusion	32	12
Intracerebral hematoma	8	3
	57	25
Normal CT scan	34	
CT scan not done	2	
Compound depressed fracture	2	2
	95	27

Table 31.2: Systemic illness in 97 elderly head injured

Illness	*No.*
Diabetes	13
Hypertension	9
Ischemic heart disease	4
Chronic airway disease	2
Total	28

CLINICAL PRESENTATION

Normally 70 to 85 percent of all head injuries are minor or moderate and only 15 to 20 percent are severe. In a study from AIIMS, Sinha et al[7] reported on 36 percent incidence of severe head injury in elderly. This is in contradiction to the fact that atrophic brain provides much more space for hematoma in elderly as compared to younger patients. However, hypotension and hypoxia can damage ageing neurons easily and quickly. Hence, elderly patients are likely to be affected by hypoxia and hypotension. Likewise, older people are likely to have unstable, cardiovascular and respiratory system, which render them more susceptible to hypotension and hypoxia.[6] In general, they have a poor reserve. Thus, during clinical evaluation proper history of systemic illness and evaluation of other systems are mandatory (Table 31.2). Evaluation of cardiac status is necessary by performing an electrocardiography. Roy et al[11] studied 146 head injury patients above 65 years of age, and reported medical illness in 117 (80%). Cardiovascular problem was the most frequent and was observed in 24 percent. Sinha et al[7] in 1993 reported systemic illness in 15 of the 37 elderly patients with mild head injury. Hence, systemic examination is an important step in elderly, as the systemic illness significantly influence the ultimate outcome in patients with head injury. Prostatic problem, arthritis, visual and hearing loss are common in old age. Some of these factors may contribute to fall in road accidents. Hearing and visual impairment also affect recovery.[1,8]

Associated injury in body adversely affects the outcome. A significant number of elderly patients with head injury, do have associated injuries.[7,12] Sinha et al[7] reported associated in 27 (Table 31.3). Fracture ribs with hemothorax, and fracture limb bones were more frequent. In 4 patients, vertebral fracture was observed. Five patients had shock. A patient with D_6 fracture had paraplegia. Van-Aalst et al[12] reported a higher incidence of multiple injury in elderly patients as compared to younger patients. According to their observation, shock was associated with poor outcome.

Table 31.3: Associated injury in elderly patients observations at AIIMS

A. **Chest Injuries**
   1. Fracture ribs alone
   2. Fracture ribs with pneumothorax
   3. Fracture ribs with hemothorax
B. **Fracture Limb Bones**
   1. Femur
   2. Tibia
   3. Elbow joints
   4. Hand bones
C. **Fracture Clavicle**
D. **Fracture Spine (Vertebra)**
   1. C_1-C_2
   2. C_5
   3. D_6
   4. Sacrum

MANAGEMENT

Management of elderly patients with head injury is important from several angles. First, the management of associated disease such as diabetes, hypertension, cardiac problem, renal problem and prostatic enlargement. These factors create problem and reduce chances of recovery. Secondly, use of analgesic and sedative should be administered carefully as the effect of the medicine may have unpredictable results. Similarly, use of mannitol to reduce brain swelling and raised ICP, may lead to profound fluid electrolyte imbalance. Thirdly, elderly patients are poor risk candidates for anesthesia and surgery, hence, require anesthetic expertee and quick surgery. Fourthly, associated injury and shock must be managed promptly to prevent ischemic damage to aging neurons.

Fluid electrolyte imbalances are frequent problem.[7] Study by Sinha et al[7] from AIIMS, revealed biochemical abnormality in serum in 57 percent. Twenty-six patients out of 97 had renal dysfunction as the urea was between 60 to 90 mg percent. Electrolyte abnormalities like, hypokalemia and hyponatremia must be prevented, or if developed, must be treated carefully.

Elderly patients have poor respiratory reserve. Lack of oxygenation can lead to hypoxic brain damage. Hence, adequate oxygenation is mandatory. Frequently, elderly patients have bronchial asthma, chronic bronchitis and chronic obstructive airway disease. These conditions reduce oxygenation, hence necessitate in artificial ventilation. Associated rib fracture also affects the respiration, due to reduction of chest movement. Study conducted at AIIMS[7] revealed half of the elderly patients with head injury required ventilatory support. Eight patients had poor respiration on arrival at casualty, hence, intubated in casualty itself. It is also important to realise that the adequate oxygenation is also required following surgery, when the patients are also on the effect of muscle relaxant and analgesic. Postoperative ventilation was necessary in 22 of 27 operated patients.[7]

Large number of head injury patients in coma, both pre- and postoperatively, altered consciousness, old age, systemic disease and above all the poor resistance, make them high-risk candidate for infection. Hence, prophylactic antibiotics is necessary. Large number of antibiotics available today may have damaging effect on the kidney. Hence, adequate proper antibiotic therapy along with frequent assessment of liver and kidney function is necessary, which not only helps in preventing infection but also helps in preventing kidney dysfunction.

Surgery for Intracranial Hematomas

Overall, aim of the surgery in intracranial hematoma removal is to reduce the raised intracranial pressure. Luckily, elderly patients with brain atrophy can accommodate large hematoma without manifesting raised ICP. Hence, these patients may not need surgery. When required surgery, patients need experienced anesthetist and quick surgery to prevent anesthetic complication. Considering above points one must not rush for surgical evacuation of the hematomas. Study of AIIMS[7] had shown large number of patients with intracranial hematoma were managed conservatively. Only 25 of 57 intracranial hematomas needed surgical evacuation.

Patients with chronic subdural hematoma, do not require general anesthesia, as liquid subdural blood can easily be drained or aspirated through drill holes or by burr holes,[10] under local anesthesia.

OUTCOME

Old age is one of the significant factor for poor outcome in patients with head injury.[1,3,5,7,13,15,16] Amacher and Baybee in 1979[1] reported as high as 84 percent mortality in patients above 80 years of age. Carlson et al[13] reported overall mortality of 78 percent in patients above 60 years of age with severe head injury. Katz et al[15] reported uniformly poor recovery in elderly patients whom GCS was lower than 13 (moderate and severe injury), as the patients were dependant and could not go back to their pre-injury employment.

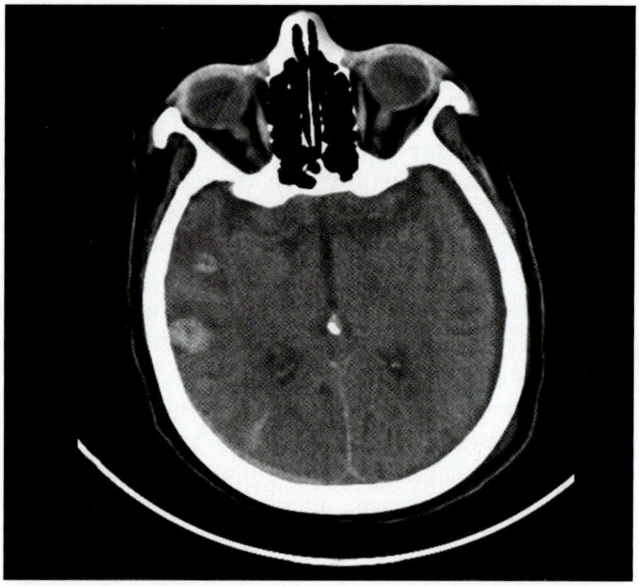

Fig. 31.1: CT showing right temporal clots and contusions in elderly female depicting post-traumatic subdural effusion on left side

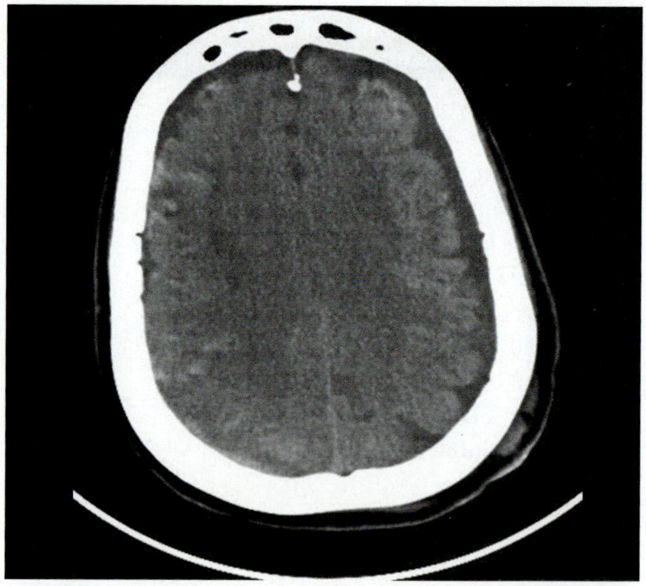

Fig. 31.3: CT showing multiple diffuse parenchymal bleed in right hemisphere and subdural effusion on left side in an elderly patient

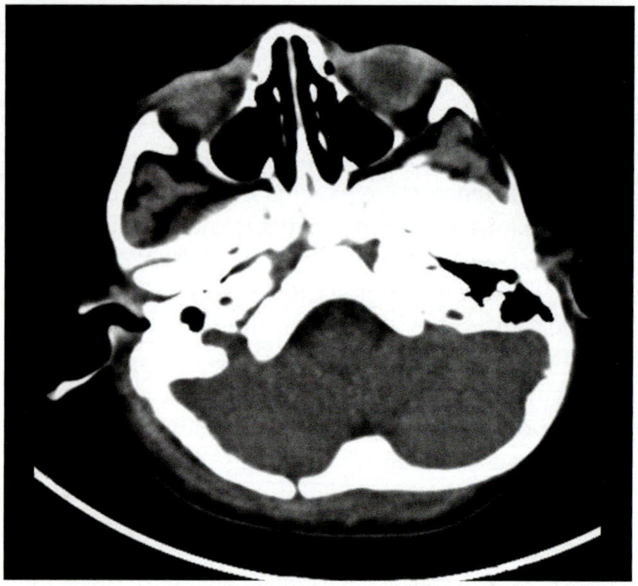

Fig. 31.2: CT shows fracture of right occipital squama

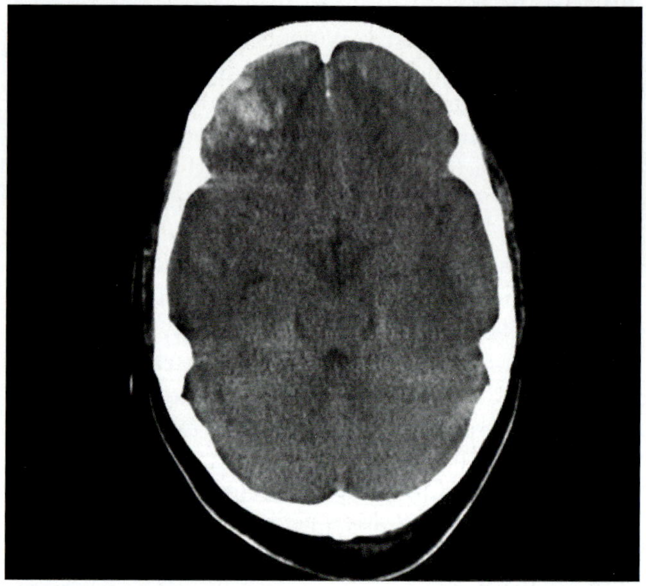

Fig. 31.4: CT showing multiple basifrontal contusions and diffuse clot on right side without mass significant mass effect

Knowing the high mortality in severe head injury in elderly Hernesienni[14] suggested no aggressive ICU care for the elderly patients with severe head injury when, the patients are in deep coma. In a study from the AIIMS,[7] mortality in 60 patients in whom GCS was less than 13 was a 37 percent, while patients with severe head injury, mortality was 79 percent (Table 31.4). Overall mortality of the patients above 80 years of age was 67 percent. Ritche et al[16] had reported high mortality and very poor functional outcome in elderly patients with head injury. Associated injury, shock and pretrauma systemic illness significantly influence the immediate and long-term outcome.

A low velocity fall was a frequent cause of admission (Canadian Tertiary Trauma Center) in elderly. Despite apparent benign mechanism, a low velocity fall is associated with more severe injuries and worse outcome.[19]

Table 31.4: Outcome of head injury on elderly observation at AIIMS[7]

(A) Age in years	No. of patients	Good outcome %	Mortality %
i. 60–70	74	50	39
ii. 71–80	17	50	23
iii. Above 80 years	6	25	67
(B) GCS	**No. of patients**	**Good outcome %**	**Mortality %**
i. 13–15 (Minor)	37	68	3
ii. 9–12 (Moderate)	27	30	37
iii. 8 or less (Severe)	33	Nil	79

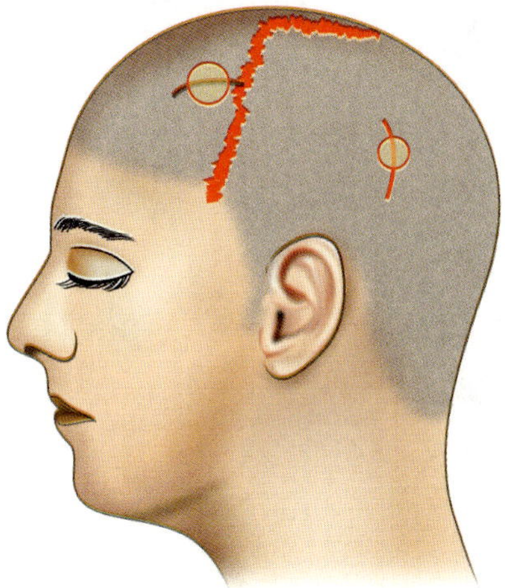

Fig. 31.5: Leteral view of head showing sites for frontal and parietal burr hole in patient with chronic SDH

An age related decline in cerebrovascular autoregulation is associated with relative deterioration in outcome in elderly patients following head trauma.[20]

Beta blockers in older patients of TBI (55 years or more) is found to be independently associated with improved survival. Older patients with severe head injury demonstrated the largest reduction in mortality with beta blockers.[21]

CONCLUSION

Head injury in elderly constitutes 5 to 10 percent of all head injuries. The most frequent cause is fall. Due to cerebral atrophy, there is more space available for expanding hematomas. Hence, raised intracranial pressure manifests late as compared to younger individuals. Extradural hematomas are rare in elderly, while chronic subdural hematomas are more frequent. Overall results are worse than young adults, with high mortality and poor functional outcome.

REFERENCES

1. Amacher SC, Baybee DC. Tolerance of head injury by the elderly. Neurol 1979;20:954-7.
2. Becker DD, Miller JD, Ward JD, et al. The outcome from severe head injury with early diagnosis and intensive management. J Neurosurg 1977;47:50.
3. Colohan A, Alves W, Gross CR, Turner JE, Mehta VS, Tandon PN, Jane JA. Head injury mortality in two centres with different emergency medical services. J Neurosurg 1989;71:202-7.
4. Wilson JA, Pentland B, Gurrie CT, et al. The functional effects of head injury in elderly. Brain Injury 1987;1: 183-6.
5. Galbraith S. Head injury in the elderly. Brit Med Jour 1987;294:325.
6. Jain SP, Kankanady VP. A study of 1500 cases of head injury in Delhi. J Indian Med Asso 1969;52:204-11.
7. Sinha AK, Mahapatra AK, Bhatia RJ. Acute head injury in elderly. JANE 2000;4:27-33.
8. Goodman H, Englander J. Traumatic brain injury in elderly individuals. Physical Medicine and Rehabilitation. Clinic of North America 1990;3(2):220-8.
9. Klashee WB, McLaurin RL, Harris SH, et al. The national head injury and spinal injury survey. Major findings. J Neurosurg 1980;53:519-31.
10. Trotter W. Post-traumatic chronic subdural haematoma. Brit J Surg 1914;2:271.
11. Roy CW, Pentland B, Millar JD. The causes and consequences of minor head injury in the elderly. Injury 1986;17:220-23.
12. Van-Aalst JA, Morris JA, Yates HK, Miller RS, Bass M. Severely injured geriatric patients return to independent living. A study of factors influencing function and independence. J Trauma 1991;31:1096-1101.
13. Carlson CA, Essen CV, Folgren J. Factors affecting the clinical course of patients with severe head injuries, Part I. Influence of biological behaviour, Part II: Significance of post-traumatic coma. J Neurosurg 1968;29:242-5.
14. Hernesienni J. Outcome following head injury in aged. Acta Neurochir (Wien) 1979;39:67-9.

15. Katz DT, Kehs GJ, Alexander MD. Prognosis and recovery from TBI: The influence of advancing age. Neurol 1990;40:276.
16. Ritche PD, Cameron PA, Ugoni AM, et al. A study of the functional outcome and mortality in elderly patients with head injuries. J Clin Neurosci 2000;7:301-14.
17. Hemlat A, Mazzon AM, et al. Intracranial epidural hematoma in elderly patients. Observation in 14 patients. Acta Neurochir 2005;147(10):1055-60.
18. Pieracci FM, Eachempati SR, Shou J, et al. Degree of anticoagulation but not warfarin use itself, predicts adverse outcome in TBI in elderly. J Trauma 2007;63(3): 525-30.
19. Bergeron E, Clement J, Lavoie A, et al. A simple fall in elderly. J Trauma 2006;60(2):268-73.
20. Czosnyka M, Balestreri M, Steiner L, et al. Intracranial pressure, autoregulation and outcome after brain trauma. J Neurosurg 2007;106(3):516-7.
21. Inabak K, Teixeira PG, David JS, et al. Beta blockers in isolated blunt injury. J Am Coll Surg 2008;206(3):432-8.

32 Chronic Subdural Hematoma

Raj Kamal, AK Mahapatra

INTRODUCTION

According to the time of onset of symptoms after the injury the subdural hematoma is classified into three types: Acute, subacute and chronic.

Acute – Within 48 to 72 hours.
Subacute – 3 to 20 days.
Chronic – > 3 weeks to several months.

Into last group are placed the cases in which either no history of trauma or the trauma described is of such trivial nature that its relationship to trauma is doubtful. About 20 to 30 percent of cases have no history of trauma. The incidence of chronic subdural hematoma is 1 to 2 per 100,000 people per year.[1] Most patients are 50 years of age or older.

PATHOGENESIS AND PATHOLOGY

Chronic subdural hematoma is seen in elderly patients in whom cerebral atrophy causes widening of the subdural space thus exposing the bridging veins to a greater risk of rupture when subjected to angular shearing forces.[2,3]

Oozing of blood is usually gradual and spreads over a large area of the surface of the brain and may extend in the interhemispheric fissure along the falx cerebri. Several hundred milliliters of blood may accumulate gradually in this space without causing symptoms. Subdural hematomas evoke a peculiar reaction largely derived from the inner surface of the dura and results in granulation tissue, referred to as "neomembranes", that encircle the hematoma.[4] The neomembrane facing the dura is called outer membrane and that facing the surface of brain is called inner membrane. The outer membrane is thick and highly vascular whereas inner membrane is thin, relatively avascular and sometimes adherent to the arachnoid. Formation of outer membrane begins as thin membrane and by four weeks it becomes thick and vascular.

Initially a fibrin layer forms around the periphery of the clot on the dural, but not the arachnoid side, this is invaded by fibroblasts and blood vessels. The outer membrane, which looks more like pigmented dura with the passage of time, is continuous with the much thinner inner membrane in which a thin layer of fibroblasts appears, presumably by migration from the edges of the outer layer.

The subdural blood clot liquefies in the center with passage of time and is resorbed. The capillaries of the neomembrane are abnormal and friables.[5,6]

Progressive enlargement of hematoma occurs due to repeated microhemorrhages from the friable capillaries of the neomembranes.[2,7]

Repeated microhemorrhages cause the enlargement of the chronic subdural hematoma by directly increasing the volume of the clot and resupplying substrates for coagulation and fibrinolysis.[8-10] Another postulation for the enlargement of a chronic SDH is that the outer and inner membrane acts as an osmotic membrane, imbibing cerebrospinal fluid into the hematoma thus increasing its volume.[11]

Sometimes, the loculated fluid is totally absorbed and the two membranes fuse.

Bilateral subdural hematomas, more common in children, may impede the free flow of CSF in the subarachnoid space and can cause hydrocephalus and dementia.[2]

Sources of nontraumatic, so called spontaneous chronic subdural hematomas are convexity angiomas, aneurysms and other cerebral vascular disorders such as inflammations, thrombosis and hemorrhagic diasthesis.

Factors which can predispose to chronic subdural hematomas:

1. Low intracranial pressure
2. Cerebral atrophy
3. All coagulopathies
4. Anticoagulants.

Low intracranial pressure can occur following over-drainage of CSF following VP shunt, dehydration and spinal anesthesia. Due to decrease in cerebral volume, tangential movements occur easily, predisposing rupture of bridging veins. Also because of reduced pressure hemorrhages are not immediately stopped.

Alcoholics are also more prone to develop chronic subdural hematoma due to higher rate of accident

Table 32.1: Symptoms and signs in chronic subdural hematoma			
Symptoms	*(%)*	*Signs*	*(%)*
Headache	81	Altered consciousness	59
Altered consciousness	47	Motor paresis	41
Confusion	38	Memory loss or confusion	59
Vomiting	30	Papilledema	22
Weakness (motor)	22	Pupillary inequality	21
Visual symptoms	13		
Seizures	9	Dysphasia	11

than general population, secondary coagulation disturbances and/or generalized vascular fragility as a result of avitaminosis.

CLINICAL MANIFESTATIONS

Chronic subdural hematoma patients may have suffered a significant head injury. However, in approximately one-third of patients there is no definite history of preceding head injury.

The incidence of chronic subdural hematoma increases steadily and more rapidly approaching the 60 to 70 age group. Chronic SDH shows male predominance. The symptoms and signs are given in Table 32.1.[12]

Classically, the patient may present without the history of head injury in one of three ways:

1. Raised intracranial pressure without significant localizing signs. The patient presents with headache, vomiting and drowsiness.
2. Fluctuating level of consciousness.
3. A progressive dementia.

INVESTIGATION

CT is the investigation of choice for evaluation of chronic subdural hematoma. A chronic subdural hematoma is hyperdense in first week after injury. It becomes isodense in about ten days to two weeks and thus could be over-looked on the CT scan examination. After three weeks, chronic subdural hematoma usually appears hypodense on CT (Fig. 32.1). It is often difficult to distinguish isodense chronic SDH from cerebral parenchyma. Isodense subdural hematoma displaces surface sulci of the brain away from inner table. They have been often misdiagnosed as cerebral swelling or tumor. Chances of missing bilateral isodense subdural hematoma is still higher.

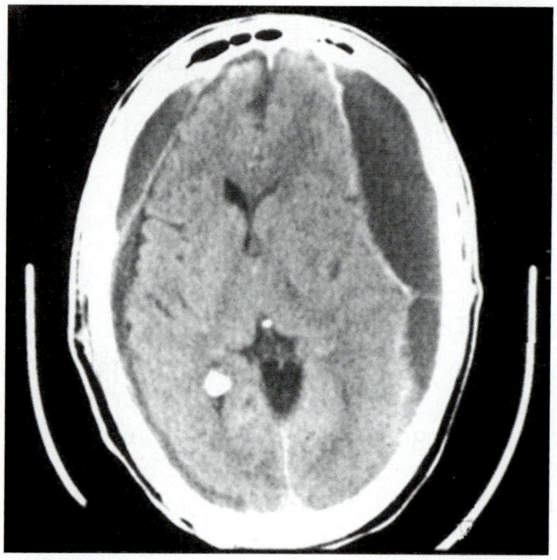

Fig. 32.1: CT head shows bilateral septated chronic subdural hematomas

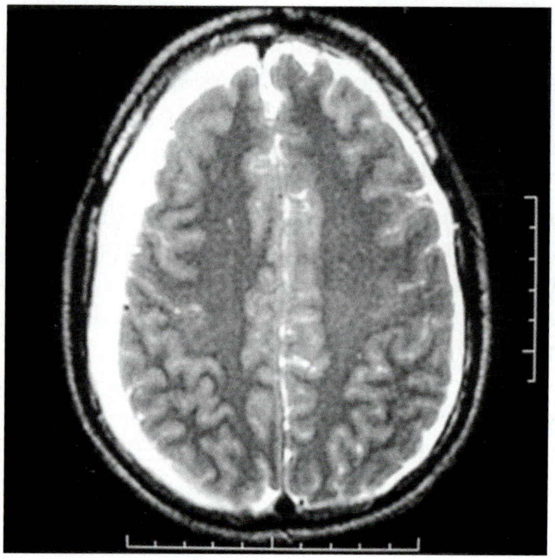

Fig. 32.2: MRI showing subdural hematoma, who was on acitrom following cardiac surgery

Large chronic subdural hematomas resulting in subfalcine and transtentorial herniations. Associated subfalcine and transtentorial herniation can be diagnosed very well on CT scan.

Subacute subdural hematoma (1-2 weeks) have high signal on both T_1 and T_2 weighted images due to presence of extracellular methemoglobin.

Chronic subdural hematomas may be hyperintense relative to brain and CSF in both short TR and long TR images due to presence of extracellular methemoglobin.

MRI can also demonstrate acute hemorrhage within chronic SDH. MRI is more sensitive than

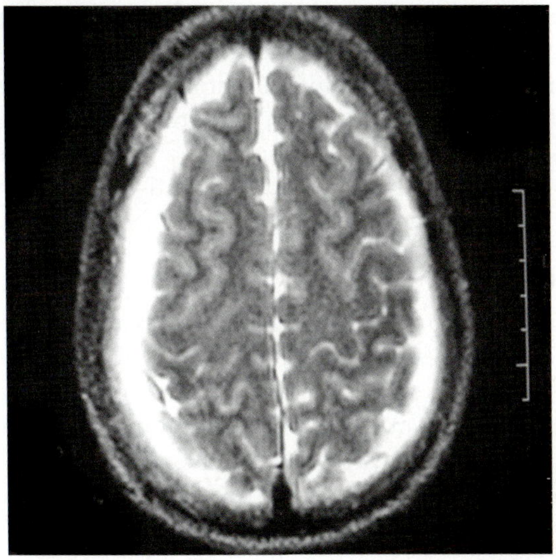

Fig. 32.3: MRI showing chronic subdural hematoma of right hemisphere

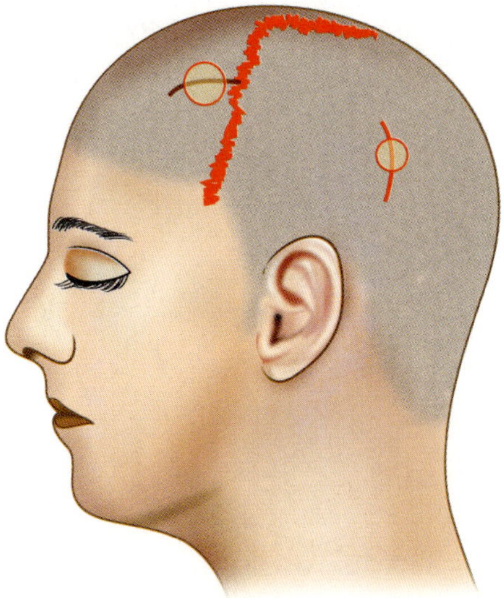

Fig. 32.4: Frontal and parietal burr holes with skin incision

CT in identifying isodense SDH. Subacute subdural hematomas are bright on T_1 weighted images (hyperintense) and relatively dark (hypointense) on T_2 weighted images (Figs 32.2 and 32.3).

The presence of beta trace protein (beta TP) has been documented in majority of chronic (CSDH) and subdural hygroma cases (SH). The patients who have recurrence of CSDH and SH had higher concentration of beta TP in CSF and beta trace protein in serum (Beta TPSF) at initial presentation than patients not requiring reoperation for recurrence. It signifies leakage of CSF in subdural space.[22]

TREATMENT

The following treatment modalities are available for chronic subdural hematoma:

1. *Medical management*: Bed rest, osmotic diuretics, corticosteroids.
2. *Surgical management*:
   a. Twist drill craniostomy
   b. Burr holes
   c. Craniotomy.

Medical Management

Suzuki and Takakua[13] treated 23 chronic subdural hematoma patients with 20 percent mannitol, 500 to 1000 ml daily. The average duration of treatment was 31 days. Most of their patients became asymptomatic within 1 to 2 months from the beginning of treatment. Unfortunately, these good results could not be verified in a control series by Gjerris and Schmidt[14] in which mannitol regime failed in first seven patients and the study has to be abandoned.

Conservative treatment may be tried in patients with minimal neurological signs and small chronic subdural hematoma found incidently or those who refuse surgery. In these cases, ultimately surgery may be required. Conservative treatment alone either is not effective or requires very long hospitalization.

Twist Drill Craniotomy

This procedure is performed under local anesthesia. Complete head shaving is mandatory for twist drill aspiration. Head is prepared meticulously with povidone iodine after cleaning with savlon. About 1 cm long incision is placed 3 cm away from midline and anterior to coronal suture or should be placed adjacent to the thickest part of subdural hematoma as determined by the CT scan. The twist drill hole should be placed accordingly. The direction of twist should be posteriorly and inferiorly usually making an angle of 45° to the perpendicular.

The drainage of chronic subdural hematoma should be slow and controlled otherwise intracerebral hemorrhage may occur following rapid decompression. A catheter may be passed into subdural space and connected to closed sterile drainage system.

Burr Holes

Two burr holes (Fig. 32.4) are usually placed under local anesthesia after preparing the head as described for twist drill aspiration.

Burr holes are guided by the site and size of chronic SDH on CT scan. Posterior burr hole is placed just posterior to the thickest portion of hematoma which

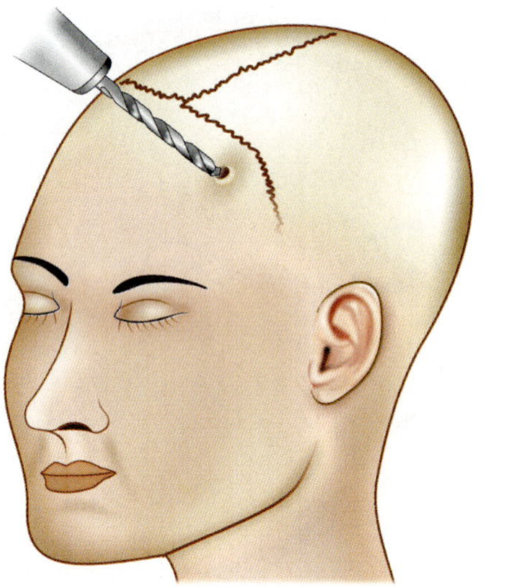

Fig. 32.5: Direction of twist drill posteriorly inferiorly making an angle of 45° with the skull vault

is parietal eminence in most cases. The anterior frontal burr hole is placed anterior to the coronal suture 3 cm lateral to the midline (Fig. 32.5).

Dura is incised in cruciate manner identifying outer membrane. Outer membrane is incised separately with slow and controlled drainage of hematoma. The second burr hole is made to facilitate irrigation with isotonic saline. A drain can be placed in the subdural space postoperatively for 24 to 48 hours for drainage of residual hematoma. Care should be taken while inserting pediatic feeding tube inside subdural space, drain-tip should be soft and directed over the convexity of the brain.

The proximal end of drain should be taken out from separate incision. Drain is not necessary if the brain expands adequately after the drainage of subdural hematoma. If brain fails to expand following evacuation of chronic subdural hematoma then measures recommended by various authors are:

Lumbar puncture and intrathecal infusion of 40 to 300 ml isotonic or Ringer's lactate solution. Favorable results shown by La Londe and Gardner,[15] Cameron,[16] Grisoli et al.[17]

COMPLICATIONS

1. Recurrence: Twist drill 5 to 24 percent
   Burr hole 0 to 26 percent
2. Subdural empyema occurs in < 2 percent[16,17] of burr hole evacuation of chronic subdural hematoma
3. Intracerebral hemorrhage is 1 to 5 percent.[18,19]

The role of local inflammation in the pathogenesis and postoperative recurrence of chronic subdural hematoma is established. The brain trauma causes inflammatory process within the dural border cell layer; high level of inflammatory cytokines were significantly correlated with recurrence and layering of chronic subdural hematoma. The concentration of both IL-62 and IL-8 were significantly higher in the cases of recurrence of chronic SDH.[23]

CONCLUSION

Chronic subdural hematoma is a common neurosurgical problem which produces symptoms from three weeks to several months after injury. Subacute subdural hematoma, produces symptoms, from 3 to 20 days. Most patients are over 50 years of age. History of trauma is absent in 25 to 50 percent of cases. Chronic alcoholism, brain atrophy, epilepsy, and coagulopathies are important precipitating factors.

Headache, altered sensorium are most common presenting symptoms. For evaluation, CT scan is investigation of choice. After three weeks the vast majority of SDH will be hypodense and will assume lenticular appearance but because of recurrent bleeding from hematoma membranes, chronic SDH can also appear hypo- and hyperdense.

Isodense SDH on CT scan are easily diagnosed by MRI.

For symptomatic chronic subdural hematoma treatment should be in favor of operation. Recurrence in chronic subdural hematoma is not uncommon.

REFERENCES

1. Fogdholm R, Waltimo O. Epidemiology of chronic subdural haematoma. Acta Neurochir (Wien) 1975;32:247-50.
2. Giuffre R. Physiopathogenesis of chronic subdural hematomas: A new look to an old problem. Riv Neurol 1987;5:298.
3. Yamashima T, Friede RL. Why do bridging veins rupture into the virtual subdural space? J Neural Neurosurg Psychiat 1984;47:121.
4. Powers JM, Horoupian. Central Nervous System. In Damjanov I, Linder J (Eds). Anderson's Pathology; 10th edn, Mosby 1996;10:2693-793.
5. Yamashima T, Yamamoto S. How do vessels proliferate in the capsule of a chronic subdural haematoma? Neurosurg 1984;15:672.
6. Yamashima T, Yamamoto S, Friede RL. The role of endothelial gap junctions in the enlargement of chronic subdural haematomas. J Neurosurg 1983;59:298.
7. Kawakami Y, Chikama M, et al. Coagulation and fibrinolysis in chronic subdural haematoma. Neurosurg 1989;25:25.

8. Markwalder TM, Reulen HJ. Influence of neomembraneous organization, cortical expansion and subdural pressure on the postoperative course of chronic subdural haematoma, an analysis of 201 cases. Acta Neurochir (Wien) 1986;79:100.
9. Weir B. Oncotic pressure of subdural fluids. J Neurosurg 1980;53:512.
10. Ito H, Komai T, Yamamoto S. Fibrinolytic enzymes in the lining walls of chronic subdural haematoma. J Neurosurg 1978;48:197-200.
11. Zollinger R, Gross RE. Traumatic subdural haematoma: An explanation of the late onset of pressure symptoms. JAMA 1934;103:245-9.
12. Mc Kissock W, Richardson A, Bloom WH. Subdural haematoma: A review of 389 cases. Lancet 1960;1:1365.
13. Suzuki J, Takakua A. Non-surgical treatment of chronic subdural haematoma. J Neurosurg 1970;33:548.
14. Gjerris F, Schmidt K. Chronic subdural haematoma. Surgery or mannitol treatment. J Neurosurg 1974;40:639.
15. La Londe AA, Gardner WJ. Chronic subdural haematoma. Expansion of compressed cerebral hemisphere and relief of hypotension by spinal injection of physiological saline solution. N Eng J Med 1948;239:493.
16. Cameron MM. Chronic subdural haematoma: A review of 114 cases. J Neurol Neurosurg Psychiat 1978;41:834.
17. Grisoli F, Graziani N, et al. Perioperative lumbar injection of Ringer's lactate solution in chronic subdural haematomas: A series of 100 cases. Neurosurg 1988; 23:616.
18. D' Arella D, De Blasi F, et al. Intracerebral haematoma following evacuation of chronic subdural haematomas: Report of two cases. J Neurosurg 1986;65:710.
19. Modesti LM, Hodge CJ, et al. Intracerebral haematoma after evacuation of chronic extracerebral fluid collections. Neurosurg 1982;1:689.
20. Al Hani Q, Gupta PK, Mahapatra AK, Lad SD. Development of chronic SDH. A reminder of its pathogenesis. Oman Medical Journal 2001;17:20-4.
21. Satyarthee GD, Mahapatra AK. Delayed appearance of subdural haematoma following radiation for Corpus Callosum GBM (in Press).
22. Kristof RA, Brimm JM, Stoffel Wagener B. CSF leak in to subdural space; Possible influence on pathogenesis and recurrence frequency of chronic SDH and subdural hygroma. J Neurosurg 2008;108(2):275-80.
23. Frati A, Salvati M, Mainiero F, et al. Inflammation markers and risk factors for recurrence in 35 patients with a post-traumatic chronic subdural hematoma–prospective study. J Neurosurg 2004;100(1):24-32.

33 Traumatic Cerebellar Hematomas

AK Mahapatra, Raj Kumar

INTRODUCTION

Traumatic posterior fossa lesions are rare[1-3] as compared to supratentorial pathology of any nature. Among the posterior fossa hematomas, extradural hematomas are more frequent.[4-6] Traumatic intracerebellar pathology, be it contusion/hematoma are indeed very rare, and reported as small series, in the literature.[1,7-11] In spite of being a well recognized clinicoradiological entity, posterior fossa traumatic lesions have received little attention. Because of rarity of lesion, no single series has vast experience. Recently, d' Avella et al,[7] published a multicentric study dealing with 81 patients with cerebellar hematoma. Considering the clinical uncertainity and unpredictable course, these lesions require careful evaluation and monitoring.

A study aiming to see the frequency of tentorial hematomas revealed traumatic subarachnoid hemorrhage and cerebral contusion in 60 percent patients, subdural hematomas in 45 percent, intracerebral hematoma in 31 percent, pathology in posterior fossa in 12 percent and epidural hematomas in 8 percent.[28]

The present chapter is a brief review on the traumatic cerebellar hematoma.

PATHOLOGY OF TRAUMATIC CEREBELLAR LESIONS

Traumatic cerebellar hematoma is a rare condition and exact incidence is not known (Fig. 33.1). Except the multicentric study published by d' Avella et al[12] no other large series is published in the literature. The above authors could collect 81 cases over a three years period and provided detailed clinicoradiological profile. Overall, cerebellar pathology is noticed in three percent of all head injury.[13,14]

Pathologically, traumatic cerebellar lesions could be primary or secondary. It can be isolated cerebellar lesion or could be a part of diffuse axonal injury (DAI). Posterior fossa lesions can result from both high velocity motor vehicular accidents or low energy[12,15,16] injury, due to fall from the height. Patients can also have coup or center coup lesions. Hemorrhagic contusion of the cerebellum constitute a fourth of the all traumatic lesions of the posterior fossa.[13]

Various mechanisms are hypothesized contributing to the formation of traumatic posterior fossa lesion (TPFL). Most common mechanism is direct injury or coup injury over the occipital region.[3,16] This type of injury is more frequent due to fall, leading to low energy trauma.[12] Contrecoup injury is relatively rarer phenomenon.[15,17,18]

Other mechanism which produce cerebellar hematoma is the shearing strain. First rotational propulsion of the brain within cranial cavity leads to widespread axonal injury and scattered foci of hemorrhage at the junction of white and gray matter junctional area, in both cerebrum and cerebellum.[19] Thus, in 25 percent of DAI cerebellum may be involved. This type of injury results from high velocity vehicular injury with rotational force. Fifty percent patients reportedly had high velocity injury.[12]

Rarely, cerebellar hematomas could be delayed in onset.[12,20,21] Cerebellar contusions are prone to increase in size. Hematoma may develop at site of previous contusion or even in area which looked normal on the first CT scan.[22] The delayed hematoma may be the result

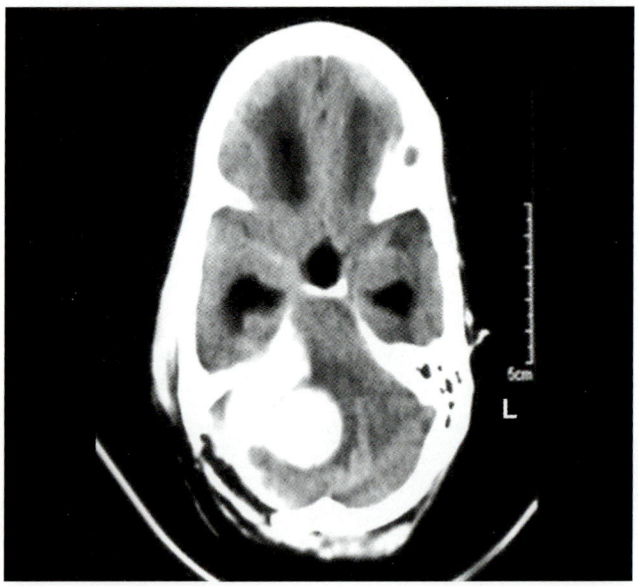

Fig. 33.1: CT showing acute subdural hematoma of posterior fossa along with large midline hematoma and secondary hydrocephalus

Table 33.1: Classification of traumatic cerebellar lesion

A. Primary cerebellar hematoma – Hemispheric – Vermian – Both	Delayed cerebellar hematoma
B. Primary cerebellar hematoma associated with	a. Supratentorial pathology b. Post-fossa hematoma – EDH – SDH
C. Cerebellar hematoma as a part of diffuse axonal injury	
D. Cerebellar contusion/laceration – Part of compound injury – In closed head injury	

of coagulopathy[22] (Table 33.1). Hemorrhagic contusion can slowly grow in size up to 4 days, as noticed by d' Avella et al[12] While posterior fossa EDH is more common in children, cerebellar hematomas are very rare in pediatric age group.[23] Surprisingly, d' Avella et al[12] reported uniform incidence in all age groups.

CLINICAL PRESENTATIONS

Clinical presentations of patients with cerebellar hematomas are varied. It depends on the size and the location of hematoma.[2,12,25] The associated supratentorial pathology and DAI also influence the clinical presentation. Overall, 50 percent patients are admitted in coma.[12] As in some cases hematomas may grow in size over a period of time, there is a high possibility of deterioration of conscious state and development of raised ICP due to hydrocephalus. When a patient is in coma from the beginning, it is natural to think a high velocity impact and higher chance of having DAI. In the series presented by d' Avella et al,[12] 81 percent of patients in coma had an associated supratentorial lesion and 19 of 34 had DAI. A total of nine patients out of 81 had evolving clinical course, which suggest progressive deterioration. In conscious patients, headache, confusional state and presence of cerebellar signs would raise the possibility of posterior fossa mass lesion. A significant number of patients may have occipital scalp hematoma or scalp laceration.

INVESTIGATIONS

As usual CT scan is the investigation of choice.[12,25] In significant number of patients X-ray skull may show occipital bone fracture. In CT scan posterior fossa lesions are reported in three percent cases.[13,14,25] CT scan also delineate the presence of associated supratentorial pathology, DAI and development of hydrocephalus. According to CT scan findings, hematomas can be classified as midline or hemispheric, and small or large depending on the size more than 3 cm in diameter or less. In small percentage of patient may have initial normal CT and when repeated may show delayed development of cerebellar hematoma.[12,21,22,25] Hence, d' Avella et al[12] suggested repeated CT scan daily for first 4 days, depending on need.

MANAGEMENT POLICY (TABLE 33.2)

Surgical treatment of cerebellar hematoma is still a topic of considerable controversy. As the clinical course

Table 33.2: Some series on cerebellar lesions

Series authors	*Year*	*Number of patients*	*Other lesions*
1. Pozzati et al[9]	1982	7	Nil
2. Zuccarello et al[23]	1982	5	Nil
3. St John & French[3]	1986	3	One EDH, one SDH
4. Karasawa et al[13]	1997	13	11 had supratentorial 2 had post-fossa SDH
5. d' Avella et al[7]	1998		7 had associated lesion
6. d' Avella et al[12]	2002	81	–

Flow chart 33.1: Treatment option

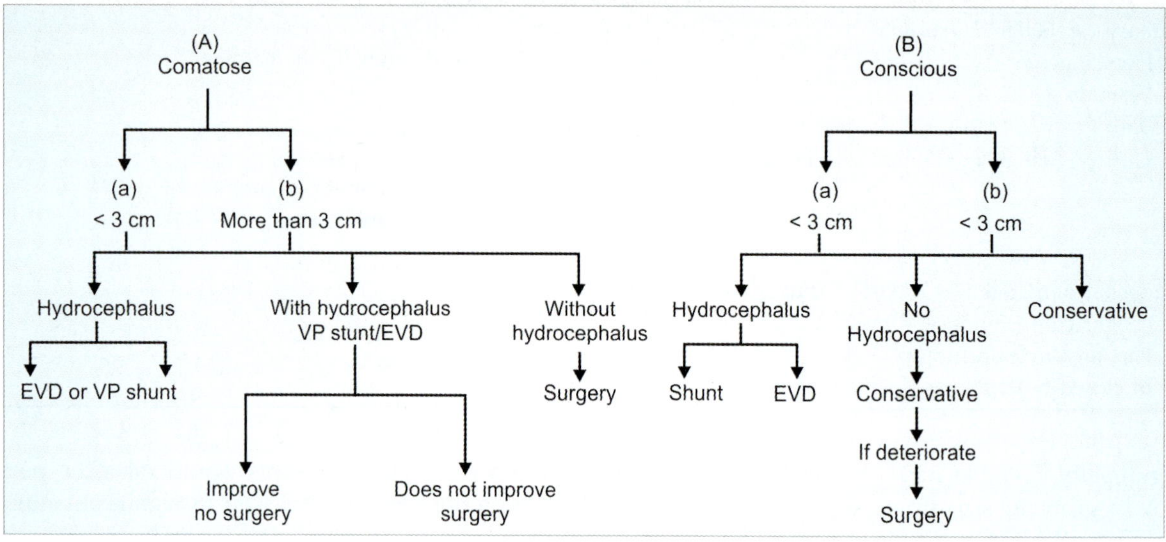

is unpredictable, and there is a possibility of rapid clinical deterioration, some authors advocate early surgery in traumatic cerebellar hematoma to prevent sudden deterioration and death.[13,14] However, few of the above studies are pre CT scan era. Recently, with accumulating evidence, it is convincing that large number of patients do run a benign course which were not appreciated earlier.[8,9,24,26] Not all hematomas of the cerebellum require surgery.[12,24,26] Surprisingly, no clearcuts guidelines are available, however, there are several points which favor surgical evacuation. In 1994, Kobayashi et al[27] had laid down the criteria for surgical treatment of hypertensive cerebellar hematoma. In absence of clearcut guidelines for traumatic cerebellar hematoma, criteria laid down by Kobayashi[27] et al can serve as a guideline.

Size and site of the cerebellar hematomas are two major radiological parameters help for surgical decision. Clinical criteria, state and raised ICP are also important (Flow chart 33.1). There is a general consensus that conservative treatment is a logical option for the noncomatose patients with clots less than 3 cm in diameter, when there is associated EDH or SDH in posterior fossa. Surgery is indicated in all patients with clot larger than 3 cm in diameter. Large number of patients do need EVD or VP shunt to reduce the ICP, in those patients who develop hydrocephalus[12,13] which is noticed in 20 percent cases.

Pathological lesions and hematomas of middle cerebellar peduncle can be approached through cerebellomedullary fissure approach. It provides greater access to dorsal surface of middle cerebeller peduncle and to lateral part of pons. However, complication can be ataxia and 6th and 7th nerve pareses.[29]

ICP monitoring helps in decision-making for the surgical evacuation. In conscious patients with large hematoma or in unconscious patients with small hematoma it acts as a good indicator. Associated supratentorial hematomas need management according to their own merit.

OVERALL

Overall poor outcome is reported in around 60 percent cases (Table 33.3). However, poor outcome is reported between 42 to 85 percent.[9,12,13,25] d' Avella et al[12] in a multicentric study of 81 cases of cerebellar hematoma reported 44.6 percent mortality. Mortality is low in patients with hematomas smaller than 3 cm and patients who are not in coma. In conscious patients favorable result are reported in as high as 85 percent patients.[2] Patients with brainstem signs, obliteration of basal cistern in CT and with associated supratentorial lesion also have poor prognosis. Thus, large number of factors influences the overall outcome (Table 33.4).

Table 33.3: Overall poor outcome

Authors	*No. of patients*	*percent*
1. Tsai et al[25]	14	85
2. Pozzati et al[19]	7	42
3. Sato et al[24]	8	50
4. Karasawa et al[13]	13	54
5. d'Avella et al[12]	81	44

Table 33.4: Factors influencing the outcome

	Good outcome	*Poor outcome*
1. Age	Less than 50 years	Above 50 years
2. Type of injury	Low velocity injury	High velocity injury
3. Associated hematoma	Nil	Present
4. Size of clot	Less than 3 cm	More than 3 cm
5. GCS	9 or above	8 or below
6. Hydrocephalus	Absent	Present
7. Basal cistern	Normal	Obliterated

CONCLUSION

Traumatic cerebellar hematomas are rare and probably occur in less than one percent of head injury patients. Often, this lesion is associated with other lesions in posterior fossa, supratentorial pathology and with DAI. Significant number of cases may have small hematoma and patients are conscious and neurologically static. This group of patients run a benign course and only a small percentage of patients may deteriorate if hematoma is vermian and there is associated hydrocephalus. By and large cerebellar hematoma patients in coma have hematoma larger than 3 cm in diameter or have associated injury. Small percent of patients have delayed development of cerebellar hematoma and deteriorate 3 to 4 days following injury. CT scan is still the investigation of choice, and required repeatedly in first 3 to 4 days to assess the progression of hematoma or development of the hydrocephalus. Conscious patients with small hematomas by and large managed conservatively, while surgery is indicated in unconscious patients with large hematoma. Management of patients of coma with hematoma less than 3 cm remains debatable. Around 20 percent patients develop hydrocephalus and need either VP Shunt or EVD. Overall the outcome is poor in 50 to 60 percent of the patients.

REFERENCES

1. Cassinari V, Dorizzi A, Pauli P, et al. Expansive traumatic lesions of the posterior cranial fossa. On 4 cases cerebellar contusion and laceration. Minerva Neurochir 1967;11:230-9.
2. Servadei F, Staffa G, Vorgoni G, et al. Post-traumatic acute subdural haematoma of the posterior fossa extending towards the cerebellopontine region. Report of a case. J Neurosurg Sci 1995;39:187-90.
3. St John JN, French BN. Traumatic haematomas of the posterior fossa. A clinicopathological spectrum. Surg Neurol 1986;25:457-66.
4. Mahapatra AK, Bhatia R, Banerji AK. Posterior fossa extradural haematoma—A report of 5 cases. Neurology India 1982;30:239-44.
5. Gupta PK, Mahapatra AK, Lad SD. Posterior fossa extradural haematomas—a study of 29 cases (In press).
6. Mahapatra AK. Posterior fossa extradural haematoma in children. Indian Pediatr 1990;27:989-92.
7. d' Avella D, Salpietro FM, Angileri FF, et al. Management of traumatic cerebellar haemorrhagic contusions and haematomas. Acta Neurochir Suppi (Wien) 1998;71:410.
8. Pozzati E, Piazza G. Benign traumatic intracerebellar haematoma. Neurosurg 1981;8:102-3.
9. Pozzati E, Grossi C, Padoveni R. Traumatic intracerebellar haematomas. J Neurosurg 1982;56:691-4.
10. Yokota H, Nakazawa S, Kobayashi S, et al. Clinical study of two cases of traumatic cerebellar injury (In Japanese) No Shinkei Geka 1990;18:67-70.
11. Sokol JH, Rowed DW. Traumatic intracerebellar haematomas. Surg Neural 1978;10:340-1.
12. d' Avella D, Servadei F, Scerrati M, et al. Traumatic Intracerebellar Hemorrhage: Clinicoradiological Analysis of 81 patients. Neurosurg 2002;50:16-27.
13. Karasawa H, Furuya H, Naito H, et al. Acute hydrocephalus in posterior fossa injury. J Neurosurg 1997; 86:629-32.
14. Wright RL. Traumatic haematomas of the posterior-cranial fossa. J Neurosurg 1966;25:402-09.
15. Stone JL, Ladenheim E, Wilkinson SB, et al. Haematoma in the posterior fossa secondary to a tangential gunshot wound of the occiput: Case report and discussion. Neurosurg 1991;28:603-6.
16. Vrankovic D, Splavski B, Hecimovic I, et al. Anatomical intracerebellar protection of contrecoup haematoma development: Analysis of the mechanism of 30 posterior fossa coup haematomas. Neurosurg Rev 2000;23:156-60.
17. Olin MS, Young HA, Schmidek HH. Contrecoup intracerebellar hemorrhage: Report of a case. Neurosurg 1980;7:271-73.
18. Isla A, Alvarez F, Manrique M, et al. Posterior fossa subdural haematoma. J Neurosurg Sci 1987;31:67-9.

19. Adams JH, Doyle D, Ford I, et al. Diffuse axonal injury in head injury: Definition, diagnosis and grading. Histopathol 1989;15:49-59.
20. Nagata K, Ishikawa T, Shigeno T, et al. Delayed traumatic intracerebellar haematoma: Correlation between the location of the haematoma and the pre-existing cerebellar contusion—case report. Neural Med Chir (Tokyo) 1991;31:792-6.
21. Tibbs PA, Goldstein SJ, Smithson JR. Delayed traumatic intracerebellar haematoma. Surg Neural 1982;16:309-11.
22. Stein SC, Young GS, Taluci RC, et al. Delayed brain injury following head trauma: Significance of coagulopathy. Neurosurg 1992;30:160-5.
23. Zuccarello M, Andrioli GC, Fiore DL, et al. Traumatic posterior fossa haemorrhage in children. Acta Neurochir (Wien) 1982;62:79-85.
24. Sato K, Hinokama IC, Matsuzawa Y, et al. Clinical study of traumatic cerebellar contusion (In-Japanese) No Shinkei Geka 1987;15:1285-9.
25. Tsai FY, Teal JS, Itabashi HH, et al. Computed tomography of posterior fossa trauma. J Comput Assist Tomogr 1980;4:291-305.
26. Koziarski A, Frankiewich E. Medical and surgical treatment of intracerebellar haematomas. Acta Neurochir (wien) 1991;110:24-28.
27. Kobayashi S, Sato A, Kageyama Y, et al. Treatment of hypertensive cerebellar hemorrhage: Surgical or conservative management? Neurosurg 1994;34:246-51.
28. Moskala M, Polak J, Moskala A, et al. Hematoma in tentorium cerebelli, new pathology or new prognostic factor in neurotraumatology? A preliminary report. Neurol Neurochir Pol 2007;41(3):234-40.
29. Majchrzak H, Tymowski M, Majchrzak K, Stepien T. Surgical approach to pathological lesions of middle cerebellar peduncle and lateral part of pons clinical observation: Neurol, Neurochir Pol 2007;41(5):436-44.

34 Traumatic Basal Ganglia Hematomas and Infarcts

P Sarat Chandra, AK Mahapatra

INTRODUCTION

Traumatic basal ganglion hematomas (TBGHs) are observed in approximately 3 percent of patients admitted to a neurosurgical unit following a closed head injury.[1] However, the incidence in autopsy series of closed-head injuries, including the pediatric population, is higher in the range of 10 to 12 percent.[2] As these are deeply located hemorrhages developing in the parenchyma between coup and countrecoup injuries, they have been considered as intermediary contusions. Traumatic basal ganglia hematomas account for less than two percent of post-traumatic intracerebral contusions. They are believed to rise from shearing of the lenticulostriate or anterior choroidal blood vessels caused by acceleration/deceleration forces at the time of injury. This shearing occurs as a result of high-velocity trauma, thus placing TBGHs into a distinctive category.[2,3]

MECHANISM (FLOW CHART 34.1)

Traumatic basal ganglia hematomas occur mainly in young persons, however, the clinicopathological profile of these lesions is still poorly understood.

The mechanism of formation of TBGH is unique as it involves formation of blood clot within the parenchyma and is also known to increase with time. Traumatic basal ganglia hematomas are dynamic lesions that tend to enlarge during acute post-traumatic period. The patient's in whom volume of hematoma is larger than 25 ml and in those in whom hematoma enlarges or raised intracranial pressure occurs have worst outcome, perhaps indicating more aggressive surgical treatment.[29]

Formation of TBGH: Courville and Blomquist believed that TBGHs were small, usually multiple, and located in the zone of the lenticular nucleus and external capsule, on either one or both the sides.[4] In contrast, spontaneous hemorrhages in this area were large, usually single, and located in the region of the thalamus and internal capsule. Therefore, solitary deep-seated intracerebral hematomas with mass effect were always deemed spontaneous, and, thus, when a patient suffered a head injury it was considered to be the consequence rather than the cause of the hematoma.

Flow chart 34.1: Mechanism and effects of head trauma

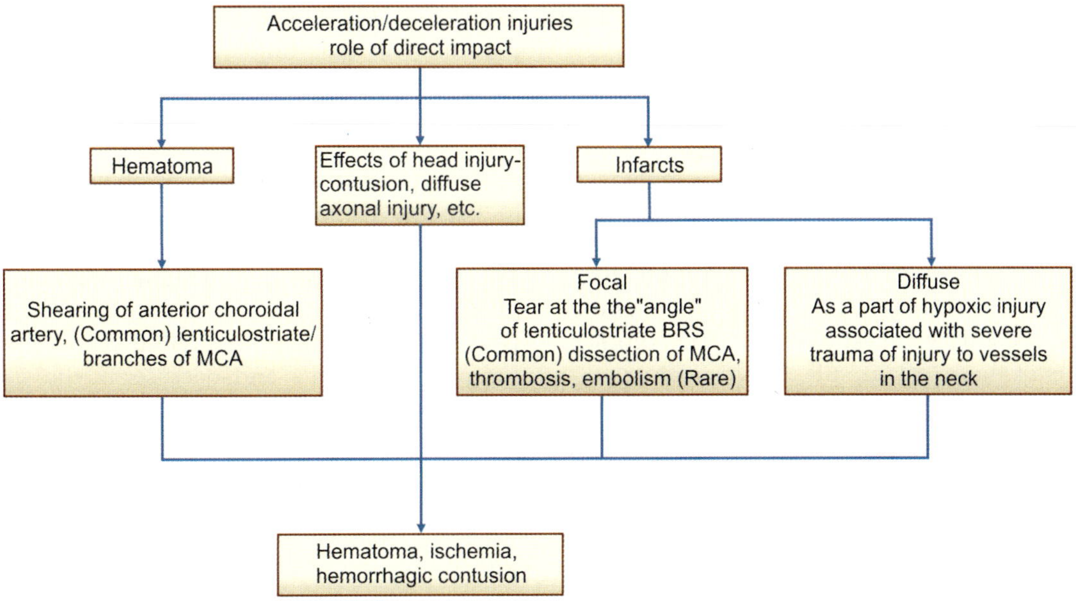

The above view was considered true till in 1959. Mossberg and Lindenberg[3] reported on one patient whose clinical condition progressively deteriorated and died following a head injury. In their patient, a massive hematoma in the pallidum and a ruptured arterial twig of the anterior choroidal artery within the clot was found at autopsy. After histological examination of the vessel, the arterial tear was found to be traumatic in origin, demonstrating that massive hematomas in the basal ganglia can result following head injury. According to these authors, traumatic hemorrhage in the region of the basal ganglia should be diagnosed in cases where trauma occurs while the head is in motion (coup and countrecoup) and the impact, sufficient to deform the skull, is applied to the vertex; forehead, or occipital area and directed toward the tentorium. Under these circumstances, there would be a shift of the brain through the tentorial notch, producing shearing forces among different tissues, which in turn would produce stretching and tearing of the pallidal branches of the anterior choroidal artery, and occasionally, of the striate branches of the MCA, resulting in hemorrhages within the basal ganglia region.[3,5] Because other brain structures might also be displaced through the tentorial notch, contusions and/or small hemorrhages in areas such as the corpus callosum, thalamus, hypothalamus, hippocampus, and midbrain are not uncommonly associated with the TBGH. Thus, previous occurrence of a head injury and the evidence of other typically traumatic lesions in the same patient would suggest a traumatic origin of the hemorrhage in the basal ganglia. It should also be noted that TBGHs might rarely be accompanied by ventricular hemorrhage, simulating hypertensive intraventricular hematoma.[6]

Mossberg and Lindenberg[3] also suggested that the compression of vessels supplying the basal ganglia region might cause not only hemorrhage but also infarcts, and considered the traumatic hemorrhages of the basal ganglia to be hemorrhagic contusions, in contrast to Courville and Blomquist,[4] who labeled them hematomas. Whether TBGHs should be considered contusions or, by contrast, intracerebral hematomas remains a secondary question, and the ultimate mechanisms of these lesions still remain unclear.

In 1980, Maki and Colleagues[7] reported on a 6-year-old girl who after suffering severe head injury presented with a massive unilateral hemorrhage measuring 20 ml and located contralateral to the side of impact; the lesion required surgical aspiration through a craniotomy. The authors postulated that the anterior stretch of the lateral branch of the perforating vessel of the MCA, secondary to the opposite direction of rotation of the skull and the brain after injury, plays a major role in the pathogenesis of these lesions. This mechanism could also explain the occurrence of TBGHs located contralateral to the side of impact, which was observed in 76 percent of the patients in our series. Recently, Fujioka, et al,[8] have demonstrated that traumatic dissection of the MCA produces infarction and hemorrhage in the basal ganglia. On the other hand, the basal ganglia and the thalamus are the most frequent places in which hypoperfusion is detected using single-photon emission a brain perfusion scanning after mild and moderate head injury.[9]

In an autopsy series of 635 fatal nonmissile head injuries, Adams, et al[12] found 63 patients with basal ganglia hematomas; the lesion was defined as an intracerebral hemorrhage involving the striatum, pallidum, or thalamus. Most patients were involved in traffic accidents. They rarely experienced a period of lucidity and they exhibited a high incidence of diffuse axonal injuries (DAIs) gliding contusions, and large contusions, suggesting that these deep-brain hematomas were a primary event that occurred the moment of injury and arose from the shear strains elicited by acceleration/deceleration forces.[2,10,11] Patients with this type of injury have a relatively low incidence of skull fractures, in contrast with those suffering falls, in whom TBGHs rarely develop.[1-12] However, it should be noted that TBGHs can occur in the absence of DAI, and not all patients with DAI have TBGHs.

In a recent review of 37 cases of TBGH, in severe head injuries, 73 percent of the patients had an associated DAI, and skull fracture was present in 43 percent. This was unlike previous studies where the incidence of skull fractures was quoted quite low.[13]

ENLARGEMENT

A unique feature of TBGH is that they are known to expand with time. They may evolve into large hematomas as early as 30 to 60 minutes after injury. The rate and extent of volume increase has been related to factors such as the caliber of the injured vessel, the reduction in cerebral blood flow causing secondary ischemia and necrosis in the surrounding white matter leading to hematoma enlargement by coalescence, the occurrence of blood dissection, the presence of hypoxia or systemic arterial hypertension, and a bleeding tendency, which occurs in persons suffering from alcohol abuse.[14] A recent study[13] has shown that 65 percent of TBGHs enlarged during the acute post-traumatic period and 86 percent of the patients exhibited some type of coagulation disorder that might have contributed to the development of delayed hematomas or the enlargement of a pre-existing one.

The formation of hematoma has also been shown to have a bimodal peak. In a study by Okada et al[15] reporting 83 cases of traumatic intracerebral hematomas, 49 were delayed; 10 hematomas (four of them delayed) were located in the basal ganglia. According to this author, completion of hematoma formation displays two incidence peaks, the first within 6 hours postinjury and the second between 12 and 24 hours postinjury.

Bilateral TBGHs

Another interesting aspect is the occurrence of bilateral TBGHs. Yanaka et al[16] reported on two cases of bilateral TBGHs. Ozgun and Castillo[17] described a case of bilateral TBGH occurring after a lightning strike to the head. Boto et al[13] have shown petechiae in the basal ganglia contralateral to the TBGH in three patients.

Basal Ganglionic Infarcts

These are uncommon and more commonly found in children. Oharker et al have described a series of 23 cases that presented with sudden onset of hemiparesis since the time of head injury. Most of the cases were not associated with loss of consciousness. CT scan showed presence of small infarcts within the region of basal ganglia extending into the posterior limb of internal capsule. They have postulated that head injury could have resulted in damage at the level of the angle of the lenticulostriate branches as they enter the perforating substance leading to shearing, thrombosis or embolism.[18,19] Basal ganglionic infarcts may occur in isolation or they may be associated with diffuse axonal injuries, hematoma or contusions[18,20] or as a part of global ischemia seen in severe head injuries or due to injury to the vessels in the neck.

MANAGEMENT

Mossberg and Lindenberg[3] first published the case of a severe head injury patient in whom a hematoma located in the region of the pallidum and was successfully aspirated through a brain cannula. Apart from such anecdotal reports, most of cases of TBGH in the past were managed non operatively. Boto et al[13] showed that in their series only one patient with a TBGH larger than 25 ml survived without surgery and all the other patients with raised ICP as well as 73 percent of the cases showing hematoma volume enlargement died. This shows that a more aggressive approach should be directed towards patients with TBGH at least in patients in whom ICP is difficult to control. Traumatic basal ganglia hematomas may be evacuated by means of open surgery, CT-guided stereotactic aspiration surgery or ultrasound-guided aspiration surgery. Endoscopic evacuation is a more recent technique; previously being applied for spontaneous intracerebral hematomas may also be used for TBGH.[21] It has been recently published that early treatment with citalopram, a selective serotonin reuptake inhibitor, may have a beneficial effect on the extent of morbidity associated with TBGHs.[22]

Lobar hematoma with their extension to basal ganglion can be treated by endoscopic surgery. Complete removal of hematoma can be obtained.[27]

OUTCOME

Smaller intermediary contusions of the basal ganglia may cause extrapyramidal signs secondary to changes in the substantia nigra, motor paralysis due to involvement of the pyramidal tracts in the internal capsule, visual deficits as well as language and sensory impairments due to injury to the lateral geniculate bodies and the thalamus[7,8,20] respectively, and prolonged unconsciousness due to involvement of the reticular activating system.[23] Lucid intervals have been demonstrated especially in those cases where the hematoma has expanded.[13-23]

Studies have shown that TBGH are generally associated with a worse prognosis than other types of post-traumatic intracranial hematomas.[1,13,23,24] However, TBGH are associated with good recovery especially when they occur in isolation, and their final prognosis is related to the extent of the related DAI.[13]

The predictive critical score of GCS should be set at 5 for pediatric TBI. Because it strongly correlates with outcome in this age group. Subarachnoid hemorrhage with brain swelling and edema, subdural, intracerebral hemorrhage and basal ganglion lesions are associated with sever injury and poor outcome ($P<0.05$). However, cortical lesions do not effect severity outcome.[28]

Some authors have correlated the prognosis with the size and found poorer outcome in massive hematomas,[25] while others have not found any correlation with the size or location.[26] Lee and Wang[12] have shown that advanced patient age (> 60 years), the presence of abnormal pupillary changes, impaired oculocephalic and motor responses, and intraventricular and brainstem hemorrhage correlated with poor prognosis. The prognostic factors are summarized in Table 34.1.

Table 34.1: Summary of the prognostic factors in TBGH

Poor prognostic factors	*Good prognostic factors*
• Age > 60 years	• Age < 60 years
• Impaired brainstem reflexes	• Preserved brainstem reflexes
• Poor GCS score	• GCS score above 9
• Intraventricular/brainstem hemorrhage	• TBGH in isolation
• Associated DAI	• Immediate medical surgical intervention
• Massive TBGH	

CONCLUSION

These are summarized below:

1. TBGH are dynamic lesions and tend to expand in volume during the acute post-traumatic period, hence there is importance of serial CT scanning.
2. The pathogenesis and the biomechanics of these lesions is still unclear and further studies are necessary.
3. Surgical intervention is necessary in lesions more than 25 ml. In patients being managed conservatively, a very close monitoring is essential in the ICU and ICP monitoring is mandatory.
4. The overall mortality is high and morbidity considerable in survivors. Some patients with isolated hematomas may do well.

REFERENCES

1. Macpherson P, Teasdale E, Dhaker S, et al. The significance of traumatic hematoma in the region of the basal ganglia. J Neurol Neurosurg Psychiatry 1986;49:29-34.
2. Adams JH, Doyle D, Graham DI, et al. Deep intracerebral (basal ganglia) haematomas in fatal non-missile head injury in man. J Neurol Neurosurg Psychiat 1986;49:1039-43.
3. Adams JH, Doyle D, Graham DI, et al. Deep intracerebral (basal ganglia) haematomas in fatal non-missile head injury in man. J Neurol Neurosurg Psychiat 1986;49:1039-43.
4. Courville CB, Blomquist OA. Traumatic intracerebral hemorrhage with particular reference to its pathogenesis and its relation to "delayed traumatic apoplexy." Arch Surg 1940;41:1-28.
5. Lindenberg R. Significance of the tentorium in head injuries from blunt forces. Clin Neurosurg 1964;12:129-42.
6. Hara M, Shiogai T, Tamagawa T, et al. Three cases of traumatic intracerebral hematoma with ventricular hemorrhage. No Shinkei Geka 1980;8:295-9.
7. Maki Y, Akimoto H, Enomoto T. Injuries of basal ganglia following head trauma in children. Childs Brain 1980;7:113-23.
8. Fujioka M, Maeda Y, Okuchi K, et al. Secondary change in the substantia nigra induced by incomplete infarct and minor hemorrhage in the basal ganglia due to traumatic middle cerebral arterial dissection. Stroke 1999;30:1975-7(Letter).
9. Abdel-Dayem HM, Abu-Judeh H, Kumar M, et al. SPECT brain perfusion abnormalities in mild to moderate traumatic brain injury. Clin Nucl Med 1998;23:309-17.
10. Crooks DA. Pathogenesis and biomechanics of traumatic intracranial hemorrhages. Virchows Arch A Pathol Anat Histopathol 1991;418:479-83.
11. Denny-Brown D, Russell WR. Experimental cerebral concussion. Brain 1941;64:93-164.
12. Lee W, Wang ADJ. Post-traumatic basal ganglia hemorrhage: Analysis of 52 patients with emphasis on the final outcome. Trauma 1991;31:376-80.
13. Boto GR, Lobato RD, Rivas JJ, et al. Basal ganglionic hematomas in severely head injuries: Clinicoradiological analysis of 37 cases. J Neurosurg 2001;94:224-32.
14. Lindenberg R. Trauma of meninges and brain. In: Minckler J (Ed): Pathology of the Nervous System. New York: McGraw Hill 1971;2:1705-65.
15. Okada T. (Clinical aspects of traumatic intracerebral hematomas. Pathogenesis of delayed traumatic intracerebral hematomas). Nippon Ika Daigaku Zasshi 1989;56:545-58 (Jpn.).
16. Yanaka E, Egashira T, Maki Y, et al. Bilateral traumatic hemorrhage in the basal ganglia: Report of two cases. No Shinkei Geka 1991;19:369-73 (Jpn.).
17. Ozgun B, Castillo M. Basal ganglia hemorrhage related to lightning strike. AJNR 1995;16:1370-71.
18. Dharker SR, Mittal RS, Bhargava N. Ischaemic lesions in basal ganglia in children after minor head injury. Neurosurg 1993;33:863-5.
19. Dharker SR. Traumatic ischaemic lesions in children. Neurol India (Suppl)1995;43:61-3.
20. Mahapatra AK, Bhatia R. Basal ganglionic hematomas in head injuries: Review of 26 cases. Neurol India (Abstr) 1986.
21. Auer LM, Deinsberger W, Niederkom K, et al. Endoscopic surgery versus medical treatment for spontaneous intracerebral hematoma: A randomized study. J Neurosurg 1989;70:530-5.

22. Andersen G, Stylsvig M, Sunde N. Citalopram treatment of traumatic brain damage in a 6-year-old boy. J Neurotrauma 1999;16:341-4.
23. Katz DI, Alexander MP, Seliger GM, et al. Traumatic basal ganglia hemorrhage: Clinicopathologic features and outcome. Neurol 1989;39:897-904.
24. Gean AD. Imaging of Head Trauma. New York: Raven Press 1994;165-6.
25. Munemoto S, Komai T, Aizumi S, et al. (Traumatic hemorrhage in the basal ganglia in the child. Five cases). No Shinkei Geka 1985;13:1027-33.
26. Jayakumar PN, Kolluri VRS, Basavakumar DG, et al. Prognosis in traumatic basal ganglia haematoma. Acta Neurochir 1989;97:114-6.
27. Stachura K, Libionka W, Czepko R. Endoscopic treatment of spontaneous intracerebral hematoma. Neurol Neurochir Pol 2004;38(6):489-94.
28. Chung CY, Chen CL, Chang PT, See LG, et al. Critical score of GCS for pediatric traumatic brain injury. Pediatr Neurol 2006;34(5):379-87.
29. Boto GR, Lobato RD, Rivas JJ, Gomez PA, et al. Basal ganglion hematomas in severely head injured patients: Clinicoradiological analysis of 37 cases. J Neurosurg 2001;94(2):224-32.

35 Post-traumatic Meningitis and Brain Abscess

Aditya Gupta, AK Mahapatra

INTRODUCTION

Meningitis and brain abscess following trauma constitute the most common infective complications of head injury.[1-8] The rare ones are subdural empyema, extradural abscess, osteomyelitis and infection in a hematomas.[8] Infective complications not only add to the secondary morbidity of head injury, but also substantially increase the cost associated with its management. Infective complications may affect the ultimate outcome of the patient, and are also known to affect the propensity for developing post-traumatic epilepsy.

The infective complications mostly, but not without exception, affect patients who have sustained compound head injuries (Fig. 35.1). Uncommonly, patients are affected by these complications who have sustained closed injuriess.[8,9] Even those patients are affected who have sustained injuries many years ago, even at sites remote from the site of impact. Certainly, closed head injury patients that have been operated can be subject to these complications like any other patient after a neurosurgical procedure.

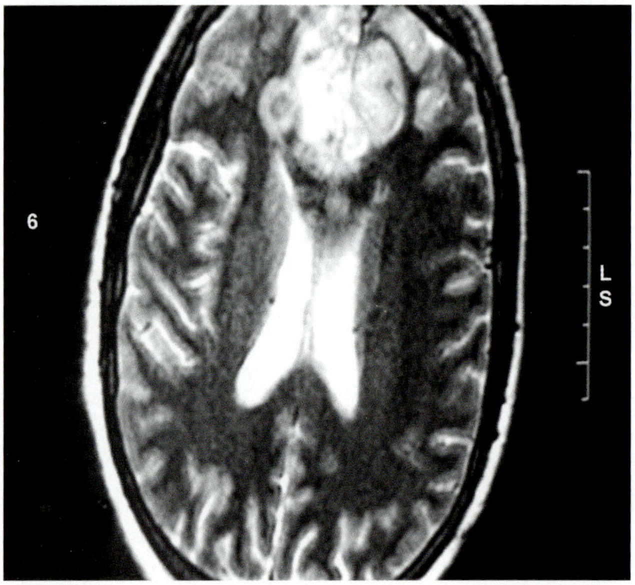

Fig. 35.1: MRI of a patient with compound frontal fracture with basifrontal and midline bleed, who developed abscess and septicemia by 8th day

Infective complications and their impact have certainly lessened after introduction of effective prophylactic antibiotics, but in most areas of the world these complications are still regularly encountered. Surprisingly, we found that the literature relating to post-traumatic brain abscesses was rather scant. As the incidence of high-velocity vehicular accidents rises, neurosurgeons would more regularly encounter compound injuries with skin, bone and soft tissue loss and thus the urgent need to be aware of these infections occurring in the background of trauma. The particular aspects of etiopathogenesis of these complications, the latency, the different microbial spectrum and specific issues related to patient investigation and management necessitate separate mention.

POST-TRAUMATIC MENINGITIS

Meningitis taking place in the post-traumatic setting is usually bacterial in etiology, with incidence widely varying. After an exhaustive review, Kaufman and Colleagues[1] arrived at a reported incidence of 0.2 to 17.8 percent of head injuries. The incidence following compound head injury (external or internal) is much higher. For example, the estimated incidence of meningitis after CSF leak is 3 to 50 percent.[1,2] A recent study concluded that the presence of a CSF leak increased the probability of meningitis by tenfolds.[3] This risk appears to be greater if the leak persists for more than a week following injury.[4,5] In clinical practice, CSF fistula seems to be the most commonly encountered antecedent of post-traumatic meningitis. Acute purulent meningitis complicated by chronic subdural hygroma is rare, but may occur in infant and small children.[62]

A point to note is that the spectrum of causative organisms in the post-traumatic setting is certainly quite distinct from that of community acquired meningitis at different ages of life.[6] One should remember that till recently, the overall case fatality rate for bacterial meningitis is in the range of 25 percent.[7]

It is learnt that craniocerebral trauma is a major risk factor for development of meningitis. Alcohol abuse is significant risk factor in trauma patients with meningitis presenting in 50 percent in one series. Most common pathogen is *Strep. pneumoniae*. Mortality is however low (5%) but neurological sequelae may be more.[61]

Pathogenesis

The pathogenesis of meningitis after head injury may be direct or indirect. The direct course of events follow direct penetrating injury, compound injuries (internal or external) or CSF leaks. The cribriform plate is the most common site of dural fistula as bone is thin in this region, with the adherent dura predisposing to a dural breach at the time of fracture. Also to be considered in this category are cases of meningitis following neurosurgical procedures in head injury patients. The indirect method involves spread of infection from an adjacent compartment. In this group would be cases of meningitis following skull osteomyelitis, intracranial suppurative phlebitis, and brain abscess. The further sequence of events is the same as for meningitis in general,[18] thus not deserving separate mention here.

Microbiology

In general the common organisms responsible for post-traumatic meningitis are the following,[8,9] in the respective clinical settings (Table 35.1).

Sometimes, other unusual organisms may also be isolated, such as *Listeria*.[9] This emphasizes the importance of using specific culture media according to the organisms expected.

Clinical Features

The onset of meningitis is usually within 3 to 5 weeks after the head injury, but is well known to occur even months to years later. This is generally true for those cases associated with initial CSF leak that temporarily stops, only to recur and lead to an attack of meningitis for the first time many months or years later. This underscores the importance of taking a detailed history of events that may have occurred months to years before the patient presents with meningitis. Indeed, the patient may have dismissed the trauma as "trivial" with some minor "nosebleed". Of course, it could occur much earlier in a patient with an external or internal compound injury or in whom the CSF leak persists.[4,5]

Table 35.1: Common organisms responsible for post-traumatic meningitis

Organism	Clinical setting
1. *Strep. pneumoniae* 2. Other streptococci 3 *H. influenzae* 4. *Neisseria* sp.	CSF fistula or Internal compound injuries
5. *Staph. aureus* 6. Enteric gram-negative bacilli 7. *Staph. epidermidis*	Penetrating or external compound injuries

For the patient presenting in the acute phase after trauma, the diagnosis is usually straightforward. In addition to an obvious CSF leak from nose/ear often admixed with blood, other evidence of a basilar fracture may be present, such as anosmia, periorbital and retroauricular ecchymoses. Petrous compound fractures are notorious in that they may result in facial nerve paresis, meningitis and at times present with paradoxical rhinorrhea.

Reccurent episodes of meningitis in a patient should always warn against the possibility of a dural fistula (of whatever etiology); reccurent pneumococcal meningitis is extremely suggestive of an otherwise occult dural fistula.[10]

CSF Analysis

The important objective is to establish that the leaking fluid is, in fact, CSF. Routine bedside estimation of glucose in the fluid may be helpful in confirming that the fluid is CSF, but a negative test may not rule out the possibility. Glucose concentration of more than 30 mg/dl is usually considered confirmatory, whereas concentrations below that may be occasionally observed in lacrimal fluid or mucus.[11] β2-Transferrin is a specific indicator of the presence of CSF in the leaking fluid.

Usual microscopic and biochemical analysis of CSF is mandatory as soon as meningitis is suspected. Of course, in the acute post-traumatic setting, one must ensure absence of significant mass effect prior to perform a lumbar puncture. Also, the presence of traumatic subarachnoid hemorrhage may confound interpretation of CSF findings due to presence of pleocytosis and hypoglycorrhachia. In this context, Gram stain and rapid diagnostic modalities for bacterial detection and isolation are quite useful.[12,13] These are also quite useful in patients who have partially treated meningitis.

Culture of the fluid should be routinely carried out in consultation with a microbiologist to ensure that proper media are available for plating. A sample of CSF should always be obtained prior to start any antibiotic therapy.

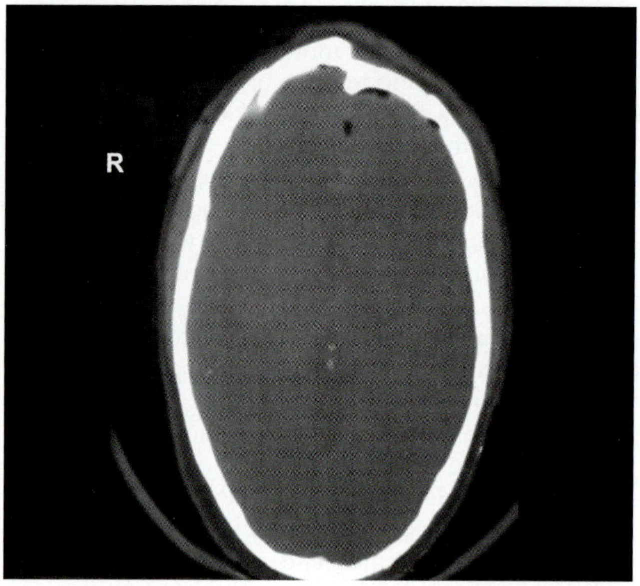

Fig. 35.2: Bone window of compound frontal fracture shows small intracranial air pockets

Radiological Evaluation

Plain radiographs do not provide any substantive information, hence do not serve any useful purpose in this setting. However, the presence of intracranial air, air-fluid levels or even opacity in the paranasal sinuses are the common findings (Figs 35.2 and 35.3).

CT remains the mainstay of radiological evaluation of patients having post-traumatic meningitis. It provides useful information depending on the clinical situation:

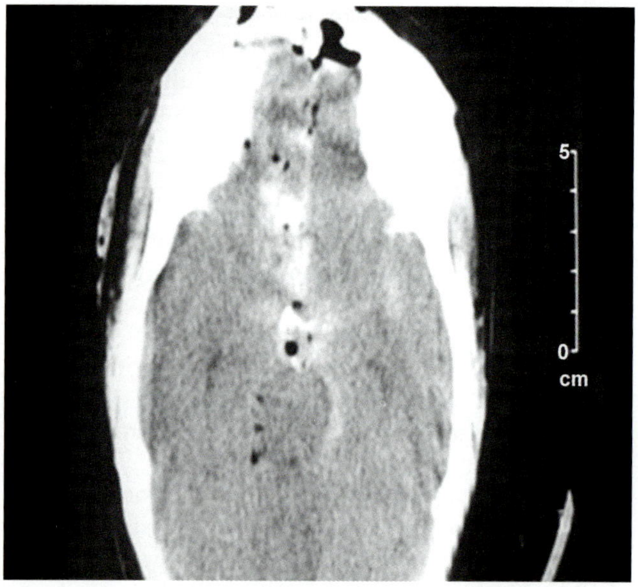

Fig. 35.3: CT of a compound fracture of frontal bone showing diffuse basifrontal bleed

1. *In the acute post-traumatic setting:* CT provides valuable information regarding the presence of fracture, injury to underlying brain and presence of internal or external compounding. Fluid or blood in the sinuses indicates the presence of otherwise occult basilar fractures. Thin-slice axial and coronal studies of the skull base (with bone window) may be required in some cases to demonstrate basilar fractures.[10,14]
2. *In the delayed setting:* Routine CT study may show the presence of intracranial air, which is diagnostic. CT with studies of the skull base is required to delineate basilar fractures responsible for CSF leak. In addition, high-resolution CT cisternography using a water-soluble contrast medium should be used[1] to identify the exact site of leak in patients requiring operative closure of the dural fistula.

The above studies may also be required in patients presenting with reccurent meningitis (especially pneumococcal).[10]

Contrast CT may be necessary on occasion in patients who do not respond or deteriorate despite of adequate treatment. In these situations, one may expect to find development of a subdural empyema or even a brain abscess.

MR imaging is also of help, especially in the delayed setting. In the acute setting, blood and blood products may obscure the delineation of dural breach. In the delayed phase, thin-slice coronal imaging is of great value in delineating a dural fistula. This is visualized best in the T_2-weighted images as a continuation of the subarachnoid space reaching extradurally across a bony gap or fracture. CSF may also seen in the contiguous air sinuses. An encephalocele may also be seen to accompany this tract in some cases. The advantage of MR imaging here is its non-invasive nature, when compared to the alternative of CT cisternography, which requires intrathecal contrast administration.

Isotope studies at the present time certainly help in documenting a CSF leakage but the poor spatial resolution precludes a useful delineation of the site of leak. Thus, ultimately one has to choose between MR and CT cisternography for identification of the site of CSF leakage.

Management

The management of post-traumatic meningitis involves three aspects:

- Optimal antimicrobial treatment
- Symptomatic and adjunctive measures
- Treatment of the cause.

Antibiotic Treatment

Treatment with parenteral antibiotics effective against the causative organism in adequate dosage for optimal duration is the key to proper treatment. No time should be lost in initially instituting empirical antibiotic therapy[15] after taking the CSF sample for the various analyses. The initial empirical antibiotic should fulfill the following criteria:

1. It should have good penetration into the CSF.
2. It should be able to reach a minimum bactericidal concentration (MBC) in the CSF.[15]
3. It should be effective against the probable causative organisms, i.e. must be broad-spectrum.
4. The choice should be in accordance with the emerging sensitivities of the expected groups of organisms.

As indicated in the section on microbiology, one can consider two broad clinical groups in order to determine the effective empirical antibiotic regime.

In the group having meningitis secondary to CSF fistulae or internal compounding, the likely organisms indicated would likely respond to a third generation cephalosporin and an aminoglycoside together with metronidazole. Of there three, metronidazole and the third generation cephalosporin have excellent CSF penetration, and are quite effective.

For the group having penetrating or external compound injuries, a better empiric choice of antibiotics would be a combination of vancomycin (or a penicillinase resistant penicillin) and a third-generation cephalosporin with good activity even against *Pseudomonas* organisms (such as ceftazidime).

The clinical response should be closely monitored and results of CSF cultures obtained as soon as possible. One should convert to the specific antibiotic therapy quickly in adequately high doses. Curtailing the duration of broad-spectrum antibiotics would also help in preventing the rapid development of resistance in these organisms.

The duration of the antibiotic therapy should be at least 14 days, and should continue till at least 7 days after defervescence.[15,16] Gram-negative bacillary meningitis requires antibiotics to be continued at least 2 weeks beyond sterilization of CSF.[8] Nonresponding patients should be evaluated with contrast CT to exclude pus collection elsewhere (such as abscess or subdural empyema). If present, these should be drained. Repeat CSF analysis should also be done, so as to ascertain the response of antibiotics on the cytological and biochemical CSF parameters (decline in cell counts, rise in sugar levels) also to repeat CSF cultures and evaluate for other unusual pathogens causing meningitis solely or in combination.

Symptomatic and Adjunctive Measures

Antipyretics, analgesics and hydrotherapy may be required for the control of fever. Anticonvulsants are indicated from the point of view of head injury, or if patient has a seizure during the illness.

Corticosteroids have been shown to have a role in preventing the development of sensorineural deafness in children with meningitis due to *H. influenzae*.[17] However, routine use in children is still controversial.[18] Some reports suggest that the use of corticosteroids may be beneficial in adults with pneumococcal meningitis,[19] high CSF bacterial load and in those with high CSF pressure.[20]

Adjunctive surgical measures may be indicated in the following clinical situations:

1. Hydrocephalus (requiring ventricular drainage).
2. Development of subdural empyema or abscess.
3. Persistent hydrocephalus after successful treatment of meningitis.
4. Treatment of the cause.

Treatment of Cause

The underlying cause if managed optimally would in fact prevent the occurrence of meningitis in the first place. Adequate debridement and removal of foreign material in compound head injuries and proper management of CSF fistulas would certainly help in this regard.

CSF fistulas need specific operative management in case the leak persists more than 7 to 10 days after injury, or if there is another episode of meningitis. Even a single episode of delayed meningitis is considered an indication for undertaking operative obliteration of the fistula.

POST-TRAUMATIC BRAIN ABSCESS

The earliest available record of successful drainage of a post-traumatic brain abscess was by Dupuytren in 1839, who opened a compound skull fracture to drain the abscess in a soldier who later survived. Intracranial infections occurring after head injury are among the most dreaded complications.[21] Fortunately, the occurrence of a brain abscess after head injury is a rather uncommon sequel.[22] Most cases, as mentioned, occur following a compound head injury. There are also reports of several cases of post-traumatic abscess following closed head-injury,[23,25] including a report from our institution.[26] The reported incidence of abscess following head trauma has ranged from 3 percent of 203 cases of penetrating head injuries sustained during World War II, to 16.7 percent of 42 cases of compound brain injuries in various reports.[27-29]

As a percentage of all brain abscesses, traumatic brain abscesses constitute anywhere from 4.1 percent in an autopsy series and 30 to 12 to 20 percent in other retrospective series.[29,31,33] Clearly, this entity cannot be put aside as a rare occurrence. Further, the mortality rate for brain abscesses has declined in the antibiotic era, but still remains high at 10 to 30 percent.[8]

Pathogenesis

The pathogenesis can be conveniently thought of as being direct or indirect. The direct pathway of genesis of a post-traumatic abscess involves direct penetration of the cranial vault and the dura at the time of injury. This results in the following components being present intracranially, all of which individually predispose to formation of the abscess:

1. *Foreign material:* Dust, skin and soft tissue debris, hair, bone fragments, and metallic or nonmetallic fragments of various kinds. These different agents have varying propensity for leading to abscess formation: a high-speed bullet fragment may remain inert for prolonged periods of time, whereas the same is not true of other organic and nonorganic fragments such as glass, wood, etc. Furthermore, these nonviable agents lead to the formation of a nidus as described below.
2. *Contused and lacerated brain tissue:* Like the above agents, provide an areas of low oxygen tension and variably low blood supply. This promotes the formation of an infectious nidus.[34]
3. Hematoma around the area of brain injury.

The indirect pathway results in abscess formation after any of the following events have taken place:

1. Meningitis.
2. Osteomyelitis.
3. Suppurative intracranial phlebitis.
4. Hematogenous spread of infective organisms from a focus to a foreign body.

It should be noted that traumatic CSF fistulae also predispose to the development of an abscess,[35] usually as a sequel to meningitis.

The further sequence of events proceeds in much the same way as for any other abscess and the evolution, particularly in a head injury setting may be influenced by various factors such as virulence of the organism, type and duration of the antibiotic therapy apart from others.[8]

At times, organisms may be of low enough virulence or the host reaction may be sufficient to wall these off for prolonged periods, resulting in unusually long latency. An interesting case reported[36] that of coexistent chronic pyogenic abscess and glioblastoma multiforme developing after 37 years at the site of a metallic splinter injury.

The above discussion would not be complete without commenting on those unusual cases of post-traumatic brain abscesses that occur following supposedly closed injury.[23-25] These abscesses seem to have a predilection for frontal and temporal regions, as was evident from the study from our institution.[26] A review of three other cases cited revealed that steroid therapy may have played a role in one patient. In another report,[24] exploration of the abscess that followed supposedly closed head injury revealed a basifrontal fracture. Moreover, the abscess was contiguous and bone splinters were found within the orbitofrontal cortex. This suggests that in many cases of abscess following seemingly "closed" head injury the cause may actually be internally compound head injury. This would also explain the proximity to frontal and temporal regions, where the air sinuses are contiguous.

Microbiology

In one of the earliest reports, Cairns reported that staphylococci and streptococci were the commonly isolated organisms.[28] From our institution, the published data revealed that *Staphylococcus aureus* was the most common organism in 12 (33%) cases.[26] Other microbes isolated were almost equally distributed among the gram-negative enterobacteria (*E. coli, Pseudomonas, Klebsiella* and *Proteus*) and anaerobe groups (*Clostridia, Bacteroides,* and *Bacillus* species). *Streptococcus pneumoniae* (earlier called *Pneumococcus*) is particularly associated with post-traumatic abscesses especially those following CSF rhinorrhea.[35] Gas-containing abscesses, though rare, have been described in other reports, with *Clostridia* being the most common species responsible for gas-containing intracranial abscesses.[37] So far, a total of 38 *clostridial* abscesses have been described, of which 32 (84%) were related to a penetrating head injury.[37] There are also solitary reports of other unusual organisms such as *Nocardiae,*[38] *Bacillus* species,[39] *Propionibacterium,*[36] among others. As a rare occurrence, fungal organisms may concommitantly be isolated in pus from post-traumatic brain abscess.[37] Only a total of 6 such cases have been reported so far, with *Aspergillus* and Mucoraceae being the main offenders.[37]

It is clearly advisable to obtain an adequate pus sample prior to instituting any antimicrobial therapy.[40]

However, circumstances may be extenuating, and the patient may already have received broad-spectrum empiric therapy prior to reach neurosurgical attention. Fastidious organisms may still result in a sterile culture despite all above precautions. To prevent this, appropriate culture media should be readily available. For example, specific culture media should be used for plating when suspecting *Haemophilus* or *Clostridia* species as the causative organisms.

Sampling of CSF may be potentially dangerous in the presence of an abscess with mass effect, and should be avoided.[8]

Latency

Post-traumatic abscesses can form as early as 5 weeks after injury. In some cases of penetrating injuries, this may be even sooner. For example, in the case reported by Tekkok et al[37] a gas-containing tract was seen in a CT study 5 days after a penetrating injury with a rusted nail. A well-defined ring-enhancing abscess could be seen 4 weeks post-injury. Despite the occasional exception, 5 weeks seem to be required for the chain of the pathogenetic steps to take place and sequentially result in the formation of an abscess.

The usual latency for a post-traumatic abscess to form is 3 to 4 months. This seems to be the general experience from various reports, and also in the series reported by Dinakar Rao[2,29] and also from our institution.[26] The latency may at times be unusually long.[36,41,42] The most illustrative example to this effect was the case reported by Robinson et al.[42] They operated a patient suspected to have a meningioma, which turned out at operation to be a chronic abscess containing viable gram-positive cocci even 36 years after sustaining a compound head injury. In the post-antibiotic era, such a delayed presentation is more common, with patients receiving potent antibiotics for suspected compound head injury.

Clinical Features

The affected population seems to be more commonly young males.[26,29] The most important point is the history of penetrating head injury, which is usually present in a majority. One must insist on a thorough description of the events, especially from any witness, as the patient may be amnesic regarding the actual sequence of events. This is important as gauged from numerous reports wherein this information was initially lacking. In children, seemingly innocuous injuries with pencil-tips[43] around the periorbital region have resulted in brain abscesses. This point is to be kept in mind, as the bony walls of the orbit are thin in children (especially the roof) predisposing to penetrate injuries with otherwise harmless objects. A definite subgroup of patients would not have any history of compound or penetrating head injury.[23-36] For example, in the report from our institution,[26] 13 of 36 patients had no evidence of compound head injury among them 3 had been operated for closed head injury.

Seizures and focal neurological deficits may be seen depending on the severity of the initial injury and location of the developing brain abscess. The other relevant manifestations are that of a wound discharging pus, brain fungus and signs of raised intracranial pressure. In our experience, the signs of raised intracranial pressure were the most common manifestations, followed by seizures. An interesting finding was that patients with closed head injuries seemed to have fresh focal deficits more commonly, which was statistically significant.[26]

Location

By and large, post-traumatic abscesses are confined to the supratentorial compartment. Not only is this because compound injuries and air sinuses usually relate to this compartment, but also because penetrating wounds when occurring in the posterior fossa are commonly fatal.[44] The above observations not withstanding, Webster and Gurdjian[33] encountered one case of abscess in the mid-cerebellar region. Another report by Kepes et al[38] illustrated a fatal case in which the patient survived the trauma but later succumbed to an abscess located in the medulla.

Frontal and parietal regions are the favored locations in compound head injuries, are also the leading sites for traumatic brain abscesses.[26,29]

Radiological Evaluation

Plain radiographs at the present time do not seem to much value in the evaluation for a post-traumatic brain abscess. These may demonstrate intracranial air in gas-containing abscesses in 75 percent of cases,[37] which has important management implications.

CT constitutes the mainstay of radiological evaluations.[8] A contrast-enhanced CT study is able to demonstrate brain abscess, with the appearance depending on the evolutionary stage of the abscess. A CT study would be expected to demonstrate important findings related to a post-traumatic brain abscess, as depicted in Table 35.2.

CT serves as a baseline for initial evaluation as well as a medium for objective assessment of the response

Table 35.2: Things to look for in contrast CT study for post-traumatic brain abscess

1. Location
2. Size of the abscess
3. Stage of evolution of the abscess
4. Mass effect due to the abscess and the surrounding edema
5. Wall thickness
6. Number of loculi
7. Communication with ventricular system or ventriculitis
8. Hydrocephalus
9. Air in the abscess cavity
10. Presence of foreign body

to the chosen modality of management (medical, aspiration or surgical excision). As mentioned above, in cases supposedly following closed head injury, thin-slice axial and coronal sections should be taken to rule out the basal fractures that may be otherwise missed. In situations wherein a CSF fistula is thought to result in meningitis leading to brain abscess, a CT cisternography study after administering intrathecal contrast is often of help.

MR imaging is not of much value in this setting, but may occasionally be required for delineation of rare posterior fossa abscesses, or when the diagnosis itself is in doubt. Pyogenic acute abscesses have fairly striking and specific MR appearances,[45,46] but one should always exclude the possibility of a metallic foreign body prior to MR imaging in a case of post-traumatic brain abscess.

MANAGEMENT

Overall Strategy

The overall management strategy for post-traumatic brain abscesses has undergone changes, but controversies still abound as to the best initial treatment for these patients and whether solely conservative treatment has any role at all.

The best treatment of post-traumatic abscess is still its prevention. Compound injuries need to be treated with adequate debridement, all foreign material must removed and proper dural closure should be done, together with prophylactic antibiotics.

Treatment with antibiotics is certainly an important part of the overall regime. In fact, Sandermann et al[47] advocated that as the sole treatment for post-traumatic abscesses. It has been realized that antibiotics in general penetrate the blood-brain barrier poorly. In fact, they may be able to reach therapeutically important levels in the abscess only in the presence of cerebritis and hyperemia.[48-51] In this regard, another finding has been that clinical response may be lacking despite higher-than-MIC concentrations of antibiotics in the abscess pus presumably owing to unfavorable local factors such as local pH and bacterial loads.[2]

The first report of successful conservative treatment of brain abscesses was by Heinemann and Braudes,[53] who treated 6 patientss.[53] However, all the lesions were in the cerebritis stage. Other studies[47-50,54] followed. Sandermann and Colleagues[47] considered surgical options such as aspiration or excision only in extreme situations of raised intracranial pressure. In an analysis of 67 cases of conservatively treated encapsulated abscesses reported in literature, Rosenblum and Colleagues[55,56] demonstrated that the mean diameter of abscesses that responded to medical treatment was 1.7 centimeters and no abscess larger than 2.5 centimeters responded to medical treatment alone. Another important result of this study was that in as many as 28 percent patients, there was no certainty of diagnosis. This fact is important as many lesions can mimic the ring-enhancing appearance of an abscess. Further, a totally conservative approach does not allow us to identify the organism or its particular antibiotic sensitivity. In fact, if a purely medical approach does not yield results, even later conversion to a surgical approach may preclude this identification owing to broad-spectrum empiric antimicrobial therapy.

At the present time, with availability of precise localization techniques and low-risk for aspiration performed under local anesthesia, there is little justification for purely medical treatment of an abscess. Possible exceptions are an uncontrolled bleeding diathesis, or a deep seated or small lesion (less than 1.5 cm) in a neurologically intact patient. These situations are rarely encountered in brain abscesses following trauma. For multiple abscesses (rarely seen after trauma), antibiotics can be used for the smaller lesions if a culture has been obtained after aspiration from the larger one or from any of the lesions.[57]

Antibiotic Therapy

In general it is advisable to start empiric antibiotic treatment with broad-spectrum parenteral antibiotics. The usual recommended combination[35,58,59] is either a third generation cephalosporin with anti-*Pseudomonas* activity plus a penicillinase-resistant penicillin or vancomycin plus an aminoglycoside in proper dosage. If compound injury has involved an air sinus, intravenous metronidazole should be added for the first 3 to 5 days. The cultures should be expeditiously obtained and specific antibiotic therapy started depending on the sensitivity of the organism isolated. Parenteral antibiotics need to be given for a minimum of 4 to 6 weeks, and longer in some cases depending on whether aspiration of the abscess has been undertaken or excision.

In cases where the abscess cavity contains gas, the possibility is either an abscess with a coexistent CSF fistula or the causative organism being gas producing. If a CSF fistula can be excluded, the preferred agent in combination is Penicillin G, keeping in mind that the most common of fenders are usually *Clostridia* species.[37] However, it should be noted that a significant number of clostridial abscesses are polymicrobial,[37] hence the need for other broad-spectrum agents as part of the combination. The use of polyvalent gas gangrene antiserum and hyperbaric oxygen therapy has not shown any clear benefit.[37] In case of a CSF fistula with coexistent brain abscess, the likely organisms to be targeted are as mentioned in the previous section on post-traumatic meningitis.

Surgical Treatment

Surgical options seem to have some evident advantages (Table 35.3). Surgery achieves rapid decompression, which may be of crucial importance in patients with raised intracranial pressure. At the same time, it enables us to identify the offending organism and subject it to sensitivity testing. Occasionally, this may completely alter the antibiotic regimen when a typical organisms are cultured such as Nocardiae[38] or Fungi.[37]

Two broad surgical options exist: aspiration of the abscess and excision. With availability of ultrasonic or stereotaxic (frame based or frameless) guidance, aspiration has become even for smaller lesions and those located in functionally dense regions. Additionally, one can target the desired lesion in case there are multiple abscesses or take a biopsy of tissue even in the cerebritis stage (when an open procedure may be more hazardous). Aspiration is likely to succeed if there is no retained foreign body, the pus is of fluid consistency, there is a single locule, and the wall is thin. All these increase the likelihood of the penetration of antibiotics, drainage of a significant amount of purulent material with probability of collapse of abscess walls. With precise localization and performance of the procedure under local anesthesia, the surgical risk is quite low.

Table 35.3: Indications for surgery
1. Abscess containing foreign material[35]
2. Abscess containing gas (CSF fistula or gas-producing organisms)[34]
3. Abscess with concommitant CSF fistula[34]
4. Abscess following operation for closed head injury[8,26]
5. Cerebellar abscess (failure of decompression may be fatail[58]
6. Abscess caused by fungi[58]

Excision may entail a slightly higher surgical morbidity, but has definite advantages in many situations. Overall, there is a general opinion that post-traumatic abscesses should more often be subjected to excision rather than aspiration.[8,26] In the study from our institution, 14 patients were initially managed with aspiration of the abscess. This was sufficient in only 3, as 8 patients required excision of the abscess and remaning 3 required repeated aspirations.[26] Excision should be strongly considered as the primary modality of surgical treatment in the following situations:

In addition, abscesses may need to be secondarily excised:

1. No response to antibiotics and aspiration attempts.
2. Hematoma following attempted abscess aspiration.
3. Non-improvement in clinical condition after aspiration (e.g. after aspiration of a temporal abscess in a comatose patient).

Patients with abscesses rupturing into the ventricular system may require the use of an external ventricular drain till the infection subsides.

Use of Anticonvulsants and Steroids

Majority of the patients would already be on anticonvulsant treatment given the background of prior significant head injury. Some may have uncontrolled seizures, requiring multiple antiepileptic drugs. In a study by Legg et al,[60] 72 percent of their patients reported seizures when followed up without anticonvulsants. This indicates the rationale of routinely prescribing anticonvulsants to all patients with post-traumatic brain abscesses. There may be a beneficial response as regards seizure frequency after excision, but intractable cases would require formal evaluation to spatially define the epileptogenic focus, and subsequently may have to undergo excision of the focus.

Steroids should be used only in situations where the edema surrounding the abscess poses a danger to the survival of the patient, and then too, for the shortest permissible duration. Though the steroids lessen edema, their effect on lessening both the degree and extent of encapsulation[35] may increase the amount of adjacent tissue destruction.

REFERENCES

1. Kaufman BA, Tunkel AR, Pryor JC, et al. Meningitis in the neurosurgical patient. Inf Dis Clin N Am 1990;4:677-701.
2. Leech PJ, Patterson A. Conservative and operative management for cerebrospinal fluid leakage after closed head injury. Lancet 1973;1013-6.
3. Tenney JH. Bacterial infections of the central nervous system in neurosurgery. Neurol Clin 1986;4:91-114.
4. Mincy JE. Post-traumatic cerebrospinal fluid fistula at the frontal fossa. J Trauma 1966;6:618-22.
5. Raaf J. Post-traumatic cerebrospinal fluid leaks. Arch Surg 1967;95:648-51.
6. Durack DT, Perfect JR. Acute bacterial meningitis. In: Rengachary SS and Wilkins RH (Eds): Neurosurgery, Vol III. New York, McGraw-Hill Book Company 1985;1921-28.
7. Durand ML, Calderwood SB, Weber DJ, et al. Acute bacterial meningitis in adults: A review of 493 episodes. N Engl J Med 1993;328:21-8.
8. Gormley WB, del Busto R, Saravolatz LD, Rosenblum ML. Cranial and intracranial bacterial infections. In: Youmans JR (Ed): Neurological Surgery, Vol V. Philadelphia, WB Saunders Company 1996;3195-3220.
9. Hirschmann JV. Bacterial meningitis following closed cranial trauma. In: Sande MA, Smith AL, Root RK (Eds): Bacterial meningitis. New York, Churchill Livingstone 1985;95-103.
10. Sponsel C, Park JW. Recurrent pneumococcal meningitis. Search for occult skull fracture. Postgrad Med 1994;95(1):109-10.
11. Hyslop NE, Montgomery WW. Diagnosis and management of meningitis associated with cerebrospinal fluid leaks. In: Remington JS, Swartz MN (Eds): Current clinical topics in infectious diseases, Vol 3. New York, McGraw-Hill 1982;254-85.
12. Kaplan SL, Feign RD. Clinical presentations, prognostic factors and diagnosis of bacterial meningitis. In Sande MA, Smith AL, Root RK (Eds): Bacterial meaningitis. New York, Churchill Livingstone 1985;83-94.
13. Wilson CB, Smith AL. Rapid tests for the diagnosis of bacterial meningitis. In: Remington JS, Swartz MN: Current clinical topics in infectious diseases, Vol 7. New York, McGraw-Hill 1986;134-56.
14. Rath SA, Knoringer P. Late abscess after severe craniocerebral trauma with fronto-orbital fracture. Childs Nerv Syst 1989;5:121-3.
15. Roos KL, Tunkel AR, Scheld WM. Acute bacterial meningitis in children and adults. In: Scheld WM, Whitley RJ, Durack DT (Eds): Infections of the central nervous system. New York, Raven Press 1991;335-410.
16. Overturf GD. Bacterial meningitis. In: Hoeprich PD, Jordan MC Ronald AR: Infectious diseases. Philadelphia, Lippincott Company 1994;1111.
17. Lebel MH, Freij BJ, Syrogiannopoulos GA, et al. Dexamethasone therapy for bacterial meningitis: Results of two double-blind, placebo-controlled trials. N Engl J Med 1988;319:964-71.
18. Word BM, Klein JO. Therapy of bacterial sepsis and meningitis in infants and children: 1989 poll of directors of programs in pediatric infectious diseases. Ped Inf Dis J 1989;8:635-37.
19. Girgis NI, Farid Z, Mikhail IA, et al. Dexamethasone treatment for bacterial meningitis in children and adults. Ped Inf Dis J 1989;8:848-51.
20. Quagliarello VJ, Scheld WM. New perspectives on bacterial meningitis. Clin Inf Dis 1993;17:603-10.
21. Jennett B, Miller JD. Infection after depressed fractures: Implications for management of non-missile injury. J Neurosurg 1972;36:333-39.
22. deTribolet N, Guiguard G, Zander E. Brain abscess after intracranial penetration of a paint brush. Surg Neurol 1979;11:187-89.
23. Bhatia R. Brain abscesses in children. Ind J Pediat 1983;50:91-597.
24. Rath SA, Knoringer P. Late abscess after severe craniocerebral trauma with fronto-orbital fracture. Childs Nerv Syst 1989;5:121-3.
25. Moskopp D. Septic brain abscess following closed craniocerebral trauma with steroid therapy. Neurochirurgia (Stuttg) 1985;28:147-51.
26. Patir R, Sood S, Bhatia R. Post-traumatic brain abscess: Experience of 36 patients. Br J Neurosurg 1995;9:29-35.
27. Gillingham FJ. Neurosurgical experience in Northern Italy. Br J Surg. War Suppl no. 1: Wounds of the head. Bristol, John Wright and Sons 1947;80-87.
28. Cairns H, Calvert CA, Daniel P, Northcroft GB. Complications of head wounds with special reference to infection. Br J Surg War Suppl no. 1: Wounds of the head. Bristol, John Wright and Sons 1947;198-243.
29. Dinaker I, Rao B. Post-traumatic brain abscess. J Post Grad Med 1971;17:137-141.
30. Ewans W. Brain abscess, Pathology and Etiology. Lancet 1931;1:1231-5.
31. Kerr FW, King RB, Meagher JN. Brain abscess, a study of 47 consecutive cases. J Am Med Assoc 1958;168:868-72.
32. Webster JE, Gurdjian ES. The surgical management of intracranial suppuration. Surg Gynec Obst 1950;90:209-34.
33. Gurdjian ES, Webster JE. Experiences in the surgical management of intracranial suppuration. Surg Gynec Obst 1957;104:205-14.
34. Young RF, Frazee J. Gas within intracranial abscess cavities: An indication for surgical excision. Ann Neurol 1984;16:35-39.
35. Osenbach RK, Loftus CM. Diagnosis and management of brain abscess. Neurosurg Clin North Am 1992;3:403-20.
36. Sabel M, Felsberg J, Messing-Junger M, Neuen-Jakob E, Piek J. Glioblastoma multiforme at the site of metallic splinter injury: A coincidence? Case report. J Neurosurg 1999;91(6):1041-4.

37. Tekkok IH, Higgins MJ, Ventureya EC. Post-traumatic gas containing brain abscess caused by *Clostridium perfringens* with unique simultaneous fungal suppuration by Myceliophthora thermophila: Case report. Neurosurgery 1996;39(6):1247-51.
38. Kepes JJ, Schoolman A. Post-traumatic abscess of the medulla oblongata containing Nocardia asteroides. J Neurosurg 1965;22(5):511-14.
39. Bert F, Ouahes O, Lambert-Zechovsky N. Brain abscess due to Bacillus macerans following a penetrating periorbital injury. J Clin Microbiol 1995;33(7):1950-53.
40. Mampalam TJ, Rosenblum ML. Trends in management of bacterial brain abscess: A review of 102 cases over 17 years. Neurosurg 1988;23:451-8.
41. Marquardt G, Scick W, Moller-Hartmann W. Brain abscess decades after a penetrating shrapnel injury. Br J Neurosurg 1999;13:246-8.
42. Robinson EF, Model RH, Gol A. Brain abscess 36 years after head injury: Case Report 1997;1:11.
43. Foy P, Sharr M. Cerebral abscesses in children after pencil-tip injuries. Lancet, 1980.
44. Grant FC. Post-traumatic brain abscess. In: Brock S (Ed). Injuries of the brain and spinal cord 4th edn. London, Cassel 1960;4:187-202.
45. Haimes AB, Zimmerman RD, Morgello S, et al. MR imaging of brain abscesses. AJNR 1989;10:279-91.
46. Sze G, Zimmerman RD. The magnetic resonance imaging of infections and inflammatory diseases. Radial Clin North Am 1988;26:839-59.
47. Sandermann JE, Harse J, Bartholdy NS, Udison H. Nonsurgical treatment of brain abscesses in the child. Childs Nerv Syst 1986;2:49-51.
48. Donald FE, Ispahani P. Use of cefotaxime in brain abscess. Br J Neurosurg 1988;2:539-40.
49. George B, Roux F, Pillon M, et al. Relevance of antibiotics in the treatment of brain abscesses: Report of a case with eight brain abscesses simultaneously treated and cured medically. Acta Neurochir (Wien) 1979;47:285-91.
50. Kammin M, Biddle D. Conservative management of focal intracerebral infections. Neurol 1981;31:103-6.
51. Levy RM, Gutin PH, Baskin DS, et al. Vancomycin penetration of a brain abscess: Case report and review of the literature. Neurosurg 1986;18:632-6.
52. Black PM, Graybill JR, Charache P. Penetration of brain abscess by systemically administered antibiotics. J Neurosurg 1973;38:705-9.
53. Heinemann HS, Braude Al. Intracranial suppurative disease. JAMA 1971;218:1542-7.
54. Rousseaux M, Lesion F, Destee A, et al. Developments in the treatment and prognosis of multiple cerebral abscesses. Neurosurg 1985;16:304-8.
55. Rosenblum ML, Mampalam TJ, Pons V. Controversies in the management of brain abscess. Clin Neurosurg 1986;33:603-2.
56. Rosenblum ML, Hoff JT, Norman O, et al. Nonoperative treatment of brain abscess in selected high-risk patients. J Neurosurg 1980;52:217-25.
57. Mamelak AN, Mampalam TJ, Rosenblum ML. Improved management of multiple brain abscesses: A combined surgical approach based on a review of 16 cases. Neurosurg 1995;36:76-86.
58. Wispelwey B, Scheld WM. Brain abscess. In: Mandell CL, Douglas RG, Bennett JE (Eds): Principles and Practice of infectious disease. New York, Churchill Livingstone 1990;777-88.
59. Britt RH. Brain abscess. In: Wilkins RH, Rengachary SS (Eds): Neurosurgery. New York, McGraw-Hill 1985; 1928-56.
60. Legg NJ, Gupta PC, Scott OF. Epilepsy following cerebral abscess: A clinical and EEG study of 70 patients. Brain 1973;96:259-68.
61. Holeckova K, kolenova A, Lensnakova A, et al. Bacterial meningitis after craniocerebral trauma in community, Neuroendocrinol Lett 2007;28(Suppl.)3:12-3.
62. Imataka G, Miyamoto K, Fujiyama Y, et al. Acute purulent meningitis associated with chronic subdural hematoma and subdural hygroma. Turk J Pediatr 2007; 49(4):437-40.

36 Post-traumatic Hydrocephalus

AK Mahapatra, Raj Kumar

INTRODUCTION

Post-traumatic hydrocephalus (PTH) is a rare but well recognized condition. The incidence is reported 2 to 8 percent cases of all closed head injury.[1-4] Surprising, only few large series are published.[3,6] Delayed dilatation of ventricles, following severe head injury is not uncommon. It is the result of brain atrophy following head injury, which of no consequences in long run and merits no specific treatment. On the contrary, PTH is a distinct clinical entity and needs precise treatment so as to help the patient from further brain damage. Thus, there is a need for differentiating ventriculomegaly from the PTH. This chapter highlights the pathogenesis, diagnosis and management of PTH.

Ventriculomegaly is common after severe head injury but destinction between atrophy and potentially treatable hydrocephalus cannot be made on the basis of conventional CT or MRI, scanning alone. Physiological measurement of ICP and CSF outflow resistance may be helpful. These factors together with limited literature effect CSF diversion in outcome of vegetative patients.[17]

PATHOGENESIS

Pathogenesis of (Table 36.1) PTH is many folds. By and large time required from injury to the development of hydrocephalus ranges from 3 to 8 weeks.[1,3,4] Rarely, ventricle can also enlarge rapidly.[7] The genesis of hydrocephalus is either due to obstruction to CSF flow in the ventricle, leading to obstructive hydrocephalus or due to blockage of arachnoid granulation, resulting communicating hydrocephalus.[8] Acute obstructive hydrocephalus is common in patients with traumatic intraventricular hemorrhage (Figs 36.1 to 36.3)[4] contusion or and hematomas of the posterior fossa, which can easily block the IV ventricle, leading to obstructive hydrocephalus.[1,10,12] Grcevic in 1983[11] reported an unusual case, in whom tear of tela choroidea, followed by intraventricular bleed and SAH leading to impairment CSF absorption and communicating hydrocephalus. Supratrentorial clot can lead to acute hydrocephalus of the contralateral ventricle.[1] Chronic PTH can also be a result of post-trauma meningitis[1] or decompressive craniectomy.[1,3,9,13] However, pathogenesis of hydrocephalus following a decompressive craniotomy is not very clear. Blockage of CSF absorption in the cerebral convexity, following the craniectomy is presumed to be the cause of the hydrocephalus.

Hydrocephalus or ventriculomegaly can also be the result of birth trauma.[4,12] Brain injury and intraventricular hemorrhage are more frequent in preterm infants.[12] However, the differentiation of hydrocephalus

Table 36.1: Post-traumatic hydrocephalus etiology

	Obstructive	*Communicative*
• Acute	IVH Posterior fossa hematomas	– SAH
• Chronic	Gliosis of aqueduct Ventriculitis due to EVD	– Postcraniectomy – Meningitis – SAH

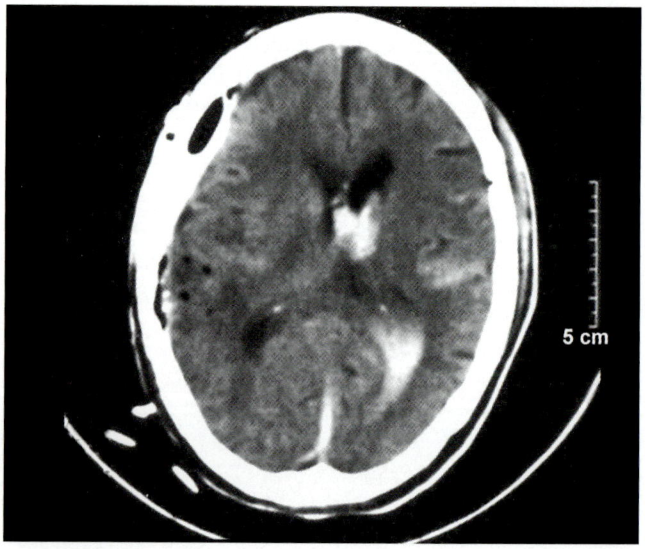

Fig. 36.1: CT showing right frontal extradural clot, multiple diffuse parenchymal bleed and a frank intraventricular bleed to cause hydrocephalus

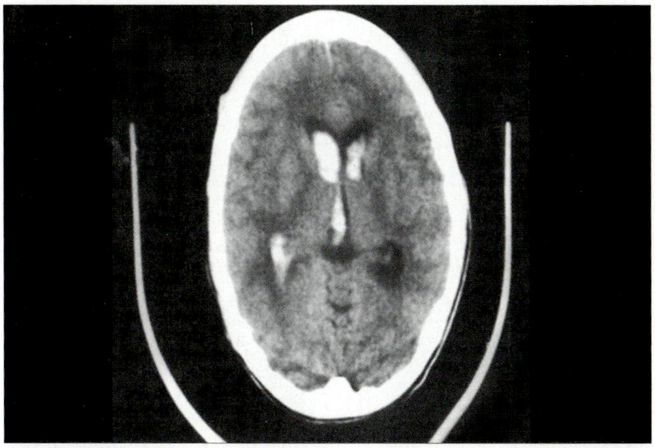

Fig. 36.2: CT shows post-traumatic intraventricular hemorrhage (acute stage), no ventriculomegaly is seen at this stage, which may occur later

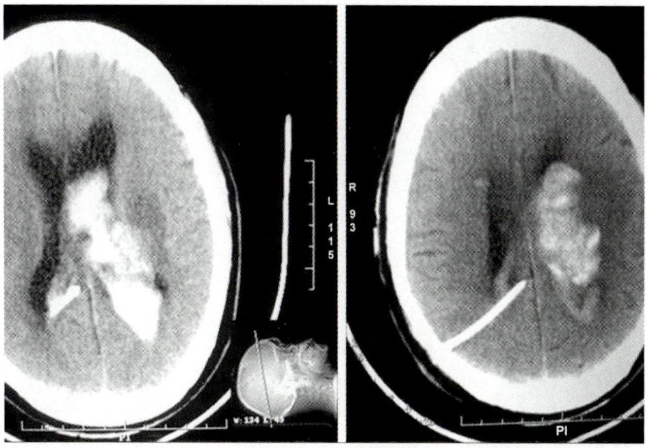

Fig. 36.3: CT showing post-traumatic intraventricular bleed and drain

from the compensatory ventricular dilatation, in infants is more difficult. The animal models have demonstrated that the ventricular distention may cause direct parenchymal injury. Similarly, secondary parenchymal injury in premature infants can occur, however, precise impact of secondary parenchymal injury is not clear.

CLINICAL SYMPTOMATOLOGY

Post-traumatic hydrocephalus (PTH) may lead to various syndromes[9,14] depending on rapidity of ventricular dilatation age of the patient and initial brain damage. The symptoms could be early[1,3,7] or late neurological deterioration can be seen.[1] The symptom could start even within few hours, as reported by Takagi et al.[6] There explanation was acute SAH, and raised ICP, aggravated by frequent seizure leading to hydrocephalus due to obstruction to CSF pathways. Also, chronic problem such as neuropsychological deficit in closed head injury is dependant on ventricle brain ratio (VBR),[15] and ventricular dilatation was related to duration of coma and speed of the vehicle at the time of injury.

Raised intracranial pressure, failure to improve and psychomotor retardation are the usual symptoms. Patients with severe head injury who are already in coma may not manifest clinical signs except for lack of improvement. In such situation fundi may reveal papilledema.[1,3,5] Some patients may present like normal pressure hydrocephalus in whom, memory loss, gait disturbances and urinary incontinence may be the predominant features.[1,9]

PTH is a rare condition in children with birth trauma.[1,9,12,16] Intraventricular hemorrhage due to birth trauma is the frequent cause of hydrocephalus in preterm infant. Rapid enlargement of head size, inability to thrive and lathergy are the common features. Many of these infants do have evidence of secondary brain damage. However, it is difficult to determine neurological outcome and long-term neurodevelopmental disability.

DIAGNOSIS

Post-traumatic ventricular dilatation is observed in 30 to 85 percent of severe head injury, however, the incidence is almost nil in minor head injuries and 5 to 10 percent in moderate head injuries.[1,3,4] The problem is the differentiation between ventricular dilatation and hydrocephalus, ventriculomegaly may be present in 39.3 percent of severe head injury patients and in 27.3 percent of these with moderate head injury. Increased ventricular size is evident in 4 weeks after injury in 57.6 percent and at 2 months after injury in 69.7 percent. No relationship is found with age, initial GCS, presence of SAH and type of lesion (focal or diffuse), it significant correlation with outcome,[18] still remains difficult to establish in several situations. With the availability of CT scan the diagnosis of ventricular dilatation is easy, however, it may not be always symptomatic. Hence, there is a need for serial CT scan to prove not only the progression of the ventricular size or ventricle brain ratio (VBR) but also the association of periventricular lucency.[1,6,8,12,16,17] Significant ventricular dilatation may require further evaluation by radionuclide cisternography.[9,17] Other investigations necessary to establish the presence of symptomatic ventricular dilatation are overnight ICP recording, lumbar or ventricular infusion test, or even

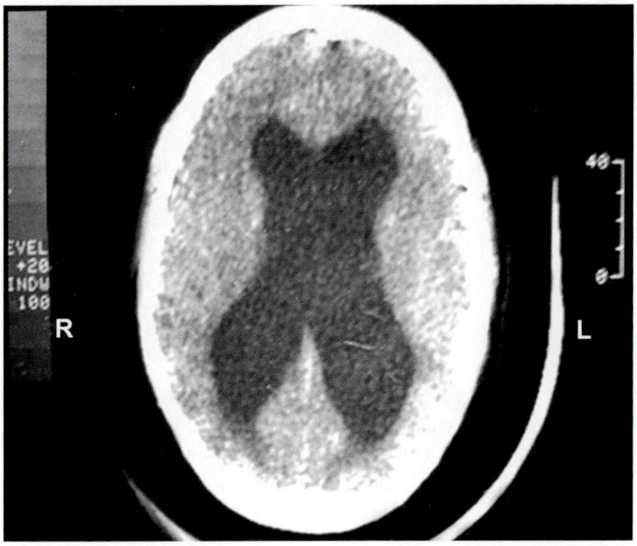

Fig. 36.4A: CT showing post-traumatic hydrocephalus (CT 3 months following trauma)

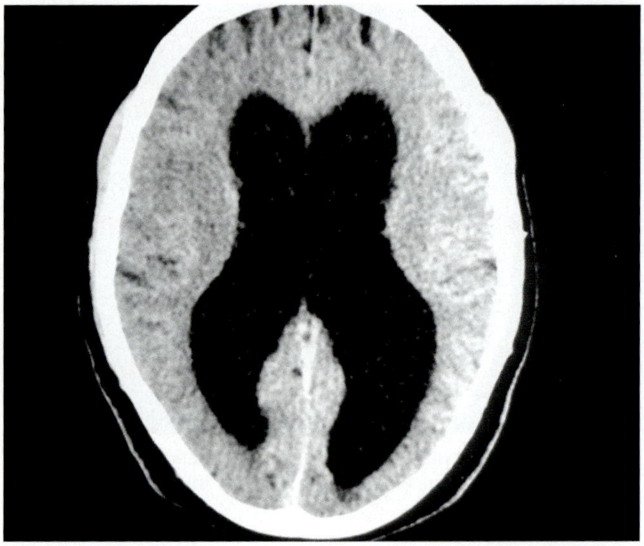

Fig. 36.4B: CT showing post-traumatic hydrocephalus

diagnostic LP drainage.[1,3,9,16,17] Some authors have suggested lumbar computerized infusion test to a certain normal or low resistance to CSF outflow and degree of cerebral compliance.[13] CSF dynamics were correlated to the change in ventricular size during the first three months post-trauma in patients with severe head injury (GCS 8 or low) to distinguish between atrophy and hydrocephalus as two possible causes of ventriculomegaly. The baseline ICP and pressure volume index and resistance for CSF absorption (RO) provided a three-dimensional profile of CSF dynamics that was correlated with ventricular size and Glasgow outcome scale (GOS) at post 3,6 and 12 months trauma. It concluded that 44 percent head injury survivor may develop post-traumatic ventriculomegaly. Post-traumatic hydrocephalus as indicated by abnormal CSF dynamics was designed in 20 percent of survivors and their outcome was significantly worse.[16]

Thus, particular care must be taken to evaluate the need for shunting (Figs 36.4A to 36.6) procedure as large number of patients with ventriculomegaly do not need shunting procedure.[6,9,13] Kishore et al[6] reported hydrocephalus in four patients out of 29 patients in whom CT scan had shown significant ventricular dilatation.

TREATMENT

Treatment of PTH is relatively simple, provided the diagnosis is accurately established. In obstructive hydrocephalus, the ventriculoperitoneal shunt is the procedure of choice.[1,3,4,14,18] In communicating hydrocephalus, repeated lumbar punctures or even lumboperitoneal shunt is a good enough treatment.[4]

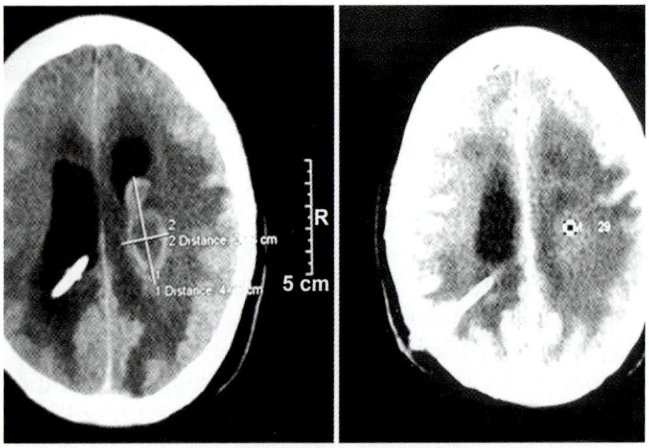

Fig. 36.5: CT showing shunt in post-traumatic hydrocephalus

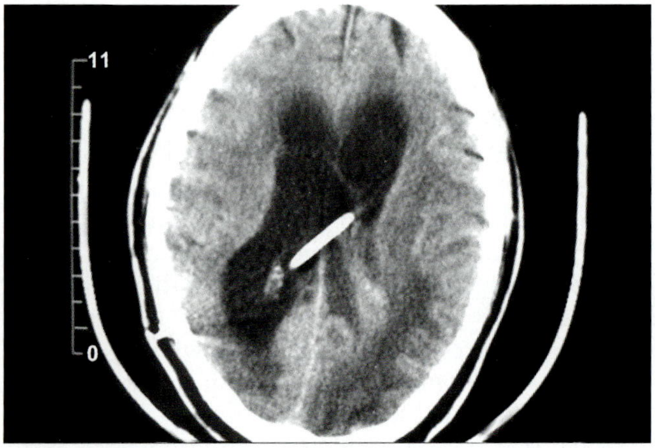

Fig. 36.6: CT showing 4th shunt block of same case as Figures 36.3 to 36.5

Table 36.2: Overall outcome in PTH

Authors and year	*No. of cases*	*Good outcome %*	*No. improvement %*
• Cardoso and Galbraith[1] 1998	17	50%	25%
• Padetti et al[5] 1983	36	45%	22%
• Xie et al[18] 1997	32	70%	30%
• Rodrigues et al[4] 2000	22	45%	36%

In acute hydrocephalus an external ventricular drainage may be adequate enough in many cases.[4,10] In some cases external ventricular drainage (ventriculostomy) need VP shunt procedure subsequently.[4,10] Fleischer et al[10] reported two cases of IVH with acute obstructive hydrocephalus, among them ventriculostomy resulted in complete recovery in one patient, while the second patient required ventriculostomy followed by VP shunt after sometime. Placement of Ommaya reservoir is an another alternative to ventriculostomy, as there is a higher incidence of ventriculitis in patients with ventriculostomy as compared to insertion of Ommaya reservoir. Both the procedure ultimately may require VP shunt. Rodrigues et al[4] in a study of 22 cases of PTH reported EVD followed by shunt in four patients, Ommaya reservoir insertion followed by VP shunt in four patients and reported LP drainage in one patient. Lumboperitoneal shunt was good enough to relieve raised ICP.

OUTCOME

Outcome of the treatment for PTH depends upon several factors. Few important factors are age of the patients, cause of hydrocephalus, degree of ventricular dilatation, associated parenchymal damage and condition of the patients. Patients in coma, neonates with IVH and patients with significant brain damage fair badly.[3,12,16] With proper diagnosis and timely performed shunting procedure, good outcome is reported in 45 to 70 percent cases[1,4,5,18] (Table 36.2). Rarely, ventriculostomy may result in good outcome in patient with acute hydrocephalus due to IVH.[10] Overall effectiveness of shunt depends upon evidence of increased ICP. In patients with no raised ICP or asymptomatic ventriculomegaly, shunting procedures are likely to fail.

CONCLUSION

Ventricular dilatation following severe head injury is the result of cerebral atrophy, however, small percentage (3–5%) do develop PTH, which need surgical procedure. The presentation can be varied and in comatose patient diagnosis is difficult. Baring acute hydrocephalus, due to IVH or posterior fossa hematoma, PTH by and large develop three to eight weeks following injury. A careful evaluation is necessary to establish PTH and to determine the need for shunting procedure. Serial CT scanning, radionuclide cisternography, ICP monitoring and therapeutic lumbar CSF drainage help in establishing the need for a shunting procedure. When shunt is performed in patients with proper indications, good results are reported in 45-70 percent cases. Patients with birth trauma, significant primary or secondary brain damage or patients with coma do badly, even if shunts are performed with proper indications.

REFERENCES

1. Cardoso ER, Galbraith S. Post-traumatic hydrocephalus: A retrospective review. Surg Neurol 1985;23:261-4.
2. Guyot LL, Micheal DD. Post-traumatic hydrocephalus. Neurol Res 2000;22:25-8.
3. Pheupathow N, Ratanalert S, Seheng S, Sripanojkul B. Post-traumatic hydrocephalus, experience in 17 cases. J Med Asso Thai 1999;82:46-53.
4. Rodrigues D, Sharma RR, Sousa J, Pawar SJ, Mahapatra AK, Lad SD. Post-traumatic hydrocephalus in severe head injury. Series of 22 cases. Pan Arab J Neurosurg 2000;4:63-7.
5. Padetti P, Pezzotta S, Spanu G. Diagnosis and treatment of post-traumatic hydrocephalus. J Neurosurg Sci 1983; 27:171-5.
6. Kishore PR, Lipper MH, Miller JD, et al. Post-traumatic hydrocephalus in patients with severe head injury. Neuroradiol 1978;16:261-5.
7. Takagi H, Tanaka Y, Moru S, Okwada T. Rapid enlargement of the ventricles after head injury. Surg Neurol 1981;16:103-5.
8. Groswasser Z, Cohen M, Reider-Groswasser I, Stern MJ. Incidence, CT findings and rehabilitation outcome of patients with communicating hydrocephalus following severe head injury. Brain Injury 1988;2:267-72.
9. Fleisher AS, Huhn SL, Meislen H. Post-traumatic acute obstructive hydrocephalus. Ann Emerg Med 1988;17: 165-7.
10. Beyerl B, Black PM. Post-traumatic hydrocephalus. Neurosurg 1984;15:257-61.

11. Grcevic N. Traumatic tear of the tela choroidea as an unrecognized cause of post-traumatic hydrocephalus. Act Neurochir'Suppl (Wien) 1983;32:79-85.
12. duPlessis AJ. Post-hemorrhagic hydrocephalus and brain injury in the preterm infants. Dilemmas in diagnosis and management. Sem in Pediatr Neurol 1998;5:161-79.
13. Czosnyka M, Copeman J, Czosnyka Z, et al. Post-traumatic hydrocephalus. Influence of craniectomy on the CSF circulation. J Neurol Neurosurg Psychit 2000;68:216-8.
14. Spanu G, Knerich R, Messina AL, et al. Post-traumatic hydrocephalus. Riv Neurol 1985;5:185-96.
15. Levin HS, Meyers CA, Grossman RG, Sarwar M. Ventricular enlargement after closed head injury. Arch Neurol 1981;38:623-9.
16. Brye S, Zlomaniec J, Gradzinski S, Kaluzynski F. Post-traumatic hydrocephalus in children in CT image. Ann Univ Manae Curie SK odowska 1993;48:163-78.
17. Gudeman SK, Kishore PR, Becker DP, et al. Radiol 1981;141:397-402.
18. Xie J, Yang C, Hu C. Ventriculoperitoneal shunts for thirty-two patients with traumatic hydrocephalus. Hunan Ta Hsuesh Hsuch Pao 1997;22:431-3.
19. Marmaron A, Foda MA, Bandoh K, et al. Post-traumatic ventriculomegaly: Hydrocephalus or atrophy: New approach for diagnosis using CSF dynamics. J Neurosurg 1996;85(6):1026-35.
20. Pickard JD, Coleman MR, Czosnyka M. Hydrocephalus ventriculomegaly and the vegetative state. Neuropsychol Rehabil 2005;15(3-4):224-36.
21. Pocca MA, Sahuquillo J, Mtario M, et al. Ventricular enlargement after moderate and severe head injury. A frequent and neglected problem. J Neurotrauma 2005;22 (11):1303-10.

37 Post-traumatic Epilepsy

Raj Kamal, AK Mahapatra

INTRODUCTION

The relationship between head injury, early post-traumatic epilepsy and late post-traumatic epilepsy represents perhaps the best studied of all causes of epilepsy. Only specific types of head injury carry a significant risk of post-traumatic epilepsy. The more severe the head injury, greater is the risk of post-traumatic epilepsy.[1,2] Post-traumatic seizures occur clinically in approximately 4 percent within the first week of head injury. However, continuous EEG monitoring had disclosed incidence as high as 22 percent.[2a] Recently it has been proved, clinically probable hippocampal sclerosis was associated in patients those who sustained moderate to severe head injury aged between 10 and 30 years.[2]

Jennett classified post-traumatic epilepsy (PTE) into two groups:[2]

1. **Early epilepsy:** Occurring within first week following head trauma.
2. **Late epilepsy:** More than one week after injury.

Seizures occurring during first 24 hours are called immediate seizures.[3]

Early Post-traumatic Epilepsy

Incidence of early seizures in patients with closed head ranges from 2 to 5 percent. The presence of risk factors will further increase the incidence of early post-traumatic epilepsy (Table 37.1).

Table 37.1: Risk factors and incidence of early PTE

Risk factors	*Incidence of early PTE (Percentage)*
1. Severe head injury GCS < 8	~35%
2. Intracranial hematoma (Higher with subdural or intracerebral hematoma)	20–30%
3. Post-traumatic amnesia > 24 hours	11–14%
4. Depressed fractures	10–11%
5. Children < 5 years	9.8%

Jennett[2] and others have used post-traumatic amnesia as an indicator of severity of injury (Table 37.2). For patients with post-traumatic amnesia of more than 24 hours, a 10 percent overall incidence of early epilepsy was found in patients under 16 years of age. It was 12 percent for older patients. Patients with hematomas, focal neurological deficit, and depressed skull fracture were prone to early epilepsy. Of these factors, intracranial hematoma is the most significant. Intradural hematoma carries more risk than extradural hematoma does.[2] Early seizures are focal in 56 percent of patients with depressed fracture and in 57 percent of patients with non-depressed fractures.[2]

A common post-traumatic location of epileptogenesis is the medial temporal lobe despite evidence of associated diffuse or remote cerebral injury. The favorable outcome is obtained following surgery in this group attest to the commonality with other risk factors in genesis of epilepsy in this location.[20]

Late Post-traumatic Epilepsy

Incidence of late post-traumatic epilepsy in non-missile head injury ranges from 1.85 to 9 percent (Table 37.3). Late post-traumatic epilepsy occurred in 5 percent of all patients admitted to hospital after non-missile head injury.

Table 37.2: Influence of PTA on incidence of early epilepsy (Jennett[2])

	PTA < 24 hours	*PTA 24 hours*	*Probability*
< 16 years	5%	10%	NS
> 16 years	2%	12%	0.001
Depressed			
Fracture	9%	14%	NS
Hematoma	26%	30%	NS
Focal signs	9%	14%	NS
No depressed			
Fracture or hematoma	2%	9%	0.001

Table 37.3: Incidence of late epilepsy

Series	*Total cases*	*Epilepsy %*
Jennett (1975)		5
Annegers et al (1980)	2747	1.85
De Santis et al (1983)	472	4.44

Late epilepsy are significantly more common in patients who have suffered early seizures. In Jennett's series, a patient's risk of developing late seizures is 25 percent, if the patient had an early seizure. Seizures occurring immediately do not necessarily imply a risk of recurrence. However, seizures developing more than 1 hour after injury convey an increased rate of late seizures. Amongst the early post-traumatic seizures 58 percent occur within 24 hours of trauma. Risk factors for developing non-excellent outcome included the patients who undergo surgical intervention and presence of late provoked seizures during the acute phase of TBI.[22]

Other risk factors for late seizures include focal lesions (hematoma, contusion) focal neurological signs, depressed skull fracture with dural laceration, and prolonged coma or amnesia.[1,2,5,6] With penetrating missile injuries the risk of seizures also increases with the volume of brain tissue destroyed, with lesions located centroparietally, and if metal fragments are retained.[7,8] Important risk factors for late epilepsy are given in Table 37.4.

Fifty percent of patient, having late post-traumatic epilepsy experience their first seizure within 1 year of head injury and 70 to 80 percent within 2 years. Patients with the onset of seizures more than 4 years after injury were more likely to have persistent epilepsy.

Table 37.4: Risk factors for late epilepsy (Pagni, 1990)

	Incidence of late PTE (%)
1. Penetrating missile head injury	53
2. Intracerebral hematoma	39
3. Focal brain damage on early CT	32
4. Early seizures	25
5. Depressed fracture-torn dura	25
6. Extradural or subdural hemorrhage	20
7. Focal signs	20
8. Depressed skull fracture	15
9. Loss consciousness of 24 hours	5
10. Linear fracture	5
11. Mild concussion	

The most common type of late PTE was generalized seizures (focal attacks becoming generalized secondarily) found in 60 to 70 percent of cases followed by partial seizures in 30 to 40 percent of cases.

Hereditary Factors Associated with Early and Late Epilepsy

Heredity plays little influence on risk of post-traumatic seizures. No genetic influence was found by Salazar[8] in a long-term following study of missile injuries incurred in Vietnam. In Jennett's series[2] of non-missile injuries hereditary factors did not play any role in early PTE. However, in patients younger than 16 years, a family history played significant role who had late seizure. In adult patient, family history did not play any role in occurrence of late PTE.

In a study by Hanser[9] recurrence of seizure was higher in patients with a family history of seizures or a history of prior neurologic insult. Suri et al[9a] had shown familial incidence of post-traumatic epilepsy.

PATHOPHYSIOLOGY

The degree of parenchymal brain damage is related to risk of post-traumatic seizures. Contusional hemorrhage results in deposition of hemoglobin and iron in the brain tissue. Several experimental studies[10-12] have shown hemoglobin and iron to be epileptogenic and this has been attributed to free radical formation and lipid peroxidation thus destroying neuronal membranes.[13,13a]

Ferric ions decrease the release of GABA (gamma-aminobutyric acid) and increase levels of excitatory neurotransmitters such as glutamate and aspartate.[10] Decreased release of GABA and increased release of excitatory neurotransmitters result in paroxysmal depolarization shift (PDS) and neuronal synchronization which is necessary for seizure genesis and spread.[14]

Recently, many authors have proved the possibility of non-convulsive seizures following head injury.[14a,14b] The abnormal electrical discharge can be recorded by continuous EEG recording.[14a] Towne et al[14b] in 2000 had reported non-convulsive status epilepticus in head injury patients.

Prophylaxis of Early and Late Post-traumatic Epilepsy

Drug prophylaxis: Two good randomized double blind placebo controlled study of phenytoin for the prevention of post-traumatic epilepsy have been done by Young et al[15] (1983) and Tempkin et al.[14c,16]

Young et al[15] randomized 204 patients into two groups. One group received phenytoin within 24 hours of admission and plasma concentration of at least 10 μg/ml was achieved. No significant reduction in the early or late post-traumatic seizures was found between the treated and placebo group.

Tempkin et al[3,16] randomized 404 patients with severe head trauma. Patients were randomly assigned to receive either phenytoin or placebo. Treatment was given for the first year and phenytoin serum levels maintained in the optimum therapeutic range in most patients. Patients were followed for 2 years. The results showed that phenytoin was effective in preventing seizures for the first week after cerebral injury (3.6% treated versus 14.2% control) but was no better than placebo in exerting a protective effect during the remainder of the study period. It was, therefore, concluded that phenytoin should be given to patients at risk of post-traumatic seizures during the first week after trauma and then discontinued unless further seizures occur.

Compilation of the available data supports prophylactic administration of phenytoin for prevention of early seizures. A meta-analysis done by Tempkin[16] of the controlled studies found that the phenytoin can prevent early seizures but has no beneficial role in preventing late post-traumatic epilepsy. Other antiepileptic drugs such as sodium valproate, phenobarbital have not been adequately evaluated for their use as prophylactic anticonvulsant in head injury patients.

However, the EEG study with spectral coherent analysis allows to predict post-traumatic epilepsy and to use differential approach in prescribing appropriate anticonvulsant therapy to the patients after TBI.[21]

Surgical Prophylaxis

The incidence of post-traumatic seizures has not decreased significantly even with gradual improvement in medical and surgical management of head injury patients.[7]

Depressed fracture and penetrating injuries of head are important risk factors in post-traumatic seizures. No study done till now, shows elevation of depressed fracture decreases the incidence of PTE.

In the study of penetrating injuries by Salazar et al[8] which was done during Vietnam war, the presence of retained intracerebral bone fragments did not correlate with post-traumatic seizures, whereas retained metal fragments did show a relationship to seizure occurrence.

Treatment of Post-traumatic Seizures

Acute post-traumatic seizures should be treated aggressively with benzodiazepine and a loading dose of phenytoin. Inadequate control of early post-traumatic seizure results in severe hypoxic and secondary metabolic damage of the already injured brain. Uncontrolled seizures should be treated as status epilepticus. Status epilepticus is defined as repeated seizures without recovery of consciousness between attack. Post-traumatic status epilepticus if controlled within 1 to 5 hours is unlikely to cause any significant morbidity, whereas status epilepticus of more than 10 hours has severe morbidity and mortality.[17]

Hypoxia may be the cause and result of seizures. Hypoxia may result from airway obstruction or improper ventilation. Seizures also lead to inadequate respiration and ventilation. As metabolic demand of cerebral tissue during seizures is increased, the effects of hypoxia on brain is compounded. Release of excitatory neurotransmitters and decreased level of inhibitory neurotransmitters cause significant neuronal damage.[18]

Hence, during seizures airway patency and ventilation are of prime importance. Patients having multiple fits (status epilepticus) with deteriorating level of consciousness, endotracheal intubation and ventilation may be required. Non-convulsive status epilepticus may be missed in comatose patients.[14b] Hyponatremia or hypocalcemia in such patients should be ruled out.

Post-traumatic seizure should be treated initially with benzodiazepines followed immediately by a loading dose of maintenance anticonvulsant.

For benzodiazepine commonly used are diazepam, lorazepam.

Dose of diazepam: 0.25 mg/kg body given as IV bolus @ 2-5 mg/min. This can be repeated after 10 minutes. IV infusion dose 8 mg/hour.

Lorazepam: Given as IV bolus 0.1 mg/kg adult usually 4 mg can be repeated after 10 minutes.

Status epilepticus can be divided into following stages:

1. Premonitory stages
2. Early stage
3. Established stage
4. Refractory stage.

Premonitory stage is prodromal period during which there is gradual increase in frequency of seizures. Acute administration of AEDs may stop the progression of status. The initial stage of status

Table 37.5: Protocol for the treatment of convulsive status epilepticus in adults

Premonitory stage	Diazepam 10 mg rectally repeated once after 15 min.
Early status epilepticus	Lorazepam 4 mg or alternatively diazepam 10 mg IV repeated after 10 min.
Established status	Phenytoin 15–18 mg/kg IV @ 50 mg/min with Lorazepam if not already given and/or
	Phenobarbital 10 mg/kg IV @ 100 mg/min.
Refractory status	GA with concomitant EEG monitoring continued for 12–24 hours after last clinical seizure/ electrographic seizures.

epilepticus is called early stage. Once the seizures have continued for 30 min, the stage of established status epilepticus, is entered. Walker and Shorvon[19] suggest the following alternatives at the stage:

1. Diazepam or lorazepam with intravenous phenytoin.
2. Phenobarbital.

If the seizures still continue, then the stage of refractory status epilepticus is reached.

A protocol suggested by Walker and Shorvon[19] for the treatment of convulsive status epilepticus in adults is given in Table 37.5.

CONCLUSION

Post-traumatic epilepsy may occur within first week following head trauma (early epilepsy) or may occur more than one week after injury (late epilepsy). Incidence of early PTE ranges from 2 to 5 percent and that of late PTE ranges from 2 to 9 percent of all patients admitted to hospital after non-missile head injury. Risk factors for early PTE are severe head injury, intracranial hematoma, PTA > 24 hours, and depressed fractures. Risk factors for late PTE are more common in patients who have suffered early seizures. Hereditary factor probably dose not play any role in PTE. Iron and Hb are epileptogenic as they decrease the release of inhibitory neurotransmitters such as GABA. Phenytoin is most frequently used anticonvulsant which can prevent early seizures but has no beneficial role in preventing late PTE. Autopost-traumatic seizures should be treated with loading dose of phenytoin and benzodiazepines.

Uncontrolled seizures should be treated as status epilepticus. Prevention of early PTE in patients with internal hematoma would prevent rise in ICP and brighten the chance of survival.

REFERENCES

1. Annegers JF, Grabow JD, et al. Seizures after head trauma: A population study. Neurol 1980;30:683-9.
2. Jennett B. Epilepsy after non-missile head injuries. 2nd edn. Chicago: Heinemann-Year Book, 1975. 2a. Olson DA. Head Injury, Medicine. 21st October 2003;1-32.
3. Tempkin NR, Dikmen SS, et al. A randomized, double-blind study of phenytoin for the prevention of post-traumatic seizures. N Engle J Med 1990;323:498-502.
4. Hahn YS, Fuch S, et al. Factors influencing post-traumatic seizures in children. Neurosurg 1988;22:864-7.
5. Pagni CA. Post-traumatic epilepsy incidence and prophylaxis. Acta Neurosurg Suppl 1990;50:38-47.
6. Weiss GH, Salazar AM, et al. Predicting post-traumatic epilepsy in penetrating head injury. Arch Neurol 1986;43:771-3.
7. Caveners WF, Meirowsky AM, et al. The nature of post-traumatic epilepsy. J Neurosurg 1979;50:545-53.
8. Salazar AM, Jabbari B, et al. Epilepsy after penetrating head injury. Clinical correlates: A report of the Vietnam Head Injury Study. Neurol 1985;35:1406-14.
9. Hauser WA, Anderson VE, et al. Seizure recurrence after a first unprovoked seizure. N Engl J Med 1985;307:522-8.

9a. Suri A, Mehta TS, Mahapatra AK, Singh VP, Jain S. Factor affecting post-traumatic epilepsy. Neurosurg 1998;90:20-8.

10. Mori A, Hiramatsu M, et al. Biochemical pathogenesis of post-traumatic epilepsy. Pav J Bid Sci 1982;25:54-62.
11. Rosen AD, Frumin NV. Focal epileptogenesis after intracortical hemoglobin injection. Exp Neurol 1979;66: 277-84.
12. William LJ, Hurd RW, et al. Epileptiform activity initiated by pial inotophoresis of ferrons and ferric chloride on rat cerebral cortex. Brain Res 1978;152:406-10.
13. Willmore LJ, Hiramatsu M, et al. Formation of superoxide radicals after Fe Cl_3 Injection into rat isocortex. Brain Res 1983;277:393-6.

13a. Willmore LJ, Triggs WJ, Gray JD. The role of iron-induced hippocampal peroxidation. In acute epileptogenesis. Brain Res 1986;382:422-6.

14. Matsumoto H, et al. Cortical cellular phenomenon in experimental epilepsy. Exp Neurol 1964;9:305-26.

14a. Vespa PM, Nuwer MR, New V, et al. Increased incidence and impact of non-convulsive and convulsive seizures after traumatic brain injury as detected by continuous electrocence phalographic monitoring. J Neurosurg 1999;91:50-60.

14b. Towne AR, Waterhouse EJ, Boggs JG, et al. Prevalence of non-convulsive states epilepticus in comatose patients. Neurol 2000;25:340-5.

14c. Temkin NR, Dikmen SS, Adevsin GD, et al. Valproate therapy for prevention of post-traumatic seizure: A randamized tricel. J Neurosurg 1999;91:593-600.

15. Young B, Rapp RP, et al. Failure of prophylactic administered phenytoin to prevent late post-traumatic seizures. J Neurosurg 1983;58:236-41.

16. Tempkin NR, Dikman SS, Winn HR. Post-traumatic seizures. Neurosurg Clin N Am 1991;2:425-35.
17. Delgado-Escueta AV, Wasterlain C, et al. Management of status-epilepticus. N Engl J Med 1982;306:1337-40.
18. Wasterlain CG, Fujikawa DG, et al. Epilepsia, 1993;34(suppl 1):537-53,1993.
19. Walker MC, Shorvon SD. Treatment of status epilepticus and serial seizures. In: The Treatment of Epilepsy. Shorvon SD, Dreifuss F, Fish D, Thomas D (Eds) Blackwell Science, 1996.
20. Hartzfeld P, Elsevich K, Pace M et al. Characteristics and surgical outcomes of medial temporal post-traumatic epilepsy. J Neurosurg 2008;22(2):224-30.
21. Kurbanova SA, Oleinikova OM, Avakian GN. The neurophysiological analysis of symptomatic post-traumatic epilepsy. Zh Neurol Psikhiatr IM SS Korsakova 2007;107(6):50-3.
22. Wang HC, Chang WN, Chang HW, et al. Factors predictive of outcome in post-traumatic seizures. J Trauma 2008;64(4):883-8.

38 Post-traumatic Cerebrospinal Fluid Fistula—CSF Rhinorrhea

Raj Kamal, Raj Kumar

INTRODUCTION

Leakage of cerebrospinal fluid from the nose is called CSF rhinorrhea and leakage of cerebrospinal fluid from the ear is called CSF otorrhea. Post-traumatic leakage is the evidence that a basal fracture communicates with the subarachnoid space. When rhinorrhea, otorrhea or recurrent meningitis follow a head injury, the causative breach in the dura mater and/or skull base may be difficult to identify with enough precision to enable surgical repair. CSF can escape from one nostril, for example, as a result of a dural defect on the same side, anteriorly or posteriorly, on the opposite side or even, via the eustachian tube, as the result of a fracture of the petrous bone. The range and number of imaging techniques have been proposed. Thin section CT through the affected region after intrathecal injection of water soluble contrast medium is the technique worth attempting.[1]

INCIDENCE AND ETIOLOGY

According to Lewin,[2] post-traumatic CSF rhinorrhea occurs in 2 percent of unselected closed head injuries. The risk of CSF leak is higher in penetrating head injuries. Meirowsky[3] reported 9 percent patients with penetrating head injuries had CSF leak. Post-traumatic CSF leaks are not related to age and sex.

Meningitis, the most dreaded complication of CSF leak occurs in about 21 percent of post-traumatic leaks, as reported by Wehrle.[4]

In about 2/3rd of patients with CSF leak, it started within 48 hours of trauma, while in most of the remainder delayed leaks occurred up to 3 months after head injury.[2] It can appear up to several years after injury.

Ommaya[5] and McCoy[6] classified CSF leaks into traumatic and non-traumatic origins (Flow chart 38.1). Traumatic is further classified into acute and delayed types. Non-traumatic CSF leaks are classified into high pressure and low pressure leaks depending on the etiology (Flow chart 38.1).

Fifty percent of post-traumatic CSF leaks will cease within one week and almost all stop by 6 months.[5] This occurs due to adhesions or herniation of brain into bony defects and regenerative qualities of meninges. As post-traumatic basal dural tear communicates with paranasal air sinuses, risk of meningitis is considerable even in absence of demonstrable CSF leak.

Most cases of traumatic CSF rhinorrhea are secondary to the fractures involving anterior cranial fossa. The roof of ethmoid, the cribriform plate are the most frequent sites of CSF rhinorrhea because of thin bone and tight adherence of dura to bone in this area.[10]

Flow chart 38.1: Classification of CSF leaks (from Ommaya AK: Clin Neurosurg 1976;23:363)

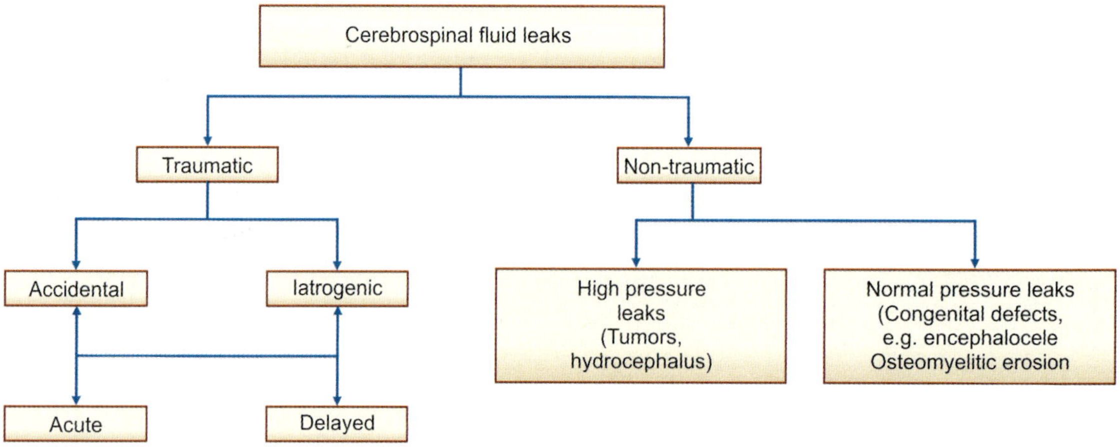

Fracture of frontal sinus are also common sites dural tear leading to CSF rhinorrhea. Rarely CSF rhinorrhea is reported due to aqueductal stenosis and pulsion diverticulum of lateral ventricle into frontal air sinus.[33]

The appearance of CSF may be apparent immediately after trauma or days to weeks later. Delayed appearance of CSF leak may be due to delayed elevation of intracranial pressure following trauma, lysis of a clot in an area of bone and dural dehiscence, resolution of soft tissue edema, maturation and contraction of wound edges, or loss of vascularity and necrosis of soft tissue and bone around the wound.[11-13] Also, during or following dural healing, dura may herniate through a fracture line. The constant physiologic changes in CSF pressure may result in progressive dural herniation with its eventual dehiscence and CSF leakage.[10]

CSF otorrhea is defined as leakage of CSF through external auditory canal which requires a pathologic communication between subarachnoid space and the pneumatized areas of the temporal bone. In addition, there must be damage to the tympanic membrane or a defect in the external auditory canal wall. CSF otorrhea results from fracture of middle cranial fossa with damage to tympanic membrane.

Fracture can be longitudinal or transverse to the long axis of petrous bone. Hicks and Wright[7] studied 40 temporal bone fractures and noted that CSF leak occurred in 29 percent of the longitudinal fractures and 44 percent of the transverse. Ghorayeb and Rafie[8] reported a 21 percent incidence of CSF otorrhea in 123 cases of temporal bone fractures.

If the tympanic membrane heals rapidly or if it is not damaged then CSF leaks through eustachian tube resulting in CSF rhinorrhea. Hence, fracture of middle cranial fossa can result in both CSF otorrhea and rhinorrhea. CSF otorrhea ceases spontaneously in almost all cases. Raaf[9] reported persistent CSF otorrhea in only one case in a series of 79 patients with otorrhea.

CLINICAL FEATURES

Traumatic CSF rhinorrhea can be present in two ways:

1. Watery fluid discharge from nose
2. Meningitis.

In majority of cases they present as watery fluid draining from the nose. CSF leak can be from either nostril but may be ipsilateral to the defect site. Post-traumatic rhinorrhea develops within 48 hours in approximately 55 percent of all patients who ultimately develop CSF rhinorrhea as a result of trauma. This frequency increases to 70 percent by the end of the first week as edema, which may be temporarily preventing CSF leakage, resolves.[11]

Sixty to eighty percent of patients with CSF rhinorrhea will have anosmia and hyposmia due to olfactory nerve damage resulting from fracture of cribriform plate. Meningitis can be presenting symptom in about 20 percent of patients with CSF rhinorrhea.[11] The chances of developing meningitis within first 3 weeks in patients with CSF rhinorrhea following head injury has been reported to be 3 to 11 percent.[11] Wehrle reported meningitis in 21 percent of patients having CSF rhinorrhea following head injury.[4] Headache due to presence of intracranial air has been reported in 1/5th of patients with traumatic CSF leakage.[13,14] Postoperative CSF rhinorrhea results from transsphenoidal removal of pituitary tumors and anterior skull base surgeries. Incidence of CSF rhinorrhea following transsphenoidal surgery is approximately 3 to 6 percent.

Non-traumatic CSF rhinorrhea have following features.

Age >30 years, female preponderance (2:1), insidious at onset, present for longer duration (in years) and profuse nasal drainage.

Aerocele, anosmia and meningitis are rare. Laun reported that CSF otorrhea occurred immediately in 94 percent of those who ultimately developed CSF otorrhea following head trauma.[15] CSF rhinorrhea or a sensation of postnasal discharge may occur if the tympanic membrane is intact as the CSF finds its way into nasopharynx through eustachian tube.

DIAGNOSTIC STUDIES

The diagnosis of CSF fistula depends on:

1. Demonstration that the leaking fluid is CSF.
2. Localizing the site of leakage.

Demonstration that the leaking fluid is CSF:

a. Profuse persistent clear nasal discharge.
b. 'Halo sign' or 'Target sign' in which a clear fluid area surrounds a blood stain when CSF mixed with blood is absorbed on a filter paper. This may differentiate between CSF mixed with blood or other nasal secretions and serosanguinous fluids.
c. *'Reservoir sign':* When patient is about to voluntarily produce CSF it will be correct positioning of the head. This is because ethmoid and sphenoid sinus acts as CSF reservoir.
d. *Glucose content:* If glucose content of discharging fluid is >30 mg/ml then probably it is CSF. Nasal secretions have glucose content <10 mg/ml.
e. Immunoelectrophoretic identification of β_1 and β_2 transferrin. The presence of β_2 fraction, which is characteristic of CSF, is diagnostic of CSF fluid.[16,17]

f. Other techniques to demonstrate CSF leakage: Injection of colored dyes and radioactive tracer into subarachnoid space be retrieved extra-cranially for accurate demonstration of CSF leak. It has little localization value. Injection of colored dyes has been abandoned because of morbidity it produces. Radioactive tracers are preferred methods because demonstration of even small amount of radioactive tracer is easier. Isotope cisternography is performed using DTPA (diethylenetriamine pentaacetic acid). Pledgets placed in anterior roof of nose, middle meatus, posterior roof will be contaminated accordingly. This method is useful in patients with small and intermittent CSF leak.

Intrathecal fluorescein injection can decipher the site of CSF leak from skull base but a complication of delayed absence seizure is reported in case report.[34]

Localizing the site of leakage: Following investigations may be done to localize the leak and sites of leak:

1. Plain X-ray
2. CT scan
3. MRI

Plain X-ray skull with patient in supine position, the presence of air fluid level in the frontal, ethmoidal and sphenoid sinuses indicate that a fracture exists in anterior cranial fossa.

The CT scan head is the preferred method for investigating CSF rhinorrhea. Thin section (1 to 1.5 mm) through anterior and middle cranial fossa in both axial and coronal planes, fracture of cribriform plate (Fig. 38.1), sella turcica, of ethmoid of frontal sinuses, particularly when associated with an air fluid level in the adjacent sinus, are presumptive evidences of a leak and help to guide subsequent investigation.[18]

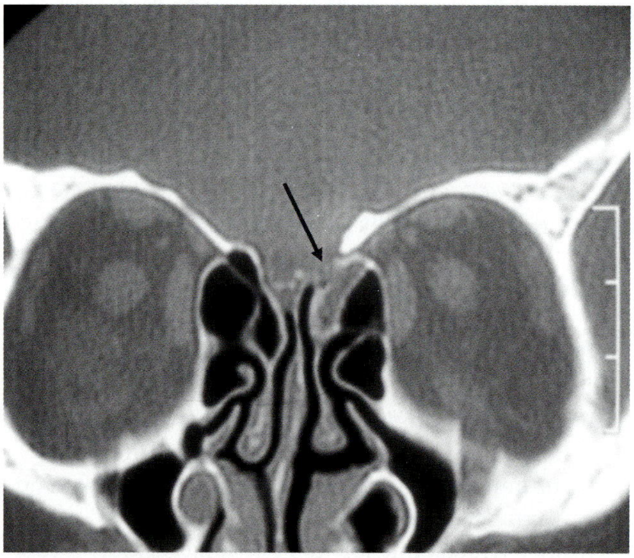

Fig. 38.1: CSF rhinorrhea with defect at anterior skull base

Metrizamide Computed Tomography Cisternography (MCTC)

Metrizamide, which is water soluble, nonionic contrast medium, is injected by lumbar puncture and positioned in the cranial subarachnoid space by tilting the patient head down (60°) for about a minute. Contiguous 1.5 mm sections in both axial and coronal sections are taken to demonstrate bony defect and site of leak. In majority of patients with acute leak contrast can be seen passing through the bony defect[10] in contrast cisternography followed by CT may provide useful data on CSF flow patterns and dynamics. However, a study revealed that a noncontrast high resolution CT could show the defect in 70 percent cases of patients with CSF leak. Hence, CT cisternography and radionuclide cisternography may be reserved for patients in whom initial high resolution CT does not identify a bone defect in patients with multiple fractures or postoperative defects.[32]

MRI has also been used to investigate CSF rhinorrhea. Gammal and Brooks[19] have reported the use of MR cisternography in cases with CSF rhinorrhea for localizing the site of CSF leak. MRI has not proved equal to CT for bony detail. It can image soft tissue lesions that are 2 to 3 mm in diameter. However, complex CSF leaks may remain under diagnosed on conventional MRI or CT imaging. A use of intrathecal Gadopentetate dimeglumine (Gd-DTPA) for MR cisternography and ventriculography has shown no side effects and is potentially useful method to diagnose selected pediatric cases.[31]

However, only a few cases have been reported and it remains to be proven whether these modalities can replace other investigations.

MANAGEMENT

The majority of traumatic CSF fistula heal without surgical intervention. Hence, the initial management of CSF leaks should be aimed at supporting the factors which stops CSF leak and prevents meningitis. In non-traumatic CSF rhinorrhea, conservative treatment has no role to play. Following conservative measures can be taken to promote cessation of CSF leak;

1. **Position:** Head should be elevated in the range of 30 to 45 degrees from horizontal. This decreases ICP by improving venous outflow.

2. **Continuous lumbar drainage:** Continuous lumbar drainage reduces the ICP, thus reducing the CSF leak. This can be tried for 3 to 5 days, draining about 150 ml of CSF daily. A 19 G catheter is threaded rostrally (~10 cm) percutaneously through 17 G Tuohy needle. The proximal end of catheter is connected to closed sterile drainage system. Complications of lumbar drainage are infection (meningitis), pneumocephalus, headache and vomiting. Headache, vomiting and pneumocephalus results from over drainage.
3. **Drugs:** Drugs which reduces the production of cerebrospinal fluid such as acetazolamide (Diamox) may be helpful in reducing CSF leak.
4. **Antibiotics:** Prophylactic antibiotics have not been shown to be effective in the prevention of meningitis and are no longer given for closed post-traumatic leaks.[20-23] They are given only postoperatively.

Operative Treatment

Indications for surgery in traumatic CSF leak:

1. Persistent and profuse CSF leak by the end of one week.
2. CSF leaks resulting from penetrating missile injuries, e.g. bullet injury.
3. Recurrent meningitis. Even an attack of meningitis with CSF leak is an indication for operating such patients.
4. The presence of an intracranial aerocele.

Operative approaches can be divided into: Intracranial and Extracranial approach.

Intracranial approach

- Extradural
- Intradural

Intracranial

The first successful repair of CSF rhinorrhea was done by Dandy in 1926.[24] Dandy described the intracranial approach in detail. For anterior fossa, two approaches have been described: the intracranial intradural and the intracranial extradural.

The intracranial intradural approach is recommended by many authors as preferred method.[25,26] The intracranial extradural approach allows wide exploration with visualization of both sphenoid wings, both cribriform fossa, and both orbital roofs. The most important factor is proper identification and repair of dural defect. The advantage of intracranial extradural approach is that, there is very little brain retraction and damage because of intervening dura. The disadvantages include inevitable dural tears and areas of cerebral tissue herniation into bony defects cannot be easily visualized.[25] Damage to olfactory nerves is inevitable in both intracranial intradural and intracranial extradural approaches.

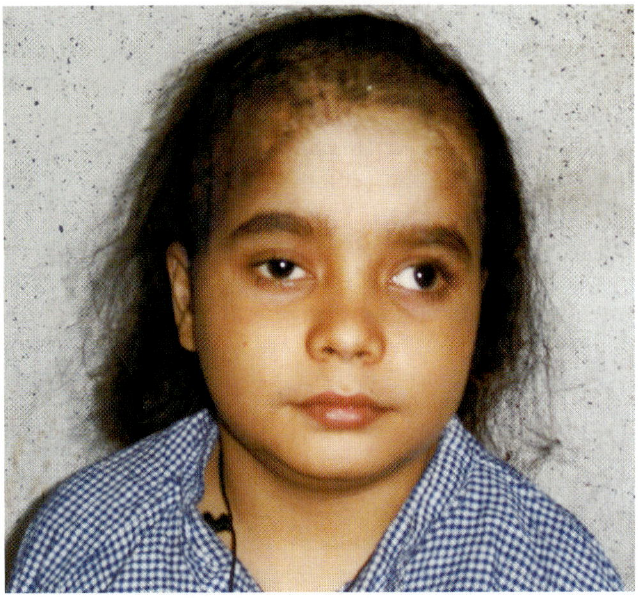

Fig. 38.2: Clinical print of child operated for post-traumatic CSF rhinorrhea

Closure of dural defect can be done by: (i) Autografts of fascia, fat and muscles, (ii) Tissue adhesives.

Fascia can be taken from temporalis muscle, pericranium or fascia lata (Fig. 38.2). Tissue adhesives such as cyanoacrylates have been used to achieve water tight closure. Disadvantages include porosity, biodegradability and meningitis.[28,29]

Recent introduction of human fibrin tissue glues is gaining popularity to achieve water tight closure of defect.[30] Large bone defects can be closed by using methyl methacrylate.

Extracranial

The extracranial approaches which are done in collaboration with ENT surgeons, has less morbidity as compared to craniotomy. The common extracranial approaches available are:

i. Transnasal transsphenoidal for sellar and parasellar leaks.
ii. Transethmoidal transsphenoidal approach.
iii. Extranasal approach through frontal and ethmoidal sinuses.

McCormack et al reported that extracranial approaches have success rate equal or superior to intracranial approach with comparatively low morbidity. However, Lewin[2] and Ommaya[26] did not find any difference in success rate or morbidity between intracranial and extracranial approaches. Ommaya recommends that extracranial techniques should be reserved for sellar and parasellar leaks in carefully selected patients. He argued that repair of meninges is more important than closing bone defect which is rarely possible with extracranial approaches except for the lower part of sella turcica as exposed through transsphenoidal route. Hence, leaks through sella turcica are best approached via the transsphenoidal route.

CSF Otorrhea

Leaks from posterior fossa dura into the mastoid are approached through mastoidectomy. The mastoid approach also allows for obliteration of mastoid cavity and, if necessary, middle ear cleft and eustachian tube orifice. A small extradural craniotomy via the temporal squama, in combination with a mastoidectomy provides the advantages of limited craniotomy and to those of a mastoidectomy.[27] Herniated brain tissue should be gently excised by means of bipolar coagulation. The dural defect is packed with fat and fascia. A pedicled temporalis muscle flap can be used for further support.

CONCLUSION

Post-traumatic CSF rhinorrhea occurs in about 2 percent of closed head injuries admitted to hospital and in 9 patients with penetrating head injuries. In majority of patients the CSF leak occurs soon after the injury or within 48 hours of trauma. In most cases CSF leak stops spontaneously within one week. The roof of ethmoid, the cribriform plate are the most frequent sites of CSF rhinorrhea. CSF otorrhea results from transverse and longitudinal fractures of petrous bone. The risk of meningitis is 3 to 11 percent in patients who have post-traumatic CSF rhinorrhea. Isotope cisternography can be done to demonstrate CSF leak. Metrizamide cisternography and MRI can localize the site of CSF leak in most cases. Most cases of CSF rhinorrhea leak stop spontaneously in one to two weeks. Indications for surgery are profuse and persistent rhinorrhea, meningitis, and CSF leak following penetrating injuries. Repair of CSF fistula can be done through an intracranial, extracranial or combined approach. Recently, endoscopic repair of CSF rhinorrhea has been reported with good result. In 10 percent patients there is risk of recurrence of CSF rhinorrhea.

REFERENCES

1. Lane B, Moseley IF, Stevens JM. The skull and brain. Methods of examination: Diagnostic approach. In Grainger RG, Allison DJ (Eds). Grainger and Allison's Diagnostic Radiology. A Textbook of Medical Imaging. 3rd edn. Churchill Livingstone 1997;2039-65.
2. Lewin W. Cerebrospinal fluid rhinorrhea in non-missile head injuries. Clin Neurosurg 1996;12:237-52.
3. Meirowsky AM, Caveness WF, et al. Cerebrospinal fluid fistulas complicating missile wounds of the brain. J Neurosurg 1981;54:44.
4. Wehrle PF, Mathies AW Jr, Leedom JM. Management of bacterial meningitis. Clin Neurosurg 1967;14:72-85.
5. Ommaya AK. Cerebrospinal fluid rhinorrhea. Neurol 1964;14:106.
6. Mc Coy G. Cerebrospinal fluid rhinorrhoea. Laryngoscope 1963;73:1125.
7. Hicks GW, Wright WJ Jr, Wright WJ III. Cerebrospinal fluid otorrhea. Laryngoscope 1980;80(Suppl 25):1-25.
8. Ghorayeb BY, Rafie JJ. Fracture of the temporal bone. Evaluation of 123 case J Radio (Fr) 1989;70(12):703-10.
9. Raaf J. Post-traumatic cerebrospinal fluid leaks. Arch Surg 1967;95:648.
10. Calcaterra TC. Diagnosis and management of ethmoid cerebrospinal rhinorrhea. Otolaryngol Clin North Amie 1985;18:99.
11. Loew F, et al. Traumatic, spontaneous and postoperative CSF rhinorrhea. Adv Tech Stand Neurosurg 1984;11:169.
12. Myers DL, Sataloff RT. Spinal fluid leakage after skull base surgical procedures. Otolary Clin North Am 1984;17:601.
13. Park JI, Strelzow VV, Friedman WH. Current management of cerebrospinal fluid rhinorrhea. Laryngoscope 1983;93:1294-1300.
14. Ommaya AK. Spinal fluid fistula. Clin Neurosurg 1976; 23:363.
15. Laun A. Traumatic cerebrospinal fluid fistulas in the anterior and middle cranial fossa. Acta Neurochir 1982; 60:215.
16. Ryall RG, Peacock MK, Simpson DAD. Usefulness of beta 2-transferrin assay in detection of cerebrospinal fluid leaks following head injury. J Neurosurg 1993;77(5):737-9.
17. Oberascher G. A modern concept of cerebrospinal fluid diagnosis in oto- and rhinorrhea. Rhinol 1988; 26(2):89-103.
18. Douglas AG. Intracranial trauma. In Puturan CE, Ravin CL (Eds). Textbook of diagnostic imaging. 2nd edn, WB Saunders Company, 1994.
19. EL Gammal T, Brooks BS. MR cisternography initial experience in 41 cases. AJNR 1994;15:1647-54.
20. Klatersky J, Sadeghi M, et al. Antimicrobial prophylaxis in patients with rhinorrhea or otorrhea: A double blind study. Surg Neurol 1976;6:111.
21. Eden K. Traumatic cerebrospinal rhinorrhea. Repair of a fistula by a transfrontal intradural operation. Br J Surg 1941;29:299-303.

22. Appel Baum E. Meningitis following trauma to the head and face. JAMA 1968;173:116-20.
23. Dagi TF, Neyer FB, et al. The incidence and prevention of meningitis after basilar skull fracture. Am J Emerg Med 1983;3:295-8.
24. Dandy WE. Pneumocephalus (intracranial pneumatous cele or aerocele). Arch Surg 1926;12:949-82.
25. Dagi TF, George ED. Surgical management of cranial cerebrospinal fluid fistulas. In Schmidek HH, Sweet WH (Eds). Operative Neurosurgical Techniques, Indications, Methods, and Results, 3rd edn, Volume 1. WB Saunders Company 1995;117-31.
26. Ommaya AK. Cerebrospinal Fluid Fistula and Pneumocephalus. In Wilkins RH, Rengachargy SS (Eds). Neurosurgery, 2nd edn. McGraw Hill 1996;2773-82.
27. Adkins WY, Osguthrope JD. Minicraniotomy for management of CSF otorrhea from tegmen defects. Laryngoscope 1983;93:1038.
28. Lehman RA, Hayes GJ. The toxicity of alkyl 2-cyanoacrylate tissue adhesives: Brain and blood vessels. Surgery 1967;61:915.
29. Mickey BE, Sampson D. Neurosurgical applications of the cyanoacrylate adhesives. Clin Neurosurg 1982;29:429.
30. Ferrante L, Palatinsky E, et al. Intradural extracranial repair for cerebrospinal otorrhea with human fibrin glue: Technical note. J Neurol Neurosurg Psychiat 1988;51:1438.
31. Munoz A, Hinojona J, Esparza J. Cisternography and ventriculography gadopentetate dimeglumine- Enhanced MR imaging in pediatric patients: preliminary report. AJNR 2007;(28):889-94.
32. Stone JA, Castillo M, Heelon B, Mukheris SK. Evaluation of CSF leak: High resolution CT compared with contrast enhanced CT and radionuclide cisternography. AJNR 1999;20:706-12.
33. Barazi S, Choom M, Martin A. CSF rhinorrhoea due to pulsion diverticulum of frontal horn, by J. Neurosurg 2008;22(4):580-1.
34. Anari S, Waldron M, Carrie S. Delayed absence seizure: A complication of intrathecal fluorescein injection. A case report literature review. Auris, Nazus Laryne 2007; 34(4):515-8.

39 Post-traumatic CSF Otorrhea

Abrar Ahad Wani, Raj Kumar

CEREBROSPINAL FLUID OTORRHEA

Cerebrospinal fluid (CSF) leak fistula is a common, occasionally serious, and potentially fatal condition whose successful management requires a fundamental understanding of the anatomy and pathophysiology of the problem. Such leaks can occur from the nose (CSF rhinorrhea), or from the ear (CSF otorrhea) or in many of postoperative leaks through the incision sites. The primary danger of CSF leakage has been framed in terms of potential for meningitis which occurs in approximately 25 percent of traumatic CSF leaks of all types.[1] CSF otorrhea occurs in the presence of a perforated tympanic membrane in the following settings: (a) fractures of the petrous temporal bone,[18] (b) translabyrinthine and/or mastoid surgery, (c) developmental defects of the tegmen tympani or petrous apex with meningocele formation and spontaneous or post-traumatic meningeal laceration, (d) perilymphatic fistula from trauma with stapes fracture and torn round or oval window membrane, (e) translabyrinthine fistula due to the Mondini developmental defect of the cochlear modiolus and/or lamina cribrosa,[19] and (f) wide cochlear aqueduct syndrome.

EPIDEMIOLOGY, CLASSIFICATION AND FREQUENCY

Because this problem is so rare, the exact frequency with which it occurs is unknown. Leaks as a postoperative complication of skull base surgery represent the bulk of cases. This complication has been reported to occur in 6 to 12 percent of such cases. Leakage as a result of temporal bone fracture is the second most common etiology and occurs in 21 percent of patients with temporal bone fractures. Spontaneous leakage is rare, with less than 500 cases having been reported in the literature worldwide. Such leakage is more common in children (72%) than adults. Although rare, spontaneous leakage represents the greatest challenge to the clinician because the source of the leakage is not readily obvious.[21]

CSF otorrhea like all other transcranial CSF leaks fall into two major categories: traumatic and spontaneous or non-traumatic leaks.

TRAUMATIC LEAKS

They usually complicate about one-third of temporal bone fractures.[2,3] When the fractures tears the dura, CSF leaks into the tympanomastoid space. If the tympanic membrane has been disrupted, otorrhea occurs. If the membrane is intact, the fluid can leak down the eustachian tube into the nasopharynx, leading to rhinorrhea. CSF otorrhea can occasionally occur with a laceration of external auditory canal via fractured mastoid air cells without tympanic membrane disruption. CSF otorrhea occurs in equal proportions among the patients with transverse, longitudinal and oblique type of petrous bone fractures. However, classifying such fractures as otic capsule-violating and otic-capsule sparing types, the former was eight times more likely to have CSF otorrhea than the latter type.[4]

The traumatic group is further divided into two groups: acute or early leaks that present within one week of injury and delayed leaks that occur months or years later. It is a recognized complication of acoustic neuroma removal and other skull base surgery. These leaks are usually evident in the early postoperative period. They rarely occur more than 2 months postoperatively.

NON-TRAUMATIC LEAKS

Cerebrospinal fluid (CSF) fistulas of the temporal bone without preceding trauma are rare, they usually present as otorrhea but just like traumatic fistulas they may present as rhinorrhea via the eustachian tube. Otorrhea is often unrecognized especially if the tympanic membrane is intact and may simulate serous otitis media. They have been described in congenital defects of temporal bone,[5] temporal bone encephaloceles[6] and pituitary tumors.[7]

With a translabyrinthine fistula, CSF mixes with perilymph in the cochlea or vestibule and forms perilymphatic hydrops with displacement or perforation of the maldeveloped stapes footplate; the fluid leaks into the middle ear.[20] Wide cochlear aqueduct syndrome is a controversial and doubtful entity in adult patients because the aqueduct is filled with fibrous tissue and not functional beyond childhood.

APPROACH TO THE PATIENT

In a patient with known temporal bone fracture, clear or serosanguinous fluid running out of ear is pathognomonic. However, if the drainage is slight or intermittent, the diagnosis can be difficult to establish. Delayed leaks may present as obvious CSF leak or as an attack of meningitis without an obvious leak. Furthermore, meningitis may promote inflammatory changes at the site of leak with resulting cessation of leak, if there was already an obvious leak.

The 'halo sign' is a clear ring around a bloody center on absorbent paper or cotton gauze or pillow and if present implies the presence of CSF. Attempts to demonstrate the leak can be aided by the Valsalva's maneuver or jugular vein compression.

DIAGNOSIS

Involves two steps—first being to confirm that the leaking fluid is really CSF and second delineating the site of fistula. Identification of CSF is done with biochemical tests which must show values for glucose > 30 mg/dl to be conclusive. It should be noted, however, that a test with glucose oxidase paper has a 45 to 75 percent chance of positive results with nasal and other sources (e.g. middle ear) or serous or serosanguinous drainage and therefore, a negative test with such strips is more helpful particularly in traumatic cases with serosanguinous leaks.[8] If the diagnosis remains in doubt, some laboratories are capable of performing immunoassays for the presence of CSF-specific substance beta 2-transferrin.[9] This test, although rarely needed, is diagnostic. Another surrogate marker for CSF is beta trace protein (prostaglandin beta synthase) which is reported to offer an overall accuracy of 95.7 percent, a specificity of near 100 percent and a sensitivity of 91.2 percent.[10]

To localize site of fistula, following modalities are utilized:

i. Plain radiography and multiplanar tomography detects basal fractures and pneumocephalus. These are helpful in only 21 percent and 53 percent, respectively.
ii. High resolution CT scan with 3D-reconstruction leads to better detection and definition of temporal bone fractures. With IV contrast, leak site is usually associated with enhancement of adjacent brain parenchyma.
iii. *CT-cisternography:* An intrathecal injection of metrizamide is followed by CT scan and yields excellent visualization of active leaks.[11] It is essentially recommended if leak site is not identified on plain CT or if bony defect seen on plain CT does not have associated changes of abnormal enhancement of adjacent brain parenchyma or when multiple bony defects are identified and it is essential to determine which site is actively leaking. Smaller fistulas have been demonstrated by having the patient cough or carry out a Valsalva's maneuver. The risk of provoking seizures and aseptic or chemical meningitis following cisternography should be kept in mind.
iv. *Tracers:* The categorized proof of CSF fistula is the ability to retrieve extracranially a tracer substance injected into the CSF. The nonradioactive substances injected are the visible dyes like fluorescein and indigocarmine.[12] Radioactive tracers,[11] In-DTPA and 99Tc-Albumin are commonly used.[13] These are injected intrathecally and in the presence of an active leak, cotton pledgets placed in the ear can be used to confirm that a leak exists.
These tracer techniques have been used for CSF rhinorrhea mostly and these too have been abandoned in favor of CT and MR techniques.
v. *MR cisternography:* Utilizes MRI technologies to visualize CSF flow.[14] Heavily T_2-weighted fast spin-echo studies with fat suppression are reported to yield high sensitivity and specificity.

TREATMENT

Observation: Vast majority of post-traumatic CSF fistulas with otorrhea close spontaneously within two weeks of trauma.[2]

Prophylactic antibiotics: Their role in patients with CSF fistula has not been firmly established. In most studies, there was no difference in the incidence or morbidity of meningitis between treated and untreated patients.[2,15] Furthermore, the risk of selecting resistant strains appears real and is therefore, usually avoided.[16] Still many centers prefer to use prophylactic antibiotics depending on sensitivity of prevalent strains.

Nonsurgical treatment: Bedrest, stool softeners, modest fluid restriction and acetazolamide aims to reduce ICP are used as conservative treatments and help in stoppage of leakage. In profuse or long lasting leaks a continuous lumbar subarachnoid drainage can be helpful.[2,17] Drainage should be continued for 3 to 5 days after stoppage of leak to allow healing. If leakage recurs, operative repair is indicated.

Surgical treatment: Indications for surgical repair include persistence beyond two weeks, persistent or enlarging pneumocephalus, recurrent leak and meningitis.[2] Meningitis should be treated with antibiotics before surgical therapy.

The usual choice for surgical closure of a CSF fistula with otorrhea is subtemporal craniotomy, followed by dural repair via an extradural approach as this approach provides better access to leaks involving petrous bone and posterior margin of temporal fossa. However, intradural repair is preferred by some. The dura can sometimes be closed primarily but more frequently requires a dural substitute graft such as free pericranial graft, temporalis muscle fascia or commercially available grafting material. If the patient has lost hearing in the ipsilateral ear, the temporal bone air cells may be obliterated and packed with fat along with eustachian tube ligation.

REFERENCES

1. Schlosser RJ, Bolger WE. Nasal cerebrospinal fluid leaks: Critical review and surgical considerations. Laryngoscope 2004;113(2):255-65.
2. Brodie HA, Thompson TC. Management of complications from 820 temporal bone fractures. Am J Otol 1997;18:188-97.
3. Ghorayeb BY, Yeakley JW, Hall JW, et al. Unusual complications of temporal bone fractures. Arch Otolaryngol Head Neck Surg 1987;113:749-53.
4. Little SC, Kesser BW. Radiographic classification of temporal bone fractures. Clinical predictability using a new system. Arch Otolaryngol Head Neck Surg 2006;132:1300-4.
5. Kramer SA, Yangisawa E, Smith HW. Spontaneous cerebrospinal fluid simulating serous otitis media. Laryngoscope 1971;181:1083-9.
6. Landy LB, Graham MD, Kastush JM, et al. Temporal bone encephalocele and cerebrospinal fluid leaks. Am J Otol 1996;17;461-69.
7. Piziak VK, Gilliland PF, boyd G, et al. Pituitary tumour initially seen as serious otitis media. JAMA 1984;251: 3131-2.
8. Gadehott H. The reaction of glucose—oxidase test paper in normal nasal secretion. Acta Otolaryngol (Stockh) 1964;58;271-2.
9. Obserascher G, Arrer E. First clinical experience with beta-2 transferrin in cerebrospinal fluid oto- and rhinorrhea. INH 1986;34:151-5.
10. Backmann G, Nekic M, Michel O. Clinical experience with beta trace protein as a marker for cerebrospinal fluid. Ann Otol Rhinol Laryngol 109(12pt.1) 2000;1099-1102.
11. Ahmadi J, Weiss MH, Segall HD, et al. Evaluation of CSF leak by metrizamide CT cisternography. Neurosurg 1985;16:54-60.
12. Strauss H. Fluorescein als indikator fuer die nierenfunktion. Berliner Klin Wchschr 1913;50:2226-7.
13. Stab EV, Shirkoda A. Cerebrospinal fluid scanning. Clin Nucl Med 1981;6:103-9.
14. El Jamel MS, Lidgeon CN, Toland J, et al. MRI cisternography and the localization of CSF fistula. Br J Neurosurg 1994;8:433-7.
15. Klastersky J, Sadeghi M, Brihaye J. Antimicrobial prophylaxis in patients with rhinorrhoea or otorrhoea: A double blind study. Surg Neurol 1976;6:111-4.
16. Spetzler RF, Zabaramaski JM. Cerebrospinal fluid fistula. Contemp Neurosurg 1986;8:1-7.
17. Lee D, Honrado C, Har-El G, et al. Pediatric temporal bone fractures. Laryngoscope 1998;108;816-21.
18. May JS, Mikus JL, Matthews BL, et al. Spontaneous cerebrospinal fluid otorrhea from defects of the temporal bone: A rare entity?. Am J Otol. Nov 1995;16(6):765-71.
19. Burton EM, Keith JW, Linden BE, Lazar RH. CSF fistula in a patient with Mondini deformity: Demonstration by CT cisternography. AJNR Am J Neuroradiol. Jan-Feb 1990;11(1):205-7.
20. Rajkumar KT, Orabi AA, Timms MS. Spontaneous cerebrospinal fluid leak presenting as unilateral (left-sided) middle ear effusion. Ear Nose Throat J. Feb 2008;87(2):79-80.
21. Hanson MB, kwarljer JA. Skull base, CSF Otorrhea, emedicine.medscape.com 2006.

40 Skull Base Fractures

Abrar Ahad Wani, Raj Kumar

INTRODUCTION

Fractures of the skull base are relatively common. They have been reported to occur in 3.5 to 24.0 percent of head injury patients. This wide variation results from differences in studied patient populations and from difficulty of obtaining radiographic verifications of the fracture.[1] The traumatic Coma Data Bank in a prospective series of severe head injury reported that 25 percent had basilar skull fractures.[2]

BIOMECHANISM OF THE FRACTURE AT SKULL BASE

Basilar skull fracture basically is a linear fracture in skull base. These fractures are often part of a convexity fracture that has extended into skull base, though they also occur alone. They occur chiefly due to either direct impact or because of propagation of stress waves through the skull as a result of remote impact. They also occur as a consequence of impact to facial bones.[3] The skull base is prone to fracture at certain anatomical sites like sphenoid sinus, foramen magnum, petrous temporal ridge, inner potion of sphenoid wings at skull base. The middle cranial fossa is weakest with thin bones and multiple foramina which predispose it to fractures.

The unique anatomical relationship of the base of skull is responsible for the particular problems that may arise after injury. The dura being firmly adherent to skull base makes it vulnerable to laceration by a fractured bone. Such a fracture places the subarachnoid space in direct contact with the sinuses, middle ear structures or mastoid cells providing a pathway for CSF leak, infection (Meningitis, abscesses) and/or persistent fistula.[4-7] Basal fractures often traverse foramina and thereby may damage cranial nerves[3,6,8] and blood vessels.[6,9]

ANATOMY OF SKULL BASE

Skull base can be divided into three subtypes:[6]

1. *Anterior skull base:* It is related to paranasal sinuses, cribriform plate, and orbital roof.
2. *Middle skull base:* Includes major parts of sphenoid bone and temporal bone.
3. *Posterior skull base:* Includes clivus, condylar as well as portion of petrous temporal bone (Fig. 40.1).

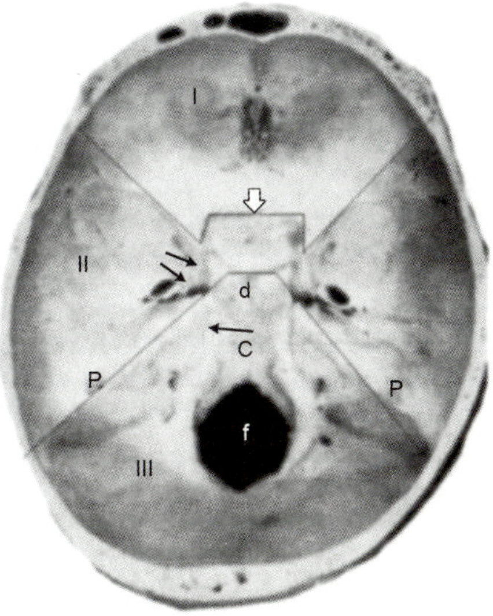

Fig. 40.1: I—Anterior cranial fossa base, II—Middle cranial fossa III—Posterior cranial fossa base, d—Dorsum sellae, C—Clivus, P—Petrous temporal bone, f—Foramen magnum

RADIOGRAPHIC DIAGNOSIS

Although, plain X-ray skull in anterior-posterior, lateral and basal projections may sufficiently demonstrate the extent of fractures, however, modern CT scans with bone windows, thin section cuts of up to 1 to 1.5 mm and coronal cuts provide improved detection and resolution of even tiny fractures without increased exposure to radiation.[2,10] Occasionally the fractures may be misinterpreted. False-positives may result when normal sutures are misdiagnosed as fracture lines. False-negatives may occur with subtle fractures or when suboptimal technique is utilized (as when the study is performed using section thickness >1.25 mm collimation or without employing a bone algorithm). The most common differential diagnosis of fracture is normal suture; hence one has to differentiate between the two. These can be differentiated in Table 40.1.

Helical CT is helpful in occipital condylar fractures and 3-D reconstruction in temporal bone fractures[11] in addition to providing useful information in other basal skull fractures.[12]

Table 40.1: Differences between fracture and sutures in radiology

Suture	*Fracture*
• Less than 2 mm in width	• Greater than 3 mm in width
• Same width throughout	• Width at the center and narrow at the ends
• Lighter on X-rays compared with fracture lines	• Runs through both the outer and the inner lamina of bone, hence appears darker
• At specific anatomic sites	• Usually over temporoparietal area
• Does not run in a straight line	• Usually runs in a straight line
• Curvaceous	• Angular turns

Indirect radiographic findings (on CT scan or plain X-ray film) that suggest a basal skull fracture include pneumocephalus in the absence of an open fracture of cranial vault and air-fluid level within or opacification of air sinuses with fluid.

MRI is of supplementary value for suspected vascular injuries and when cranial nerve palsy occurs in order to recognize neural compression. Moreover, early and late complications of basal skull fractures due to infection, brain contusion and herniation require CT scan to visualize the osseous prerequisites of complication and MRI to define the adjacent brain and soft tissue involvement.[13] Ligamentous injuries are best seen on MRI.

ANTERIOR SKULL BASE FRACTURES (RHINOBASAL)

Includes fractures of posterior wall of frontal sinus, roof of anterior and posterior ethmoid cells, cribriform-ethmoid junction, and the orbital roof. Such patients present with CSF rhinorrhea, bilateral periorbital ecchymosis (Raccoon's eyes), anosmia and damage to optic nerves and orbital contents.[14]

The anterior and posterior ethmoid foramina are located at the superior aspect of the ethmoid bone in the frontoethmoid suture. Shearing of the corresponding arteries that traverse these foramina may result in orbital hematoma. The optic canal is positioned farther posterior and is less commonly distorted by the fracture lines. However, local edema within the optic canal or free bone fragments may lead to a disturbance in the vascular plexus of the optic nerve, leading to temporary or permanent blindness. CSF leak being of high significance because of association of meningitis, abscess, and persistent fistula, needs to be actively searched for by the attending physician, especially in the presence of craniofacial or high mid facial fractures (Le Fort II and III).[13,15] Further, a CSF leak may be first detected several days to weeks after trauma due to the fact that CSF leak was initially hidden in bloody nasal discharge from facial fractures or less frequently, due to delayed development of hydrocephalus with rupture of arachnoid at fracture site. A 'double-ring' sign of bloody nasal discharge which is CSF mixed with blood, can be seen on patient's pillow and is a useful bedside test. Further, association with anosmia and salty taste in mouth is highly suggestive.

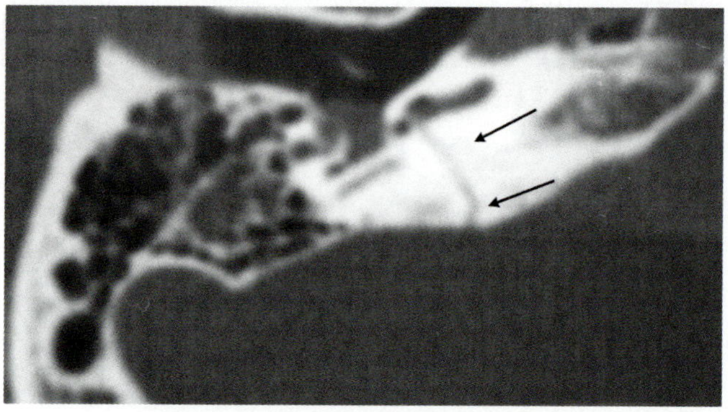

Fig. 40.2A: CT scan showing transverse fracture of temporal bone

Temporal Bone Fractures

One of the common basal skull fractures is categorized as transverse or longitudinal, depending on the axis of fracture in relation to petrous ridge[16] (Figs 40.2A and B).

Approximately 80 to 90 percent of temporal bone fractures are longitudinal, 10 to 20 percent are transverse and 8 to 10 percent are mixed.[17] A longitudinal fracture

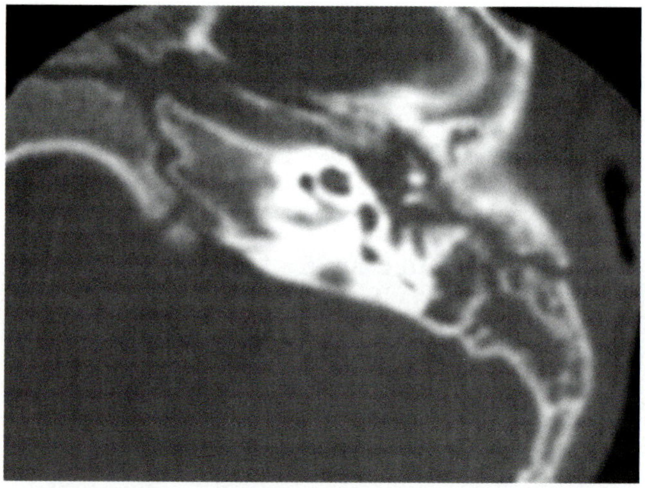

Fig. 40.2B: CT scan showing longitudinal temporal bone fracture

typically runs parallel to the external auditory canal (EAC), through the middle ear, anterior to otic capsule and parallel to petrous ridge extending to the foramen ovale. Transverse fractures run perpendicular to petrous ridge, from the foramen magnum margin across the petrous pyramid, often including the internal auditory canal and into the foramen spinosum or lacerum. Longitudinal fractures typically result from lateral blows to the temporal or parietal skull, while transverse fractures are more often associated with frontal or occipital blows. However, high resolution CT has shown that the most common fracture has elements of both types and is called mixed or oblique fracture, given its slanting course across the petrous pyramid.[18]

Longitudinal temporal bone fractures cause blood and CSF otorrhea (Tympanic membrane disruption), hemotympanum, a bony step-off in EAC, retromastoid ecchymosis (Battle's sign), conductive hearing loss due to disruption of ossicular chain, and in about 20 to 30 percent a facial nerve paralysis usually due to geniculate ganglion dissipation. In transverse temporal fractures, tympanic membrane and EAC are usually spared making hemotympanum and CSF otorrhea relatively infrequent. Vertigo, severe sensorineural hearing loss (SNHS) and nystagmus are commonly present because of disruption of internal auditory canal. Approximately 50 percent of the patients present with facial paralysis with the nerve usually injured in the geniculate ganglion or in the tympanic segment superior to oval window.[16,17]

In order to make it clinically more relevant and predictable, another classification divides these fractures into 'otic capsule sparing' and 'otic capsule violating' types,[19,20] the latter type was more likely to have complications like facial nerve injury, SNHL, vestibular dysfunction and CSF fluid otorrhea than those with the former. Thin section CT is diagnostic and 3-D reconstruction is helpful.[11]

The common complications are:

i. *CSF leak and fistulas:* Occur in 1/3rd of temporal bone fractures. When the fracture tears the dura, CSF leaks into tympanomastoid space. If the tympanic membrane has been disrupted, otorrhea occurs. If membrane is intact, fluid can leak down the eustachian tube into the nasopharynx, leading to rhinorrhea. Vast majority close spontaneously within 2 weeks of trauma.
ii. *Hearing loss:* Twenty to eighty percent of patients with temporal bone fractures demonstrate some degree of hearing loss. Patients with known or suspected temporal bone fractures should have their hearing evaluated as soon as possible with clinical and audiological (Pure tone audiometry, speech discrimination) tests. Patients with an altered level of consciousness may be tested using auditory evoked potentials.
iii. *Vestibular dysfunction:* Usually ranging from transient non-specific dizziness to episodic vertigo with nystagmus occurring from several weeks to months after injury. It has been attributed to vestibular concussion and is generally self-limited with no permanent sequelae. However, trauma can also lead to benign paroxysmal positional vertigo (BPPV) and development of hydrops of endolymphatic sac which need treatment on their own merits.
iv. *Facial nerve injury:* Complicates about 3 percent of all head injuries and practically all cases of post-traumatic facial palsy occur in the setting of temporal bone fractures, with >90 percent located in the perigeniculate region. It is caused by a hematoma within the nerve, anatomic disruption, contusion or an impinging bony fragment. Clinical assessment and electrophysiological testing in the form of electroneuronography (ENoG) must be regularly performed to determine the timing of onset of facial weakness (i.e. immediate or delayed) and whether injury is partial or complete.

Sphenoid Bone Fractures

It includes fractures of body of sphenoid (via sphenoid sinus, sella turcica and upper clivus), fractures of greater wing (through orbital, basal and temporal surfaces), fractures of lesser wing (via planum and anterior clinoid) and fractures passing through pterygoid process (Fig. 40.3).

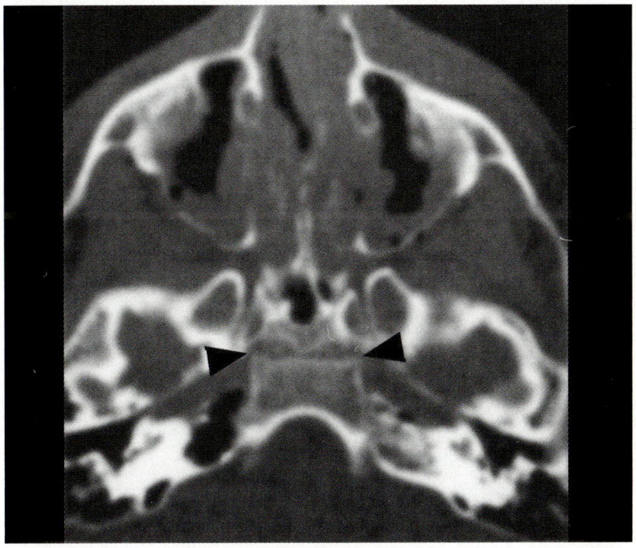

Fig. 40.3: CT scan transverse fracture through body of sphenoid

Considering all fractures of sphenoid bone, they exceed in number to all other basal skull fractures including anterior basal and temporal bone fractures.[21] Such fractures may result in:[6,21]

i. CSF rhinorrhea.
ii. Injury to cranial nerves III, IV, VI: Causing ophthalmoplegia.
iii. Optic nerve injury.
iv. Chiasmal injury and endocrine abnormalities (in sellar fractures).
v. Injury to ICA: Supraclinoid portion with a potential to cause cerebral ischemia, pseudoaneurysm formation and carotico-cavernous fistulas. Carotid injury can also occur when a fracture line runs across carotid canal. CT angiography should, therefore, be done as soon as fracture running in proximity to course of internal carotid artery is detected on a thin slice CT and it becomes more worthwhile since appropriate and expeditious treatment of carotid injury and its complications has become safely available after enormous developments in endovascular treatments.

Clivus Fractures

These rare fractures have been described in high speed motor vehicle accidents and attributed to high energy impacts therein. Longitudinal, transverse, and oblique types have been described in the literature. These are rarely diagnosed on conventional X-rays.

Longitudinal fractures are associated with injuries of vertebrobasilar system and brainstem trauma or both and are usually highly lethal. The abducent nerve may be directly damaged in these fractures. The transverse fractures extend through the carotid canal and petrous temporal bone. While less frequently contributing directly to mortality, transverse fractures are associated with CSF leaks, cranial nerve injuries, diabetes insipidus and carotico-cavernous fistulas.[22]

Occipital Condylar Fracture

Very uncommon, these result from a high energy blunt trauma and are divided into three types:

Type I: Secondary to axial compression resulting in communition of occipital condyle.

Type II: Result from a direct occipital blow, where condylar fracture is an extension of linear basal skull fracture.

Type III: Avulsion of condylar fragment occurs during rotation, lateral bending or a combination of mechanisms. This is an unstable fracture.

They should be suspected in any blunt trauma with craniocervical injuries causing altered mental status/coma, quadriparesis, occipital pain or tenderness, lower cranial nerve palsies or retropharyngeal soft tissue swelling. They are rarely diagnosed on plain X-rays and CT scan is recommended for establishing the diagnosis. MRI is recommended to assess the integrity of craniocervical junction.[23]

MANAGEMENT

Ethmoid Fracture

Use of antibiotics has not proven effective in changing the incidence of meningitis in post-traumatic CSF leaks and therefore, they are no longer recommended routinely.[24,25] Most acute post-traumatic leaks stop spontaneously within 10 days of injury. This is also true of leaks or dural tears associated with midface fractures when they are reduced.[26] The use of lumbar drainage may further increase the rate of healing. Persistence of CSF leak beyond 10 days, recurrent CSF leak, a bout of meningitis and pneumocephalus are indications for neurosurgical intervention. CT cisternography or MRI is done to precisely localize the fistula, followed by obliteration of fistula by dural patch graft or fat plus or muscle pledgets or injection of fibrin or other glues or tissue transfers may be needed. Usually, subfrontal or frontobasal approaches with intradural or extradural repair (intracranial) or combination of two is done.[5,6] Endoscopic repairs have also been a common practice at many centers.[27]

Regarding optic nerve injury following anterior basal fractures, it has been seen that there is no difference in improvement of vision in patients treated with surgical decompression versus nonsurgical methods (steroids and expectant management).[28] The recovery of VEPs from no response to abnormal wave or abnormal wave to normal VEP is both indicators of relatively good visual prognosis. The surgical decompression is indicated for documented deterioration of initially good vision following head trauma especially in case of retrobulbar hematoma and CT/MRI documented bone fragment dislocation into the orbit, comprising retrobulbar part of optic nerve.[6,28]

Temporal Fracture

Most of the patients can be managed conservatively. Mortality in the setting of temporal bone fracture typically occurs from an associated injury (like, closed head trauma, abdominal or thoracic injury) caused by blunt trauma. Mortality may also result, rarely, from delayed complications of fracture, such as meningitis.

CSF leak: Bedrest, elevating head 30 degrees, stool softeners and occasionally fluid restriction are used as conservative treatment. Lumbar subarachnoid drainage is helpful. Prophylactic antibiotics are controversial and many centers have policy of using these and many do not. Surgical therapy is indicated for persistent (>2 weeks) fistulas, persistent or enlarging pneumocephalus, and meningitis. Through a subtemporal extradural or intradural approach, dura can be closed primarily or more commonly a dural substitute graft is placed.[5,6]

Hearing loss: Conductive hearing loss can result due to injury to the auricle, external auditory canal, tympanic membrane, or ossicular chain. About 80 percent of such patients improve spontaneously. Conductive hearing loss greater than 30 decibels persisting beyond 3 months in a patient with intact tympanic membrane is highly suggestive for ossicular chain disruption and an otolaryngologist should be consulted for a possible ossicular chain reconstruction. SNHL can result due to trauma to cochlea, cochlear nerve or central auditory pathways. The prognosis of recovery of significant SNHL is poor. Most authors recommend amplification with a hearing aid.[29,30]

Vestibular dysfunction: Electronystagmography or MRI can be valuable in the work up of a patient with post-traumatic vestibular dysfunction to identify or exclude central lesion. Leakage of perilymph from inner to middle ear (perilymphatic fistula) can cause both hearing loss and vestibular dysfunction. Surgical exploration and repair of fistula with muscle, fat, autologous or allograft material will be needed.[30]

Facial nerve injury: Approximately 90 percent of patients with delayed onset of facial paralysis or those who have partial weakness will fully recover spontaneously. Thus, conservative treatment is indicated in these patients which includes short-term oral corticosteroid therapy to reduce edema of the nerve within the fallopian canal. Surgical intervention is warranted in patients with penetrating injury or in whom radiography (high resolution CT) demonstrates an obviously discontinuous fallopian canal with immediate complete facial paralysis. In case of delayed facial palsy, if ENOG drops to less than 10 percent of the contralateral side, surgical decompression may be considered. Removal of hematoma and bone fragments (decompression) facilitates nerve regeneration. Severely contused or disrupted nerves require resection of the damaged portion with end-to-end anastomosis, in case resulting nerve is not under tension or cable grafting with sural or greater auricular nerves in case segment loss is significant. Facial nerve grafting, when successful, can require up to 2 years for full regeneration.[6,30,31]

Sphenoid Fracture

CSF rhinorrhea: In sphenoid sinus fracture is managed like an anterior basal fracture. In addition repair can be done via transsphenoidal route.

Injury to ICA: Supraclinoid portion with a potential to cause cerebral ischemia, pseudoaneurysm formation and carotico-cavernous fistulas. Carotid injury can also occur when a fracture line runs across carotid canal. CT angiography should, therefore, be done as soon as fracture running in proximity to course of internal carotid artery is detected on a thin slice CT and it becomes more worthwhile since appropriate and expeditious treatment of carotid injury and its complications has become safely available after enormous developments in endovascular treatments.[21]

Endocrinopathy: Usually responds to hormonal replacement.

Clivus fracture: These are invariably fatal. However, in the surviving patients basic management is as in other basal fractures.[22,32]

Occipital Condylar Fracture

These are treated with external cervical immobilization (hard cervical collar/halo) for 6 to 8 weeks; however, those type III injuries that involve total ligamentous disruption are best managed with a posterior occipitocervical arthrodesis.[23]

REFERENCES

1. Willberry J, Chu DA. Management of head injury. The skull and Meninges. Neurosurg Clin North Am 1991;2(1):341-50.
2. Eisenberg HM, Gary HB, Aldrich EF, et al. Initial CT findings in 753 patients with severe head injury: A report from INH traumatic coma data bank. J Neurosurg 1990;73(5):68-81.
3. Thibault LE, Gennerelli TA. Biomechanics and craniocerebral trauma: Central Nervous System Trauma Research Status Report-1985, Bethesda: National Institute of Neurological and Communicative disorders and stroke. NIH 1985;379-89.
4. Park JI, Strelzow VV, Freidman WH. Current management of CSF fluid rhinorrhoea. Larynoscope 1983;93:1294-6.
5. Spetzler RF, Zabramski JM. Cerebrospinal fluid fistula. Contemp Neurosurg 1986;8:1.
6. Samii M, Tatagiba M. Skull base trauma: Diagnosis and management. Neurol Res 2002;24(2):147-56.
7. Abuabara A. Cerebrospinal fluid rhinorrhea: Diagnosis and management. Med Oral Patol Oral Cir Bucal 2007;12(5):397-400
8. Rovit RL, Mumti R. Injuries of the cranial nerves. In: Cooper PR (Ed). Head Injury, 3rd edn. 1993;183-202.

9. Aarabi B, M Queen JD. Traumatic internal carotid artery. Occlusion at the base of the skull. Surg Neurol 1978;10:233-6.
10. Conor SE, Tan G, Fernando R, Chaudhury N. Computed tomography pseudofractures of the mid face and skull base. Clin Radiol 2005;60(12):1268-79.
11. Girish M, Amish H, Motul Dugar, et al. Role of 3D CT in the evaluation of temporal bone. Radiographics 2006;26:S117-S132.
12. Three-dimensional (3-D) image reconstruction of the facial skull and skull base in computerized tomography. Radiology 1987;PMID:3423258.
13. Schuknecht B, Graetz K. Radiologic assessment of maxillofacial, mandibular, and skull base trauma. Eur Radiol 2005;15(3):560-8.
14. Kienstra MA, Van Loveren H. Anterior skull base fractures. Facial Plast Surg 2005;21(3):180-6.
15. Management of cerebrospinal fluid leak associated with craniomaxillofacial trauma. J Oral Maxillofac Surg 2004;PMID:15170277.
16. Ishman SL, Friedland DR. Temporal bone fractures: Traditional classification and clinical relevance. Laryngoscope 2004;114(10):1734-41.
17. Canon CR, Jahrsdocrfer RA. Temporal bone fractures: Review of 90 cases. Arch Otolaryngol 1983;109:285-8.
18. Ghorayeb BY, Yeakley JW. Temporal bone fractures: Longitudinal or oblique? The case of oblique temporal bone fractures. Laryngoscope 1992;102:129-34.
19. Fisch U. Facial paralysis in fractures of petrous bone. Laryngoscope 1974;84:2141-4.
20. Steward CL, Bradley WK. Radiographic classification of temporal bone fractures. Clinical predictability using a new system. Arch Otolaryngol Head Neck Surg 2006;132:1300-4.
21. June MU, Lindell RG, Jeffrey EG. Sphenoid fractures: Prevalence, sites and significance. Radiol 1990; 175:175-80.
22. Joslyn JN, Mirvis SE, Markowitz B. Complex fractures of the clivus: Diagnosis with CT and clinical outcome in 11 patients. Radiol 1988;166:817-21.
23. Anderson PA, Moutesano PX. Morphology and treatment of occipital condyle fractures. Spine 1988;13:731-6.
24. Villalobos T, Arango C, Kubilis P, Rathore M. Antibiotic prophylaxis after basilar skull fractures: A meta-analysis. Clin Infect Dis 1998;27(2):364-9.
25. Brodie HA. Prophylactic antibiotics for post-traumatic cerebrospinal fluid fistulae. A meta-analysis. Arch Otolaryngol Head Neck Surg. 1997;123(7):749-52.
26. Bell RB, Derks EJ, et al. Management of cerebrospinal fluid leak associated with craniomaxillofacial trauma. J Oral Maxillofacial Surg 2004;62(6):676-84.
27. Hughes RGM, Jones NS, Robertson IJA. The endoscopic treatment of CSF rhinorrhoea. The Nottingham experience. J Laryngol Otol 1997;111:125-8.
28. Wang BH, Robertson BC, Girotto JA, et al. Traumatic optic neuropathy: A review of 61 patients. Plast Reconst Surg 2001;107(7):1655-64.
29. Hickman MJ, Cote DN. Temporal bone fractures. J La State Med Soc 1995;147:527-30.
30. Brodie HA, Thompson TC. Management of complications from 820 temporal bone fractures. Am J Otol 1997;18:188-97.
31. Coker NJ. Management of traumatic injuries to the facial nerve. Otolaryngol Clin N Am 1991;24:215-27.
32. Menku A, Koc RK, Tucer B, et al. Clivus fractures: Clinical presentations and courses. Neurosurg Rev 2004;27(3):194-8.

41 Traumatic Carotico-cavernous Fistula

AK Mahapatra

INTRODUCTION

Carotico-cavernous fistula (CCF) is among rare consequences of head trauma. Approximately 1 to 2 in 40,000 hospital admissions are patients of CCF.[1] About 75 to 80 percent of all CCF are post-traumatic in origin due to blunt (acceleration-deceleration)/penetrating (foreign body, bony spicule) injury. Occasionally CCF can be iatrogenic following surgical procedures.[2-5] The most important implication of CCF are related to hemodynamics and anatomic characteristics. Parkinson and Barrow et al[9] has proposed classification based on these aspects.[6-9] Barrow's type A or Parkinson type I fistulas are usually traumatic, high flow, high pressure fistulas and in these cases clinical presentation is generally abrupt and severe.[10] As many as 66 percent of these patients present within one week of trauma.[11] Spontaneous resolution of these high flow fistula is very rare and thus they require treatment, that should ideally close the fistula and maintain the patency of ICA to avoid cerebral ischemia.

Traumatic CCF is most common in young males (75–80%), involved in high speed/penetrating trauma. Severe closed head injury, with basal skull fracture and penetrating trauma are the most common types of head injury resulting in CCF. Cavernous part of ICA is predisposed to injury as ICA proximal and distal to cavernous sinus (CS) is mobile but ICA in cavernous sinus is fixed to dura and is immobile in response to injury. Head injury occasionally results in partial or complete tear of intracavernous ICA (Parkinson type I) or avulsion of intracavernous branch of ICA (Parkinson type II) resulting in CCF. Radiologically, classification by Barrow et al[9] divides CCF into four groups. Types A and B are most likely traumatic in origin.

PATHOPHYSIOLOGY

Pathophysiological effects of CCF on different organs (eye, nerves and cerebral circulation) need to be understood because it affects the management.[11]

Effects on Eye

Although most patients present with ipsilateral proptosis, a careful examination will reveal proptosis in other eye because of interconnection between CS. There is expansion of CS and the venous channels which drain into it. Superior ophthalmic veins (SOVs) and sphenoparietal sinus get distended. Engorgement of SOV leads to venous congestion of orbital contents and proptosis, chemosis and later corneal ulceration. Diminished vision is because of variety of reasons and more than one may be responsible in a given patient. Different causes for visual loss in traumatic CCF are:

1. Direct optic nerve injury during trauma (up to 20% incidence in literature).[11]
2. Decreased perfusion pressure in ophthalmic artery.
3. Increased intraorbital pressure and increased venous pressure leading to retinal ischemia.
4. Vitreous hemorrhage, papilledema and glaucoma in chronic stage.
5. Presenile cataract due to decreased perfusion.
6. Corneal damage due to excessive proptosis and exposure.

Rarely, if SOV on the ipsilateral side is absent/hypoplastic and CS are interconnected, contralateral proptosis may occur.

Effect on Other Cranial Nerves

Increased CS pressures stretches the nerves leading to III, IV, VI palsy. These signs are more prominent when the anterior drainage is absent.

Effect on Cerebral Circulation

Due to fistula, large amount of blood is diverted away from circulation leading to chronic cerebral ischemia (steal phenomena). Back pressure changes can lead to venous hypertension and engorgement of cortical veins. These veins can rupture due to increased pressure and weak walls leading to SAH or intracerebral hemorrhage. Therefore, early filling of cortical veins is one of the indications for immediate treatment of CCF.

CLINICAL FEATURES

Signs and symptoms of fistula can be due to abnormal venous drainage, vascular steal, mass of dilated venous channels secondary to venous congestion.[12-15a] Interval

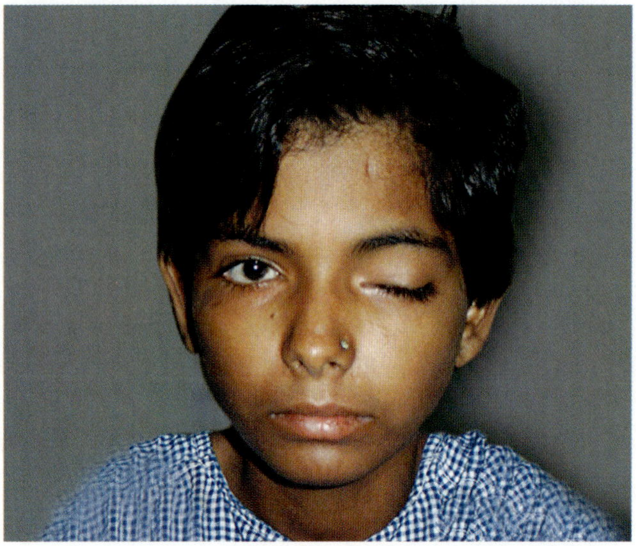

Fig. 41.1: Clinical print of a child having post-traumatic CCF with mild proptosis and lid edema of left eye

between the trauma and presentation varies from a day to several years. One-third of patients presenting within the first day and one-third about a week after the trauma. Initial symptoms of CCF may be missed because of post-traumatic eye swelling and altered sensorium. However, unresolving eye swelling should alert the physician the possibility of CCF. Proptosis is the most common (Fig. 41.1) presentation present in almost all cases (in our series 97 percent incidence), but occasionally patient may have a loud bruit/tinnitus.[16] Other occasional presentations are severe epistaxis, CSF rhinorrhea or unilateral blindness. Bruit is best heard over eye/temporal region/retromastoid region. Bruit in traumatic CCF is synchronous with pulse and is reduced by ipsilateral ICA compression. Details of clinical presentation in our series of 73 cases is given in Table 41.1.

Table 41.1: Clinical profile of 73 patients at AIIMS

Clinical features	*No. of patients*
Proptosis	73
Ocular palsy	50
Chemosis	51
Fruit	43
Tinnitus	17
Visual loss	25
Ptosis	08
Papilledema/optic atrophy	12
Facial hypoesthesia	06
Epistaxis	08
Prominent veins on the forehead	04

INVESTIGATIONS

CT scan: All patients at our institute underwent CECT/NCCT head to see for basal skull fracture and distended SOV and cortical veins. Bulbous CS can also be a frequent finding. In our series[16] dilated SOV was seen in all cases and giant cavernous sinus was seen in 49 percent cases.

Digital subtraction angiography (DSA) is the basic investigation for precise localization of CCF. Also DSA gives information about collaterals and adequacy of the circle of Willis. In patients where ipsilateral ICA injection fails to localize the site of CCF, vertebral angiogram with ipsilateral carotid compression can be used for identifying the site of fistula (Fig. 41.2). Various authors have quoted different ICA segments to be most commonly involved in their series.[17,18] In our series C-5 segment was most commonly involved. Steal phenomenon, total or partial steal (diversion of blood away from cerebral circulation), can be seen on DSA. Total steal does not mean that ICA is occluded. Ipsilateral vertebral injection with carotid compression reveals site of CCF in these cases. Details about steal phenomenon in our series (Tables 41.2A to C), venous drainage—anterior, posterior and cortical drainage can be observed. About 50 percent of patients have more than one type of drainage. Exclusive contralateral and exclusive cortical drainage can be seen occasionally.

Radiological classification of CCF was given by Barrow et al in 1985.[9]

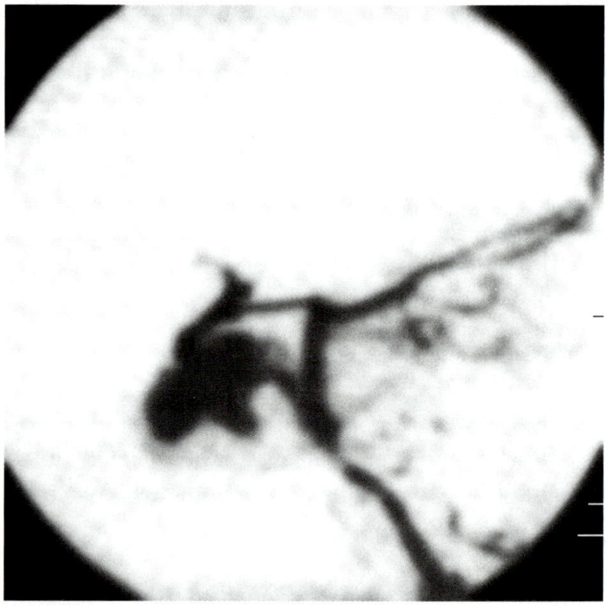

Fig. 41.2: DSA posterior circulation showing filling of CCF

Tables 41.2A to C: Traumatic carotid cavernous fistula

Table 41.2A

Radiological features		*No.*
Giant cavernous sinus		20
Intercavernous communications		07
Venous drainage	Anterior	34
	Posterior	14
	Inferior	03
	Cortical	15
	Contralateral	04
	Combined	20

Table 41.2B

Radiological features	*No.*
C2	02
C2-3	03
C3	05
C3-4	02
C4	05
C4-5	03
C5	19
Steal phenomenon	
Mild	14
Moderate	05
Severe	07

Table 41.2C

Treatment modalities	*No.*
Balloon	30
Coils	02
IBCA	01
Ivalon	01
Balloon + coil	01
Surgery	01

Type A: Direct shunts between ICA and CS.
B: Shunts between meningeal branches of ICA and CS.
C: Shunts between meningeal branches of ECA and CS.
D: Shunts between meningeal branches of ICA, ECA and CS.

Type A includes traumatic and aneurysmal rupture and B, C, D include dural AVMs.

TREATMENT

The first description of direct CCF was given by Travers,[2] who incorrectly thought that pulsating exophthalmos is caused by "aneurysm by anastomosis" of the orbit. He successfully treated the case by CCA ligation. Usually there is one site of communication between ICA and CS which is short, tangential and arterialized.[7] Unique anatomy of ICA in CS region is that ICA is fixed to dura at the skull base, limiting

Table 41.3: Indications for treatment
1. Progressive visual failure*
2. Intolerable bruit
3. Disfiguring progressive proptosis*
4. Extension into air sinus*
5. Early filling of cortical veins*
6. Repeated TIA
7. Pseudoaneurysm formation
8. Intracerebral bleed*
9. SAH*

*Indication for early treatment

its mobility and, therefore, predisposing it to blunt and penetrating trauma. Treatment of traumatic CCF remains a challenging job for an interventionist as well as treating neurosurgeon. Treatment strategy depends upon a number of factors including clinical condition, arterial and venous anatomy, availability of various techniques, skills of interventional neuroradiologist and patient preference.[12] Various indications of treatment are given in Table 41.3.[21-24]

Treatment modalities (Table 41.4) varies from manual compression of ICA[19] to direct surgery.[6] Daily intermittent compression can result in closure of 15 percent CCF but spontaneous resolution has been reported in up to 20 percent cases of traumatic CCF. Mullan and Debrun[20] advocated treatment/intervention in cases which do not close within 6 months spontaneously. Transvenous/arterial are two routes used.

Transvenous Occlusion[20]

The aim is to achieve complete thrombosis of CS by packing it with thrombogenic materials (gelfoam, surgicel, copper/phosphor bronze wires, etc.). Anterior approach uses SOV and posterior uses superior petrosal sinus. Both endovascular and direct surgical exposure can be used for transvenous routes.

Table 41.4: Treatment modalities		
1. Conservative		– Intermittent manual compression
2. Surgical	A.	– Transvenous packing of cavernous sinus
	B.	– Direct exposure and ligation of CCF under cardiac bypass and deep hypothermia
	C.	– Carotid ligation
3. Endovascular	A.	– Transvenous
	B.	– Transarterial

Advantages

1. No intra-arterial manipulation and, therefore, no risk of embolism, occlusion of ICA or hemispheric dysfunction.
2. Decreased pressure in ophthalmic vein may help in restoring vision.
3. Can be used in case where ICA has been ligated earlier.
4. Transcranial approaches for trans-sinusal endovascular therapy of dural atriovenous fistula (DAVF) has been sporadically reported by large craniectomies but selective image guided craniectomy is efficient and safe for direct percutaneous transvenous embolization of dural AVF in a single anesthetic session. It has the advantage of leaving a bone beside the sinus to prevents a parenchymal traumatic puncture.[36]

Disadvantages

1. Incomplete packing can lead to pseudoaneurysm formation which can raise CS pressure and worsen cranial nerve palsy.
2. Occlusion of posterior drainage without complete obliteration of the CCF can lead to worsening of ocular signs.

Transarterial Embolization

Intravascular occlusion has been widely used for CCF treatment and detachable balloon embolization remains the preferred treatment. In cases of failure of balloon embolization for internal carotid artery occlusion on affected side if not contraindicated, hydrocoil occlusion is a safe and effective alternative. However, it is an expensive and stable method of maintaining high carotid patency.[38]

Parkinson[6] described direct surgical approach based on anatomical studies. Under deep hypothermia (8–10°C), circulatory arrest and cardiac bypass, he was able to open CS, isolate the fistula site and occlude it with a clip. But this technique did not gain popularity because of inherent difficulty and operative mortality.

ICA ligation today has almost no role in CCF (traumatic) management and traping of ICA leads to opening of collaterals and recurrence of CCF. Serbinenko[25] introduced detachable balloon technique with preservation of ICA and this changed the management of direct CCF. Debrun and Lacour[26,27] described a similar technique in 1975. Successful closure of CCF is accomplished by transarterial route in 85-100 percent case (Table 41.5) with carotid preservation in 70 to 87 percent cases[28,29] (Fig. 41.2). At our institute

Table 41.5: Traumatic carotid cavernous fistula, experience at AIIMS—73 cases

Results	*No.*
Complete closure	57
Partial closure	07
Carotid preserved	30
Carotid occluded	05
Spontaneous occlusion	01

we achieved successful closure of fistula in 85 percent cases and ICA was patent in 85 percent patients after embolization.[16] CCF recurs in 1.3 to 9 percent of patients and responds to additional treatment.[30] Higashida et al[31] has the largest experience with this technique. Procedure is done under local anesthesia, femoral artery is cannulated, balloon is steered into mouth of fistula at the minimum inflation that secures total obliteration—the balloon is detached, total closure and carotid patency is checked on angiogram and clinically noticed by absent bruit.

In a series of CCF pre- and post-embolization, TCD was carried out and was observed that it, on complete occlusion, TCD, value increased and subsequent angiogram showed complete closure of fistula. On the contrary if TCD value did not rise following embolization, an incomplete closure was always observed in angiogram (Table 41.6).[31a]

Advantages

1. Procedure carried out under LA and can be aborted if patient develops deficit.
2. Advances in balloon type leads to improved closure rates.

Complications reported are premature detachment of balloon, dislodgement of previous balloon, intracranial migration, thromboembolism.[9,32] As many as 30 percent develop transient 6th nerve paresis and permanent deficit is reported in 0 to 5 percent.[9,17] Pseudoaneurysm or venous pouch formation is more after latex balloon embolization and, therefore, some recommend balloon to be filled with permanent agent (e.g. silicone/hydroxymethyl methacrelate).[33] Others recommend against permanent agents as they tend to produce permanent cranial nerve palsies and have prolonged mass effect.[34,35] We use only latex balloons in order to avoid permanent deficit and prolonged mass effect and treat pseudoaneurysm/venous pouch if it is extending beyond CS. Some patients especially children have smaller ICA and are difficult candidates for transarterial route. We prefer to wait in these and once carotid enlarges, we plan embolization with balloons.

Table 41.6: TCD finding in CCF

a. **Complete closure**—TCD value increases and angio showed complete obliteration.
b. **TCD velosity do not increase**—Partial embolization and repeat angio shows fistula, need re-embolization.

When standard treatments for CCF are failed, a covered stent grafts can be used as valid alternative in treatment of CCFs, but a long-term follow of more data is required to validate the option. A good patency in most cases was documented at angiographic follow-up of a small series of 7 cases.[37]

CONCLUSION

Traumatic CCF is a rare complication of head injury. Most of these patients present within few days of trauma and require treatment. Endovascular treatment is the safest mode of treating these cases. Complete closure of CCF with preservation of ICA is the goal of treatment. Successful closure can be achieved in about 85 percent cases with minimal complications.

REFERENCES

1. Parker L. Neuro-ophthalmological aspects of carotid-cavernous fistula: Smith R, Armin F, Russell W (Eds.) In: Seminars in neurological surgery, vascular malformations and fistulas of brain. New York: Raven Press 1982;181-98.
2. Debrun GM, Vinuela F, Fox AJ, et al. Indications for treatment and classification of 132 carotid-cavernous fistulas. Neurosurg 1998;22:285-9.
3. Fleishman JA, Garfinkel RA, Beck RW. Advances in the treatment of carotid-cavernous fistulas. Int Ophthalmol Clin 1986;26:301-11.
4. Miller NR. Carotid Cavernous fistulas. In: Miller NR (Ed). Walsh and Hoyt. Clinical Neuro-ophthalmoneurology. 4th edn, Batimore, William William Publisher William 1991;2165-209.
5. Gaston A, Combes C. Bilateral post-traumatic carotid-cavernous fistula: Anatomical-radiological correlations on a case treated with detachable balloon. J Neuroradiol 1986;13:55-61.
6. Parkinson D. Carotid-cavernous fistula, direct repair with preservation of carotid artery; technical note. J Neurosurg 1973;38:99-106.
7. Parkinson D. A surgical approach to cavernous portion of carotid artery. Anatomical study and case report. J Neurosurg 1965;23:474-83.
8. Parkinson D. Transcavernous repair of carotid-cavernous fistula, case report: J Neurosurg 1967;26:420-4.

9. Barrow DL, Spector RH, Braun IF. Classification and treatment of spontaneous carotid-cavernous fistula. J Neurosurg 1985;62:248-56.
10. Isamat F, Ferrer E, Twose J. Direct intracavernous obliteration of high flow carotid-cavernous fistula. J Neurosurg 1986;65:770-5.
11. Viswanathan R. Manual of neurosurgery, Neuro-96. Carotid-cavernous fistula 1996;480-6.
12. Morrein LH, Rigamonte D. Cerebral arteriovenous shunting—direct carotid-cavernous fistula. Neurosurg Quat 1996;6(4):251-66.
13. Parkinson D, Ramsay RM. Carotid-cavernous fistula with pulsating exophthalmos: A fortuitous cure. Can J Surg 1963;6:191-5.
14. Miller N. Carotid-cavernous fistulas. In: Clinical neuro-ophthalmology, vol 4, Baltimore: Williams and Wilkins 1991;2165-209.
15. Henderson JW, Scheider RC. The ocular findings in carotid-cavernous fistula—a series of 17 cases. Am J Ophthalmol 1959;48:585-97.
15a. Kurve AS, Mahapatra AK, Mishra NK. Traumatic CCF. A 17 years Experience at AIIMS. Annual Neurotrauma conference at Pune-August 2003.
16. Jindal A, Mishra NK, Mehta VS, Mahapatra AK. Clinical profile, radiological findings and results—a series of 41 cases: Data presented at 6th National Neurotrauma Conference, at Varanasi, August 1997.
17. Debrun, et al. Treatment of 54 cases of traumatic carotid-cavernous fistula. J Neurosurg 1981;55:678-92.
18. Debrun, et al. Detachable balloon and calibrated leak balloon technique in treatment of cerebral vascular lesion. J Neurosurg 1978;49:635-49.
19. Higashida RT, Hieshima GB, Halbach VV, Bentson JR. Closure of carotid-cavernous sinus fistulae by external compression of carotid artery and jugular vein. Acta Radiol Suppl 1986;369:580-3.
20. Mullan S. Fistulas and vascular malformations of the dura and dural sinuses. In Apuzzo MLJ (Ed). Brain Surgery: Complication avoidance and management, New York, Churchill Livingstone 1993;1117-246.
21. Halbache VV, Hieshima GB, Higashida RT. Carotid-cavernous fistulae: Indications for urgent treatment. AJNR 1987;8:627-33.
22. Gelbert F, et al. Severe epistaxis by rupture of the internal carotid artery into the sphenoidal sinus. J Neuroradiol 1986;13:163-71.
23. Debrun GM, Nauta JH, et al. Combining the detachable balloon technique and surgery in imaging carotid-cavernous fistulae. Surg Neurol 1989;32:3-10.
24. Debrun GM, Vinuela F, et al. Indications for treatment and classification of 132 carotid-cavernous fistulas. Neurosurg 1988;22:285-9.
25. Serbinenko FA. Balloon catheterization and occlusion of major cerebral vessels. J Neurosurg 1974;41:125-45.
26. Debrun GM, Lacour P, et al. Inflatable and released balloon technique. Experimentation in dogs. Applications in man. Neuroradiol 1975;9:267-71.
27. Debrun GM, Lacour P. Experimental approach of treatment of carotid-cavernous fistulas with an inflatable and isolated balloon. Neuroradiol 1975;9:9-12.
28. Lasjaunias P, Berenstein A. Arteriovenous fistulas (AVFs). In Surgical neuroangiography. 2 Endovascular treatments of craniofacial lesions. Berlin: Springer-Verlag 1987;175-233.
29. Kendall B. Results of treatment of arteriovenous fistula with Debrun technique. AJNR 1983;4:405-8.
30. Hedges TR, Debrun G, Sokol S. Reversible optic neuropathy due to carotid-cavernous fistula. J Clin Neuro-ophthalmol 1985;5:37-40.
31. Higashida RT, Halbach VV, Tsai FY. Interventional neurovascular treatment of carotid and vertebral artery lesion: Results of 234 cases. AJR 1989;153:577-82.
31a. Arora T. TCD blood flow study before and after embolization of carotico-cavernous fistula. A study at AIIMS M.Ch thesis deposited in 2000.
32. Chalif DJ, Flamm ES, Berenstein A, Choi IS. Microsurgical removal of a balloon embolus to the internal carotid artery. Case report. J Neurosurg 1983;58:112-116.
33. Kwan E, Hieshima GB, Higashida RT, Halbach VV. Interventional neuroradiology in neuro-ophthalmology. J Clin Neuro-ophthalmol 1989;9:83-97.
34. Debrun G. Carotid-cavernous fistulas. In: Taveras J Ferrucci JT (Eds). Radiology, diagnosis-imaging-intervention. Vol 43 Philadelphia: Lippincott 1992;1-11.
35. Sabates FN, Tsai F, et al. Transient cranial nerve palsies after cavernous sinus fistula embolization. Am J Ophthalmol 1991;111:771-3.
36. Bruneau M, Lubic ZB, Pirotte B, et al. Selective image guided venous sinus exposure for direct embolization of dural arteriovenous fistula, technical case report. Surg Neurol 2008;69(2):192-6.
37. Archondakis E, Pero G, Valvassori L, et al. Angiographic fallow-up of traumatic CCF treated with endovascular stent graft placement. AJNR AM J Neuroradiol 2007; 28(2):342-7.
38. Zhi-Gang W, Xuan D, Ji-oing Z, et al. Hydrocoil occlusion for treatment of traumatic CCF: Preliminary experience. Eur J Radiol 2008;14 abstract ahead of print.

42 Traumatic Dural Venous Sinus Thrombosis

Deepak Agarwal, AK Mahapatra

INTRODUCTION

Intracranial dural venous sinus thrombosis remains a poorly understood condition with unpredictable course and outcome. The first description of dural sinus thrombosis was made by Ribes, who in 1825 reported on a 45-year-old man with malignancy, headache, seizures and delirium. Postmortem examination revealed superior sagittal sinus, transverse sinus, straight sinus, and cortical vein thrombosis. Overall, since 1942, fewer than 250 cases of intracranial venous sinus thrombosis have been reported.

EPIDEMIOLOGY

The incidence of dural venous sinus thrombosis has been reported to be up to 4 percent with penetrating trauma and to be extremely rare with closed head injuries.[1] The mortality ranges from 5.5 to 50 percent.[2] Even amongst the survivors, 15 to 25 percent demonstrate lasting abnormalities.

PATHOPHYSIOLOGY

Dural venous sinus thrombosis has been described in association with trauma in a number of entities, including penetrating and closed head injuries, cranial fractures, disseminated intravascular coagulopathy (DIC), and after neurosurgical and non-neurosurgical operations. With penetrating trauma, thrombosis occurs due to trauma to the sinus or compression of the sinus from adjacent structures. Extension of the thrombosis from the scalp injuries or injured emissary veins has also been described. Although dural venous sinus thrombosis has been described in association with both mild and severe head injuries,[1] the mechanism of dural venous sinus thrombosis with closed head injury remains unknown till date.

Dural puncture with corticotherapy could be predisposing factors for cerebral venous thrombosis (CVT). CVT has been reported with spinal and epidural anesthesia with accidental punctures. It is reported following lumbar puncture and oral corticoid treatment. Corticosteroids can be considered as procoagulant stimuli.[6]

Superior sagittal sinus is most often occluded by trauma, tumor or coagulopathy. Delay in diagnosis may lead to life-threatening hyperpyrexia, elevation in ICP, venous infarction, seizure, coma, and death. However, the third of patients with nonseptic occlusion may survive untreated with few residue. The little data that exist suggest that rapid control of infection, seizure prophylaxis and anticoagulation must be achieved early so as to prevent progression of thrombosis and intracranial venous hypertension. In recent years direct retrograde venous thrombolysis has become increasingly available and has produced remarkable results that it is likely to become primary modality of choice for nontraumatic and non-tumoral occlusions.[7]

CLINICAL FEATURES

Signs and symptoms of dural venous sinus thrombosis are numerous, with a variable time course. Thrombosis of the nondominant sinus may remain asymptomatic. Symptoms include headache, stroke, visual loss, seizures and pulmonary embolus.[2] Headache is found in approximately 75 percent of cases and is thought to result from elevated intracranial pressure.[3] Protracted vomiting, increases intracranial pressure, hydrocephalus and papilledema are particularly described with thrombosis of the sigmoid and transverse sinuses.[4]

INVESTIGATIONS

CT, MRI and angiography are all used to assist in the diagnosis of dural sinus and cerebral vein thrombosis. CT images of the brain may be normal in 10 to 20 percent of the patients with venous thrombosis (Figs 42.1 and 42.2). Findings may include hemorrhagic or nonhemorrhagic venous infarcts, cerebral edema, small ventricles, hydrocephalus, contrast enhancement of the tentorium and falx, thrombosed cortical veins (cord sign), a dense triangle sign representing fresh thrombus in the posterior SSS, and an empty delta sign on contrast studies that represents enhancement of collateral veins in the SSS wall surrounding a nonenhancing thrombus. The 'empty

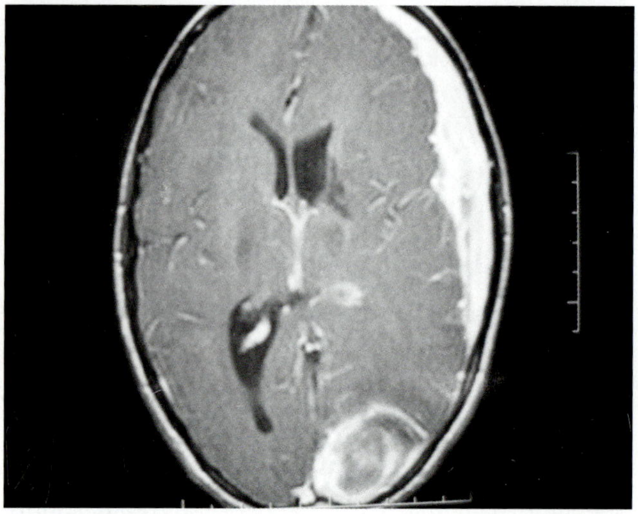

Fig. 42.1: CT showing acute subdural hematoma and enhancing posterior thrombus in left parieto-occipital region

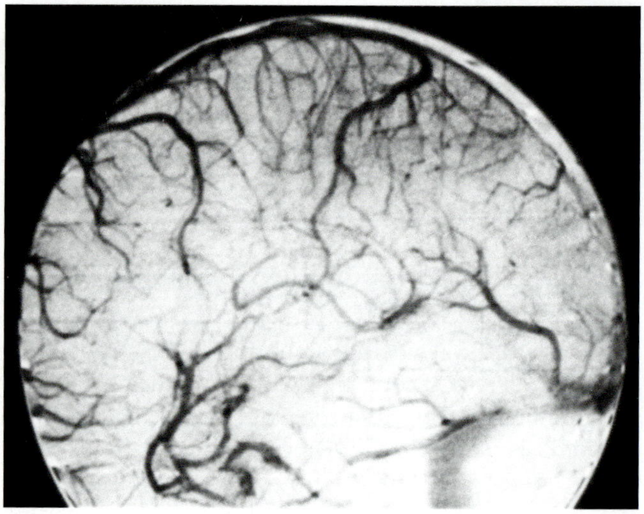

Fig. 42.3: DSA showing superior sagittal sinus thrombosis

delta sign' may be confused with the 'pseudodelta sign', the latter seen on unenhanced CT scans and caused by parafalcine interhemispheric hemorrhage or posterior parafalcine subarachnoid hemorrhage after head injury. Angiographic findings include partial or complete nonopacification of venous sinuses and veins, dilated cortical collateral veins and cork-screw appearance, increased cerebral circulation time, and reversal of flow away from the obstructed sinus or vein (Fig. 42.3).[2] MRI and MR angiography present noninvasive means of assessing the presence of thrombosed sinuses and veins[2] and are currently considered investigations of choice in cases of suspected dural venous sinus thrombosis.

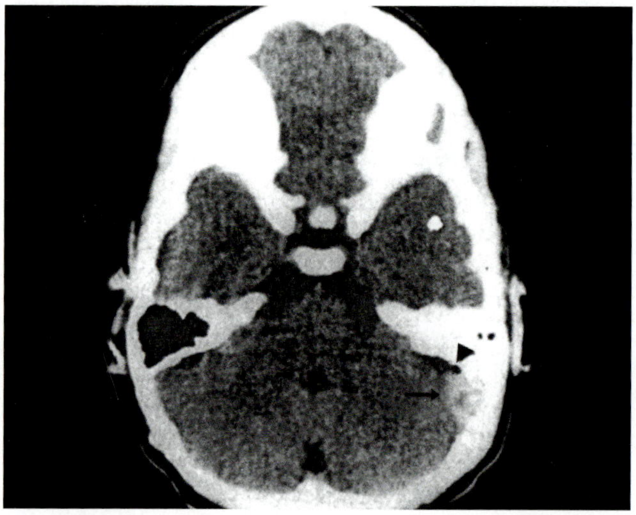

Fig. 42.2: Plain CT head showing hyperdensity in left sigmoid sinus, consistent with sigmoid sinus thrombosis

TREATMENT

Treatment of dural venous sinus thrombosis in the setting of closed head injury remains difficult. Treatment options include cerebral dehydrating agents, steroids, acetazolamide, cerebrospinal fluid, drainage, barbiturates, decompressive craniectomy, sinus thrombectomy, heparin/warfarin, urokinase and tissue plasminogen activator. Since the thrombosis leads to the formation of hemorrhagic infarctions, there has been much concern over the use of anticoagulation in the treatment of superior sagittal sinus thrombosis.[3] Einhaupal et al performed the only randomized, blinded study of adjusted dose of heparin in patients with venous sinus thrombosis and concluded that treatment with heparin was not only safe, but also beneficial, even in the setting of intracerebral hemorrhage.[3,5] Typically anticoagulation is reserved for those with early, partial or propagating thrombosis without evidence of hemorrhagic venous infarction. In patients with progressive neurological decline, treatment must be instituted to prevent progression of the thrombus, and in severe cases, treatment is directed at restoring flow through the sinuses. More aggressive treatment, including endovascular thrombolysis or surgical thrombectomy, is reserved for those patients with serious neurological sequelae. Thrombolysis has been performed either percutaneously (via the femoral vein) or by a small craniotomy over the SSS and directly injecting thrombolytic drugs such as urokinase into the sinus. In general, a conservative treatment regime that may be used includes an initial administration of 100,000 units urokinase during 30 to 45 minutes and than an infusion in the range of 40,000 to 60,000 units per hour is preferred. This regime must be adjusted based on the patients' neurological condition and response to treatment. Following thrombolysis patients are usually kept anticoagulated for at least six months.

CONCLUSION

While neurologic changes following head trauma may result from concussion or more life-threatening injuries such as subdural or epidural hematomas, intracerebral hemorrhage, arterial dissection, and diffuse axonal injury, venous sinus thrombosis should be considered when other etiologies are eliminated. Only prompt identification and treatment can help in avoiding secondary complications that can at times be life-threatening.

REFERENCES

1. Kuether TA, O'Neill O, Nesbit GM, Barnwell SL. Endovascular treatment of traumatic dural sinus thrombosis: Case report. Neurosurg 1998;42:1163-7.
2. D' Alise MD, Fitchel F, Horowitz M. Sagittal sinus thrombosis following minor head injury treated with continuous urokinase infusion. Surg Neurol 1998;49:430-5.
3. Ferrera PC, Pauze DR, Chan L. Sagittal sinus thrombosis after closed head injury. Am J Emerg Med 1998;16:382-5.
4. Brors D, Schafers M, Schick B, Dazert S, Draf W, Kahle G. Sigmoid and transverse sinus thrombosis after closed head injury presenting with unilateral hearing loss. Neuroradiol 2001;43:144-6.
5. Einhaupl KM, Villringer A, Meister W. Heparin treatment in venous sinus thrombosis. Lancet 1991;338:597-600.
6. Milhaud D, Heroum C, Charif M, et al. Dural puncture and corticotherapy as risk factors for cerebral venous sinus thrombosis. Eur J Neurol 2000;7(1):123-4.
7. Buonanno FS. Cerebral sinovenous thrombosis. Curr Treat Option Cardiovasc Med 2001;3(5):417-27.

43 Cranioplasty

Raj Kumar, Arun Kumar Srivastava

Cranioplasty as name suggest is the method for the reconstruction of the skull defect. Cranioplasty is an important part of the neurosurgical methods and especially in neurotrauma.

BACKGROUND

Cranioplasty is a procedure that dates to antiquity. Incas performed cranioplasty using precious metals and gourds.[1] In 1668, there is reported case of bone graft from a canine skull,[1-3] over the years many metals known to human being has been used for the cranioplasty.[4-7] Autogenous bone graft become popular in the early 1900s, iliac bone graft was reported in the year 1908[8] while first rib cranioplasty was reported by the Kappis in 1915s.[9] The world wars has been the era of using different prosthetic materials and maximum failure is also noticed during that period due to the infection and exposure.[10]

INDICATION/CONSIDERATION FOR CRANIOPLASTY

1. Location of the defect; cosmetic consideration was taken in account in cases of defect below the hair line.
2. Size of the defect; in children below 12 to 18 months any sizable defect can be followed as there dura and periosteum has a great strength of reossifying the sizable defect.[11,12] In older children and adults cranioplasty is advocated in the defect more than 10 cm^2 though, no absolute criteria has been laid down.[13]
3. Possibility of infection; in presence of past history of defect site infection or when the defect is in close proximity of the frontal and ethmoid sinus, there is always high-risk of defect site infection and to avoid the same the cranioplasty is mandatory.

Table 43.1 compares alloplastic vs autogenous cranioplasty.

ALLOPLASTIC CRANIOPLASTY

1. Polymethyl methacrylate (PMMA): It is inexpensive, easily moldable, can be made prior to the surgery using 3-D CT reconstruction technique for better cosmetic result. Steel mesh can be incorporated into the PMMA,[14,15] which gives extra strength and fixation.
2. Hydroxyapatite (HA); they are more biocompatible and with minimal tissue response. They are available in various forms like granules, blocks and paste. Unlike PMMA the paste hardening reaction is isothermic as well as they have got osteoconductive properties, due to these properties they are preferred over PMMA.[16,17]
3. Cadaveric demineralized bone.

AUTOGENOUS CRANIOPLASTY

1. Autologous bone graft in case of decompressive craniectomy; they are stored at the temperature

Table 43.1: Alloplastic vs autogenous cranioplasty

	Advantages	*Disadvantages*
Synthetic material	• Better cosmesis • No resorption • No added morbidity	• Infection • Chance of fracture • No osteoconductive properties • Irradiated area • With skin graft
Autogenous	• Low infection rate • Grows with craniofacial growth	• Cosmesis • Resorption • Donor of morbidity

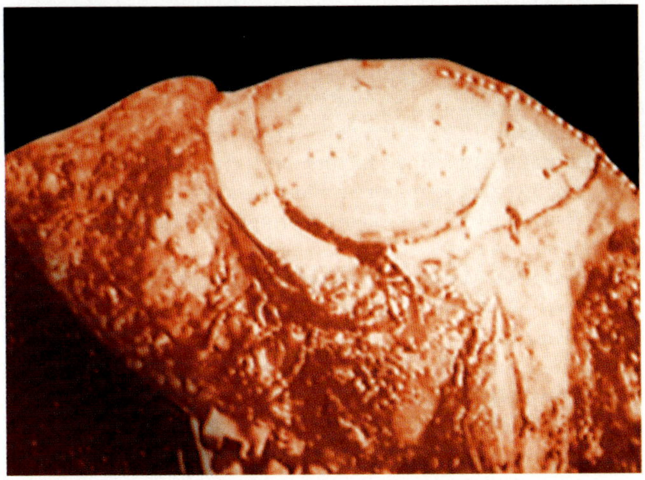

Fig. 43.1: Cranioplasty using cranium bone split graft

of –70 degree Celsius and best timing after initial surgery is 6 to 8 months.

2. Autologous bone graft preserved in the abdominal subcutaneous pocket; this is the method we commonly used in cases of decompressive craniectomy with good GCS.
3. Cranial bone; they are the best donor site and has several advantages over rib and iliac crest graft. It is already in the operative field. Cranial bone has the appropriate curvature. Donor site morbidity is minimal. Finally there is evidence that bone of membranous origin (cranium) undergoes less resorption than bone of endochondrial origin (rib and iliac crest) (Fig. 43.1).
4. Rib; this donor site is capable of supplying a large amount of bone for cranioplasty, they have tremendous capacity of regeneration when harvested subperiosteally (Figs 43.2 and 43.3).
5. Iliac crest; there is relatively small amount of cortical bone present in the iliac crest which limits its use as an donor for the cranioplasty, however its provides an abundant source for cancellous bone which can be used to obliterate frontal sinus.

TECHNIQUE OF CRANIOPLASTY

1. *Acrylic (PMMA) cranioplasty:* The scalp flap is elevated, the edges of the defect are identified, and the dura was dissected from the undersurface of the margin, taking care not to perforate the dura once the defect is encountered. Multiple holes are drilled in the adjacent bone margin and 26 G wires are placed through these holes, spanning the defect to form scaffolding for the acrylic. The acrylic in the powder form then mixed with the resin to form a thick paste. Once the consistency is such that the paste barely moves in the mixing container, it is placed in the defect, onto the wire scaffolding, and shaped. As the process of PMMA hardening is exothermic, it is helpful to irrigate the cranioplasty with cool saline while it is drying. During this time, applicator stick can be used to perforate small holes in the cranioplasty to permit extradural blood to drain into the subgaleal spaces. Drains should be placed prior to the closure and closure is done in layers.
2. *Cranial bone cranioplasty:* The recipient site is prepared as described above. A bone rongeur is used to debride the sclerotic bone margin until the healthy bleeding bone is identified. Once

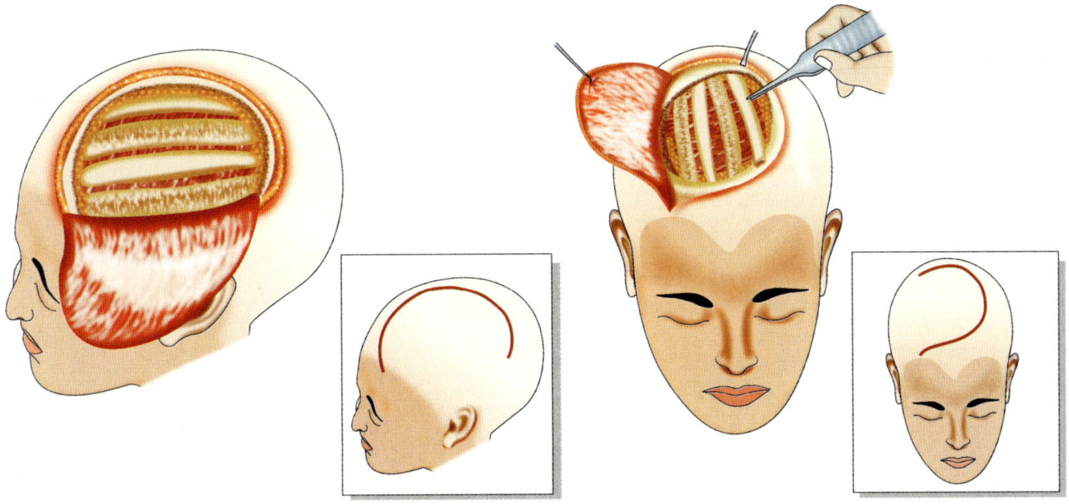

Fig. 43.2: Cranioplasty using rib graft

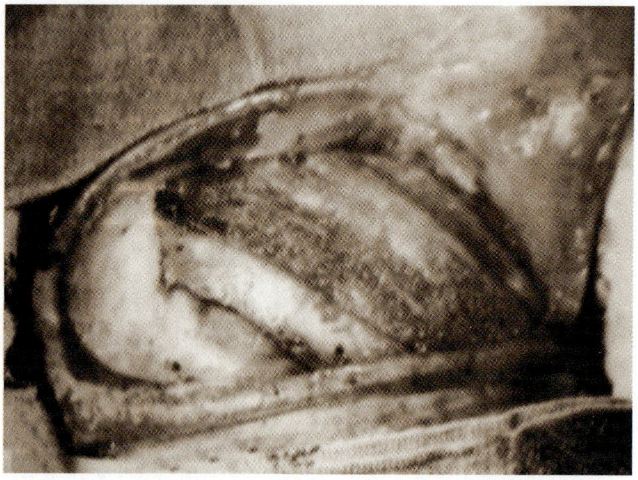

Fig. 43.3: Operative photograph after rib bone cranioplasty

the full size of the defect is known a template is made. The skull of the parietal region is generally chosen as the donor site, because the bone here is thickest. The template of the defect is traced on the parietal skull. A small olive burr is then used to burr through the outer cortex, the entry in the diploic space is heralded by the marked increase in the bleeding. With the help of osteotome the outer table is removed and shaped accordingly.

An alternative method is to performed a full thickness craniotomy. The inner and outer table is split *ex vivo* using a slow saw or an osteotome. The inner table is generally returned to the donor site and outer table is harvested.

REFERENCES

1. Sanan A, Haines SJ. Repairing holes in the head: A history of cranioplasty. Neurosurgery 1997;41:999.
2. Munro I, Guyuron B. Split rib cranioplasty. Ann Plast Surg 1981;7:341.
3. Van Meekren J. Observationes Medicochiurgical Amsterdam, Henrici and T. Bloom,1682.
4. Courville CB. Cranioplasty in prehistoric times. Bull Los Angeles Neurol Soc 1959;24:1.
5. Manson PA, Crawley WA, Hoopes JE. Frontal cranioplasty: Risk factors and choice of cranial vault reconstructive material. Plast Reconstr Surg 1957;20;281.
6. Reeves DL. Cranioplasty. Springfield Charles C. Thomas, 1950.
7. Scott M, Wycis HT. Experimental observation on the use of stainless steel for cranioplasty. J Neurosurg 1946;3;310.
8. Mauclaire H. Bbreche cranienne restauree par la prosthese metallique: Comments on article by Rouvillois. Bull Mem Coc Chir Paris 1908;34:232.
9. Kappis A. Zur decking von schadelfekten. Zentralbl Chir 1915;42:897.
10. Tessier P. Autogenous bone graft taken from the cranium for facial and cranial application. Clin Plast Surg 1987; 79:531.
11. Hobar PC, Masson JA, Wilson R, et al. The importence of the dura in craniofacial surgery. Plast Reconstr Surg 1996;98:217.
12. Marchac D. Radical forehead remodeling for craniostenosis. Plastr Reconstr Surg 1987;61:823.
13. Rish B, Dillon J, Meinonsh D. Cranioplasty: A review of 1070 cases of penetrating head injury. Neurosurgery 1979;4:381.
14. Hammon WM, Kempe LG. Methyl-methacrylate cranioplasty: 13 years experience with 417 patients. Acta Neurochir (Wein) 1971;25:69.
15. Vaandrager JM, Van Mullem PJ, Wijn JRDE. Craniofacial contouring and porous acrylic cement. Ann Plast Surg 1988;26:583.
16. Hobar PC. Implantation: Bone, cartilage, and alloplastic. Selected readings in plastic surgery 1922;7:22.
17. Costantino PD, Friedman CD, Jones K, et al. Hydroxy-apatite cement. Basic chemistry and histologic properties. Arch Otolaryngol Head and Neck Surg 1991;117:379.

44 Visual Problems Following Head Injury

AK Mahapatra

INTRODUCTION

Visual abnormalities are uncommon findings following closed head injury. In some large series, the problems are reported in 1 to 5 percent case.[1-4] Mahapatra and Bhatia had reported a figure of 1.5 percent incidence of optic nerve injury in head injury. Jennett et al in 1981 had reported a 13 percent incidence of optic nerve injury in severe head injury patients. Surprisingly, however, an incidence as high as 44 percent was reported by Crompton,[5] among them 24 percent had bilateral pathology. In a study Mahapatra published 32 cases of bilateral injury.[5a] Exact incidence is difficult to determine, as many unconscious patients may die and autopsy is not carried out. The pathogenesis of optic nerve injuries, is by and large not clear and the management is controversial. Hence, this chapter highlights the visual problems in head injury and rationalize the treatment of optic nerve injury.

ANATOMICAL AND PATHOLOGICAL CONSIDERATION

Visual pathway is divided into anterior and posterior parts. The anterior visual pathway includes, optic nerves and chiasma. The posterior visual pathway includes rest of the visual system distal to the chiasma. Barring the occipital infarction due to herniation, the pathology of posterior visual pathway in head injury is rather rare.

Most important pathology, in optic pathway injury is the optic nerve involvement.[1,3,6,11] Optic nerve extends from the globe to the chiasma and is approximately 5 cm long. The optic nerve is divided into four parts: (a) Intraocular part, (b) Intraorbital part is the longest around 25 to 30 mm, (c) Intracanalicular part is 4 to 10 mm long and lies in optic canal where the nerve is fixed to the periosteum, and (d) The intracranial part, which is 10 to 15 mm long (Fig. 44.1). Near the intracranial opening to the optic canal there is a strong and sharp dural edge. There is a potential risk of damage of the optic nerve against sharp edge. The blood supply to the nerve is important. The intracanalicular part is relatively avascular and derives blood supply from the centripetal branch of the pial vessels. The intracranial optic nerve is supplied by the small pial vessel of the anterior cerebral and anterior communicating artery. These small vessels play an important role in optic nerve injury and lead to ischemic neuropathy.

PATHOLOGY

Visual problem following head injury can involve: (a) anterior, or (b) posterior visual pathways. According to the site of injury the lesion can be at various places (Table 44.1).

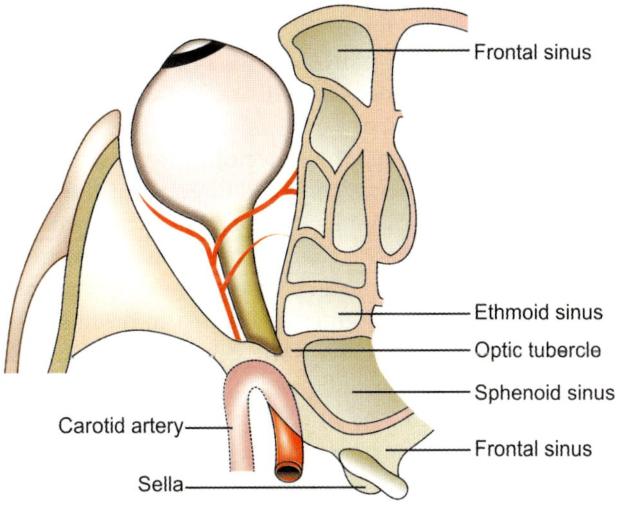

Fig. 44.1: Anatomy of optic nerve and its relation to other structure

Table 44.1: Sites of visual pathway injury

A. Anterior visual pathway injury
- Optic nerve injury
  - Anterior marginal tear
  - Intraorbital optic nerve injury
  - Intracanalicular injury
  - Intracranial optic nerve injury
- Chiasmal Injury

B. Posterior visual pathway injury
- Optic tract and geniculate lesion
- Optic radiation or calcarine lesion

INDIRECT OPTIC NERVE INJURY

Optic nerve is the most frequent site of visual pathway injury, in head injury. It was first described by "Hippocrates". Probably the 1st case of optic nerve injury was described by Dutonchel in 1822. However, in 1879, Berlin described the optic nerve lesion at autopsy.[12] Battle in 1890[13] had distinguished the direct optic nerve injury from indirect optic nerve injury. Callon in 1892[14] had postulated the mechanism of optic canal fracture leading to optic nerve injury and reviewed 80 cases of optic nerve injury reported in the literature.

Involvement of the optic nerve is reported in 0.6 to 3 percent of all head injury. The most frequent site of the injury is the optic canal. Hughes in 1962[2] described the various types of optic nerve injury, depending on the site: (a) anterior marginal tear, (b) anterior optic nerve injury and (c) posterior optic nerve injury, which can be intraorbital, intracanalicular and intracranial.

(a) Anterior marginal tear occurs at the optic nerve head in retina. It was first described by Lowenstein in 1943.[15] Hughes reported 13.3 percent of anterior marginal tear in his patients with optic nerve injury. This type is also associated with retinal and choroidal injury. Ophthalmoscopy reveals hemorrhage and irregular disk margins, (b) Anterior optic nerve injury involves the optic nerve behind the globe till the entry of central artery of retina. 12.3 percent incidence was reported by Hughes.[2] The retinal vessel spasm is reported in 30 to 35 percent cases, (c) Posterior optic nerve injury is more frequent. Traumatic orbital apex syndrome is a rare condition, occurring in muscle cone. In this situation optic nerve gets involved along with proptosis, III, IV and VI cranial nerve palsy. Intracanalicular optic nerve injury occurs in optic canal, where nerve is relatively fixed as the nerve sheath is firmly adherent to periosteum. This type of injury can occur in anterior cranial fossa fracture. Hughes[2] reported bilateral optic nerve injury in patients with Le Fort Type III fractures.

Pathophysiology of Optic Nerve Injury

The exact mechanism of optic nerve damage is not understood. However, large number of hypothesis have been put forward. Walsh and Lindenberg in 1963[16] classified the optic nerve injury into: (a) Primary, and (b) Secondary depending on nature of the pathology, as observed at autopsy (Table 44.2). The concussion of optic nerve was first described by Walsh in 1979.[9] Secondary involvement of the optic nerve is due to edema and ischemia leading to the infarction of the nerve, as a result of microvascular thrombosis. This hypothesis has been suggested by many authors.[2,16,17] The most likely mechanism leading to microvascular thrombosis is probably due to shearing strain on the nerve as a result of acceleration and deceleration injury to the orbit. It is also likely that midline forehead injury can produce bilateral optic nerve injury[18] while blow over supraorbital area, temporal area produces unilateral optic nerve injury. The shearing and stretching forces can lead to rupture of optic nerve axons.

One of the most favored mechanism of optic nerve damage in head injury is vascular insufficiency.[1-3] The vascular injury is generally at pial vessel, which could be immediate. Delayed onset of visual involvement is due to edema and ischemia. In patients with irreversible visual loss, the most important cause is probably optic nerve infarction.[2,19,20] In two of Hughes's cases, histology of intracanalicular optic nerve revealed infarction. Infarction was also reported by Ramsey,[20] in both intracanalicular and intracranial portion of the optic nerve.

The fracture of the anterior cranial fossa, orbital roof, anterior clinoid process and the optic canal can produce optic nerve injury. These fractures can produce tear or compression of the nerve. Contusion of the nerve is a form of primary injury, which results from shearing force to the nerve. Hooper in 1951[21] had reported contusion of intracranial optic nerve in a patient with anterior clinoid fracture. Rarely, an optic sheath hematoma has also been reported.[22,25] Intraneural hemorrhage occurs due to the rupture of small veins or capillaries, resulting in a perivascular hematoma. Imachi et al[23] had reported few cases of

Table 44.2: Pathology of optic nerve injury

A. Primary pathology
   a. Concussion
   b. Avulsion or tear (partial/complete)
      – Partial
      – Complete
   c. Contusion
   d. Hemorrhage
      – Intraneural
      – Extraneural

B. Secondary pathology
   a. Edema
   b. Ischemia
   c. Microvascular thrombosis
   d. Infarction of the nerve

intraneural hematoma. Mahapatra et al[26] observed one case of optic nerve hematoma among 100 patients. Tandon et al[24] observed a single case among 27 patients subjected to optic nerve decompression.

Inspite of normal looking nerve at surgery or at autopsy histopathological abnormalities are consistently reported.[2,3,21,24] Pathological entities such as degeneration of myelin, loss of axons, chronic inflammation with phagocytosis are found at microscopic examination. Vascular involvement in the form of thromboischemia and infarction are also seen.

Clinical Features

In conscious patients diagnosis is not difficult. Typical history of unilateral visual loss or rarely bilateral visual loss is the main complaint. The visual loss could be immediate or delayed type.[1,3,4,11,18] In 90 percent cases, patients do have history of loss of consciousness. In severe head injury, when a patient is unconscious, unilateral fixed dilated pupil with retained consensual light reflex raised the possibility of unilateral optic nerve injury. This phenomenon is described as "Marcus Gunn's Pupil". By definition eyeball is intact and there is no ocular injury, however, external injury over forehead or temporal region with black eye may be present. In unconscious patients it is difficult to determine the timing of onset of visual deterioration. In 15 to 20 percent patients, visual loss may be partial and patients may also have visual field cuts. In patients with optic nerve concussion, patients have transient visual loss. Hence, it may be possible to have some visual recovery by the time patients reach the ophthalmologist or neurosurgeon.[9,19,25]

Table 44.3: Investigations in patients with optic nerve injury
– X-ray skull
– VEP
– Field charting
– CT scan with orbital cut
– MRI scan
– Orbital ultrasound

Examination usually reveals normal cornea, lense and vitreous. In anterior marginal tear, ophthalmoscopy may show retinal hemorrhage.[1,3,21] In vast majority of cases fundi reveals no abnormality. Rarely, congestion of the disk may be observed. Optic disk atrophy is observed 4 to 6 weeks following injury (Table 44.3).

Field Defects

Various types of field defects have been reported in patients with optic nerve injury.[1-3,11,18,27] Surprisingly, only few authors have described visual field problem in their patients with optic nerve injury. Traquair et al[27] had reported central or parcentral scotoma and altitudinal field cut. Hughes[2] in 1962 had reported lower field was involved. Mahapatra et al,[11] Mahapatra and Tandon[26] had reported all possible field defects (Figs 44.2A and B) including nasal field. However, temporal field was most frequently involved. The

A

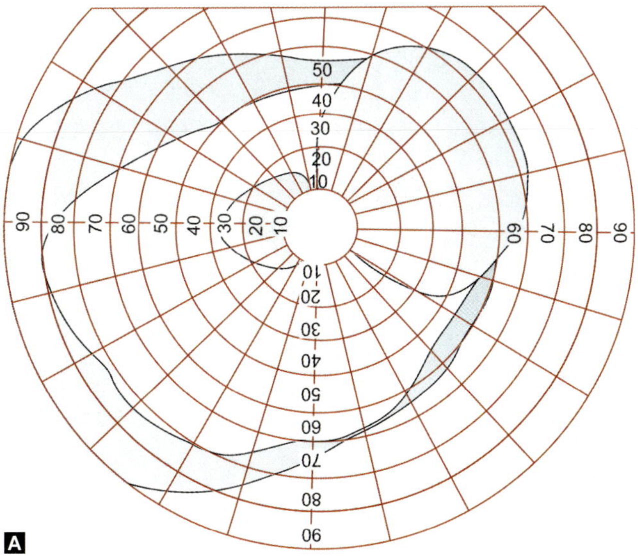

B

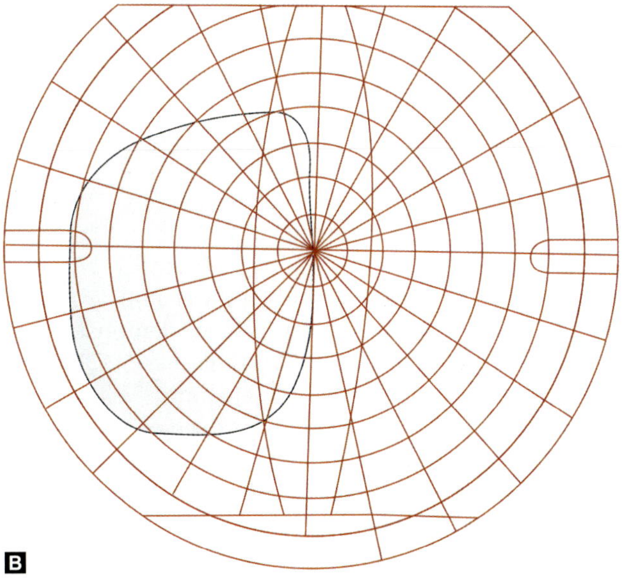

Figs 44.2A and B: Field defects in patients with optic nerve injury

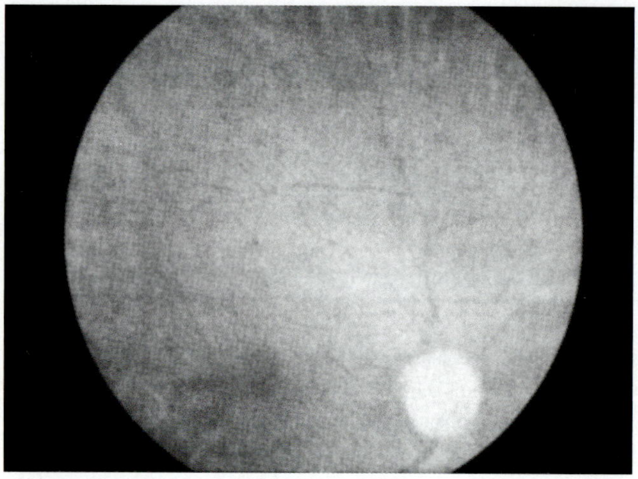

Fig. 44.3: Color photography of fundus showing primary optic atrophy in a patient with optic nerve injury

exact reason is difficult to explain. One of the possible explanation is the selective involvement of nasal fibers as the bone in the medial side of the orbit is thin and is likely to fracture more frequently.

Fundus Finding

Fundus finding varies according to the site of the injury and the degree of damage to the nerve. Except anterior marginal tear, immediate or early examination may not shows any abnormality. In anterior marginal tear, fundus examination few hours later usually show edema and hemorrhage. In anterior optic nerve injury, when the site of damage is nearer to the eyeball, fundus changes occur earlier than distal optic nerve injury. Generally, optic atrophy sets in 3 to 6 weeks time[1,2,28] (Fig. 44.3).

Investigations (Table 44.3)

X-ray skull, paranasal sinus view and optic canal view are important radiological investigations. Skull fractures are reported in 50 to 80 percent patients.[1-3,11,29] A wide variation in the incidence of optic canal fracture has been reported (0–90%). This is basically because of difference in surgical, radiological and autopsy findings. With the advent of CT scan, demonstration of optic canal fracture has become easy. CT cuts with bone window helps in establishing the fracture. Recently, CT scanning is regularly used in suspected cases of optic nerve injury.[4,11,18,30-33] High resolution CT is the procedure of choice. Manfredi et al[31] reported sphenoid and ethmoid hemorrhage in PNS view and among them 5 had CT scan evidence of optic canal fracture. Grove[30] had pointed out the role of soft tissue injury. We observed optic canal fracture in 8 to 10 percent cases, in CT scan.[4,11,18,26] Tandon et al[24] had observed optic canal fracture in CT scan in 6 patients, among 29 subjected to surgery. CT scan frequently shows fracture in anterior cranial fossa and opacity in ethmoid and sphenoid sinuses. Rarely, CT scan may show optic sheath hematoma. Mahapatra et al[26] reported a single case of optic sheath hematoma among 100 patients.

Recently, MRl scans are freely available. MRl scan is a very good investigation for the orbit. However, there is limited publication on MRl in optic nerve injury. We have performed MRI over 40 patients and reported our findings[11,18,26] (Fig. 44.4). Nerve swelling and contusion is well visualized in MRl. Surprisingly, I have never seen a real transection of the optic nerve in MRl. Orbital ultrasound is a very good investigation. It can show thickening of the nerve, orbital hematoma or a bony fragment. In 20 patients repeated ultrasound examination was carried out by us. Initially optic nerves were thickened and after 3 to 4 weeks, thinning of the optic nerve was observed.

Role of Visual Evoked Potentials

Visual evoked potentials (VEPs) is a very good indicator of the integrity of visual pathway. However, till late 80s this test was not frequently used in optic nerve injury. Feinsod and Auerbach in 1973[34] had retrospectively analyzed VEP and electroretinography in 5 patients. Shaked et al 1982[35] had reported a case and highlighted the value of VEP. Nau et al 1987[36] reported poor outcome in patients having no VEP waves, however,

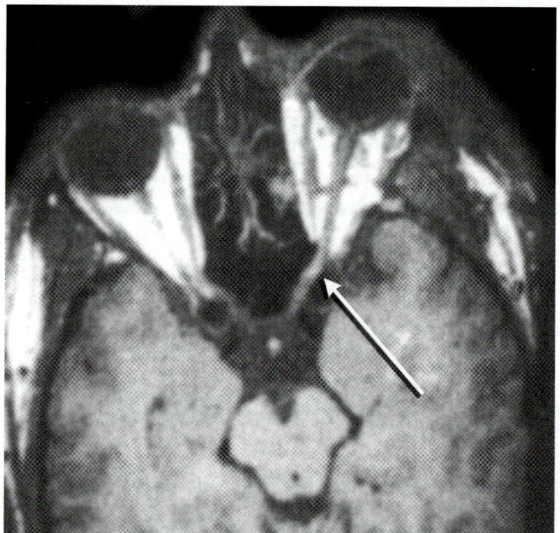

Fig. 44.4: MRI axial cut orbit in a patient with a right optic nerve injury (White arrow)

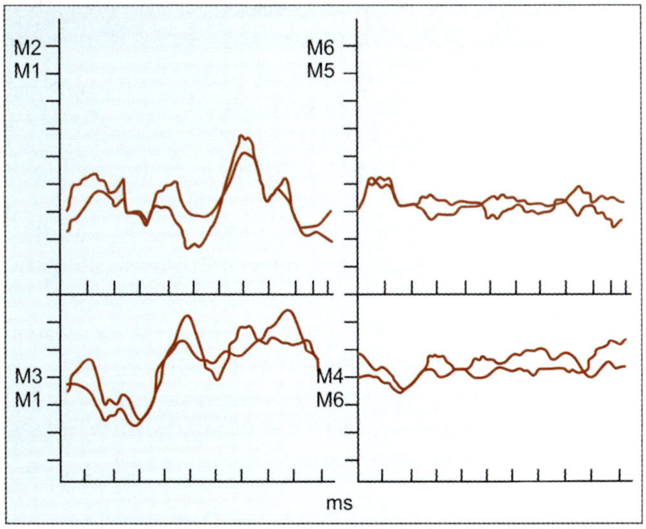

Fig. 44.5: Repeated YEP in a patient with right optic nerve injury shows no wave

they did not comment on the role of normal VEP in predicting the good outcome. Prior to our studies there was no prospective study in the world literature on the role of VEP in predicting a good or a poor outcome. Mahapatra and Bhatia,[4] Mahapatra et al[11,26] and Tandon et al[24] have repeatedly shown, 85-90% visual recovery in patients with repeated normal or abnormal VEPs (Fig. 44.5). In their experience none of the patients with repeatedly absent VEP had shown visual recovery. VEP also helps in diagnosis of visual loss in unconscious patients. We have been using Light Emiting Diode (LED) for recording VEP in unconscious paticnts.[18,37]

Treatment of Optic Nerve Injury

The treatment of optic nerve is controversial, even today. The main controversy, however, centers around the indications for surgery. Large number of studies reported in the world literature show similar results in medically managed and surgically treated group.[1,3,4,6,7,10,11,24,32,38] While many authors, from different countries have favored medical management, the Japanese authors have popularized and favored the surgical treatment.[6,7,39,40]

Medical Management

There is scanty literature on the medical treatment of optic nerve injury[4,10,33,37,38] (Table 44.4). Many authors who did not believe in surgical management, offered no treatment. Walsh (1966) stated that the "cortisone and mannitol may be helpful in patients in whom optic nerve swelling is a feature". However, establishing the swelling of the optic nerve is difficult. With the advent of ultrasound and MRI scan optic nerve swelling can be diagnosed. Delayed onset of visual deterioration also suggests, swelling or edema of the optic nerve. Not much literature is available on the role of steroid in the management of optic nerve injury. Matsuzaki et al 1982[10] treated 22 patients with a combination of prednisolone, 20 percent mannitol, urokinase and vitamin B_{12}. He reported 58.8 percent recovery in this group. Anderson et al[29] used high dose of steroid in 6 patients and 3 had shown improvement. In our study, overall improvement was observed in 53 to 58 percent patients.[4,11,24,26,37] I believe steroid must be given for a period of 3 to 4 weeks following injury. I found no significant difference using dexamethasone or methylprednisolone.

Table 44.4: Results of conservative management

Authors	*Year*	*No. of cases*	*% of recovery*
• Hooper	1951	17	29.0
• Matsuzaki et al	1982	33	58.8
• Mahapatra et al	1992	100	57.0
• Mahapatra	2002	800	58.0

Optic Nerve Decompression

Decompression of the optic nerve following injury has long been tried[1-3,6,7,24,42-45] (Table 44.5). Prior to the introduction of transethmoid surgery by Niho et al,[8] transcranial route was used for decompression. There is a great deal of controversy regarding the need for surgery and timing of optic nerve decompression. Gjerrisl[1] in 1976 stated "Comparison between two groups of patients treated with and without operation

Table 44.5: Result of surgical decompression

Authors	*Year*	*No. of cases*	*% of recovery*
Niho et al	1961	7	66.0
Impachi et al	1968	61	70.0
Fukado	1981	700	42.0
Matsuzaki et al	1982	11	42.0
Strohim and Jahnkes	1982	15	40.0
Karnik	1986	37	20.0
Tandon et al (Selected cases)	1994	39	74

Table 44.6: Result of 800 patients with optic nerve injury of AIIMS

1983–2002	
	%
Complete recovery	10%
Partial recovery	48%
No recovery	42%

reveals that the prognosis is the same in both groups, that there is no clear cut guidelines for one or the other." Walsh and Hoyt[3] considered immediate visual loss at the time of impact is a contraindication for surgery, as visual recovery is unlikely. Other authors have considered optic canal fracture as one of the indication for surgery.[6,40] Gijerris[1] had suggested against surgery in patients with immediate visual loss, having no signs of visual recovery in next few days. He also suggested conservative management when optic nerve injury is diagnosed in unconscious patients. All our studies had suggested no immediate surgery. Unless there is some spontaneous improvement[11,24,26] surgery is not indicated. Fujitani et al[38] had suggested a trial steroid therapy for 3 weeks. Patients not improving on steroid unlikely to benefit from surgery. Lessell in 1989[41] observed that the eyes with total loss of vision at the end of 3 weeks on steroid is unlikely to respond. Mahapatra in 1992[45a] reported delayed recovery from optic nerve injury. Thakar et al[45b] in 2003 reported the results of delayed optic nerve decompression for optic nerve injury (Table 44.6).

Indications for Surgery

Till recently, there was no clear cut indication for optic nerve decompression. In fact, in our first study the protocol was only conservative management.[4] Our subsequent studies showed a limited indication for surgery.[11,24,26,37] Now we manage our cases following Mahapatra's criteria (Table 44.7). Our protocol offers every patient 3 weeks of corticosteroids. VEPs are repeated and patients are closely followed up for their clinical state. Patients progressively improving or not showing any improvement, are not subjected to surgery. A group of patients those who show minimal improvement and then remain static are subjected to surgery. This situation only suggests that the optic nerve is not completely damaged and given a chance, further improvement may occur. Following this criteria patients are operated. As the group subjected to surgery is highly selective, chances of improvement is also high.[24] Thus, the role of surgery in optic nerve injury is limited.

Table 44.7: Mahapatra's criteria

a. All the patients are put on corticosteroids.
b. VEP and clinical examination repeated every 2 to 3 days for the first 3 weeks.
c. Patients showing good visual recovery do not need surgery.
d. Patients in whom visual acuity remains PL negative inspite of corticosteroid at the end of 3 weeks, do not need surgery.
e. Surgery is beneficial in those patients in whom visual improvement is marginal and then remains static.
f. One emergency indication for surgery, is delayed onset optic nerve injury, when vision rapidly deteriorates inspite of corticosteroids.

Outcome and Factors Influencing Outcome

Visual outcome in patients with optic nerve injury depends on several factors (Table 44.8). Age, mode of the injury, unilateral or bilateral involvement, presence or absence of VEP and presence or absence of vision play important role in visual recovery.[1,3,4,11,18,24,26,39,41] In two of our studies in pediatric age group we reported a recovery which was worse than adult. Similarly, presence or absence of VEP wave is of great importance.[4,11,18,34,36] Normal VEP provides a good chance of recovery in all the patients. We find time gap between injury and surgery and presence or absence of optic canal fracture are of very little significance. In one of my study, I reported better outcome in patients with bilateral optic nerve injury.[5a,18] Similar observation has not been reported in the World literature. In our experience only 10 percent patients improve to normal vision.[11,18,26] Rest 40 to 45 percent patients only have partial visual recovery. Rarely, visual recovery may start 8 to 12 weeks later. I have collected 6 patients in whom vision remained PL negative, surprisingly

Table 44.8: Factors influencing outcome in patients with optic nerve injury

Factors	*Good prognostic factors*	*Poor prognostic factors*
i. Age	Adults	Children
ii. Mode of injury	Blunt	Missile/Blast injury
iii. Unilateral/ bilateral	Bilateral injury	Unilateral injury
iv. Positive or negative VEP	VEP +ve	VEP –ve
v. Vision	PL + ve	PL–ve

visual improvement started 8 to 12 weeks later. Agarwal and Mahapatra reported 23 percent recovery rate in 100 patients with PL one vision following optic nerve injury.

CHIASMA INJURY

Introduction

Chiasmal injury is a rare condition. Except for case reports no large series is published.[8,27,46,47] Only over 100 cases have been reported in the literature. Nieden in 1833 was the first one to report chiasmal injury (quoted by Walsh & Hoyt 1969). Till 1935 only 30 cases were reported, and till 1971 the number increased to 89.[27,46] I have collected one of the largest series of chiasmal injury in the literature.[48] Hughes in 1962[2] reported 4.4 percent chiasmal injury and 7.8 percent optochiasmal injury. Elisevich et al[8] reported 5 cases of chiasmal injury while Savino et al reported 11 cases.

Pathogenesis

Pathogenesis of chiasmal injury is not clear. However, chiasmal injury can be primary or secondary as observed at operation or at autopsy (Table 44.9). Primary involvement could be tear, contusion or laceration.[1,3,5,21,27] In most of these patients, there is evidence of fracture in anterior cranial fossa. In closed head injury, due to forehead impact, there is antero-posterior distortion of the skull, which leads to mid-line chiasmal tear.[21,22] In one of the Hooper case[21] chiasma looked normal at surgery, subsequently, when the patient died, the autopsy showed atrophy of the central part of the chiasma. Crompton in 1970[5] in an autopsy study demonstrated interstitial hemorrhage and necrosis in 5 and 11 cases respectively. The usual site of the chiasmal necrosis is at the site of decussation. Review of the literature shows that the majority patients of chiasmal injury are either direct contusion or chiasmal necrosis at the central part. Chiasma also gets involved secondary to edema, ischemia leading to infraction.

Table 44.9: Chiasmal injury pathological types

A. Primary
   a. Sagittal split or tear
   b. Transverse split
   c. Contusion
   d. Laceration
B. Secondary
   a. Edema
   b. Ischemia
   c. Necrosis (Infarction).

Table 44.10: Clinical presentation in 15 cases

• Loss of consciousness	12
• Bitemporal field cut	12
• One eye blind other eye temporal cut	3
• CSF rhinorrhea	2
• Bleeding from nostril	10
• Loss of smell	11

Clinical Findings

Patients are usually adult vehicular accident victims. In my study[48] there was no children among 15 patients with chiasmal injury. History of unconsciousness is available in 90 percent patients. Chiasmal injury is also described as traumatic bitemporal hemianopia, indirect chiasmal injury or post-traumatic chiasmal syndrome. History of forehead trauma is available in 100 percent and loss of consciousness 90 to 95 percent. Head injury is by and large severe.[1,2,8,21] Bleeding from nose or CSF rhinorrhea are commonly associated.[2,8] In my series[48] most of the patients had CSF rhinorrhea. Bitemporal hemianopia is the most frequent symptoms. Laursen,[46] reviewed 89 cases of chiasmal injury and found classical bitemporal hemianopia only in 53, while 12 had nasal field cut in one or both the sides. Temporal field cut in one eye and no PL in the other eye suggest optochiasmal injury (Table 44.10). Rarely, visual deterioration may be possible due to basal meningitis and arachnoiditis.

Other, unusual symptoms associated with chiasmal injury are anosmia, pituitary insufficiency diabetes insipidus.[1-3] Rarely, there may be cranial nerve deficit, traumatic aneurysm of ICA and carotico-cavernous fistula (CCF).

Diagnosis

Clinical diagnosis is difficult in unconscious patients. However, when a patient is conscious, diagnosis is made by the history of bilateral temporal defect, confirmed by field charting (Fig. 44.6). Recently, CT scan and MRI scan have made the diagnosis easy (Fig. 44.7). The series reported by me had MRI demonstration of chiasmal injury in 5 cases.

Treatment

There is no specific treatment of chiasmal injury. As secondary involvement of chiasma can occur due to

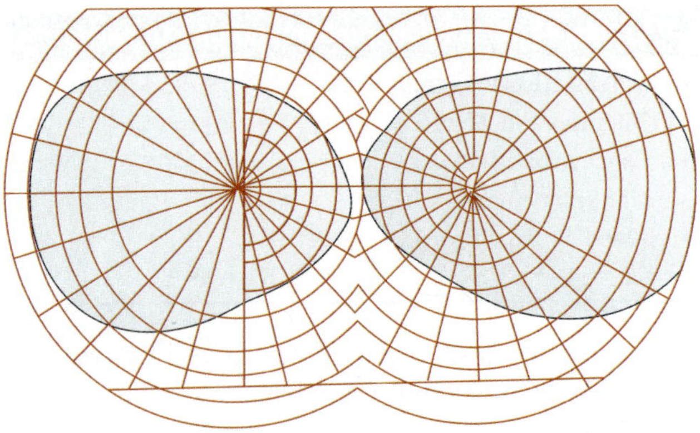

Fig. 44.6: Field charting in a patient with chiasmal injury shows bitemporal field cut

edema, it is probably rational to prescribe corticosteroid. Ten of my 15 patients[48] with chiasmal injury receive corticosteroid. In the past, several authors had explored the chiasma.[2,21,47] However, results were bad. One of Hughes'[2] patient had delayed onset visual loss, patient was operated, release of adhesion was carried out and the patient's vision improved. Hoper in 1951[21] had reported swollen chiasma at surgery.

Visual Outcome in Chiasmal Injury

Almost all patients develop varying grade of optic atrophy over a period of time. Walsh and Hoyt[3] reported a patient in whom vision improved. As the central field is retained patients can manage well. Recovery occurs over several weeks and the depth perception is regained. In my study[48] all the patients had some visual recovery. Two of my 3 patients with optochiasmal injury remain blind in one eye.

INJURY TO POSTERIOR VISUAL PATHWAY

Posterior visual pathway, is the portion distal to optic chiasma. Direct injury to these structures could result due to penetrating injury, either due to bullet or by splinters. However, rarely these structures can get involved in closed injury. Injury to posterior visual pathway occurs in patients with severe head injury.[1,3,8] Injury to optic tract, optic radiation and calcarine area is well studied in war injured patients. In closed head injury, optic tract, and optic radiation can get involved in contusion or intracerebral hematoma involving, temporal or parietal lobe. In patients with compression of posterior cerebral artery, however, many patients with transtentorial herniation may not survive.

The damage to optic tract, optic radiation and/or geniculate body is difficult to diagnose clinically in unconscious patients. In a statement Walsh and Hoyt in 1969[3] mentioned that they had not seen clinically any verifiable optic tract lesion following trauma. With the availability of CT scan, precise location of contusion and hematoma can be known. The survivors of these lesions do present with various types of homonymous hemianopia. Cortical blindness does occur with head injury and the outcome is unpredictable.

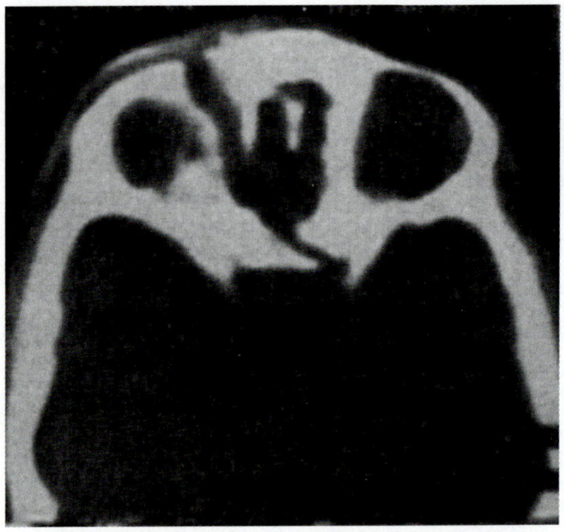

Fig. 44.7: MRI scan axial cut shows split chiasma in a patient with chiasmal injury

Monocular outcomes following severe ocular trauma are well described but little is known about effect of such injuries on binocular visual outcome. The visual field acuity did not predict the binocular outcome. A good monocular outcome does not necessarily result in satisfactory binocular visual outcome and a poor monocular visual outcome does not prevent severe binocular symptoms. A thorough orthoptic assessment is required in these cases for a good counseling regarding the risk involved in recovery.[49]

REFERENCES

1. Gijerris F. Traumatic lesions of visual pathway. In: Vinken PJ, Bruyn GW (Eds). Hand book of Clinical Neurology. North Holland Publishing Company, Amsterdam 1976; 24:27-57.
2. Hughes B. Indirect injury to the optic nerve and chiasma. Bull John Hopkin Hos 1962;111:98-126.
3. Walsh FB, Hyot WF. Involvement of optic nerve in closed head injury. In: Clinical Neuro-ophthalmology; 3rd edn, Baltimore, William and Wilkins Publishing Company 1969;3:2375-80.
4. Mahapatra AK, Bhatia R. Predictive value of visual evoked potential in unilateral optic nerve injury. Surg Neurol 1989;31:339-42.

5. Crompton MR. Visual lesion in head injury. Brain 1970;93:785-92.

5a. Mahapatra AK. Bilateral optic nerve injury. A series of 32 cases. Neurology India 1999;47:92-3.

6. Fukado Y. Result of 400 cases of surgical decompression of the optic nerve. Mod Prob Ophthalmol 1975;114:474-81.

7. Fukado Y. Microsurgical transethmoidal optic nerve decompression. Experience with 700 cases. In: The cranial nerve. Samii M, Jenetta P (Eds). Springer Verlag 1981;125-8.

8. Elisevich KV, Frod RM, Anderson DP, Strefoed JG, Richardson PM. Visual abnormalities with multiple trauma. Surg Neurol 1984;22:565-75.

9. Walsh FB. Trauma involving the anterior visual pathways. In: Ocular Trauma. HM Freeman (Ed) Appletion-Century Croft Publication, New York. 1979; pp 335-51.

10. Matsuzaki H, Kunita M, Kawai K. Optic nerve damage in head trauma. Clinical and experimental studies. Jpn J Ophthalmol 1982;26:447-61.

11. Mahapatra AK, Tandon DA. Optic nerve injury. A prospective study of 250 patients. In: Skull base anatomy, radiology and treatment. Samii M (Ed). S Karger, Basel, 1994;305-9.

12. Berlin R. Uber Seh storung nach verletzung des schadel dural stample gewalt. Ber Ophthal Ges 1979;2:9-14.

13. Battle WH. Some points relating to injuries of the head. Lancet 1890;11:57-60.

14. Callon DA. Four cases of orbital trauma. J Ame Med Assoc 1892;18:284.

15. Lowenstein A. Marginal haemorrhage on the disc. Partial tearing of the optic nerve. Clinical and histological features. Brit J Ophthalmol 1943;27:208-21.

16. Walsh FB, Lindenberg R. Die Verand ungeh ges schnervan loci indirect trauma, in Entwicklung ng sk urs tur. Augenarzte. Hamburg 1962, Ferdinand Enke Verlag.

17. Hedge TR, Gragoudas ES. Traumatic anterior ischaemic optic neuropathy. Annal of Ophthalmol 1981;13:625-8.

18. Mahapatra AK. Some more experience with optic nerve injury. Analysis of last 170 patients. In: Brain protection and Neural trauma. UK Khosla, et al (Ed). Norosa Publishing House, New Delhi 2000;269-74.

19. Bodian M. Transient loss of vision following head trauma. New York State J Med 1969;64:916-20.

20. Ramsey JH. Optic nerve injury in fracture of the canal. Brit J Ophthalmol 1979;63:607-10.

21. Hooper RS. Orbital complications of head injury. Brit J Surg 1951;39:126-38.

22. Pringle JH. Mono-ocular blindness following differential violence to the skull. Brit J Surg 1917;4:373.

23. Imachi J, Inoue K, Takahashi T. Clinical and ophthalmological investigations of optic nerve lesion in cases of head injuries. Jpn J Ophthalmol 1968;12:70-85.

24. Tandon DA, Thakar A, Mahapatra AK, Ghosh P. Transethmoidal optic nerve decompression. Clin Otolaryngol 1994;19:98-104.

25. Griffith JF, Dodge PR. Transient blindness following head injury in children. New Eng J Med 1968;278:648-51.

26. Mahapatra AK. Tandon DA, Bhatia R, Banerji AK. Optic nerve injury: A prospective study of 100 patients. Neurology India 1992;40:17-21.

26a. Agarwal A, Mahapatra AK. Outcome of patients with optic nerve injury with initial PL –ve. Indian J. Ophthalmol 1999;47:233-7.

27. Traquir HM, Dott NH, Russeu WR. Traumatic lesion of optic chiasma. Brain 1935;58:398-11.

28. Edmund J, Godtfredsen E. Unilateral optic nerve injury. Acta Ophthalmol 1963;41:693-97.

29. Anderson DP, Frod M. Visual abnormality after severe head injuries. Can J Surg 1980;23:163-65.

30. Grove AS Jr. Orbital trauma and computed tomography. Ophthalmology 1980;89:443-6.

31. Manfredi SJ, Raji MR, Sprinkle PM, et al. Computerized tomographic scan findings in facial fractures associated with blindness. Plast Recurrent 1981;68:479-90.

32. Joseph MP, Lessell S, Rizzo J, Momose KJ Extracranial optic nerve decompression for traumatic optic Neuropathy. Arch ophthalmol 1990;108:1091-3.

33. Wolin MJ, Lavin PJM. Spontaneous visual recovery from traumatic optic neuropathy after blunt head injury. Ame J Ophthalmol 1990;109:430-5.

34. Feinsod M, Auerbach E. Electrophysiological examination of visual system in the acute phase after head injury. European Neurol 1973;9:56-64.

35. Shaked A, Hadani M, Feinsod M. CT and VER follow-up of reversible vision with fracture optic canal. Acta Neurochir (Wien) 1982;62:91-94.

36. Nau HE, Gerhard L, Foerster M, Nacher HCH, Reinhardt V, Joka TH. Optic nerve trauma: Clinical electrophysiological and histological remarks. Acta Neurochir (Wien) 1987;89:16-27.

37. Mahapatra AK. Current management of optic nerve injury. In progress in clinical neurosciences. Venkataraman S, and Misra BK (Eds). Mediworld Publishing. Delhi 1997;12:241-54.

38. Fujitani T, Inoue K, Takahashi T, Ikushima K, Asai T. Indirect traumatic optic neuropathy. Visual outcome in operated and non-operated cases. Jpn J ophthalmol 1986;30:125-34.

39. Niho S, Yasuda K, Sato T, Sugita S, et al. Decompression of the optic canal by the transethmoidal route. Ame J Ophthalmol 1961;51:659-66.

40. Niho S, Niho M, Niho K. Decompression of the optic canal by the transethmoid route and decompression of superior orbital fissure. Can J Ophthalmol 1970;5: 22-40.
41. Lessell S. Indirect optic nerve trauma. Arch Ophthalmol 1989;107:382-6.
42. Naffziger HC Certain ear and eye affection in association with head injury. ophthal Rec 1916;25:502-08.
43. Karnik P. Optic nerve decompression. A new dimension of transethmoid surgery. Ind J otolaryngol 1986;10:48-51.
44. Sofferman RA. Sphenoethmoid approach to the optic nerve. Laryngoscope 1981;91:184-6.
45. Osguthorpe JD. Transethmoid decompression of the optic nerve. otolaryngol Clin North Arne 1985;18:125-37.
45a. Mahapatra AK. Delayed recovery from optic nerve injury. Report of two cases. J Neurosurgical Sciences 1992.
45b. Thakar A, Mahapatra AK. Tandon DA. Delayed optic nerve decompression for indirect optic nerve injury. Laryngoscope 2003;113:112-9.
46. Laursen AB. Traumatic bitemporal hemianopia. Acta Ophthalmol 1971;49:134-42.
47. Logan WC, Cordon DS. Traumatic lesions of the optic chiasma. Br J Ophthalmol 1973;51:258-60.
48. Mahapatra AK. Chiasmal injury—A study of 15 cases, Neuroscience today 1998;2:114-6.
49. Lam FC, Weir CR, Clearyh M; Binocularity in severe uniocular trauma, Strabismus 2008;16(2):71-5.

45 Growing Skull Fracture

AK Mahapatra, Raj Kumar

INTRODUCTION

Growing skull fracture is a rare complication of head injury, generally encountered in young children.[1-5] The condition is characterized by progressive enlargement of skull fracture over a period of time, manifesting as a visible or palpable cranial defect. Occasionally, overlying the defect there may be a scalp swelling. Surprisingly, only few large series are published in the literature.[5,6] Kingsley et al,[4] 1978 reported 10 cases from Sick Children Hospital in London. This condition was first described by Howship in 1816 (quoted by Lende and Erickson, 1961). Since, then large number of papers have been published in the literature on various aspects. Surprisingly there are only few publications from India.[5-11]

HISTORY

This condition was first described in 1816 by Howship. Subsequently this condition has been described in different heading by different authors. Traumatic leptomeningeal cyst is a term frequently used.[12-15] Other synonyms are, craniocerebral erosion and cerebrocranial erosion.[5,10,15,16] Bilroth in 1862[17] had termed this condition as meningocele spuria, while Godlee[18] in 1885 named it as cephal-hydrocele. Other names used for this condition are traumatic ventricular cyst[19] fibrosing osteitis, and craniomalacia.[8,20] The term "growing skull fracture" was originally used by Pia and Tonnis.[21] Recently, two terminologies have been used, one being expanding skull fracture[22] and evolutive fracture of the skull.[23]

Very little has been published on the histology. Probably Rokitaniky (quoted Lende and Erickson) was the first person to describe the histology. In 1987, Roy et al[10] described the detailed pathological changes in brain, bone and dura in 17 patients. From India, this condition has been reported by several authors. Rao and Subramanyam[8] had described this condition from India as early as 1963.

MECHANISM OF FORMATION OF GROWING SKULL FRACTURE

Mechanism of formation of this condition is not absolutely clear. However, it is only seen in infants and young children. The speed and morphology of evolution is variable.[5] By and large the time is between 4 to 6 weeks.

The popular concept on pathogenesis was first described by Taveras and Ransohoff.[14] They proposed the hypothesis, stating that the out pouching of arachnoid occurred through the dural laceration. The pulsation of brain is transmitted through the herniated arachnoid. The fluid enters into the arachnoid pouch. The adhesion acts as a unidirectional valve and fluid comes out. Thus, there is increase in fluid collection leading to cyst formation. The pulsation of brain and enlargement of cyst, gradually erode the bone edge leading to the enlargement of fracture and separation of dural edge more and more.

Lende and Erickson[1] did not observe the cyst in their modest series of 5 cases. They reported fibrotic bands and gliotic brain at surgery. Similar observations were made by Stein and Tenner in 1972.[3] They proposed that the cyst reported by other authors could be porencephalic cyst covered by a layer of gliosed brain.

The progressive damage to the brain and bone is not well understood. One of the possible factor leading to progressive brain damage could be interference with blood circulation. Falconer and Russell[27] in an experimental study attributed the circulatory disturbances in herniated brain leading to progressive brain damage. However, Holbourn[28] in 1944 postulated the brain damage due to stress and strain on the herniated brain. Gardner[29] presumed that the brain damage under a cranial defect could be due to altered blood flow to the part of the brain exposed to atmospheric pressure. Further, Tenner and Stein[30] observed encephalomalacia without any cyst formation. They demonstrated angiographically slow circulation due to vascular compression at the edge of bone defect. They hypothesized that the exposure of the injured brain tissue unprotected by dura, is an important cause for progressive gliosis. Gugliantini et al[31] postulated the possibility of the cyst compressing on the brain damage surface leading to progressive atrophy. Ischemic necrosis was reported in two cases by Roy et al,[10] supporting the possibility of the vascular obstruction.

Fodstal et al in 1984[32] had reviewed all the theories proposing brain damage in skull defect, the term is coined as "Syndrome of Trephined". They studied fluid dynamic in patients with skull defect and shown, cranioplasty can correct abnormal fluid dynamics to some extent.

Rarely, leptomeningeal cyst can grow in between two tables of the skull giving rise to an intradiploic cyst.[26,33,35,36] It is a rare situation and patients present with bony swelling. Mahapatra and Tandon[26] reported eight such cases. Almeida and King[36] reported, small dural tear leading to arachnoid bleb, which secretes CSF into intraosseous cyst.

PATHOLOGY

A skull fracture which continues to enlarge over a period of time is called growing skull fracture and is noticed exclusively in infants and children below 3 years of age.[37] The incidence in one study was reported to be 6 percent of all skull fractures.[37] Most common site is frontoparietal area.[5,6,37] Roekitansky in 1856 described the pathological changes. However, only scanty literature is available on microscopic pathology on this condition.[10] Lack of detailed pathological studies have led to unsatisfactory and wrong nomenclatures. Roy et al[10] reported detailed pathological changes in 17 patients.

Pathological changes are seen in skull, dura, leptomeninges and brain. Changes in bones are obvious at surgery. Grossly the edges of the fracture look ragged scalloped. In some cases, the cyst may be intradiploic expanding diploic space and thining out the outer table. There may be loculated intradiploic cysts, or posterior fossa intradiploic cyst.[10,26,33,34] Microscopic examination of the bone reveals necrotic bone even after several months after injury indicating progressive osteolysis.[10] Rarely, osteoblastic activity with formation of new bone may be observed.

Changes in meninges include both dura and leptomeninges. Generally bone covering the dura edge and dural defect is much larger than the bone defect. Probably fibrosis in dura pulls the dura away from the bone edge. Microscopically dura is thickened and hyalinied. Invariably some degree of chronic inflammation is always noticed. Rarely islands of gliosed brain may be embedded in dura and leptomeninges. Pia and arachnoid show thickening and foci of chronic inflammation with proliferating capillaries. At places, leptomeninges are adherent to the dura. The leptomeninges are also adherent to gliosed brain. In some cases island of gliosed brain may be embedded in thickened arachnoid.[10]

Changes in brain show both superficial and deeper involvement. There is varing degree of fibroglial cicatrix. There are areas of recent necrosis and accumulation of compound granular corpuscles and foci of reactive astrocytosis. Invariably, cyst of varing sizes surrounded by gliosed brain are noticed in histology. Sometimes, iron encrustation of neurons are also observed.

Overall, pathological changes show evidence of old and new changes. The changes indicate progressive damage. The case of progressive damage is not well understood.[4] Probably, most important cause of progressive damage is interference with blood circulation.[27,30] In general important factors are: (a) outward driving force, (b) rapidly enlarging brain, (c) hydrocephalus, and (d) brain edema.[34,38,39]

Association of growing skull fracture in childhood are hydrocephalus, encephalomalacia, leptomeningeal cyst, brain tissue herniation and ipsilateral ventricular dilation, the patients under age 3 years with diastatic fracture and dural tear are more prone to develop growing skull fracture.[51]

PRESENTATION

This is a condition generally observed in the infants and young children.[1,3,5-7] In the series reported by Tandon et al[5] only 4 out of 60 patients were more than 4 years. The initial injury occurs in half of the cases around 1 year of age and in 90 percent injury occurs before 3 years of age. One of the patients in Matson's[24] series was 12 years old and remaining 16 cases had a mean age of 10.1/2 months. The oldest patient reported by Tandon et al[5] was 9 years old. Moss et al[25] had reported a case of growing skull fracture in a fetus. The usual time gap between injury and noticeable gap is around 4 to 6 weeks. However, by the time they present to the neurosurgeon may be much longer. In the series reported by Mahapatra[6] only 10 patients reported within 4 weeks of injury, and 37 patients reported within 6 months. Twenty-one patients reported for surgery after 1 year and among them 7 cases after 2 years (Table 45.1). The occurrence of this condition in early childhood points to two facts: (a) dura is densely attached to bone, and (b) head grows at a rapid rate.

Table 45.1: Growing skull fracture analysis of 80 cases treated at AIIMS showing duration between injury and admission

Time gap	*Numbers*
• Less than 1 month	10
• One month to 3 months	12
• More than 3 to 6 months	15
• Six months to 1 year	22
• 1 – 2 years	14
• More than 2 years	7

Most important and frequent feature is the scalp swelling[1,5,11] overlying the fracture, aspiration usually reveals CSF mixed with necrotic brain tissue. In a large number of cases the initial scalp swelling may subside.

Other clinical features are focal or generalized seizure, recorded in a large number of patients.[4-6,15,16] In a series, reported by Tandon et al[5] 50 percent had history of seizures. In a study of 80 patients Mahapatra[6] in 1995 reported seizure in 38 patients. Infrequently, patients may come with intractable seizure.[5] Focal motor deficits, in form of hemiparesis and monoparesis is very common[5,6] and reported over 80 percent (Table 45.2).

On the basis of clinical features the patients can be divided into three groups:[5] (a) patients with associated subgaleal cyst collection, (b) patients with no cystic scalp collection, but the skin is sunken over the bone defect and pulsation of brain could be observed, (c) patients with intradiploic cyst present with a bony swelling.[5,26,34,36] Rarely, patients complain of pain or discomfort at the site of bone defect. Rarely growing fracture can involve roof of the orbit and progressive proptosis.[6a]

The natural history of this condition is not clear. Initially there is a rapid progression. In some children the defect reaches a large size within a short period. Rapid progress is then followed by slower progress or even stability. Progressive hemiparesis indicates progressive brain damage.[5,6,9] Histological changes also indicate progressive brain damage.[10] However, it is unlikely that the condition spontaneously improves with resolution of swelling and decrease in skull defect.

Table 45.2: Clinical features in 80 cases

Clinical features	*Numbers*
• Cranial defect	72
• Cranial defect with bony swelling	8
• Focal or generalized	38
• Hemiparesis or monoparesis	60
• Scalp collection	15
• Proptosis	2

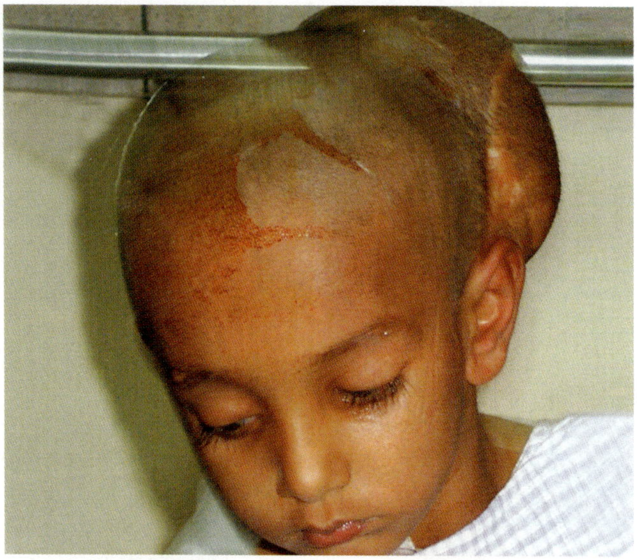

Fig. 45.1: Clinical print of a child showing large growing skull fracture. A scar of previous head injury can be seen

Growing skull fracture of anterior skull base is extremely rare. Post-traumatic pseudomeningocele or encephalocele are the part of growing skull fracture in these cases (Fig. 45.1).[50]

INVESTIGATIONS

Diagnosis of growing skull fracture is easy, and always made in a clinical ground. Investigations are directed to establish the size of the cranial defect and extent of underlying brain damage.[5,6,14,33,37] The plain X-ray skull is an important investigation (Table 45.3). Skull X-ray shows a characteristic irregular to elliptical skull defect with tapering ends.[5,12-14] The margins are sclerotic, scaloped and everted. The outer table is less affected than the inner table. Rarely, skull X-ray shows expansion of diploi.[5,26,33]

Table 45.3: Radiological findings in 80 patients

Findings	*No. of cases*
Progressive bone defect	72
Scalloping of bone edges	40
Expansion of diploic space	7
Bony swelling	7
Enlarged orbit	2

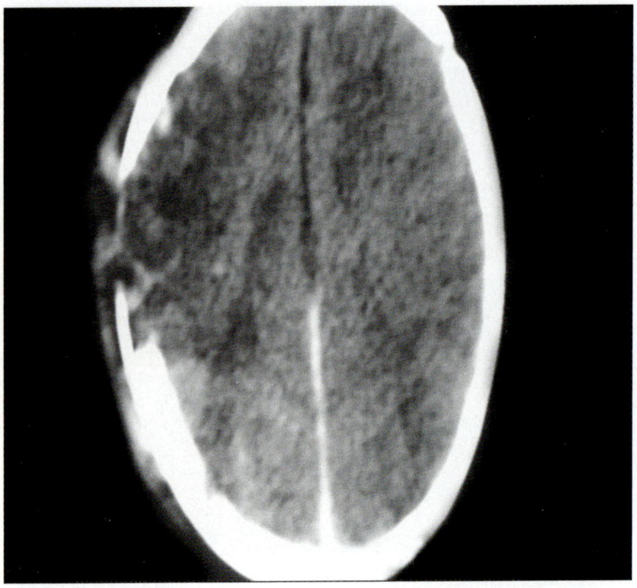

Fig. 45.2: Begining of growing skull fracture

Many investigations described in the past, such as carotid angiography,[30] pneumoencephalography[1,3-5] and RIHSA cisternography[5,40-42] are no more used as investigative modalities today. Recently, CT scan and MRI scans are routinely used to delineate the underlying brain damage.[5,6,26,33,37]

Recently, CT scans have been used.[5,6,31,33,37,43] CT scan reveals the brain damage, hydrocephalus and porencephalic cyst (Figs 45.2 to 45.4).[5,6,11,37] Amongst 80 cases reported by Mahapatra[6,45] patients had a CT scan (Table 45.4). CT scan reveals gliosed brain pulling

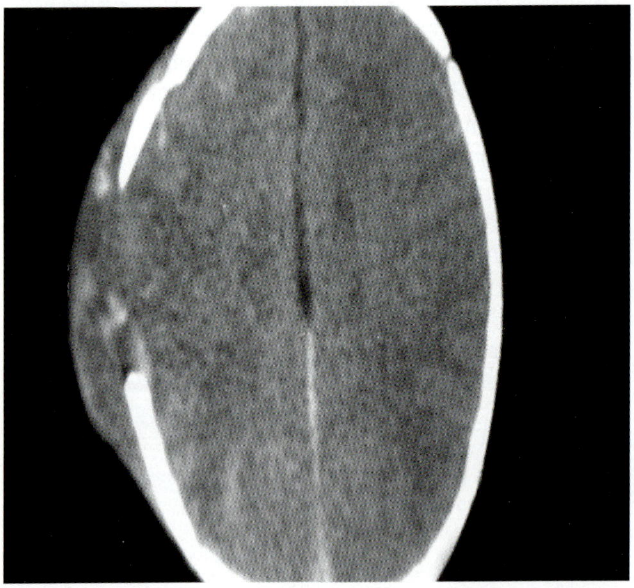

Fig. 45.3: CT showing growing skull fracture a month following trauma

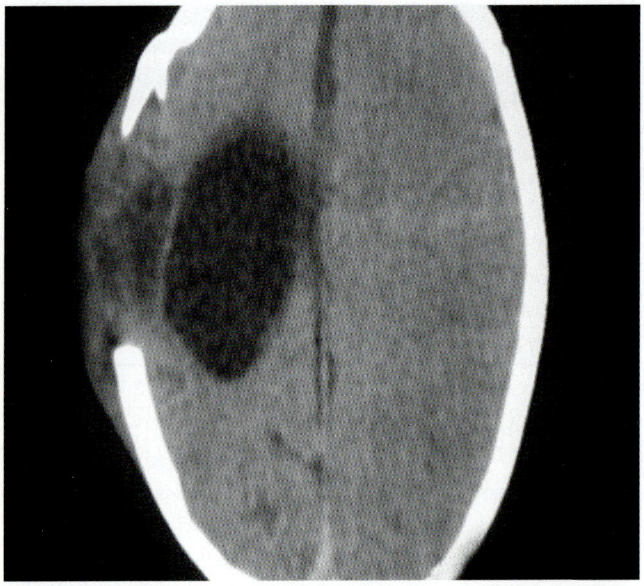

Fig. 45.4: CT of a child showing growing skull fracture of right frontoparietal bone along with adjacent encephalomalacia

of ventricle, ventriculomegaly and hydrocephalus.[5,6] In a small number of cases with intradiploic cyst, CT scan can show cyst break in inner tables.[5,26,33,34] MRI provides the best delineation of the brain and CSF changes,[11,33] however, MRI provides little information on bony changes.

Treatment of Growing Skull Fracture

The aim of the treatment of growing skull fracture is to prevent progressive brain damage and treatment of epilepsy. There is general agreement that growing skull fracture needs surgical treatment. The aim is to repair bone and dura defect.[1,3,5,6] Delay in repair may lead to progressive damage.[5,10] Hence, early surgical intervention is an important fact.

As incidence of epilepsy is high, there is a need for prophylactic anticonvulsant.[5,6,15,16] Most of the patients who developed epilepsy do so within 2 years of injury. Surgery does not prevent epilepsy, however, surgical excision of gliosed brain may reduce epileptic attacks.[1,5]

Table 45.4: CT scan finding patients in 45

Findings	*No. of cases*
Bone defect	45
Underlying cyst	45
Hydrocephalus	10
Ipsilateral ventricular enlargement	15
Intradiploic cyst	7
Orbital pseudomeningocele	2

The indications for early surgery is: (a) scalp swelling, (b) rapid and progressive hemiparesis and (c) intractable epilepsy. In such a situation excision of gliosed brain and repair of the dural defect is undertaken. A small number of cases of bony defect may be small and nonprogressive, hence surgery may not be indicated.

The usual findings at the surgery 10 are: (a) edge of fracture is scalloped, and inner table is invariably more affected than outer table, (b) dural defect is much larger than bone defect, (c) brain underlying dura defect is damaged, necrotic and gliosed, (d) occasionally, there may be porencephalic cyst and (e) gap between bone edges are occupied by fibroglial scar. For getting to the dural edges, nibbling of bone edges is necessary or there is a need for elevating a large bone flap around the bone defect. The flap is likely to expose the entire dura defect.[5] Dura is usually covered by a large pericranial, or temporalis fascia graft.

Generally, cranial defects are repaired by simultaneous cranioplasty.[1,5,6,11,44] Ribs, outer table graft and methyl methacrylate is usually used for covering the bone defect.[5,6,33,37,44] In the past-tantalum plates were used for cranioplasty.[1,29,45] In a study of 80 patients[6] of growing skull fracture, 3 patients had outer table graft and 9 had Tantalum plate cranioplasty. Methyl methacrylate (MMA) is sometimes used for cranioplasty.[6,46-48] In a study dealing with 80 patients, Mahapatra[6] had reported MMA cranioplasty in 25 patients (Table 45.5). However, 3 patients required removal of the MMA plate between 1 to 3 years. Hayashi et al[48] reported long-term follow-up in a child with MMA cranioplasty.

For large skull defects in infants which cannot be repaired by autologous graft an alternative technique can be used. A cranioplasty by interposing a titanium plate between duraplasty and bone elements without fixation with autologous bone fragments deposited over the mesh can be used. It includes osteogenesis in a growing cranial skeleton, and provides satisfactory esthetic result.[52]

Table 45.5: Material used for cranioplasty experience at AIIMS

	Numbers
Rib	43
Methyl methacrylate	25
Tantalum plate	9
Outer table of skull	3

Hydrocephalus is not a usual association with growing skull fracture. Mahapatra[6] had reported CT evidence of hydrocephalus in 10 patients. Patients with hydrocephalus need VP shunt[6,39] prior to surgery. The shunt surgery would prevent CSF leak and reduce the chance of infection.

CONCLUSION

Growing skull fracture is a rare condition and usually encountered in children under 3 years of age. Progressive neurological deficit and seizure and usual symptoms along with cranial defect and scalp swelling. Surgery is aimed to prevent brain damage and reduce the chance of epilepsy. Duraplasty and cranioplasty are the procedures undertaken during surgery.

REFERENCES

1. Lende RA, Erickson RC. Growing skull fracture of childhood. J Neurosurg 1961;18:479-89.
2. Lende RA. Enlarging skull fractures of childhood. Neuroradiol 1974;7:119-24.
3. Stein BM, Tenner MS. Enlargement of skull fracture in childhood due to cerebral herniation. Arch Neurol 1972;26:137-43.
4. Kingsley D, Till K, Hoare R. Growing fracture of the skull. J Neurol Neurosurg Psychiat 1978;41:312-18.
5. Tandon PN, Banerji AK, Bhatia R, Goulatia RK. Craniocerebral erosion (Growing fracture of the skull in children) Part II. Clinical and Radiological observations. Acta Neurochir (Wien) 1987;88:1-9.
6. Mahapatra AK. Growing fracture skull. An experience of 80 cases. Neurology India (Suppl) 1995;43:158.

6a. Suri A, Mahapatra AK. Growing fracture of the orbital roof. Pediatric Neurosurg 2002;36:96-100.

7. Banerji AK, Tandon PN. Craniocerebral erosion and post-traumatic meningocele. Neurology India 1967;15:29-32.
8. Rao BD, Subramanyam MV. Traumatic Malacia of bone in skull fracture of the childhood. Ind J Surg 1963;25:641-730.
9. Ramamurthi B, Kalyanaraman S. Rationale of surgery in growing fracture of the skull. J Neurosurg 1970;32: 427-30.
10. Roy S, Sarkar C, Tandon PN, Banerji AK. Craniocerebral erosion (growing fracture skull in children) Part I Pathology. Acta Neurochir (Wien) 1987;87:112-8.
11. Das L, Iyengar B. Craniocerebral erosion. Neurology India (Suppl) 1995;43:80-130.
12. Ducke CG. The roentgen-ray diagnosis and treatment of disease of the skull and intracranial content. In: Golden (Ed). Diagnostic roentgenology. Vol I Williams and Wilkins, Baltimore 1936;1-34.
13. Schwartz CW. Leptomeningeal cyst from a roentgenological view point. Ame J Roentgenol 1941;46:160-5.
14. Tavaras JM, Ransohoff J. Leptomeningeal cyst of the brain following trauma with erosion of the skull. A

study of seven cases treated by surgery. J Neurosurg 1953;10:233-41.
15. Penfield WP, Erickson TC. Epilepsy and cerebral localisation. Ch C. Thomas, Springer field III 1941;623.
16. Penfield WP, Jasper H. Epilepsy and function anatomy of the brain. Little Brown & Co. Boston 1954;896.
17. Billroth T (1862) quoted by Lende and Erickson 1961.
18. Godlee RJ (1885) quoted by Lende and Erickson in 1961.
19. Trolter W (1923) quoted by Lende and Erickson.
20. Pencoast HK, Pendergrass EP, Schaeffer JP. The head and neck in roentgendiagnosis. Ch C Thomas Springer field III 1940;976.
21. Pia HW, Tonnis W. Die wachsende schadelfraktur des kindesalters. Zentralbl Neurocir 1953;13:1-23.
22. Addy DP. Expanding skull fracture of childhood. Brit Med J 1973;4:338-39.
23. Kabre A, Soumare A, Badiane SB, et al. Evolutive fracture of the skull. Dakar Med 1991;36:88-93.
24. Matson DD. Neurosurgery of Infancy and childhood 2nd edn, Springfield, Charle C. Thomas 1969.
25. Moss SD, Walker ML, Ostergards S, et al. Intrauterine growing skull fracture. Child's Nervs System 1991.
26. Mahapatra AK, Tandon PN. Post-traumatic intradiploic pseudomeningocele in children. Acta Neurochir 1989;100: 120-26.
27. Falconer MA, Russell DS. Experimental traumatic cerebral cysts in the rabbit. J Neurosurg 1944;1:182-89.
28. Holbourn AHS. The mechanism of trauma with special reference to herniation of cerebral tissue. J Neurosurg 1944;1:190-200.
29. Gardner WJ. Closure of defects of the skull with tantallum. Surg Gynae Obstat 1945;80:30-312.
30. Tenner MS, Stein BM. Cerebral herniation in the growing fracture of the skull. Radiol 1970;94:351-85.
31. Gugliantini P, Caione P, Pariello G, Rivosecchi M. Post-traumatic leptomeningeal cyst in infancy. Ped Radiol 1980;9:11-14.
32. Fodstad H, Love JA, Ekstedt J, et al. Effect of cranioplasty in fluid hydrodynamics in patients with syndrome of the trephined. Acta Neurochir (Wien) 1984;70:21-30.
33. Martinez-Lange JF, Percez MM, Domingo R, et al. Post-traumatic intradiploic arachnoid cyst of the posterior fossa. Child's Nervs Syst 1997;13:293-6.
34. Patil AA, Etemadrezaie H. Post-traumatic intradiploic meningo encephalocele. Case report. J Neurosurg 1996; 84:284-7.
35. Weinards ME, Rengachary SS, McGregar DH, et al. Intradiploic arachnoid cyst. Report of two cases. J Neurosurg 1989;70:954-8.
36. Almeida ACG, King RB. Intradiploic. Cerebrospinal fluid fistula. Report of two cases. J Neurosurg 1981;54:84-8.
37. Muhonen NG, Piper JG, Menezes AH. Pathogenesis and treatment of growing skull fracture. Surg Neurol 1995;43:367-73.
38. Winston K, Beahy RM, Fischer EG. Consequence of dural defects acquired in infancy. J Neurosurg 1983;59:831-46.
39. Sharma RR, Chandy MJ. Shunt surgery in growing skull fractures. Report of two cases. Br J Neurosur 1991;5:93-8.
40. Tandon PN, Rao MAP, Basu AK, et al. 131 I RIHSA CSF scanning in paediatric neurosurgical practice. Neuro-radiol 1974;7:119-23.
41. Tandon PN, Rao MAP, Pathak SN, et al. Radioisotope scanning of cerebrospinal fluid pathways. Ind J Med Res 1974;62:281-9.
42. Front D, Minderhood JM, Beks JWF, Penning L. Leptomeningeal cysts diagnosed by isotope cisternography. J Neurol Neurosurg Psychiat 1973;36:1018-23.
43. Lye RH, Occleshaw JV, Dutton J. Growing fracture of the skull and role of computerized tomography. Case report. J Neurosurg 1981;55:470-2.
44. Longache JJ, Destefanr GA. Further observation of the behaviour of autogenous split rib grafts in reconstructions of extensive defect of the cranium and face. Plat Reconstruct Surg 1957;20:281-96.
45. Milhorat TH. Paediatric Neurosurgery. Davis. Philadelphia 1978;56-7.
46. Arseni C, Liurea AV. Clinico-therapeutic aspects in growing skull fracture. A review of the literature. Child's Brain 1981;8:161-72.
47. Scraff TB, Fine M. Growing skull fractures of childhood. In: Wilkins RH, Rengachary SS (Eds). Neurosurg Vol 2, McGraw-Hill New York 1985;1627-8.
48. Hayashi Y, Yamaki T, Odake G, et al. Long-term follow-up of a growing fracture treated by dura and cranioplasty with artificial dura mater and methylmethacrylate. Child's Nervs Syst 1997;13:349-51.
49. Milhorat TH. Paediatric Neurosurgery. Davis. Philadelphia 1978;56-7.
50. Naqata C, Katsuta T, Kenjo M, et al. Growing skull base fracture. A case report with special reference to its pathogenesis Brain Nerve 2007;59(11):1293-7.
51. Mierez R, Guillen A, Brell M, Cardona E, et al. Growing skull fracture in childhood, presentation of 12 cases. Neurocirugia (Astur) 2003;14(3):228-33.
52. Vignes JR, Jeelani NO, Dautheribes M, Sangalli F, Liquoro D: Cranioplasty for repair of large bone defect in growing skull fracture in children. J Craniomaxillofac Surg 2007;35(3):185-8.

46 Traumatic Subarachnoid Hemorrhage

AK Mahapatra, Raj Kumar, Raj Kamal

INTRODUCTION

Traumatic subarachnoid hemorrhage (TSAH) was first described by Wilkin in 1859.[1] In his autopsy study, in patients with head injury, he found hemorrhagic CSF, which he described as "Sanguineous meningeal effusion" in subarachnoid space. Surprisingly, however, till recently there have been only a few studies on traumatic SAH. Prior to the advent of CT scan antemortem diagnosis of SAH in head injury was difficult, except lumbar puncture. With the CT scan TSAH emerged as an important issue (Figs 46.1 and 46.2). Medicolegal reports frequently mention SAH in fatal head injury.[2-7] SAH associated with minor head injuries of medicolegal implication, as it is difficult to establish with certainty that SAH found at autopsy is traumatic and not spontaneous in origin.

The development of hydrocephalus in patients with head injuries were considered as delayed sequelae of traumatic SAH, due to obstruction of CSF pathways (Fig. 46.2).[8] Similarly, acute blockage of CSF pathways leads to early hydrocephalus which present acutely.[9,10] This chapter provides a bird's eye view on TSAH, realising the role of SAH in head injury management and outcome.

INCIDENCE

The exact incidence of SAH in head injury is not clear. Courville[4] in 1950, base of a series of 40,000 autopsies reported SAH as the most common intracranial pathology following head injury. Similar observations were also made by Freytag[12] in 1963, in an autopsy study on 1367 head injury deaths. Surprisingly, no large clinical study was available prior to 1990, when Eisenberg et al,[21] reported a 39 percent incidence of TSAH, in 753 patients, based on their CT scan finding, Chesnut et al[9] in 1993 reported an incidence as high as 44 percent. However, a wide range (2.44%) of TSAH is reported in the world literature[9,12-15] (Table 46.1).

PATHOLOGY

It appears that the exact mechanism of TSAH is not clear. It is highly likely that multiple mechanisms are involved in traumatic SAH. Rupture of a coincidental aneurysm (Figs 46.3 to 46.5) is proposed by several authors.[7,17-19] Lock-sley,[19] in 1966 in a cooperative study reported, 3 percent of aneurysmal (Fig. 46.6) SAH had history of head trauma preceding the SAH. Simonsen[20] reported aneurysm in 28 percent of cases of TSAH. Simonsen[20] could not demonstrate site of bleed in his autopsy study dealing with 430 cases of TSAH.

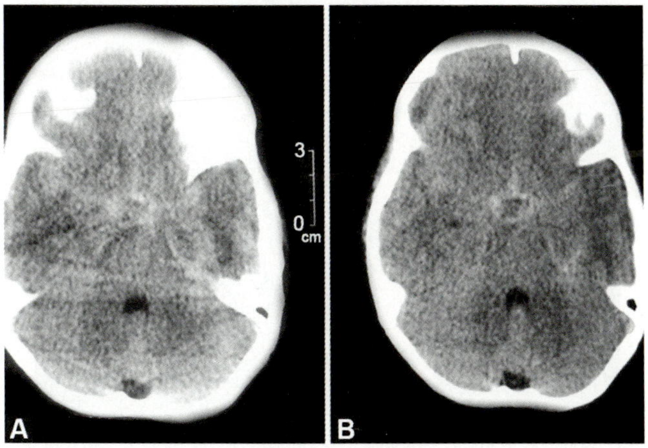

Figs 46.1A and B: CT showing post-traumatic suprasellar bleed; patient developed diabetes insipidus

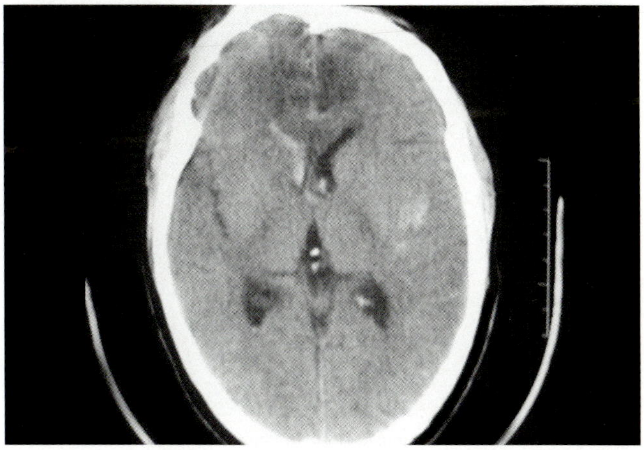

Fig. 46.2: CT of patient showing small bleed in right frontal horn

Table 46.1: Incidence of traumatic SAH

Authors	*Year*	*No. of cases*	*% TSAH*
1. De villasante and Taveras	1976	100	2
2. Takizawa et al	1984	197	12
3. Kobayashi et al	1988	414	23
4. Eisenberg et al	1990	753	39
5. Chesnut et al	1993	American Traumatic Data Bank	44

Traumatic rupture of intracranial arteries and bridging veins, identified at autopsy are also presumed to be the case of TSAH.[5,11,17] Newbarr and Courville[18] hypothesized tearing of superior cerebral veins at their entry point in superior sagittal sinus, as the site or origin of bleeding during displacement of brain following impact. Rupture of vessel in the pia-arachnoid is thought to occur during brain movement under the dura mater. TSAH is also reported in posterior fossa from rupture of the arteries of the posterior cranial fossa. Freytag[12] in 1963 reported SAH in head injured patients due to venous rupture. Thin walled veins are more liable to rupture than rupture of thick walled arteries. Overall it looks that TSAH can result in various ways from different sources. Prognosis is poor in patients with poor admission GCS scores, cisternal or fissural hemorrhage, tSAH with cerebral contusion or acute subdural hematomas.[56]

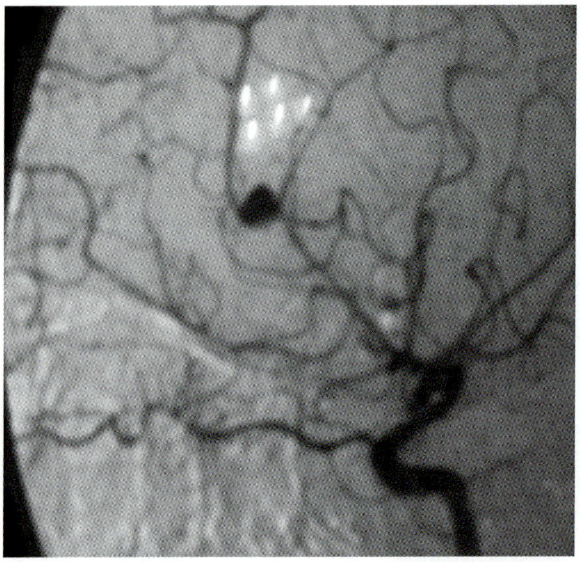

Fig. 46.3: DSA showing distal anterior cerebral artery (DACA) aneurysm

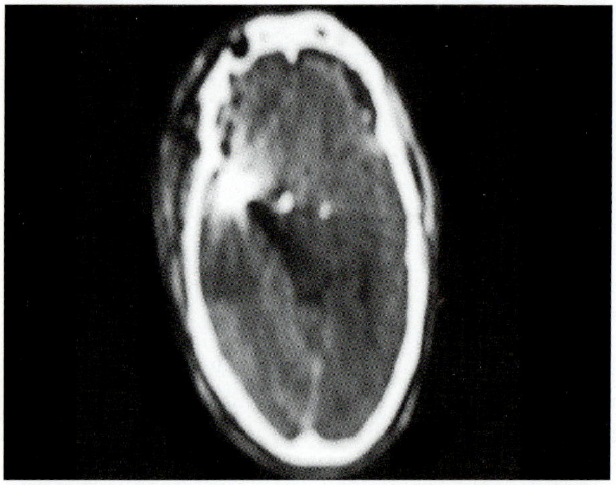

Fig. 46.4: Postoperative CT of clipped DACA aneurysm

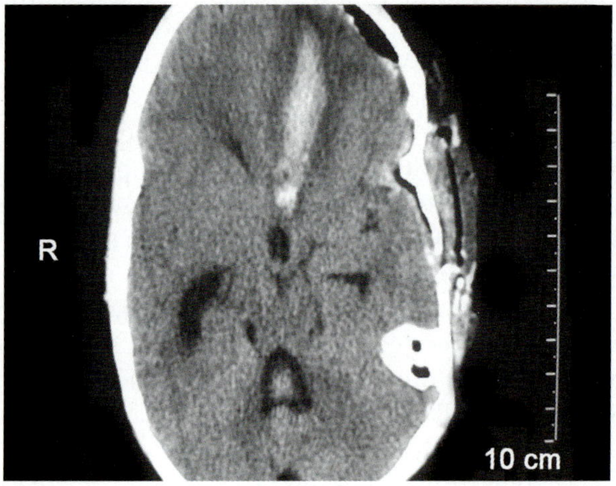

Fig. 46.5: Preoperative CT of suspected post-traumatic aneurysm

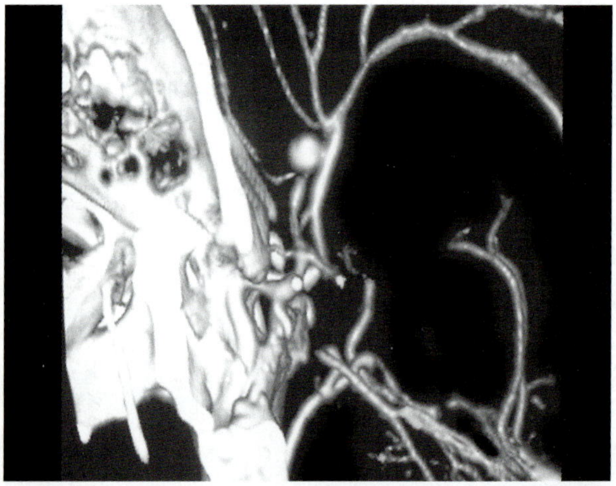

Fig. 46.6: CT angio showing A2 segment aneurysm (suspected post-traumatic), which was sucked during surgery, could be repaired with difficulty

Table 46.2: Age in traumatic SAH

	Mean age in years
1. Mean age	46 (Kakarieka 1)
2. Extensive SAH	47
3. Moderate SAH	42
4. Mild SAH	38

Table 46.3: Localization of TSAH

Sites	Percent
1. Convexity	65–70
2. Fissures-Sylvian-Interhemispheric	40–45
3. Basal cisterns	10–25
4. Tentorial edge	15–20

DEMOGRAPHIC ASPECT OF TSAH

Only a few reports are available dealing with demographic pattern of TSAH.[15,20-22] Kakarieka et al[23] in 1994 reported demographic and clinical aspect of both SAH and traumatic SAH. They reported TSAH on average 8 years older than spontaneous SAH. Mean age of their patient was 46 years. Sixty-nine percent of spontaneous SAH were below 40 years of age, women were older than men in TSAH. Incidence of TSAH increases with age[11,19] (Table 46.2). This is probably due to identification of bleed in enlarged subarachnoid space.

Alcohol intake prior to injury predisposed SAH. A strong correlation has been reported severe SAH after head injury.[2,13,23,24] In one of the study on TSAH 23 percent of patients were under the influence of alcohol. An incidence ranging from 23 to 80 percent[2,13,25] is reported in TSAH.

GRADING

Traumatic SAH (Fig. 46.7) frequently occurs in patients of TBI, but it is difficult to detect and grade. TSAH is associated with more severe CT findings and worse outcome.[54]

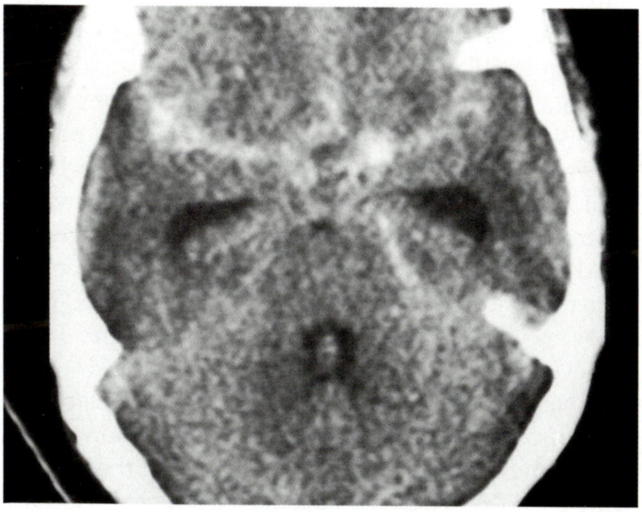

Fig. 46.7: CT showing post-traumatic subarachnoid hemorrhage

The degree of subarachnoid hemorrhage also directly influences the outcome. Patients with dilated subarachnoid space tends to collect larger amount of subarachnoid blood. Grading also becomes difficult when 1st CT is performed several days later. Brain swelling and development of contusion or hematomas tends to cause disappearance of SAH (Fig. 46.7). Grading of SAH is done in several ways.[26,27] Hijdra et al[28] scored the SAH 0-48 and average amount of blood seen in CT scan after head injury scores 10 points, while Fisher et al[27] in 1980 classified SAH from grade 1 to 4 depending on the amount of blood on CT scan. Most of the patients with TSAH were on grades 2 to 3 Fishers grading. Grade 4 TSAH is relatively rare.

LOCALIZATION (TABLE 46.3)

Convexity is the most frequent site for traumatic SAH, recorded in 70 percent in first CT scan followed by Sylvian fissure and interhemispheric fissure in around 40 to 45 percent cases. Basal cisternal blood is recorded less frequently. Bleeding into quadrigeminal cistern is most infrequent. Blood can also be seen around the tentorial edge, which is seen as hyperdense image outlining tentorium area in CT scans, indicating presence of SAH.

CLEARANCE

Clearance of TSAH depends on the amount of blood seen in initial scan. In TSAH clearance blood is faster than that described in aneurysmal SAH.[29] There are two reasons for the above observations: (a) SAH tends to be moving in aneurysmal bleed, and (b) In aneurysm rebleed can occur. Rapid clearance of blood in patients of TSAH is reported by Kakarieka 1996.[30] Reduction of subarachnoid blood to 50 percent was noticed after 2 days of initial CT and 33 percent after 3 days of initial CT scan.

VASOSPASM IN HEAD INJURY AND TSAH

Post-traumatic angiographic vasospasm was first described by Lohr in 1936. However, the correlation between TSAH and arterial spasm was reported in mid 60s.[30-33] The incidence varies from 5 to 90 percent. Leeds et al[32] 1966, reported angiographic vasospasm in 31 percent of 39 head injury patients. Wilkins and Odom[33] reported arterial spasm in 5 percent of patients with significant head injuries. They also found hemorrhagic CSF in spinal fluid and suggested pathogenesis of ischemia similar to that of spontaneous SAH. Suwanwela and Suwanwela[34] reported 19 percent incidence of angiographic vasospasm in head injured patients. Neurological deficit is related to TSAH and vasospasm.[34-37] Hence, TSAH, leading to vasospasm and ischemia play important role in morbidity and mortality in patients with head injury.

TRANSCRANIAL DOPPLER IN TSAH

Over last decade, TCD is available for the non-invasive evaluation of cerebral vasospasm. It is also hypothesized that the pathogenesis of vasospasm in SAH and TSAH are same. Vasospasm, as detected by TCD is reported in more than 40 to 68 percent of severe head injury patients.[37,44] Comptom and Teddy[38] reported 68 percent vasospasm in 25 patients with severe head injury. They also reported good correlation between vasospasm and clinical deterioration. Similar correlation was also observed by other authors.[40,41] Dorsch and Zurynski, reported 50 percent vasospasm in their severe head injured patients and reported a higher mortality in those patients. However, a varied correlation is reported between degree of subarachnoid blood, BFV (Blood Flow Velocity) and clinical outcome.[42-44]

ROLE OF CALCIUM CHANNEL BLOCKER IN TSAH

Recently calcium channel blocker has been used as a neuroprotective agent in preventing secondary brain damage. Most extensively tried calcium antagonist is nimodipine. Nimodipine has also been used in severe head injured patients,[45-48] to effectively block calcium channel and prevent ischemic damage. The results of above studies were inconclusive. Nimodipine did not improve the overall outcome in patients with severe head injury. However, in patients with TSAH there was a significantly reduced poor outcome in patients treated with nimodipine.[22,46] In a study reported by Bailey et al,[45] 352 severely injured patients were treated by intravenous nimodipine or placebo for one week. The overall outcome were similar at six months follow-up. In HIT II-study 852 patients were enrolled. Result did not favor routine use of nimodipine in severe head injured patients. The study showed improvement of favorable outcome from 59 to 61 percent and reduction of mortality from 24 to 22 percent.

In a study involving 654 patients, 210 had TSAH. Nimodipine in patients with TSAH significantly reduced the mortality and unfavorable outcome. Unfavorable outcome was recorded in 51 and 66 percent in patients with nimodipine and placebo group respectively. The incidence of post-traumatic epilepsy was lower in survivors who received nimodipine than in those who did not receive nimodipine[48,49] (03% vs 20%). Overall, nimodipine is safe and is well tolerated in patients. There is a small risk of fall in blood pressure. However, the beneficial role of nimodipine in TSAH outweigh the risk caused by drop in blood pressure.

TRAUMATIC SUBARACHNOID HEMORRHAGE AND OUTCOME

Traumatic SAH is one of the important factors influencing the overall outcome in head injured patients. The mortality is 2 to 3 times higher in patients with TSAH than those without SAH in CT scan. Eisenberg et al[22] in 1990 reported mortality among TSAH patients twice as high as in no SAH patients. In patients with TSAH unfavorable outcome is reported in 60 to 70 percent cases. TSAH patients with mild head injury showed a higher incidence of unfavorable outcome than mild head injury without SAH.[50-53] Demircivi et al[14] in 1993 had shown good outcome in the majority of cases with mild head injury despite of having TSAH in CT scan.

The outcome of patients with TSAH is directly related to clinical state and amount of subarachnoid blood seen on the first CT scan. The patients with greater amount of subarachnoid blood have a worse outcome. Patients with basal cistern SAH had poorer outcome than those who had blood found over the cerebral hemisphere.

Data from European brain injury consortium survey on head injuries revealed that 41 percent patients exhibited evidence of traumatic subarachnoid hemorrhage (TSAH) on admission CT scan. There was a strong, statistically significant association between TSAH and poor outcomes. Forty-one percent of patients without TSAH achieved the level of good recovery, while only 15 percent of patients with TSAH achieved this outcome. Patients with TSAH were significantly older (medium age 32 yr) and there was a significant tendency with TSAH to exhibit lower GCS at the time of admission. The death among the patients with TSAH is related to severity of initial mechanical damage rather than to the effects of delayed vasospasm and secondary ischemic brain damage.[55]

Table 46.4: Risk factors in TSAH

	High-risks	*Low-risks*
1.	Elderly patients	Younger patients
2.	Fisher's grade III-V	Thin layer of blood
3.	Presence of basal SAH	Convexity SAH
4.	Neurologically poor grade	Good GCS
5.	Associated vasospasm in TCD	No vasospasm

TRAUMATIC SAH AND OTHER PROGNOSTIC FACTORS

Traumatic subarachnoid hemorrhage (TSAH) is an important and independent prognostic factor in head injured patients. However, large number of factors in TSAH play important role (Table 46.4). Those include age, amount of blood, site of SAH, alcohol intoxication and associated vasospasm. As already discussed above, there is no relationship between CT findings of TSAH and initial neurological condition when seen at the first time. However, degree of SAH is directly correlated to clinical state.

CONCLUSION

Traumatic SAH is an important pathological entity. TSAH more frequent in severe head injury and in the elderly age group, due to wide subarachnoid space. With the advent of CT the diagnosis has become easy and repeated CT scan shows quick resolution. The studies have shown vasospasm in 50 to 60 percent patients. While nimodipine is not helpful in severe head injury as a whole, it is proved to be beneficial in TSAH. TSAH is an unfavorable factor in head injury, as it increases the mortality and morbidity significantly.

REFERENCES

1. Wilkin S. Sanguineous meningeal effusion. Guy Hosp Rep 1859;5:119-27.
2. Simonsen J. Fatal traumatic subarachnoid haemorrhage in alcohol intoxication. J Forensic Sci 1963;8:97-116.
3. Camaron JM, Mant AK. Fatal subarachnoid haemorrhage associated with cervical trauma. Med Sci Law 1972;12: 66-70.
4. Courville CB. Pathology of central nervous system. A study based upon a survey of lesions found in a series of forty thousand autopsies, 3rd edn, Pacific Mountain View 1950;112.
5. Dowling G, Curry B. Traumatic basal subarachnoid haemorrhage. Report of 6 cases and review of the literature. Am J Forensic Med Pathol 1988;9(1):23-31.
6. Dymock RB. Traumatic basal subarachnoid haemorrhage. Med J Aust 1977;2:216-8.
7. Ford R. Basal subarachnoid haemorrhage and trauma. J Forensic Sci 1956;1:117-26.
8. Fohz EL, Ward AA. Communicating hydrocephalus from subarachnoid bleeding. J Neurosurg 1956;13:564-6.
9. Chesnut RM, Luerssen TG, Van Berkum-Clark M, et al. Post-traumatic ventricular enlargement in Traumatic Coma Data Bank: Incidence, risk factors and influence on outcome. In: Avezaat CJJ van Ejindhover, Mass AIR, Tans JTJ (Eds). Proceedings of 8th International Symposium on Intracranial Pressure. Springer Berlin, Heidelberg, New York 1993;503-6.
10. Javid M. Current Concepts: Head injuries. N Eng J Med 1974;291:890-92.
11. Nakamura N, Taunoda M, Ohwada T, et al. Post-traumatic progressive non-obstructive hydrocephalus report of two cases. No To Shinkei 1971;23:1217-21.
12. Freytag E. Autopsy findings in head injuries from blunt forces. Statistical evaluation of 1367 cases. Arch Pathol 1963;75:402-13.
13. De Villa Sante JM, Taveras JM. Computerized tomography in acute head trauma. AJR 1976;126:146-55.
14. Demircivi F, Ozkan N, Buyukkececi J, et al. Traumatic SAH: An analysis of 89 cases. Acta Neurochir (Wien), 1993;122:45-8.
15. Levi L, Guilburd JM, Lemberger A, et al. Diffuse axonal injury: Analysis of 100 patients with radiological signs: Neurosurgery 1996;27:429-32.
16. Kobayashi S, Nakazawa S, Hiroyuki Y, et al. Traumatic subarachnoid haemorrhage in acute head injury. Noto Shinkei 1988;40:1131-5.
17. Takizawa T, Matsumoto A, Sato S, et al. Traumatic subarachnoid haemorrhage. Neurol Med Chir (Tokyo) 1984;24:390-95.
18. Newbarr FD, Courville CB. Trauma as the possible significant factor in rupture of congenital intracranial aneurysms. J Forensic Sci 1958;31:174-99.
19. Locksley HB. Report on the cooperative study of intracranial aneurysm, subarachnoid haemorrhage, and arteriovenous malformations. Based on 638 cases in the cooperative study. J Neurasurg 1966;25:219-39.
20. Simonsen J. Fatal subarachnoid haemorrhage in relation to minor head injuries. J Forensic Sci 1967;14:146-55.
21. Eisenberg HM, Garg HE, Aldrich EF, et al. Initial CT findings in 753 patients with severe head injury. A report from NIH Traumatic Coma Data Bank. J Neurosurg 1990;73:688-98.
22. Shigemori M, Tokutomi T, Hirohata M, et al. Clinical significance of traumatic subarachnoid haemorrhage. Neural Med Chir 1990;30:396-400.
23. Kakarieka A, Schakel EH, Fritze J. Clinical significance of the finding of subarachnoid blood on CT scan after head trauma. Acta Neurochir (Wien) 1994;129:1-5.

24. Marek Z. Isolated subarachnoid haemorrhage as a medicolegal problem. Am J Forensic Med Pathol 1981; 2:19-22.
25. Hillbom M, Kaste M. Does alcohol intoxication precipitate aneurysmal SAH? J. Neural Neurosurg Psychiat 1981;44:523-6.
26. Tatsun Y, Lindenberg R. Basal subarachnoid haematoma as sole intracranial traumatic lesions. Arch Pathol 1974; 97:211-5.
27. Fisher CM, Kistler JP, Davis JM. Relation of cerebral vasospasm to SAH visualised by computerized tomographic scanning. Neurosurg 1980;6:1-9.
28. Hijdra A, Brauwers PJAM, Verneulen M, et al. Grading the amount of blood on computed tomogram after SAH stroke 1990;21:1156-61.
29. Van Gijn J, Van Dongen KJ. The time course of aneurysmal haemorrhage on computed tomograms. Neuraradiol 1982;23:153-6.
30. Kakarieka A. Analysis of CT findings in TSAH. In: Traumatic Subarachnoid Haemorrhage. A Kakarieka (Ed). Springer-Verlag Berlin Heidelberg 1997;21-34.
31. Collumella F, Delzano GB, Gaist G, et al. Angiographical in traumatic cerebral laceration with special regard to some less common aspect. Acta Radiol 1963;1:239.
32. Leeds N, Reid ND, Rosen LM. Angiographic changes in cerebral contusions and intracranial Haematomas. Acta Radio Diag 1966;5:320-27.
33. Wilkins RH, Odom GL. Intracranial arterial spasm associated with craniocerebral trauma. J Neurosurg 1970;32:626-33.
34. Suwanwela C, Suwanwela N. Intracranial arterial narrowing and spasm in acute head injury. J Neurosurg 1972; 36:314-23.
35. Macpherson P, Graham DI. Correlation between angiographic findings and the ischaemic of head injury. J Neurol Neurosurg Psychiat 1978;41:122-7.
36. Marshall LF, Bruce SA, Bueno L, et al. Vertebrobasilar spasm: A significant cause of neurological deficit in head injury. J Neurosurg 1978;48:560-64.
37. Pasqualin A, vivenza C, Rosta L, et al. Cerebral vasospasm after head injury. Neurosurgery 1984;15:855-8.
38. Compton JS, Teddy. Cerebral arterial vasospasm following severe head injury: A transcranial Doppler study, Br J Neurosurg 1987;1:435-9.
39. Bakshi A, Mahapatra AK. Basilar artery vasospasm in severe head injury. A preliminary TCD study. NMJI, 1998;113:220-21.
40. Weber M, Grolimund P, Seiler RW. Evaluation of posttraumatic cerebral blood flow velocities by transcranial Doppler ultrasound. Neurosurg 1990;27:106-12.
41. Muttaquin Z, Arita K, Uozumi T, et al. Vasospasm after traumatic subarachnoid haemorrhage: Transcranial Doppler evaluation. Case report. Neurosurg Rev 1991;14:321-5.
42. Pott W, Caps M. Zerebrale vasospasmen nach traumatischer subarachnoidal blutung. Nervenarzt 1991;62: 493-5.
43. Sander D, Klingelnofer J. Cerebral vasospasm following post-traumatic subarachnoid haemorrhage evaluated by transcranial Doppler ultrasonography. J Neurol Sci 1993;119:1-7.
44. Steiger HI, Aaslid R, Stoss R, et al. Transcranial Doppler monitoring in head injury: Relations between type of injury; flow velocities, vasoreactivity and outcome Neurosurgery 1994;34:79-86.
45. Bailey I, Bell A, Gray J, et al. A trial of the effect of nimodipine on outcome after head injury. Acta Neurochir (Wien) 1991;110:97-105.
46. European study group on Nimodipine in severe head injury. A multicentre trial on the efficacy of nimodipine on outcome after severe head injury. J Neurosurg 1994; 80:797-804.
47. Kakarieka A, Harders A, Braakman R, et al. Traumatic subarachnoid haemorrhage: A clinical entity and its treatment with nimodipine. J Neurotrauma 1995;12:375.
48. Cascino GD, Meyer FB, Whisnant JP, et al. Nimodipine as an add-on therapy for intractable seizure. Neurology 1994;44(Suppl):775S.
49. Hans P, Triffaux M, Bonhomme V, et al. Control of drug-resistant epilepsy after head injury with intravenous nimodipine, Acta Anaesthesiol Belg 1994;45:175-8.
50. Rimel RW, Giordani B, Barth JT, et al. Moderate head injury: completing the clinical spectrum of head trauma. Neurosurgery 1982;11:344-51.
51. Dacey RG, Alves WA, Rimel RW, et al. Neurosurgical complications after apparently minor head injury. J Neurosurg 1956;65:203-10.
52. Williams DH, Levin HS, Eisenberg HM. Mild head injury classification. Neurosurg 1990;27:422-8.
53. Stein SC, Ross SE. The value of computed tomographic scans in patients with low-risk head injuries. Neurosurg 1990;26:638-40.
54. Matiollic C, Berelta L, Gerevini S, et al. Traumatic SAH on CT scan obtained at admission: a multicenter assessment of accuracy of diagnosis and potential impact on outcome. J Neurosurg 2003;98(1):37-42, comments J Neurosurg 2004;100(4):739-40.
55. Servadei F, Murray GD, Teasdale GM, et al. Traumatic SAH, a demographic and clinical study of 750 patients from European brain injury consortium survey of head injuries. Neurosurg 2002;50(2):261-7.
56. Okten AI, Gezercan Y, Ergin R. Traumatic SAH: a prospective study of 58 cases, Ulees Trauma Acil Cerrahi Derg 2006;12(2):107-14.

47 Craniocervical Junction Injuries

Raj Kumar

INTRODUCTION

Traumatic injuries involving the craniocervical junction (CV junction) vary widely because of the complex osseous and ligamentous anatomy. These injuries can be purely ligamentous, such as occipitocervical dislocation, or can include single or multiple bony levels. Rare, however, are occasions of isolated osseous fractures without ligamentous damage. The extent of ligamentous damage usually dictates the presence of instability and the need for surgical fixation. The most common age group to suffer an injury to CVJ is between 15 and 30 years old, motor vehicle accidents, falls and sports being the most common modes of injury.[1-5]

The complexity of the craniocervical junction mainly reflects the translational anatomy between the occiput and cervical spine. This translation enables great mobility in several planes and complements the sensory systems. The price for this mobility is vulnerability to traumatic injury of the craniocervical junction. The decision for treating these injuries includes the need to preserve this mobility, if possible. The following discussion highlights recent, innovative techniques for stabilizing traumatic cervical injuries while preserving normal physiological functions. The extent of ligamentous damage usually dictates the presence of instability and the need for surgical fixation. The details of CV junction injuries and cervical spine injuries are beyond the scope of this book, however, the screening and precautions required in cases of head injury associated with CV junction injuries are discussed here.

OCCIPITOCERVICAL INSTABILITY

Occipitocervical dislocation injuries are relatively rare and account for approximately one percent of all injuries involving the cervical spine.[6] However, these injuries are often severe and therefore tend to be fatal. In fact, they are thought to be underdiagnosed. Multiple ligaments are responsible for structural support at the occipitocervical junction. The anterior and posterior atlanto-occipital membranes attach the atlas to the occiput. The tectorial, alar, and apical ligaments attach the axis to the occiput. Finally, the transverse and atlanto-alar ligaments attach the atlas to the axis. The extent of damage to these ligaments determines the type of fixation required. There are a variety of ways to determine instability at the occipitoatlantal or atlantoaxial joints. Plain radiography is usually the first-line imaging modality. Findings related to occipitoatlantal translation, lateral atlas displacement, or atlantoaxial translation can raise suspicions of instability.[7-9] Computed tomography (CT) improves definition of these articulations and can also detect rotational subluxation. Magnetic resonance imaging (MRI) can help determine ligamentous injury, especially of the transverse atlantal ligament.[10,11] However, it should be used with caution as the sole modality for determining stability because it is highly sensitive to any type of soft tissue injury.

ATLANTOAXIAL DISLOCATION

Atlantoaxial dislocation, also known as atlantodental instability, is secondary to a laxity or rupture of the transverse ligament of the first cervical vertebrae. It is defined by an atalantodental space greater than 3 mm in adults and greater than 5 mm in children. This may result from trauma or from a variety of conditions, such as rheumatoid arthritis, ankylosing spondylitis, Down syndrome, congenital abnormalities of the odontoid, tonsillitis and pharyngitis, Marfan's syndrome, Morquio disease, and neurofibromatosis.[2,5]

CLINICAL FEATURES

Clinical manifestations vary based on the type of atlantoaxial dislocation. The classic findings in rotatory subluxation are neck and suboccipital pain, reduced range of movements at the neck, and the "cock robin" head position of torticollis. In the cock robin position, the head is tilted to one side, rotated to the opposite side, and flexed forward. Neurologic signs are rare in rotatory subluxation because the upper cervical spinal canal is capacious and rotation of C1 on C2 does not narrow canal diameter significantly. Many patients with torticollis do not have pathologic C1-C2 rotation

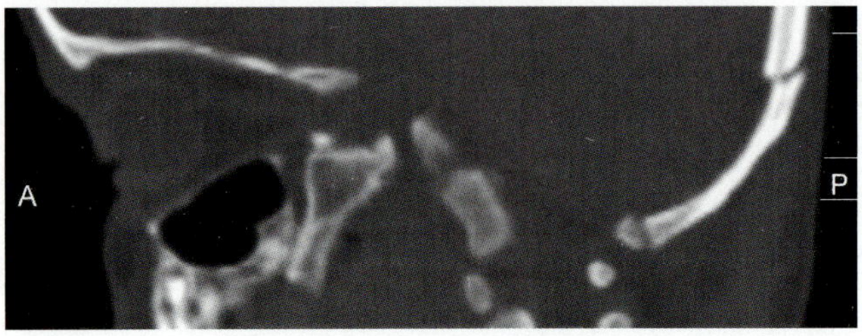

Fig. 47.1: CT bone window shows suspected post-traumatic AAD and odontoid and occipital fracture

or fixation, so the diagnosis of atlantoaxial dislocation cannot be made simply by documenting torticollis. Radiologic studies are required. It is worth noting that less severe subluxations are more likely to present in a delayed fashion than more severe subluxations.

Anterior atlantoaxial dislocation due to fracture of the base of the odontoid process (Fig. 47.1) or disruption of the transverse ligament also presents with neck pain and reduced range of motion but is more likely to have associated neurologic deficit from spinal cord compression. Bilateral disruption of the C1-C2 articulations allows forward translation of C1 on C2. This can result in spinal cord impingement by the posterior ring of C1. Neurologic deficit may range from mild sensory changes to complete paralysis. These patients may die suddenly as C1 spinal cord injury causes respiratory paralysis. Chronic dislocation and spinal cord compression can present with mechanical neck pain and myelopathic signs (e.g. hyperreflexia, proprioceptive loss).

Atlanto-occipital dislocation: There is high incidence of neurologic morbidity and even mortality in this type of dislocation, many patients dying of severe brainstem injury or respiratory arrest at the scene.[6,12-14] A useful classification describes anterior (type-1), longitudinal (type-2), and posterior (type-3) dislocation, based on the movement of the occiput with respect to the cervical spine. The preferred mode of investigating this kind of dislocation is MRI. The use of traction is controversial.[15] Effective surgical stabilization of these patient requires ORIF from the occiput to C3 or C4.[6,12-14]

Occipital condyle fracture: These fracture have been undiagnosed in the past as they are poorly visualize on the X-ray, but with increased use of CT scanning their incidence has increased to 1 to 3 percent cases of blunt CVJ injuries.[16,17]

TYPE-1 Fracture: Axial load and comminuted fracture.
TYPE-2 Fracture: Extension of a skull base fracture.
TYPE-3 Fracture: Avulsion of a condylar fragment by the alar ligament.

The types 1 and 2 are generally considered as stable if isolated and thus only symptomatic management is required and may include external immobilization.[18] Type 3 fracture are unstable and require rigid external immobilization in a collar or halo or even ORIF, if other injuries such as atlantoaxial instability is present.[18]

Atlas fracture: Fracture of atlas vertebra account for approximately 5 percent of all cervical spine injuries.[19,20] Injuries to C1 may occur in isolation but 40 percent are associated with the fracture of C2.[5,21,22] While the Jefferson's fracture, a four part ring fracture, is the most frequent fracture pattern of C1, there are many other variants like unilateral ring or lateral mass fracture.

Some authors recommended ORIF for all atlas fractures with transverse ligament disruption evident on MRI.[10] Isolated anterior or posterior arch fractures can be effectively treated with collar. Lateral mass fracture can typically be managed in a collar unless there is significant comminution, in which halo immobilization may be required for 8 to 12 weeks.[23]

TREATMENT

General principles: The clinician must maintain a high index of suspicion for potential spinal injury in all trauma patients. Proper immobilization must be maintained until the spinal injury is ruled out. Immobilization of the head and neck is of utmost importance during the resuscitation, triage and radiographic evaluation phases of the trauma patient.[4,13] As 10 percent of patients may develop the first onset of signs of cervical spinal cord injury during the evaluation phases following trauma, continued immobilization of the head and neck must be performed until a spinal fracture has been definitely excluded.[4,5]

Numerous options are available for internal fixation of the craniocervical junction after traumatic instability. New innovations in both instrumentation and imaging now often allow mobility to be preserved at the atlantoaxial joint. Image guidance facilitates performing procedures for internal fixation and increases the safety of surgery in patients with abnormal anatomical configurations. Brief surgical option has been mentioned with the respective injury or dislocation.

REFERENCES

1. Bohlman H, Boada E. Fractures and dislocations of the lower cervical spine. In: Cervical Spine Research Society. The cervical Spines. Philadelphia: Lippincott 1983:232-67.

2. Weiss J. Mid and lower cervical spine injuries. In: Wilkins R (Ed). Neurosurgery. New York: Mcgraw-Hill 1985;1708-15.
3. Hadley M, Dickman C, Browner C, Sonntag V. Acute axis fractures: a review of 229 cases. J Neurosurg 1989;71:642-7.
4. Reiss S, Raque G Jr, Shields C, Garretson. Cervical spine fractures with major associated trauma. Neurosurgery 1986;18:327-30.
5. Sonntag V, Hadley M. Management of upper cervical spinal instability. In: Wilkins R (Ed). Neurosurgery update. New York: Mcgraw Hill 1991;222-3.
6. Dickman C, Douglas R, Sonntag V. Occipitocervical spine fusion: posterior stabilization of the craniovertebral junction and upper cervical spine. BNI Quarterly 1991; 7:2-13.
7. Cohen W. Imaging and determination of post-traumatic spinal instability. In: Cooper P (Ed). Management of post-traumatic spinal Instability: Neurosurgical Topics. Rolling Meadows, IL: AANS Publication 1990;19-35.
8. Ross S, Schwab C, David E, Delong W, Boen C. Clearing the cervical spine: initial radiological ecaluation. J Trauma 1987;27:1055-60.
9. Hoffman J, Mower W, Wolfson A, Todd K, Zucker M. Validity of a set of clinical criteria to rule out injury to the cervical spine in patients with blunt trauma: National emergency X-Radiographic Utilization Study group. N Engl J Med 2000;343:94-9.
10. Dickman C, Mamourian A, Sonntag V, Drayer B. Magnetic resonance imaging of the transverse atlantal ligament for the evaluation of atlantoaxial instability. J Neurosurg 1991;75:221-7.
11. Chakers D, Flickinger F, Bresnahan J, Beattie M, Weiss K, Miller C. MR imaging of acute spinal cord trauma. Am J Neuroradiol 1987;8:5-10.
12. Bools J, Rosem B. Traumatic atlantoccipital dislocation: two cases with survival. Am J Neuroradiol 1986;7:901-4.
13. Menezes A, VanGilder J, Graf C, McDonnell D. Craniocerevical abnormalities: a comprehensive surgical approach. J Neurosurg 1980;53:444-5.
14. Ransford A, Crockard H, Pozo J, Thomas N, Nelson I. Craniocervical instability treated by contoured loop fixation. J Bone Joint Surg 1986;68B:173-7.
15. Treynalis V, Marano G, Dunker R, Kaufman H. Traumatic atlantooccipital dislocation: case report. J Neurosurg 1986;65:863-70.
16. Noble E, Smoker W. The forgotten condyle: the appearance, morphology, and classification of occipital condyle fractures. Am J Neuroradiol 1996;17:507-13.
17. Leone A, Cerase A, Colosimo C, Lauro L, Puca A, Marano P. Occipital condyle fractures: a review. Radiology 2000;216:635-44.
18. Joint Section on Disorders of the Spine and Pheripheral Nerves of thye American Association of Neurological Surgeons. Guidelines for the management of acute cervical spine and spinal cord injuries. Ch.15. Neurosurgery 2002;50:S114-9.
19. Sonntag V, Hadley M. Management of nonodontoid upper cervical spine injuries. In: Cooper P (Ed). Management of Post-traumatic Spinal Instability: Neurosurgical Topics. Rolling Meadows, IL: AANS Publications 1990;99-109.
20. Spence K, Decker S, Sell K. Bursting atlantal fracture associated with rupture of the transverse ligament. J Bone Joint Surg 1970;52A:543-9.
21. Dickman C, Hadley, Browner C, Sonntag V. Neurosurgical management of acute atlas—axis combination fractures: a review of 25 cases: J Neurosurg 1989;70:45-9.
22. Hadley M, Dickman C, Browner C, Sonntag V. Acute traumatic atlas fractures: Management and long-term outcome. Neurosurgery 1988;23:31-5.
23. Joint Section on Disorders of the spine and Peripheral Nerves of the American Association of Neurological Surgeons and the congress of Neurological Surgeons. Guidelines for the management of acute cervical spine and spinal cord injuries. Ch. 16. Neurosurgery 2002;50:S120-4.

48

Traumatic Brainstem Hemorrhage

AK Mahapatra, Raj Kumar

INTRODUCTION

Traumatic brainstem hemorrhage is a rare condition. Prior to the availability of the CT scan it was practically impossible to radiologically establish the diagnosis of brainstem hematoma (BSH). The diagnosis was generally based on autopsy[1-3] with the advent of CT scan it is possible to visualize and diagnose BSH in head injured patients.[4-8] Prior to the CT, diagnosis was made on clinical ground on findings like decerebrate rigidity and an internuclear ophthalmoplegia, however, these findings can also be present due to functional disturbances, and not always necessary to have anatomical changes in brainstem. In fact, brainstem signs are very frequently observed in head injury patients even in absence of brainstem hematoma in CT scan. This chapter highlights some aspects of traumatic BSH.

PATHOLOGY

Incidence

Incidence of brainstem hemorrhage is difficult to determine Tandon[2] in 1964 reported 69 cases of brainstem hemorrhage among 132 autopsy cases. Mahapatra et al[3] had reported 7 cases of brainstem hematoma among 62 decerebrating head injured patients (Fig. 48.1). Tsai et al[8] in 1986 reported brainstem lesions in 67 patients among 1600 head injured patients. However, the data also included indirect evidence of brainstem involvement, such as, obliteration of prepontine and perimesencephalic cisterns. Thus, only 19 patients in their study had brainstem injury and 12 of them had hemorrhage in CT scan. Zuccarello et al[9] in 1983 reported primary brainstem hemorrhage in 36 patients among 1000 patients in whom CT scans were performed. In one of our study[10] analyzing 2500 patients, 48 had brainstem hematoma. With the advent of CT scan the diagnosis has become easy and incidence of brainstem hematoma has increased. Kalyanaraman and Ramamurthy[11] reported brainstem in 4.6 percent of all head injured patients.

Mechanism of Injury

Since Duret first described this condition in 1878, there are several pathological studies describing the details of mechanism, location and pathogenesis of brainstem hematoma.[1,12-14] Acceleration and deceleration injuries involve brainstem to varying degree, depending upon several factors. Mechanical effects of stretching and distortion further aggravate the damage due to vascular injury. Involvement of brainstem can occur due to several mechanisms: (a) damage to the brainstem by direct force of impact, (b) due to flexion and distortion and (c) vascular involvement. Primary damage is also possible due to brain movement when brainstem get lacerated or contused by the tentorial edge.[1,2,15] While acute flexon is the most frequent cause, rarely hyperextension injury to the head can give rise to brainstem damage.[13] Generally primary, brainstem injury can be in the form of: (a) laceration, (b) contusion, and (c) brainstem hematoma (Table 48.1). Frequently, brainstem injury is associated with injuries elsewhere in the brain. Isolated brainstem injury/hematoma also occurs rarely.[1,2,4,13,15-17] Very rarely traumatic transection of brainstem has been reported.[18]

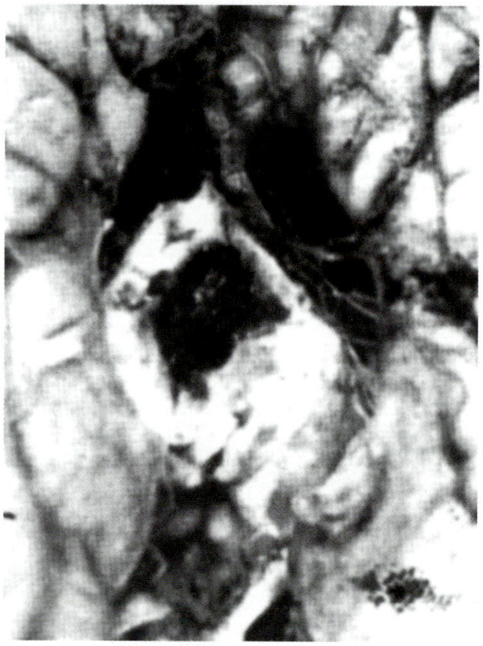

Fig. 48.1: Autopsy findings of a brain in a patient with fatal head injury shows large midbrain hematoma

Table 48.1: Pathology of traumatic brainstem lesions

A. Primary pathology
   i. Laceration
   ii. Contusion
   iii. Primary brainstem hematoma
   iv. Transection of brainstem

B. Secondary pathology
   i. Edema
   ii. Ischemia
   iii. Infarction
   iv. Secondary hemorrhage

C. Combination of primary and secondary pathology

Secondary damage to the brainstem occurs more frequently as compared to primary damage. Transtentorial herniation is most frequent cause of brainstem damage. Secondary brainstem hemorrhage is more frequent in tegmentum of midbrain and pons.[12,17-20] Multiple subependymal punctate hemorrhage can also occur secondary to transtentorial herniation. Secondary hemorrhage are often bilateral and paramedian in location.[1,13,19-22] Necrosis may occur in distorted area. Secondary medullary lesions are due to longitudinal buckling of medulla.[1] Frequently, both primary and secondary damage in brainstem may co-exist. Lesions like ischemic necrosis, small hemorrhage, microhemorrhage and degeneration of axons showing retraction bulb can also be seen.

Subthalamic lesion is prone for microhemorrhage and necrosis. Primary lesions are less common in tegmentum. In medulla, there is selective necrosis of inferior olivary nucleus and vestibular nuclei.[1,2,19] Thus, a widespread pathological lesions can be observed in brainstem, in head injury patients.

CLINICAL PRESENTATION

Typically, patients with brainstem hematoma are unconscious or in altered sensorium (Table 48.2). However, only on the basis of unconsciousness a clinical diagnosis cannot be made. Rarely, patients may have GCS more than 9.[2,4,19] In our study out of 70 patients 15 had no response to pain on admission and 35 (50%) were decerebrating. Tandon[2] in 1964 reported that only two-third cases were comatose from injury to death, while remaining were unconscious sometime during the period they survived. He also reported lucid interval in 21 percent and no initial unconsciousness in 9 percent patients. Mahapatra et al[4] in 1990 reported 5 patients who were conscious at the time of admission. In a series reported by Tandon,[2] 7 percent patients were conscious at the time of admission.

Table 48.2: Conscious state in brainstem hematoma (Experience at AIIMS)

Responses	*No*
No response	11
Decerebrating	35
GCS 5-8	15
GCS, 9 or better	5
	70

Decerebrate rigidity is commonly observed in patients with brainstem hematoma.[4,9,19] Rarely, patients can have hypotonicity.[19] However, decerebrate rigidity can occur in absence of brainstem lesion and may only be a manifestation of brainstem dysfunction.[3,23]

Other clinical findings which are sometime typical to brainstem lesions are respiratory abnormalities pupillary findings and temperature. Varieties of respiratory abnormalities are reported depending on the sites of lesion. It could be classical Chyne-Stroke breathing, hyperventilation or even shallow breathing. Some patients rapidly deteriorate to brain death with respiratory arrest. Disturbances of temperature regulation lead to hyperpyrexia. In the past, hyperthermia was considered pathognomonic of pontine hematoma. Surprisingly, Tandon[2] in 1964, reported hypothermia in 35 percent patients with brainstem hemorrhage, as compared to 48 percent patients with nonhemorrhagic brainstem involvement.

Pupillary abnormalities are well described in brainstem hemorrhage (Fig. 48.2).[2,8,24] Fixed dilated pupils were frequently observed by Tsai et al.[8] Tandon[2] in 1964 described bilateral nonreacting pupils in patients with brainstem hemorrhage, while, amongst 65 non-hemorrhagic cases, 26 had normally reacting pupils. Thus, pupillary changes are nonspecific and not diagnostic of brainstem injury. So called pin-pointed pupils are very rarely observed in patients with brainstem hematomas.[2]

Disturbance of conjugated eye movement is more frequent. This is basically because of involvement of the medial longitudinal fasciculus (MLF). The disconjugated movement and abnormal oculocephalic or Doll's eye movement is characteristic findings of brainstem damage.[8,14,25-27]

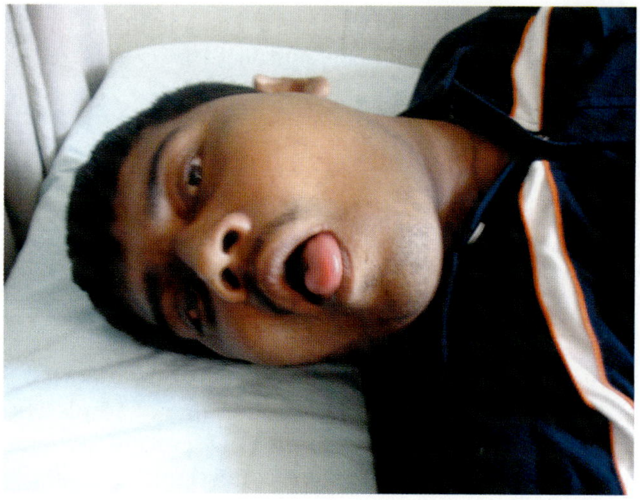

Fig. 48.2: Clinical print of a child with diffuse axonal injury and bleed of brainstem

COLD CALORIC RESPONSE (VESTIBULO-OCULAR REFLEX)

Cold caloric response is an important test assessing the brainstem integrity.[3,4,7,26-28] Its utility in predicting the outcome in severe head injury is well established.[3,7,26,28,29] It is a simple bedside test. Head is raised by 30 degrees and external auditory meatus is irrigated by ice cold saline or water which stimulate semicircular canal. The stimulus is carried by vestibular nerve to vestibular nuclei, which is connected to MLF, 3rd and 6th nerve nuclei in brainstem. Thus, stimulating vestibular nuclei, the eye movement and nystagmus are observed. Normally, there is conjugate deviation of eye with nystagmus. Depending on the site of brainstem involvement and the degree of damage there may be absent or abnormal response of varying degree[7,26,28] (Table 48.3). A complete absence of caloric response is indicative of grave prognosis.[4,7] The study must be repeated several times to assess the improvement or deterioration of brainstem function and is more predictive and reliable as compared to brainstem auditory evoked response (BAER).[4]

Table 48.3: Cold caloric response in brainstem hematoma (Experience at AIIMS—65 cases)

Responses	*No.*
1. Normal	20
2. Abnormal	24
3. Absent	21

BRAINSTEM AUDITORY EVOKED RESPONSE

Brainstem auditory evoked response (BAER) is a reliable study assessing the auditory nerve and brainstem function. BAER is frequently used as a prognostic test in severe head injury. Patients with normal BAER have a good prognosis, on the contrary, patients with repeatedly absent BAER either die or remain vegetative. Only a few studies have reported the useful value of BAER in brainstem hematoma.[4,7,30-32] Sancesario et al[30] in 1984 reported the BAER findings in 6 patients with brainstem hematomas and most frequent findings, abnormality of wave IV and V and delay in 1—V interpeak latency. In one case BAER was normal. Tsutsui et al[31] reported BAER in one patient with brainstem hematoma, prior to and following hematoma evacuation. BAER normalized following surgery and preceded clinical improvement. Mahapatra et al[4] emphasized the role of BAER in 70 patients with traumatic brainstem hematoma. Patients with repeatedly absent BAER had poor prognosis on the contrary improvement in BAER finding or repeatedly normal BAER were associated with favorable outcome.

CT Scan Findings (Tables 48.4A and B)

CT scan is a reliable imaging modality for intracranial pathology, because of its ability to demonstrate the extent, sites and nature of brain injury. Hence, today CT is the primary diagnostic method in patients with head injury. There are several reports dealing with CT findings in brainstem hematoma.[4,8,9,30-33] CT scans not only show the hematoma, it can visualize contusion, obliteration of basal cistern and blood in prepontine or perimesencephalic cistern (Fig. 48.3).[4] Tasi et al had considered direct and indirect evidence of brainstem injury. Direct evidence was the presence of hematoma. Among 67 patients diagnosed as cases of brainstem injury, only 12 had hematoma, and rest 55 were diagnosed on indirect evidences. They also described unifocal or multifocal hematoma. The hematomas may be hyperdense, isodense or hypodense, depending on hemorrhage and edema.

Table 48.4A: CT scan finding in patients with traumatic brainstem hematoma

	Midline	*Lateral*	*Total*
Midbrain	20	25	45
Pons	14	11	25
	34	36	70

Table 48.4B: Associated abnormalities along with brainstem hematoma, AIIMS experience

Nature of pathology	*Numbers*
Extradural hematoma	3*
Cerebral contusion	22(13*)
Midline shift	15

*Required surgery

Mahapatra et al[4] described their CT finding in 70 patients. Thirty-four patients had midline hematoma and 36 had laterally placed hematoma. In 45 patients hematomas were situated in midbrain and in 25 patients hematomas were in pons. Surprisingly, there was no case of medullary hematoma (Table 48.4A). CT scan also demonstrate associate hematoma, elsewhere in brain in a significant number of patients.[4,8] The study reported from our department[4] showed associated focal abnormalities in 25 patients and 16 of them required surgery (Table 48.4B).

TREATMENT

There is no specific treatment for brainstem hematoma. Associated pathology may need surgery,[4,8] depending on size of hematoma and the mass effect they produce. Overall 20 percent may have sizable hematoma elsewhere in brain needing surgery.

As the patients with brainstem hematoma are very sick and remain unconscious for a longer period, they need longer intensive care management and ventilatory support. Nursing care, management of pulmonary problems and tracheostomy care need a special mention. Moderate hypothermia and control of hyperpyrexia if present, are important factors in survival. Hypothermia definitely enhances the chance of survival.[34]

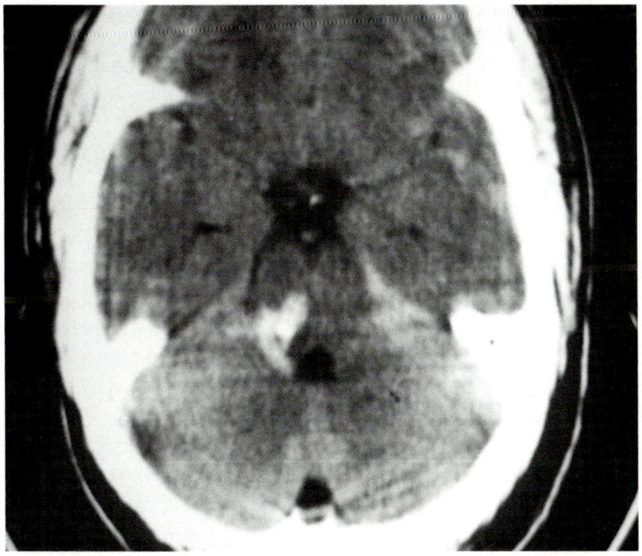

Fig. 48.3: CT of diffuse axonal injury child with dorsal midbrain and pontine bleed

Table 48.5: Outcome of patients with brainstem hematoma, 70 patients at AIIMS

Outcome	*Numbers*	
No deficit	14	good recovery
Mild deficit	8	
Moderate disability	4	poor recovery
Severely disabled	6	
Vegetative	6	
Expired	32	
Total	70	

OUTCOME IN PATIENTS WITH BRAINSTEM HEMATOMA

Outcome of patients with traumatic brainstem hematoma was considered to be grave 2 decades ago. Mostly, definite diagnosis was only made at autopsy.[1,2] With the availability of CT diagnosis and follow-up of these patients has become possible, more reports are available regarding long-term outcome and quality of survival of these patients.[4,5,8,9,17,24,30,31,34,35] Mahapatra et al[4] had reported survival in more than 50 percent cases. Among the 70 patients analyzed, 38 survived and 22 patients had a good recovery. Six patients each were severely disabled or remained vegetative (Table 48.5). Stewart et al[35] developed a prognostic model. He also studied many factors and reported age, associated skull fracture and other injuries to be significant factors. Young patients had good outcome. Gilbert and a Thierry[36] reported good recovery in an 8 years old girl. Kim et al[37] in 1985 reported long-term survival in a patient of brainstem hematoma. In a series reported by Tsai et al[8] mortality rate was 67 percent in patients with secondary brainstem injury. In another study same authors had reported 27 percent mortality in patients with transtentorial herniation, without brainstem involvement, and 61 percent had mild to moderate deficit. The survival rate in transtentorial herniation alone was 73 percent. Of the 19 patients with primary brainstem injury only 5 patients survived. Thus, in their study patients with primary brainstem hematoma had a survival rate of 25 percent, which was relatively lower survival rate.

Other significant factors which help in predicting the outcome are, findings of cold caloric response and

Table 48.6: BAER and outcome experience in 32 patients at AIIMS disability

BAER findings	*No deficit*	*Mild deficit*	*Severe deficit*	*Vegetative*	*Dead*
A. Normal[8]	4	3	1	–	–
B. Abnormal[16]	4	6	5	–	1
C. Absent[8]	–	–	–	1	7
	8	9	6	1	8

brainstem auditory evoked potential.[4,7,24,28,31] Absent cold caloric response, in patients with brainstem hemorrhage carries a grave prognosis.[4,7,28] Similarly, when repeated BAER recordings fail to show wave or absence of wave, III, IV, V denote a poor outcome[4,30,31] (Table 48.6). Presence of traumatic basal subarachnoid hemorrhage[38] associated with brainstem injury carry a poor prognosis. Thus, outcome of patients with brainstem hematoma is multifactorial, hence, these factors require time-to-time careful observation and documentation.

CONCLUSION

Traumatic brainstem hematoma is not a rare condition. With availability of CT scan more cases are diagnosed to have BSH. Common sites are pons or midbrain. Around 25 percent patients are conscious at admission. Fifty percent patients are admitted in a decerebrating state. In more than 30 percent patients there, are associated hematomas elsewhere in brain. Caloric response and BAER are two good prognostic tests. Repeated normal cold caloric response or BAER indicate good prognosis. Overall survival ranges 30 to 50 and 25 percent can have good outcome. Multiple brainstem hematoma and other associated injury reduce the chance of survival and good recovery.

Poor prognosis is common following major TBI, but is more common in those with brainstem injury. However brainstem injury is not an absolute indicator for poor outcome. Understanding the anatomy and excellent of brainstem injury as well as its relationships to supratentorial abnormalities will facilitate a more accurate use of early MRI as prognostic tool and assist in counseling of families.[39]

The flair and inversion sequences of MRI if performed in moderate to severe head injuries these detected brainstem injuries in 26.6 percent of the patients. These can present as hypertensive lesions compatible with diffuse axonal injury or the hemorrhagic lesions can be seen. In some cases these are directly related with specific neurological deficits. Unspecific consciousness disturbances can also be presentation in these cases.[40]

REFERENCES

1. Crompton MR. Brainstem lesions after head injury. Lancet 1971;1:669-73.
2. Tandon PN. Brainstem haemorrhage in craniocerebral trauma. Acta Neurol (Scand) 1964;40:375-80.
3. Mahapatra AK, Tandon PN, Banerji AK, Bhatia R. Bilateral decerebration in head injury—A study of 62 patients. Surg Neurol 1985;23:536-40.
4. Mahapatra AK, Tandon PN, Banerji AK. Brainstem haemorrhage. A review of 70 CT ventrical cases. Abstract NSI meeting 1990, Dec at Indore.
5. Bhutani AK, Singh AK, Prakash B. Post-traumatic brainstem haematoma. Neurology India (Suppl) 1993;41: 43.
6. Gentry LR, Godersky JC, Thompson B. Traumatic brainstem injury, MR imaging. Radiology 1989;171:177.
7. Mahapatra AK, Tandon PN. Brainstem auditory evoked response and vestibulo-ocular reflex in severe head injury patients. Acta Neurochir (Wien) 1987;87:40-5.
8. Tasi FY, Teal JS, Quinn MF, et al. CT of brainstem injury. AJNR 1980;134:717-23.
9. Zuccarello M, Fione DL, Triuca G, et al. Traumatic primary brainstem haemorrhage. A clinical and experimental study. Acta Neurochir (Wien) 1983;67:103-13.
10. Mahapatra AK, Tandon PN. Brainstem haematoma—study of 48 cases. Annual Conference of NSI 1988.
11. Kalyanaraman S, Ramamurthi B. Analysis of 2000 cases of head injury. Neurology India 1970;18:3-11.
12. Cooper PR, Maravilla K, Kirkpatrik J, et al. Traumatically induced brainstem haemorrhage and the computerized tomographic scan. Clinical, experimental observations. Neurosurgery 1979;4:115-24.
13. Lindenberg R, Freytag E. Brainstem lesions characteristic of traumatic hyperextension of the head. Acta Pathol 1970;90:509-15.
14. Tomlinson BF. Brainstem lesion after head injury. J Clin Pathol 1970;(Suppl)23:154-65.
15. Hooper R. Patterns of brainstem injury. In: Pattern of acute head injury. R Hooper (Ed). Edward Arnold Publisher 1971.
16. Britt RH, Herrick MK, Mason RT, et al. Traumatic lesions of pontomedullary junction. Neurosurgery 1980;6:623-5.
17. Mitchell DE, Adam JH. Primary focal damage to the brainstem in blunt head injuries: does it exist? Lancet 1973;2:215-8.
18. Harding B, Erdohazi M. Traumatic transection of the brainstem. J Neurol Neurosurg Psychiat 1981;44:1156-8.
19. Powiertowski H. Results of neurosurgical care in patients with brainstem contusion. In: Head injuries. Proceedings of an International Symposium. Gillingham FJ, Harris P, Shaw JF, Hitchcock ER (Eds). Churchill Livingstone 1971; p. 326.

20. Turazzi S, Bricolo A. Acute pontine syndrome following head injury. Lancet 1977;2:62-4.
21. Courville CB. Effect or closed cranial injuries on midbrain and upper pons. Proc Asso Res Ners Ment Dis 1945;21:131-40.
22. Cohen SI, Aronson SJ. Secondary brainstem haemorrhages. Arch Neurol 1968;19:257-64.
23. Bricolo A, Turazzi S, Alexander A, et al. Decerebrate rigidity in acute head injury. J Neurosurg 1977;47:680-95.
24. Busch EA V. Brainstem contusion: differential diagnosis, therapy and prognosis. Clin Neurosurg 1963;9:18-25.
25. Mingrino S, Molinari G, Andrioli G, et al. Some observations upon vestibular reaction in acute head injury. Excerpta Medica International Congress Series 1966;110:226.
26. Jadhav WR, Sinha A, Tandon PN, et al. Cold caloric test in unconscious patients. Laryngoscope 1971;31:391.
27. Sinha A, Tandon PN, Kacker SK, et al. Role of vestibular studies in an unconscious patient. In: J Otol 1969; 21:161.
28. Tandon PN, Bhatia R, Banerji AK. Vestibulo-ocular reflex and brainstem. Neurol (India) 1973;21:193.
29. Nelson JR. The minimal ice water caloric test. Neurology (Minneap) 1969;18:577.
30. Sancesario G, Pozzessere G, Massa R, et al. Prognostic evaluation of brainstem haematoma, the role of CT scan and brainstem auditory evoked potentials. Acta Neurol Scand 1984;70:396-406.
31. Tsutsui T, Ohno M, Symon L, et al. Combined measurement of brainstem auditory and SEP in a surgically treated brainstem haematoma. Surg Neurol 1986;25: 575-81.
32. O'Laoire SA, Crockard HA, Thomas DGT, et al. Brainstem haematoma. A report of six surgically treated cases. J Neurosurg 1982;56:222-7.
33. Texier PH, Diebler C, Bruguier A, Ponsot G. Haematoma of brainstem in childhood. Neuroradiology 1984;26:499-502.
34. Gruskiewiez J, Doran Y, Peyser E. Recovery from severe craniocerebral injury with brainstem lesions in childhood. Surg Neurol 1973;1:197.
35. Stewart WA, Lilten SP, Sheehe PR. A prognostic model for brainstem injury. Surg Neurol 1973;1:303.
36. Gilbert JJ, Thierry. Unusual brainstem findings following closed head injury. J Paediatr 1972;81:343-5.
37. Kim RC, Fagin K, Choi BH. Prolonged survival after severe traumatic injury limited to the brainstem. Surg Neurol 1985;23:525-8.
38. Patel F. Traumatic baso-brainstem subarachnoid haemorrhage. Medicine Science and the Law 1996;36: 178-81.
39. Mannion RJ, Cross J, Bradley P, et al. Mechanism based MRI classification of traumatic brainstem injury and its relationship to outcome. J Neurotrauma 2007;24(1)28-35.
40. Aguas J, Begue R, Diez J. Brainstem injury diagnosed by MRI. An epidemiological and prognostic reappraisal. Neurocirugia (Astir) 2005;16(1)14-20.

49 Management of Facial Injuries

Arun Kumar Singh, Devi Prasad Mohapatra

SURGICAL ANATOMY

The soft tissues of the face are arranged in a series of concentric layers. The most superficial layer of the face is the skin. Directly deep to the skin lies a variable amount of subcutaneous fat which sits directly above the superficial facial fascia. This fat is thicker in obese patients. The superficial facial fascia is also known as SMAS (superficial muscular aponeurosis system).[1,2] It separates the subcutaneous fat from the underlying parotido-masseteric fascia and facial nerve branches. The SMAS represents the extension of the superficial cervical fascia cephalad into the face. It is thick and dense overlying the parotid gland. As this fascial layer is traced superiorly cephalad to the zygomatic arch, it is termed temporoparietal fascia within the temporal region and the galea within the scalp. Medially into the face it overlies the masseter and the buccal fat pad and becomes less distinct. The muscles of facial expression are supplied by the branches of facial nerve. Most of these muscles lie superficial to the plane of facial nerve except for buccinator, mentalis and levator anguli oris which lie deep to facial nerve. The mimetic muscles and the SMAS function as an anatomic unit in producing movement of the facial skin. The superficial layer of the deep cervical fascia continues in the face as the parotidomasseteric fascia. The facial nerve branches and the parotid duct always lie deep to this deep fascial layer. An extension of the deep fascia superior to the zygomatic arch within the temporal region is termed as the deep temporal fascia. The facial nerve is encompassed by the parotid gland in the lateral aspect of the face. Medially it leaves the parotid to traverse the superficial surface of masseter muscle. The two principal arteries that supply the face are the facial artery and the superficial temporal artery derived from the external carotid artery. In addition, many branches of the ophthalmic and the maxillary arteries that accompany the cutaneous branches of the trigeminal nerve add to the rich vascular supply of the face. Venous drainage is through the facial vein into the external jugular vein. Venous connections of the facial veins with the cavernous sinus via the superior ophthalmic veins are an important clinical consideration for assessing routes of infection between the face and dural sinuses.

The facial skeleton consists of 14 bones. The facial skeleton is divided into region of thirds from a point of view of surgical anatomy. Fractures of the maxillae and associated bones are referred to as fractures of the middle third of the facial skeleton. This region is defined as that area bounded above by a transverse line joining the two frontozygomatic sutures passing through the frontomaxillary and frontonasal sutures and below by the incisal and occlusal plane of the maxillary teeth. The bones constituting the middle third of the facial skeleton are: (1) the two maxillae; (2) the two palatine bones; (3) the two zygomatic bones and their temporal processes; (4) the two zygomatic processes of temporal bones; (5) the two nasal bones; (6) the two lacrimal bones; (7) the vomer; (8) the ethmoid bone and its conchae; (9) the body and lesser and greater wings of sphenoid as well as the pterygoid processes. The NOE complex represents the confluence of the nasal, lacrimal, ethmoid, maxillary, and frontal bones. The paired nasal bones attach to the frontal bone superiorly and the frontal process of the maxilla laterally. The ethmoid bone is located posterior to the nasal bones. The ethmoid labyrinth separates the orbits laterally from the nasal cavity medially. The fovea ethmoidalis forms the roof of the ethmoid sinuses laterally. The cribriform plate, which is approximately 1 cm inferior to the fovea ethmoidalis, forms the roof of the nasal cavity. The upper third of the facial skeleton constitutes the frontal bone and the frontal sinuses. Mandible along with the mandibular teeth the coronoid and condyloid process forms the lower third of the face.

ETIOLOGY

Soft tissue as well as skeletal injuries of the face may arise from road traffic accidents, assaults, sports related, falls, work related, human and animal bites and gunshot wounds. Vehicular trauma is one of the leading causes of facial injuries. Trauma commonly

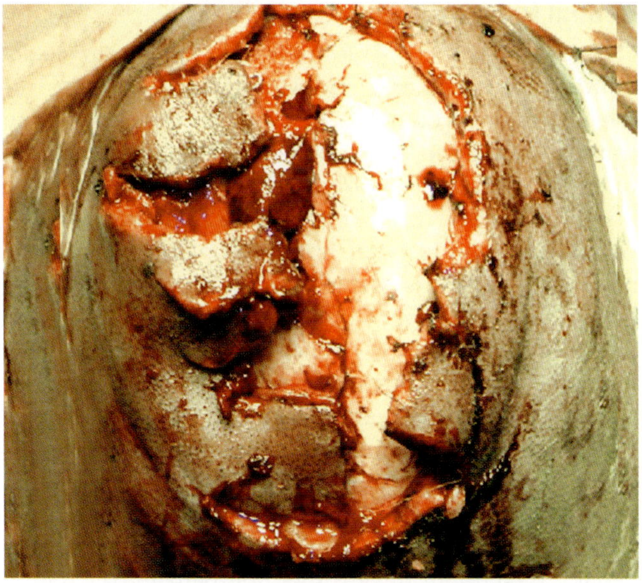

Fig. 49.1: High voltage electrical injuries can cause extensive soft-tissue and bony injuries

occurs when the face strikes a part of the vehicle's interior, such as the steering wheel. Thermal injuries from firecrackers as well as electrical injuries (Fig. 49.1) also account for maxillofacial injuries.

INITIAL MANAGEMENT OF TRAUMA PATIENT

The initial assessment and management of a patient's injuries must be completed in an accurate and systematic manner to quickly establish the extent of any injury to vital systems. Patients are assessed and treatment priorities are established based on patients' injuries and the stability of their vital signs.

Injuries can be divided into three general categories: severe, urgent, and non-urgent. Severe injuries are immediately life-threatening and interfere with vital physiologic functions; examples are compromised airway, inadequate breathing, hemorrhage, and circulatory system damage or shock. These injuries constitute approximately 5 percent of patient injuries but represent over 50 percent of injuries associated with all trauma deaths. Urgent injuries make up approximately 10 to 15 percent of all injuries and offer no immediate threat to life. These patients may have injuries to the abdomen, orofacial structures, chest, or extremities that require surgical intervention or repair, but their vital signs are stable. Non-urgent injuries account for approximately 80 percent of all injuries and are not immediately life-threatening. This group of patients eventually requires surgical or medical management, although the exact nature of the injury may not become apparent until after significant evaluation and observation. Laboratory studies, additional physical findings, radiographic examinations, and observations for several days or weeks may be required.

The goal of initial emergency care is to recognize life-threatening injuries and to provide life-saving and support measures until definitive care can be initiated. The primary goal of triage is to prioritize victims according to the severity and urgency of their injuries and the availability of the required care. Many scales and scoring systems have been developed as tools to predict outcomes based on several criteria notably, Glasgow coma score (GCS), trauma score and the revised trauma scores.[3]

The injury severity score was developed to deal with multiple traumatic injuries.[4] It compares death rates from blunt trauma using data that rate the severity of injury in each of the three most severely injured organ systems. Each injury is evaluated and categorized according to the injured organ system (respiratory, CNS, cardiovascular, abdominal, extremities, and skin) and graded according to the severity of the injury: (1) minor; (2) moderate; (3) severe non-life-threatening; (4) life-threatening, survival probable; (5) survival not probable; (6) fatal cardiovascular, CNS, or burn injuries. The three highest scores for organ systems are then squared and added. Mortality rates have been found to increase with greater severity of injury and age. The American College of Surgeons Committee on Trauma Subcommittee on Advanced Trauma Life Support has developed a schematic orderly assessment of injured patients. The advanced trauma life support (ATLS) system consists of rapid primary evaluation, resuscitation of vital functions, a detailed secondary assessment, and, finally, the initiation of definitive care.[5]

Primary Survey

ABCs during the primary survey, life-threatening conditions are identified and reversed quickly. This period calls for quick and efficient evaluation of the patient's injuries and almost-simultaneous life-saving intervention. The primary survey progresses in a logical manner based on the ABCs: airway maintenance with cervical spine control, breathing and adequate ventilation, and circulation with control of hemorrhage. Letters D and E have also been added: a brief neurologic examination to establish degree of consciousness, and exposure of the patient via complete undressing to avoid injuries being missed because they are camouflaged by clothing.

Airway Maintenance

Airway compromise is the result of either direct laryngeal injury, foreign bodies (including aspirated teeth and bone fragments), or excessive bleeding from an upper airway source. Ten percent of facial trauma patients have cervical spine injuries. Often upright positioning with cervical spine protection will improve airway function compromised by excessive bleeding or foreign bodies. Foreign bodies can be mechanically removed by the finger-sweep technique. Airway compromise can also occur when the floor of mouth and tongue lose support from a comminuted mandible fracture and can be alleviated by simple anterior traction on the mandibular symphysis. Definitive airway protection is carried out via endotracheal intubation. The use of blind nasal intubation should be carried out with caution. Endoscopic nasal or oral intubation improves safety by avoiding the cervical spine manipulation; it further provides immediate confirmation of tracheal intubation. Emergent tracheotomy is considered in the unusual circumstance of laryngeal fracture or inability to secure an upper airway route to intubation.

Hemorrhage

The dense vascularity of the head and neck can cause significant blood loss from soft-tissue injuries. Fortunately, most of these injuries allow sufficient access for direct pressure to control hemorrhage. The control of bleeding vessels should be accurate and directed. Bleeding that cannot be controlled with direct pressure requires packing. Packing in the nasal cavity is usually effective and only rarely requires augmentation with a transnasal balloon catheter in the nasopharynx. Nasopharyngeal balloon catheters only serve to impede blood from entering the oropharynx where it can more easily enter the lungs. Massive hemorrhage should be approached with emergent intubation followed by packing and direct pressure. The source of bleeding is most commonly a branch of the external carotid system, which is most appropriately controlled with angiographic embolization. The radiologist usually requires the assistance of the surgeon to remove the packing so that the source of bleeding can be more readily identified. Type-specific blood should be readily available. Surgical ligation of the external carotid artery will not control bleeding from its injured branches because of the robust collateralization present and should not be attempted.

Central Nervous System

Patients with facial trauma rarely die from facial injuries, but can die from associated injuries of the central nervous system. As part of a complete trauma evaluation most patients with facial trauma undergo computed tomography (CT) scanning to rule out head injury. Concomitant head injury is not a contraindication to facial fracture repair assuming the neurologic injury is stable and not in the process of evolution. In the event of acute brain injury, surgical repair of facial fractures generally is delayed to avoid the fluid overload associated with surgery and, most importantly, to avoid undetected decline of neurologic function during the period of general anesthesia when clinical neurologic examination cannot be performed. Once the central nervous system injury and concomitant swelling have stabilized, facial fracture repair can generally be undertaken safely. Ten percent of patients with facial trauma suffer some form of cervical spine injury. Suspicion for injury and vigilant care of the cervical spine are key elements in the care of facial trauma patients.

Definitive Clinical Examination

An accurate knowledge of how the injury occurred is of great value in indicating the likely severity and extent of damage. A thorough head and neck examination serves as the starting point and is performed in a logical and consistent manner to avoid missing something. The examiner carefully assesses the face for neurologic deficits, including the trigeminal and facial nerves. Sensory disturbances in the forehead, cheek, and lower lip should be well documented as should any deficits in facial nerve function. Undocumented preoperative nerve injuries may be attributed postoperatively to surgical intervention. Lacerations, contusions, and abrasions of the skin may focus the exam by indicating which nerves are at risk. A complete ocular examination includes the evaluation of ocular history, acuity, light and red light perception, ocular motility, pupillary exam, and examination of the conjunctiva and eyelids. Examination of the oral cavity is essential, especially in the obtunded patient who may have loose teeth, bone fragments, or foreign bodies. Identification and removal of prosthetics (e.g. dentures) is essential. The occlusion and intercuspation is carefully evaluated, as both mandibular and maxillary fractures can result in malocclusion. Proper record keeping of facial injuries includes rough sketch drawings in the medical chart and photographs to document injuries. These photographs may prove invaluable in the treatment

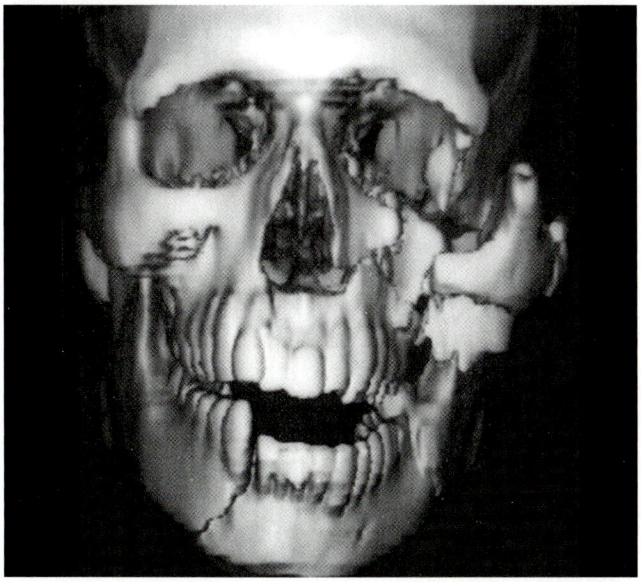

Fig. 49.2: Three-dimensional CT scans are extremely helpful in demonstrating the location and extent of facial fractures

of secondary deformities and can also be beneficial in medicolegal disputes.

Radiology

A facial trauma series consisting of plain radiographs [anteroposterior (AP), lateral, Caldwell, and Water views] are undertaken in most patients of facial trauma. In most patients with significant facial impact, CT scanning should be performed. The CT scan should be performed with axial cuts no greater than 3 mm apart, from the top of the cranium through the bottom of the mandible. In cases of complex facial trauma, it may be helpful to have a three-dimensional reconstruction of the facial skeleton formatted so as to provide for a better overall orientation (Fig. 49.2). A panoramic radiograph is helpful in the evaluation of mandibular fractures (Fig. 49.3). Certain imaging equipment allows the patient to be supine, whereas the more common equipment requires upright positioning and cervical spine clearance. These radiographs place an entire image of the mandible, condyle to condyle, on a single film. They provide excellent detail of the condyles and dentition. A supplemental posteroanterior (PA) film of the mandible complements the panoramic image by providing additional detail of the region. Lateral radiographs and CT scans can provide additional information about the regions posterior to the parasymphysis.

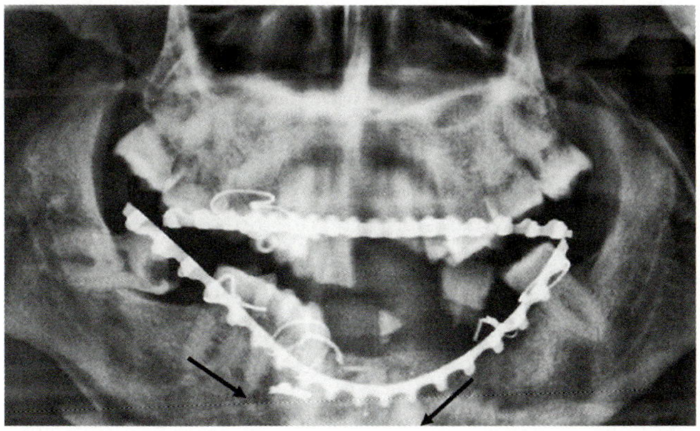

Fig. 49.3: A panoramic radiograph (OPG) showing mandibular symphyseal and parasymphyseal fracture

SOFT TISSUE INJURIES

Soft tissue wounding can have a wide spectrum of etiologic factors, from knife wound to gunshot wound, from human bites to dog mauling, from fistcuffs to motor vehicle accident, to name a few. Soft tissue injuries of the face may be clean lacerations, contused lacerations, abrasions, puncture or avulsive wounds. They may be associated with underlying bony injuries (Fig. 49.4).[6] Ballistic facial injuries are grouped by etiology: gunshot, shotgun, and high energy avulsive injuries. Gunshot wounds require careful attention and evaluation for associated facial fractures. Both entry and exit wounds should be evaluated. Exit wounds often produce marked tissue destruction and require acute debridement.[7]

Face and Scalp Injuries

Scalp wounds can occasionally cause a large amount of blood loss due to the rich vascular supply in this region and the inelasticity of the scalp preventing contraction and closure of the vessels. In patients sustaining scalp injuries it is important to evaluate for associated

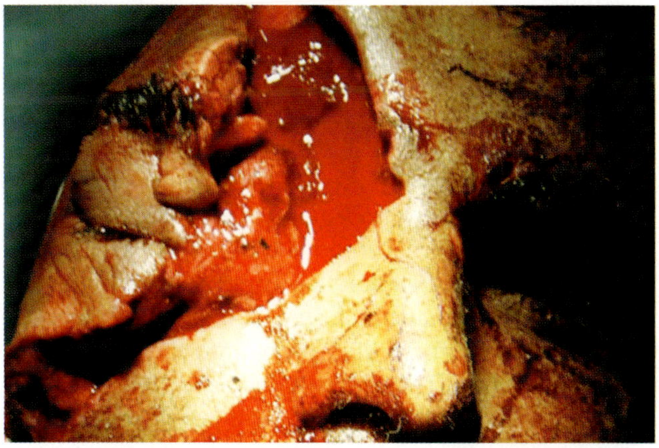

Fig. 49.4: Post-traumatic laceration over cheek, forehead and medial canthus of eye with underlying bony injuries

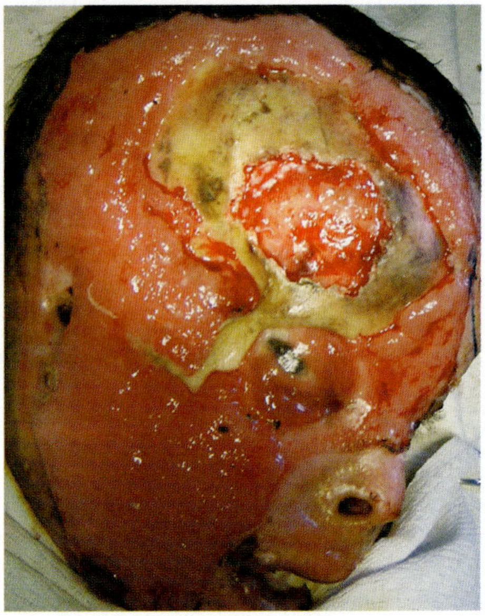

Fig. 49.5: Exposed calvaria following scalp injuries such as these require coverage with local flaps

intracranial injuries. Careful inspection should be performed to look for evidence of skull fractures. In avulsive defects in which the pericranium is intact and primary closure is not possible, a split-thickness skin graft can be used. A secondary reconstructive procedure involving various rotational and advancement flaps or tissue expansion can be undertaken after healing of the defect. If the cranial bone is exposed with large avulsive defects, then cover with various flap procedures are indicated (Fig. 49.5). Reconstruction of the eyebrow is difficult secondarily, and efforts to repair lacerations primarily without distortion are important. Eyebrows should never be shaved, as regrowth of the hair is unpredictable. Closure of lacerations should attempt to salvage as much tissue as possible.

Eyelid and Nasolacrimal Apparatus

A thorough ophthalmologic examination is important to assess for injuries to the globe and to evaluate and document visual acuity. Closure of lacerations involving the eyelids is done in a layered fashion. Care should be taken to precisely approximate the eyelid margins and the tarsus. Any lacerations that involve the medial third of the eyelid should be carefully inspected for damage to the canaliculus. Repair is accomplished by introducing a lacrimal duct probe into the puncta and into the wound. The ends of the lacerated duct are identified and approximated over a polymeric silicone tube (Crawford tube). Avulsion injuries to the eyelids are treated with skin grafts and/or local flaps. Defects of up to 25 percent of the eyelid length can be closed primarily.

Nose

The nose occupies a prominent position on the face and is often injured. Injuries of the internal nose should be evaluated using a nasal speculum. The septum should be evaluated for the presence of a hematoma, which appears as a bluish elevation of the mucosa. Hematomas involving the nasal septum should be evacuated with a small incision or needle aspiration. Nasal packing or polymeric silicone nasal splints can be placed to prevent recurrence of the hematomas and are removed in 7 to 10 days. A running 4-0 chromic gut mattress suture placed in and through the septum can prevent recurrence. Untreated hematomas can lead to infection and necrosis of the cartilage, which may cause collapse of the septum and a resultant "saddle nose". Key sutures should be placed to approximate anatomic landmarks to ensure proper orientation, especially around the nasal rim. Bone, cartilage, and/or skin grafts may be required to reconstruct avulsion defects of the nose. Skin grafts harvested from the periauricular regions provide excellent color and texture match. Local flaps may be required to restore missing tissue.

Ears

The two most prominent concerns in ear injuries are hematoma and chondritis. Collections of blood in proximity to the cartilage can result in cartilage resorption or a reactive chondrogenesis, which ultimately leads to the cauliflower ear deformity. Hematomas must be evacuated as quickly as possible to avert this adverse sequela. Chondritis is a serious complication of these injuries. As cartilage has such poor blood supply, it is difficult to treat these infections with oral antibiotics. These patients typically require admission for intravenous antibiotics and possibly debridement. Ear lacerations can usually be sutured in one layer, addressing the skin only. For larger avulsion injuries the ear should be examined for vessels for the possibility of microvascular reattachment. A more predictable method is to use the "pocket principle" described by Mladick and colleagues. The detached ear is dermabraded to remove the superficial dermis and reattached to the stump. It is then buried underneath a skin flap elevated in the posterior auricular region to provide vascular supply to the reattached ear. Approximately 2 to 3 weeks later the revascularized ear is uncovered and allowed to re-epithelialize. If salvage of the ear is not possible other alternatives include staged reconstruction with rib cartilage, skin flaps, or silicone implants. The introduction of osseointegrated implants has made prosthetic reconstruction an appealing treatment option.

Lips

The most important consideration in repairing soft-tissue injuries involving the lips involves accurate re-approximation of the injured structures, especially the vermilion. Great care must be taken to separately reapproximate the underlying orbicularis oris muscle. Avulsive defects of the lips require special attention. Up to one-fourth of the lip can be closed primarily with acceptable functional and esthetic results. Injuries that involve a greater amount of tissue loss can be reconstructed with a variety of flaps such as Abbe-Estlander or Karapandzic flaps.

Facial Nerve and Parotid Duct Injuries

Soft-tissue injuries to the face involving the facial nerve are particularly devastating. In examining the patient with facial soft-tissue injury, particularly penetrating wounds, facial motion is examined carefully. One should specifically test elevation of brow, forced closure of the eyes, voluntary smile, and eversion of the lower lip. Deficits in the presence of a penetrating injury likely represent transection of a facial nerve branch. These injuries should be repaired using microscopic magnification and 9-0 or 10-0 nylon epineural sutures. Nerve regeneration typically occurs at a rate of 1 mm per day after a 1-month lag. Involvement of the Stensen duct will result in a parotid fistula unless corrected. These injuries may be difficult to identify and may only be seen following repair of a skin lacerations with subsequent accumulation of saliva. Duct injuries should be repaired over a stent to allow healing.

Neck Injuries

Neck injuries can involve deep structures affecting the vascular, respiratory, digestive, neurologic, endocrine, and skeletal systems. The neck is divided into three anatomic zones. Zone I extends from the level of the clavicles and sternal notch to the cricoid cartilage. Zone II is from the level of the cricoid cartilage to the angle of the mandible. It is the most surgically accessible and is the easiest to evaluate intraoperatively without the aid of preoperative diagnostic testing. Zone III extends from the angle of the mandible to the base of the skull. There should be a high index of suspicion for esophageal injuries because complications can be devastating if repair is delayed. Primary repair is most often indicated in tracheal and vascular injuries.

BONY INJURIES AND THEIR MANAGEMENT

Frontal Sinus Fractures

The frontal sinus is protected by thick cortical bone and is more resistant to fracture than any other facial bone. The accurate diagnosis of frontal sinus fractures and nasofrontal recess injuries is crucial to the appropriate treatment. Improper management can result in esthetic deformity, chronic sinusitis, pneumocephalus, mucopyocele, meningitis, and brain abscess. Frontal sinus fractures can be classified by anatomic site, severity of injury, and presence of CSF leak. Appropriate treatment decisions can be made by the assessment of five anatomic parameters (Table 49.1). The goals of management are both to prevent a visible deformity and early and late complications.[8] All patients receive antibiotics tailored for upper respiratory bacterial flora at the start of treatment and for seven days after surgery, and 14 days after surgery if a CSF leak is stopped. If the anterior wall is displaced, open reduction and internal fixation best treats the fracture and avoids a frontal bone esthetic deformity. The sinus may be approached through an appropriate skin laceration or with a coronal incision. The coronal incision provides the best exposure and should be elevated with the pericranium to be utilized as a separate flap, if needed. The sinus should be explored, irrigated, and all devitalized mucosa removed. If no frontonasal duct injuries are present, the healthy mucosa is left intact and the anterior sinus wall is anatomically reduced and fixated with an absorbable or metallic microplating system. If significant bone loss is present or if fragments are judged to be too small to use, split calvarial grafts or "shavings" from the temporoparietal area are used to fill the defects. Any fracture that extends into the floor of the frontonasal duct may produce obstruction and therefore requires sinus mucosa ablation and frontonasal duct obliteration. Any evidence of frontonasal

Table 49.1: Anatomical parameters to be assessed in frontal sinus fractures
• Anterior table fracture
• Nasofrontal recess fracture
• Posterior table fracture
• Dural tear (cerebrospinal fluid leak)
• Fracture displacement/comminution

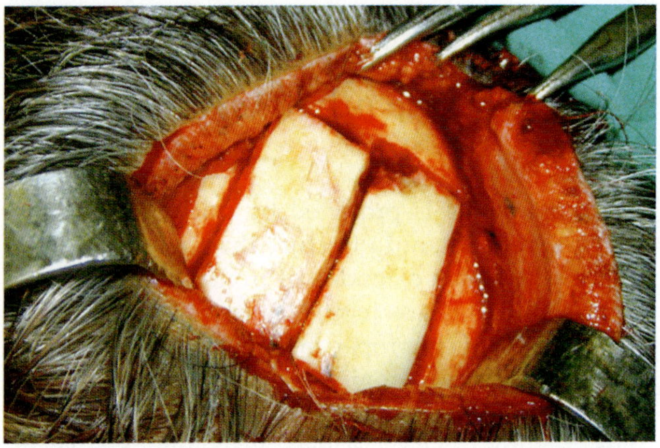

Fig. 49.6: Bone grafts harvested from outer table of calvaria can be utilized for reconstruction of frontal sinus fracture

duct obstruction makes complete removal of the sinus mucosa and obliteration of the sinus and ducts mandatory. This is performed by carefully removing all the mucosa from the sinus and burring all the bony surfaces with a high-speed round diamond burr. The burr removes a thin layer of bone from the sinus. The frontal sinus mucosa invaginates within small recesses in the bone on the inside of the frontal sinus. A pericranial flap can be elevated from the coronal flap, or from the cranium, and placed over the ducts with bone grafts to plug the duct system. Obliteration of the frontal sinus is recommended using calvarial bone grafts (Fig. 49.6) or a pericranial flap.

Spontaneous osteogenesis, galeal-frontalis flap, fat and muscle are other options. Fractures of the posterior wall of the frontal sinus are often associated with intracranial injuries. CSF leak and frontal lobe contusion may be present. Evaluation and treatment should involve neurosurgery. Management is based on the degree of displacement, duct involvement, and the presence of a CSF leak. No operative intervention is required for posterior wall fractures that are not displaced and exhibit no evidence of a CSF leak. All fractures of the posterior sinus wall that are significantly displaced require operative intervention. Displaced fractures of the posterior wall associated with a CSF leak require a cranialization procedure. Cranialization is the removal of the posterior wall of the frontal sinus, which allows the brain to displace anteriorly.

Naso-orbitoethmoid Complex Fractures

Long-term consequences of naso-orbitoethmoid complex disruption include blindness, telecanthus, enophthalmos, midface retrusion, CSF fistula, anosmia, epiphora, sinusitis, and nasal deformity.[9] Naso-orbitoethmoid

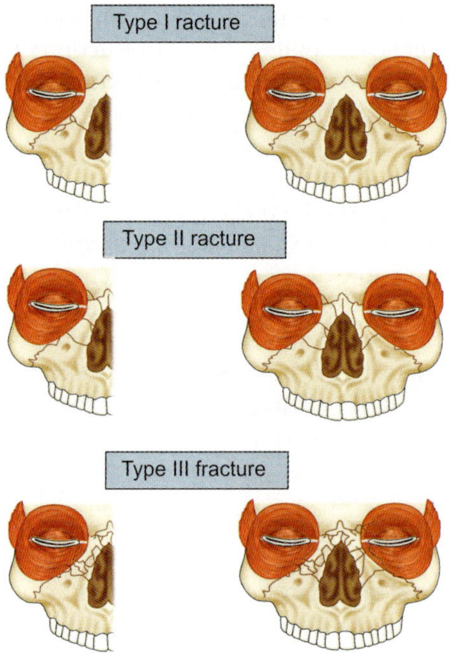

Fig. 49.7: Classification of naso-orbitoethmoid fractures

complex complex fracture is primarily a clinical diagnosis; however, thin-cut CT scans play an important role in defining the pattern and extent of injury. Telecanthus, enophthalmos, pupillary response, and extraocular muscle mobility should be assessed and documented. The nasal bones should be palpated for crepitus and comminution. Thin-cut (1.5 mm) axial and coronal CT scans should be obtained to assess cribriform plate disruption, frontal recess/sinus involvement, orbital integrity, degree of NOE complex comminution, and associated facial fractures. Markowitz et al devised a classification system describing the degree of bony injury (Fig. 49.7). Type I fractures represent a single, noncomminuted central fragment without medial canthal tendon disruption. Type II fractures involve comminution of the central fragment, but the medial canthal tendon remains firmly attached to a definable segment of bone. Type III fractures are uncommon and result in severe central fragment comminution with disruption of the medial canthal tendon insertion. Each fracture type is subclassified as unilateral or bilateral.

The goal in the treatment of the naso-orbitoethmoid complex fractures is to restore the preinjury intercanthal distance, restore nasal projection and dorsal contour, and restore normal soft tissue contours in the medial canthal area.[10] Naso-orbitoethmoid complex fractures are the most challenging fractures to treat in facial trauma. Optimum surgical treatment involves wide exposure and meticulous reduction of bony fragments with adequate stabilization. All displaced NOE fractures require operative intervention. Any instability on naso-orbitoethmoid complex manual examination requires operative intervention. Fractures that do not show any movement on examination or displacement on the CT scan do not require surgery. Management of the medial orbital rim segment, which contains the canthal tendon, is critical in the successful treatment of these injuries.

Orbitozygomatic Fractures

An orbitozygomatic fracture is another descriptive term for malar or tripod fractures. Clinical signs of an orbitozygomatic fracture include cheek and eyelid edema, loss of cheek projection, unilateral epistaxis, decreased or loss of sensation in the cheek area and upper lip, step off deformity in the infraorbital rim area, and diplopia due to displacement of the globe.[11] All patients in whom an orbitozygomatic fracture is suspected should have coronal and axial CT scans (Fig. 49.8). Analysis of the scans should focus on the degree of displacement and internal orbital injuries. The lateral orbital wall provides an excellent area to evaluate the degree of displacement. Coronal CT scans are useful in evaluating the orbital component of orbitozygomatic fractures. This evaluation is important because defects of the floor or medial wall require reconstruction to prevent enophthalmos. Orbitozygomatic fractures with no displacement require only observation. A nonchew diet will prevent the activation of the masseter from displacing the fracture segment. If the fracture is displaced, exploration with anatomic reduction and plate fixation is indicated. Repositioning of a displaced fracture in a delayed setting requires osteotomy of all buttresses and extensive craniofacial exposure. It is best to reduce and fixate fractures anatomically in the acute setting. Isolated fractures of the zygomatic arch are treated differently from true orbitozygomatic injuries.

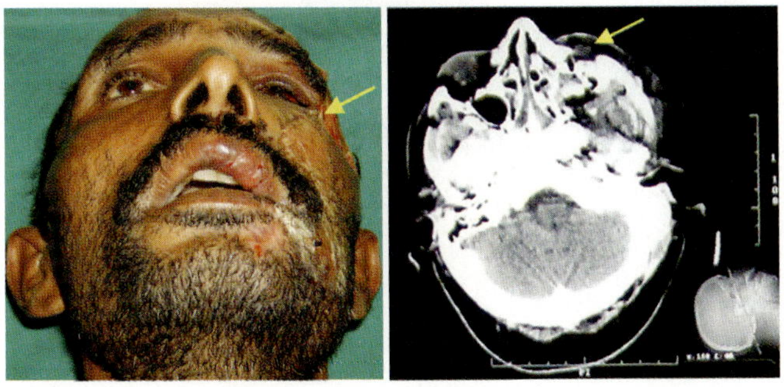

Fig. 49.8: Depressed zygomatic fractures present with loss of malar projection. Note conjunctival ecchymosis on the affected side

Isolated arch fractures frequently do not require operative reduction. Operative treatment of these fractures is indicated for severe depression of the arch causing either a cosmetically significant contour depression or impingement on the coronoid process and trismus. Diplopia is a known complication of an orbitozygomatic fracture. The complication can be caused by mechanical entrapment, contusion of the extraocular muscles, or the nerves supplying the muscles. Enophthalmos is a common, problematic complication. Enophthalmos may be caused by malposition of the zygoma, inadequate reconstruction of the internal orbit, orbital fat atrophy, loss of ligamental support, or a combination of these conditions.

Orbital Fractures

Seven bones make up the orbit: The frontal, maxilla, zygoma, lacrimal, ethmoid, greater wing of the sphenoid, lesser wing of the sphenoid, and the palatine bone. Initial evaluation includes a test of visual acuity, extraocular muscle function, and papillary reflexes. Serial examinations are performed throughout the course of treatment. The main signs of a blowout fracture are diplopia and enophthalmos. Restricted ocular movement can cause diplopia, most commonly in upward gaze. Enophthalmos, or the posterior displacement of the globe, is caused by increased orbital volume and/or a disruption of the ligamentous support of the globe (Fig. 49.9). The indications for surgery are diplopia, extraocular muscle entrapment, enophthalmos, and

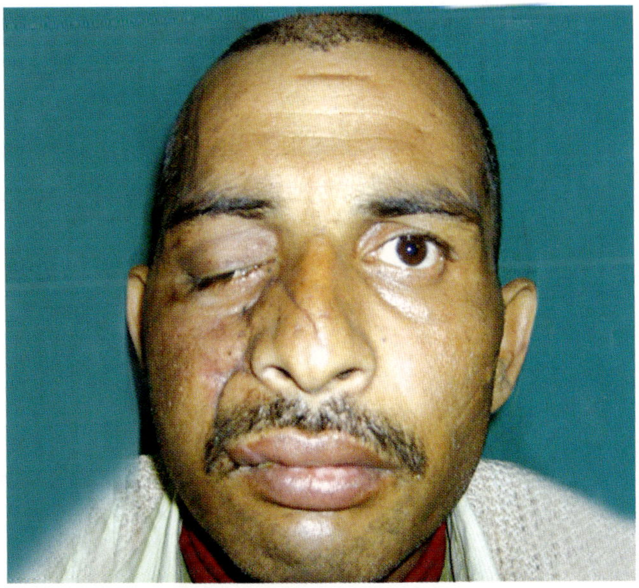

Fig. 49.9: Enophthalmos on right side following orbital floor fracture Exploration and orbital floor reconstruction with bone grafts is done for enophthalmos

large orbital floor defect (more than half of the floor). Surgery may be performed immediately or postponed until the edema has resolved, usually within a week interval from the time of the injury. Exposure of the floor is through a transconjunctival incision, with or without a lateral canthotomy. Subciliary or subtarsal incisions can be used. Reconstruction of a defect involving only the concave anterior aspect of the floor can usually be adequately accomplished with an alloplastic implant. Of the various alloplasts available, porous polyethylene (Medpor) is an ideal choice. Outer table of the skull is also a reliable option for providing autologous bone grafts.[12]

Nasal Fractures

The nasal bones are the most commonly fractured facial bones. Injuries may result from both frontal and lateral impact. Symptoms include bruising and swelling over the nose and an obvious deformity.[13] Simple fractures are treated by closed reduction. Relocation of the septum and nasal bones can be done with Ashe and Walshams forceps respectively. Secondary rhinoplasty is done for late deformities.

Maxillary Fractures

Fractures of the maxilla are often associated with fractures to the nose or other parts of the central face. Fracture patterns of the facial skeleton are well described in the trauma literature, with the most lasting contribution from René. In his classic 1901 work, Le Fort described a series of characteristic fracture patterns produced in cadaver skulls. The Le Fort I, or Guérin, fracture is a low horizontal fracture between the maxilla and palate/alveolar arch complex (Fig. 49.10). The Le Fort II, or pyramidal, fracture is the most common Le Fort fracture pattern, seen in 30 to 60 percent of cases. Classically, the fracture starts at the nasal bones and crosses the frontal process of the maxilla and lacrimal bones. The fracture line then changes direction and descends through the floor of the orbit, infraorbital rim, and the lateral maxillary sinus wall (Fig. 49.11). The Le Fort II often extends through the pterygoid plates. The Le Fort III fracture, or craniofacial disjunction, is a relatively uncommon midfacial fracture. The Le Fort III fracture typically passes through the nasofrontal suture, frontal process of the maxilla, lacrimal bones, ethmoid sinus, and lamina papyracea before crossing the orbital floor to the inferior orbital fissure (Fig. 49.12). The fracture then extends in three directions: (1) across the lateral orbital wall through the zygomaticofrontal suture, (2) through the zygomatic arch, and (3) through the pterygoid plates, thereby creating a separation of the midface from the skull base. In addition to the above, Le Fort IV fractures involving the frontal bone, have also been described. Fractures are identified clinically and confirmed radiographically. If clinical evidence strongly indicates maxillary fracture (midface mobility and malocclusion with intact mandible), then CT imaging is a confirmatory test for maxillary fractures.

Initial attention should be directed at establishing an airway and controlling hemorrhage. The most

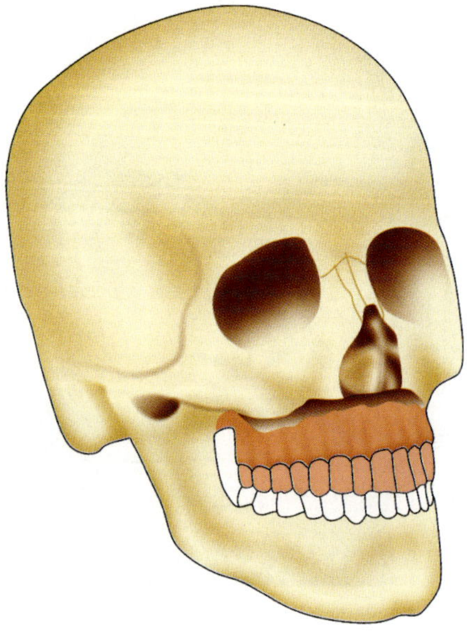

Fig. 49.10: Le Fort I fracture

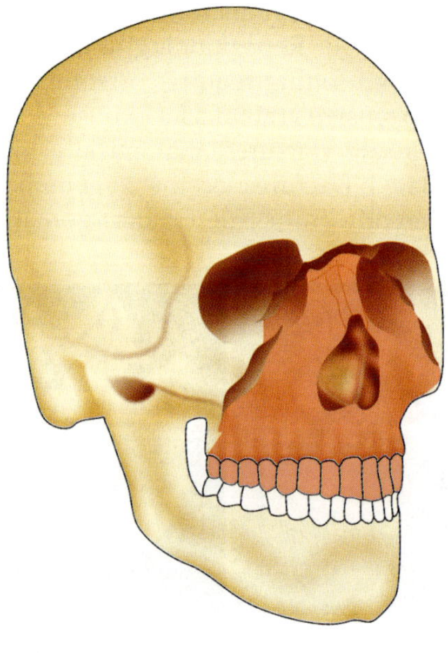

Fig. 49.11: Le Fort II fracture

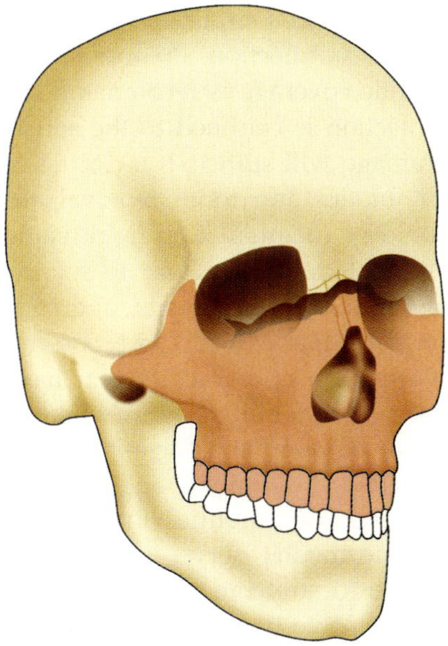

Fig. 49.12: Le Fort III fracture

frequent cause of hemorrhage in Le Fort level fractures is a fractured septum. This bleeding may be addressed by placing nasal packs. The treatment goals are to restore facial height and projection and reconstruct the preinjury occlusion. A minimally displaced, minimally comminuted fracture can either be treated with maxillomandibular fixation (MMF) or by open reduction/internal fixation (ORIF) (Fig. 49.13) if six weeks of MMF is unacceptable to the patient.[14] For more comminuted or displaced fractures, the status of the mandible is evaluated. If the mandible is intact, it serves as a guide for placing the upper dentition into occlusion. MMF is placed, and then the midface is treated with appropriate ORIF. If the mandible is

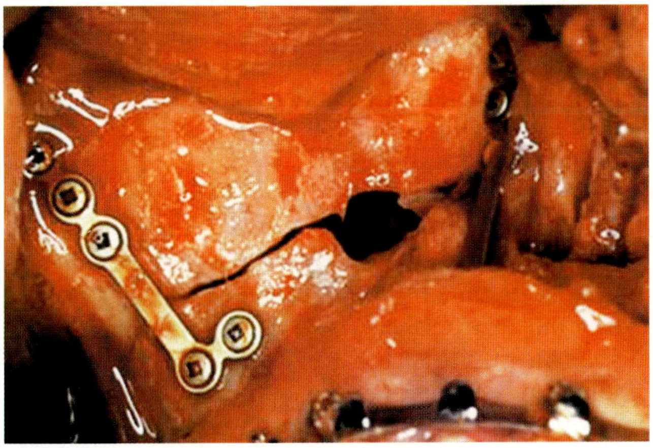

Fig. 49.13: Reconstruction of maxillary fractures with bone grafts, miniplates and screws may be required for reduction and internal fixation

Table 49.2: Complications associated with maxillary fractures
• Infraorbital nerve paresthesia
• Enophthalmos
• Infection
• Exposed hardware
• Deviated septum
• Nasal obstruction
• Altered vision
• Nonunion
• Malunion or malocclusion
• Epiphora
• Foreign body reactions
• Scarring
• Sinusitis

fractured, as long as the fracture site is not the condylar head or high condylar neck then one can place the patient in MMF, ORIF the mandible, and then proceed exactly as above. If the palate is fractured wiring of the posterior aspect of the palate is done for stability before MMF or any midfacial plating is undertaken. A number of complications are associated with maxillary fractures and their repair (Table 49.2). Although most of these may not be apparent until weeks or months of injuries, their possibility should always be borne in mind.

Mandibular Fractures

The mandible is the second most commonly fractured part of the maxillofacial skeleton after nasal bones because of its position and prominence. Mandibular fractures may be classified by the pattern of fracture present and by anatomic location (Table 49.3). Evaluation starts by questioning the patient about any bite alteration. Inspection and palpation of the face along the inferior border and temporomandibular joints may reveal point tenderness and step off deformities. Orally, malocclusion and disruptions of the teeth and dental arch form may be present. Mandibular range of motion may also be disturbed. Anterior traction on the mandible, by gently grasping the mandibular incisors and chin, will often cause pain at the fracture sites. Likewise, gently pushing inward at the angles of the mandible may also reveal fracture sites. Radiographic evaluation of the mandible is best done with a panorex or CT scan. Plain films often miss fractures of the condylar processes due to the superimposition of structures. The panorex is most helpful in evaluating the dentition before arch bars are placed. The location

Table 49.3: Classification of mandible fractures

1. Anatomic location
   a. Dentoalveolar
   b. Symphysis
   c. Parasymphysis
   d. Body
   e. Angle
   f. Ascending ramus
   g. Condylar process
2. Pattern of fracture
   a. Simple fracture
   b. Compound fracture
   c. Greenstick
   d. Comminuted
   e. Complex or complicated
   f. Telescoped or impacted
   g. Displaced fracture
   h. Dislocated fracture
3. Presence of teeth on either side of the fracture (Kazanjian and converse)
   a. Class 1: Teeth on both bony fragments
   b. Class 2: Teeth on one bony fragment
   c. Class 3: Teeth on neither bony fragment

and condition of the fracture dictates the type of reduction appropriate for any given case. Nondisplaced mandible fractures without occlusal disturbances can be treated with a soft diet until healing is complete. Closed reduction is used when a fracture is either nondisplaced or minimally displaced with occlusal disturbances. Arch bars and circumdental wires are applied to the teeth followed by maxillomandibular wires or elastics for two to six weeks to ensure stable reduction. Displaced fractures usually require open reduction with internal fixation using wires or plates. Mandibular fractures should be reduced as soon as possible to minimize pain and soft tissue injury, and reduce the risk of infection (Table 49.4).[15]

Table 49.4: Goals of therapy in mandibular fractures

1. Obtain stable occlusion.
2. Restore interincisal opening and mandibular excursive movements.
3. Establish a full range of mandibular movements.
4. Minimize deviation of the mandible.
5. Produce a pain-free articular apparatus at rest and during function.
6. Avoid internal derangement of the temporomandibular joint on the injured or the contralateral side.
7. Avoid the long-term complication of growth disturbance.

The most common complication of compound mandibular fractures is infection. Preoperative and postoperative antibiotic coverage is recommended. In cases in which the infection is confined to the soft tissues, incision and drainage will suffice. If a carious tooth causes infection, antibiotics and tooth removal are indicated. Patients should be maintained in rigid fixation until the fractures are healed (usually four to six weeks). If the infection involves bone fragments, aggressive debridement of bone, soft tissue, teeth, and loose hardware are indicated. Nonunion is a fracture that has not healed within six months. Mobility and infection are the most common cause of nonunion. Re-exploration and rigid fixation is needed. Malunions, and as a result malocclusions, may be seen. Injuries involving the inferior alveolar and the mental nerves may be present. Most injuries are due to stretching or compression and will spontaneously resolve over many months.

GUNSHOT AND PANFACIAL INJURIES

Gunshot wounds can cause any combination of soft-tissue injury and fracture within the craniofacial skeleton.[16] The goal of skeletal reconstruction must first be the restoration of the anteroposterior projection and width of the face. Primary bone grafting has proven a reliable technique in the face of bone loss and severe comminution. When a large soft-tissue component is also present, as occurs with shotgun wounds, soft-tissue reconstruction is an early priority. Stable soft-tissue coverage is vital to restoration of the skeleton, especially when bone grafting is required.[17]

SECONDARY DEFORMITIES IN FACIAL TRAUMA

Unrepaired or inadequately reduced facial fractures can result in a wide range of severe cosmetic and functional deformities (Table 49.5). Late repair or reconstruction after the soft tissue and bones have healed is much more difficult than repair at the time of initial injury. Reconstruction requires wide exposure which enables the surgeon to have direct visualization of the bony deformities.

Enophthalmos

Enophthalmos is defined as posterior displacement of the globe within the orbit. Clinically, it is noticeable when the displacement is 2 mm or greater. Inferior displacement is termed hypoglobus. The most common finding in patients with enophthalmos is diplopia, more often in peripheral than central gaze. Delayed enophthalmos is evaluated with a maxillofacial CT scan with 1.0 mm cuts through the orbits. Sagittal and coronal reconstructions are useful adjuncts to the orbital

Table 49.5: Secondary deformities in facial trauma

1. Nasal deformities
   a. Nasal deviation
   b. Nasal depression (saddle nose)
2. Naso-orbital deformities
   a. Orbitonasal angle deformity
   b. Medial canthus dystopy
   c. Decreased nasal airway patency
3. Nasofrontal deformities
   a. Reduced nasofrontal angle
   b. Decreased nasofrontal duct patency
   c. Post-traumatic meningoencephalocele
4. Nasofrontoethmoidal deformities
   a. Anosmia
   b. CSF rhinorrhea
5. Zygomatic complex deformities
   a. Facial asymmetry
   b. Eyeball dislocation
   c. Diplopia
   d. Infraorbital paresthesia
   e. Limitation in mandibular movement
6. Maxillary deformities
   a. Midface asymmetry
   b. Malocclusion
7. Mandibular deformities
   a. Malunion
   b. Nonunion
   c. Malocclusion
   d. Aesthetic deformities

analysis and comparison to the normal contralateral side is extremely helpful. Correction of enophthalmos should be directed toward correction of the orbital volume. In the case of fractures of the orbital floor or medial wall, placement of bone grafts or an alloplastic implant in the deficient areas will correct the displacement (see Fig. 49.9).

Malocclusion

Malocclusion can be related to malunion of maxillary, palatal, or mandible fractures. It is most commonly associated with poorly treated mandible fractures. When malocclusion is discovered in the immediate postoperative period, Panorex and plain radiographs can often determine if the condition is amenable to operative correction. Minor tooth interferences can be addressed by burring down teeth at the points of contact. Re-exploration and rigid internal fixation may be required.

Telecanthus

This refers to an increase in the intercanthal distance. The most common findings are tenting of the soft tissues of the medial canthus, lateral displacement of the canthus, and rounding of the medial canthal angle. The goal of revisional surgery is to correct all of the above deformities and ensure that the skeletal contour in the region is correct. Re-exploration is required.

REFERENCES

1. Mitz V, Peyronie M. The superficial musculoaponeurotic system (SMAS) in the parotid and cheek area. Plast Reconstr Surg 1976;58:80.
2. Gosain A, Yousif NJ, Madiedo G, et al. Surgical anatomy of SMAS: a reinvestigation. Plast Reconstr Surg 1993; 92:12-54.
3. Senkowski CK, McKenney MG. Trauma scoring systems: a review. J Am Coll Surg 1999;189:491-503.
4. Osler T. ICISS: an International Classification of Disease-Based Injury Severity Score. J Trauma 1996;41(3):380-6.
5. American College of Surgeons Committee on Trauma. Advanced trauma life support for doctors: student course manual. Chicago (IL): American College of Surgeons 1997.
6. Key SJ, Thomas DW, Shepherd JP. The management of soft tissue facial wounds. Br J Oral Maxillofac Surg 1995;33(2):76-85.
7. Thorne CH. Gunshot wounds to the face: current concepts. Advances in craniomaxillofacial fracture management. Clin Plast Surg 1992;19:233-44.
8. Rohrich RJ, Hollier LH. Management of frontal sinus fractures. Changing concepts. Clin Plast Surg 1992;19:219-32.
9. Sargent LA, Rogers GF. Nasoethmoid orbital fractures: diagnosis and management. J Craniomaxillofac Trauma 1999;5:19-27.
10. Gruss JS, Mackinnon SE, Kassell EE, Copper PW. The role of primary bone grafting in complex craniomaxillofacial trauma. Plast Reconstr Surg 1985;15:17-24.
11. Knight JS, North JF. The classification of malar fractures: an analysis of displacement as a guide to treatment. Br J Plast Surg 1961;13:325.
12. Manolidis S, Weeks BH, Kirby M, Scarlett M, et al. Classification and surgical management of orbital fractures: Experience with 111 orbital reconstructions. J Craniofac Surg 2002;13(6):726; discussion 738.
13. Manson P. Facial fractures. In Mathes SJ (Ed): Plastic surgery. Philadelphia WB saunders, 2006;(3):77-380.
14. Manson PN, Crawley WA, Yaremchuk MJ, et al. Midface fractures: advantages of immediate extended open reduction and bone grafting. Plast Reconstr Surg 1985;76:1.
15. Ellis E. Treatment methods for fractures of the mandibular angle. Int J Oral Maxillofac Surg 1999;28(4):243.
16. Gruss JS, Antonyshyn O, Phillips JH. Early definitive bone and soft-tissue reconstruction of major gunshot wounds of the face. Plast Reconst Surg 1991;87:436.
17. Markowitz BL, Manson PN. Panfacial fractures: organization of treatment. Clin Plast Surg 1989;16:105.

50 Nutritional Management of Head Injury

A Jindal, AK Mahapatra

INTRODUCTION

The metabolic response of normal human beings to starvation is marked decrease in energy requirements and protein utilization. After injury, the body is unable to adapt to starvation and the energy requirements rise whether feeding is instituted or not. The metabolic response to severe brain injury was systematically documented in 1980's. Up to this time, nutritional replacement was not considered very significant, by the clinicians. This was based on false assumption that due to coma/unconsciousness, metabolic requirements were reduced. Most of the work done in 1980's[1-4] was concentrated on measurements of metabolic expenditure, nitrogen loss and cardiovascular parameters. Hypermetabolism and nitrogen wasting were well documented. The mean increase noticed was in metabolic expenditure of approximately 140 percent of normal requirements in comatose patients with isolated head injury. The duration of hypermetabolic response and wide individual variation needs further investigation for better understanding.

METABOLIC REQUIREMENTS

Metabolic expenditure using indirect calorimetry was studied in 57 patients with severe head injury. By multiple regression analysis, a significant relationship was found between heart rate (HR), day since injury (DSI) and GCS in patients with GCS < 7. According to this relationship

% RME = 152 – 13 (GCS) + 0.4 (HR) + 7 (DSI)
(RME – Resting metabolic expenditure)

This formula can be used in first 2 weeks after injury. Energy requirements after first 2 weeks after brain injury have not been investigated. The duration of hypermetabolic response and the contribution of muscle tone and activity to it have been investigated. Majority of hypermetabolism is due to muscle tone and it is shown that head injured patients paralysed with pancuronium bromide or use of barbiturate come depressed the metabolic rate from a mean of 160 percent to expected 100 to 120 percent.[3] Even with paralysis, energy requirements remain elevated by considerable degree (20–30%).

NITROGEN METABOLISM

Nitrogen balance is defined as the difference between nitrogen intake and nitrogen excretion. Nitrogen excretion is urinary nitrogen + 2 to 3 g (faecal and cutaneous nitrogen loss).

For each gram of nitrogen measured in the urine, 6.25 g of protein has been catabolized in the body. Urinary nitrogen excretion normally lags behind by 3 to 8 days to the metabolic event that influenced it. Normal requirement of protein depends upon the total caloric intake and in normal human the minimal requirement of protein is about 30 g/day, if the total required calories are provided. In an injured state the energy and protein requirements increase. In head injury patients, protein contributes about 30 to 45 percent of total consumed calories as compared to 10 to 15 percent in normal state.

In starved normal human beings the loss of body mass to fat is 0.5:1, but in severe head injury and other trauma the ratio is reversed, that is 2:1 to 4:1.[5] Nitrogen excretion after severe head injury is comparable with other hypercatabolic states like sepsis, severe burns and major surgery (Table 50.1). A peak in nitrogen excretion appears to occur in the second week. With improvement in nitrogen retention by third week nitrogen balance becomes possible. Effect of steroids on nitrogen retention has been studied and it is found

Table 50.1: Urinary nitrogen excretion rate/kg/day

State	*Nitrogen excretion*
Normal	0.085 ± 0.002
Burns	0.369 ± 0.035
Sepsis	0.366 ± 0.060
Head injury (GCS < 8)	0.36 ± 0.08
Skeletal trauma	0.317 ± 0.018
Elective surgery	0.214 ± 0.027

that steroids increase the nitrogen retention by 30 percent in fasting state but their effect is lost during feeding.[6,7]

USE OF ANTHROPOMETRIC INDICES FOR ASSESSMENT OF NUTRITIONAL STATUS

Various indices used in the monitoring of nutritional status are weight, arm muscle circumference, triceps skin fold thickness, serum albumin level and transferrin level. In head injury patients, despite hyperalimentation, 15 percent weight loss occurs during first three weeks and serum albumin drops to low values.[2] By the time anthropometric changes occur, malnutrition is well advanced making these indices of limited value in acute head injury. However, they are useful after 3 weeks. It is generally believed that 10 to 15 percent weight loss is of no great importance, 20 percent loss increases susceptibility to stress and 30 percent weight loss increases morbidity and mortality appreciably.

AIMS OF NUTRITIONAL SUPPLEMENT

Complete replacement of expended calories is the aim of nutritional supplement, because without full energy replacement, protein is wasted. Since there is high individual variation in energy expenditure, investigators recommend the addition of 20 percent to the normal values of metabolic requirements obtained at rest. Feeding at levels over actual caloric expenditure is not required as it may result in hyperglycemia, uremia and increased carbon dioxide production. Recommended range of caloric intake in different neurosurgical patients is given in Table 50.2.

To achieve full caloric replacement by seven days after injury, nutritional replacement is usually began not later than 72 hours after injury because 2 to 3 days are required to gradually increase feedings to full replacement levels. Intravenous hyperalimentation may also can be used. The desired level of protein in the diet for head injury patients are not quantified and data suggest that at high range of nitrogen intake, less than 50 percent of administered nitrogen is retained.[2]

Table 50.2: Recommended range of caloric intake in different neurosurgical patients

Patient's state		*Caloric replacement k cal/kg*
Resting 70 kg male (normal)		26-30
Postoperative craniotomy		26-30
GCS = 4-5,	First week	40-50
	Second week	50-60
	Localizing/flexing	
	First week	30-40
	Second week	40-50
GCS = 8-12	First week	30-35

ENTERAL VS PARENTERAL FEEDING

There are three options for the method of feeding. Some reports indicate that jejunal and parenteral replacement produce better nitrogen retention than gastric feeding.

Advantages of enteral feeding are:

1. Less risk of hyperglycemia.
2. Lower risk of infection/septicemia.
3. Lower cost.

Maintenance of gut mucosa and mucosal barrier to bacteria is a definite advantage. It has been shown that when gut mucosal atrophy occurs, bacteria translocates to mesenteric lymph nodes and later results in septicemia. Enteral feeding can therefore reduce infection rate by ways other than avoiding central venous catheters. Feeding should be gradually increased over few days and is best administered by constant infusion. Infusion rate that should be achieved is 100-150 ml/hr.

Failure of delivery of full caloric requirement by enteral feeding by 5 to 7 days after head injury in a patient who will require prolonged nutritional support constitutes an indication for parenteral hyperalimentation. Also when diarrhea resulting from antibiotic therapy remains uncontrolled feeds can be stopped and parenteral hyperalimentation can be used. Cerebral edema is a potential contraindication to parenteral alimentation. More than 50 percent fat as caloric source can result in fat deposition in the liver.[8] Fat is preferentially used as source of energy in stressful conditions and without fat, essential fatty acid deficiences can occur. A mixed caloric source with approximately 50 percent fat in acute state and 30 percent fat as stress resolves has been recommended in head injury.[4] Prolonged parenteral alimentation is more likely to result in vitamin and mineral deficiencies. Exact increment required in vitamins and minerals are not known. The normal requirements of Sodium and Potassium (Sodium = 2 mEq/kg/day and Potassium = 1 mEq/kg/day) should be met while replacing adequate energy.

The infants with significant prenatal brain damage have increased nutritional requirement in first postnatal year and suggest that decreased postnatal brain growth may exacerbate their impairment. The axonal diameter in corticospinal tract, length and weight were found to be increased in those receiving higher energy and protein diet.[9]

In a study, the patients who were not fed within 5 to 7 days after TBI had 2 and 4 fold increased likelihood of death respectively. The amount of nutrition in first 5 days was related to death, every 10-K cals/kg decrease in caloric intake was associated with 30 to 40 percent increase in mortality rates. The helps us even after controlling factors known to effect mortality including arterial hypotension, age, papillary status, initial GCS score and CT scan findings, hence nutrition is a significant predictor of death due to TBI.[10]

CONCLUSION

It is well documented that starved head injury patients lose sufficient nitrogen to reduce rate by 15 percent per week. Secondly, nonfeeding of head injured patients by first week increases mortality rate. As complete replacement of 100 to 140 percent of resting metabolism expenditure with 15 to 20 percent nitrogen reduces nitrogen loss, full nutritional replacement should be instituted by seventh day of trauma. Early and adequate nutritional replacement is likely to reduce mortality in head injury.

REFERENCES

1. Clifton GL, Robertson CS, Choi SC. Assessment of nutritional requirements of head injured patients. J Neurosurg 1986;64:895-901.
2. Clifton GL, Robertson CS, Contant CF. Enteral hyperalimentation in head injury. J Neurosurg 1985;62:168-93.
3. Clifton GL, Robertson CS, Grossman RG. The metabolic response to severe head injury. J Neurosurg 1984;60:687-96.
4. Deutschman CS. Physiological and metabolic response to isolated head injury. Pary I: Basal metabolic state: Correlations of metabolic and physiological parameters with fasting and starved controls. J Neurosurg 1986;64:89-98.
5. Elwyn DH. Nutritional requirements of adult surgical patients. Crit Care Med 1980;8:9-20.
6. Robertson CS, Clifton GL, Goodman JC. Steroid administration and nitrogen excretion in head injured patients. J Neurosurg 1985;63:714-8.
7. Young B, Ott L, Norton J. Metabolic and nutritional sequelae in the non-steroid treated head injury patient. Neurosurgery 1985;17:784-91.
8. Stein TP, Buzby GP, Leskiw MJ. Protein and fat metabolism in rats during repletion with total parenteral nutrition (TPN). J Nutr 1981;111:154-65.
9. Adamkin DH. Nutritional rehabilitation for brain injury infants, catch up growth is good. Pediatric 2008;121(1):181-2.
10. Hartl R, Gerber LM, Ni Q, Ghajar J. Effect of early nutrition on death due to sever traumatic brain injury. J Neurosurg 2008;109(1):50-6.

51 Rehabilitation in Head Injury

AK Mahapatra, Raj Kumar

INTRODUCTION

The overall outcome of patients with severe head injury is bad. Large number of severe head injury patients die or remain vegetative.[1-5] The Glasgow outcome scale was developed by Jennett and Bond to grade the outcome of head injured patients.[6] With the availability of CT scan, ICU care and quick surgery there is a greater number of survivors and many of them do have moderate or severe disability.[7,8] With ever increasing number of head injuries, the cumulative number of disabled and vegetative patients are growing tremendously. Many of our outcome scales do not include cognitive behavioral and professional performance. In fact, to a common garden neurosurgeon or physician, successful recovery means "patient survives, patient can walk and talk". Today, the "walking and talking" are no longer considered as satisfactory measures of good recovery.

Head injury, severe or even minor, leads to large number of behavioral and cognitive problems.[9-16] Over the years, neurosurgeons have tried to bring down mortality and morbidity. Unfortunately, however, adequate attention has not been paid for the proper rehabilitation of head injured patients. Each patient represent, a unique and complex problem, which include, physical, visual, cognitive and behavioral abnormalities (Table 51.1) due to heterogeneity of neuropathology, sociocultural background and educational level. Most frequent and important abnormalities result from frontal lobe function impairment, involving higher level regulatory and problem solving capacities.[9,10]

Table 51.1: Neuropsychological abnormalities following head injury
• Physical: Paralysis, spasticity, contractures, visual or hearing problem
• Cognitive defect:
– Remediation and retaining
– Defect in arousal and attention
– Deficit in learning and remembering
– Communication deficit
– Executive deficit
– Anosognosia
• Behavioral:
– Aggressive and agitated
– Disinhibition
– Decreased initiation
– Depression
• Hypothalamic and endocrine dysfunction

REHABILITATION OF PHYSICAL DISABILITY

Large number of patients with head injury do have physical disability may be due to paralysis, or weakness of limbs, spasticity, visual or hearing problem and due to speech abnormalities (Table 51.2).[16,17] The aim of the treatment is, therefore, to see that the patient returns to a productive employment. Overall, the goal of rehabilitation is to reintegrate the patient into a supportive social system and provide a productive and active life.[18]

Weakness can be managed by repeated early mobilization and protocol based exercise. Early ambulation, mobilization in wheel chair is also important. Mackay et al[19] in a large study showed the difference in outcome in patients with formalized protocol based treatment as compared to non-formalized treatment in severe head injury.

Prevention of contracture is very important. This can be achieved by various methods such as, casting combined with stretching, different exercises, use of passive positioning with pillows, splints and special bed.[20,21] Once contractures have formed they should be treated if they are progressive by traction

Table 51.2: Physical disabilities
• Motor weakness
– Paralysis
– Spasticity
– Contractures and deformities
• Cerebellar dysfunction
– In coordination
– Ataxia
– Tremors
• Speech abnormalities
• Visual hearing impairment
• Bladder dysfunction

Table 51.3: Cognitive abnormalities in head injured patients

- Disorder or arousal
- Attention abnormality
- Inability to learn and concentrate
- Memory disturbances
- Defective communication
- Executive dysfunction
- Lack of motivation
- Anosognosia (Lack of awareness of their problems)

and prolonged stretch. Rarely, long standing severe contracture may need surgery. In severe head injury heterotopic ossification may set in giving rise to contracture.[22-24] Some authors have used different chemicals such as Disodium etidronate, aspirin and indomethacin to prevent ossification.[23,24] Prevention of spasticity is an important part in rehabilitation.[22]

Hypertonia is very common in head injury. Sometimes, spasticity may also be associated with rigidity. Spasticity also helps in development of contracture. More importantly, spasticity hampers skilled movement. Oral medication by dantrolene is the drug of choice in spasticity and it has very few side effects. Rarely, in severe hypertonia, nerve blocks may be helpful. Head injury patients do have tremor and ataxia (Table 51.3) which also influence in overall motor performance.

CARE OF EYES AND PREVENTION OF BLINDNESS

In comatose patients nursing care is important for prevention of bedsore and exposure keratitis. Facial paralysis or damage to corneal sensation can give rise to redness of eyes or even exposure keratitis. Prevention of exposure, proper use of eye drops and ointment can prevent corneal damage. Rarely, a tarsorrhaphy may be necessary to prevent keratitis.

In 2 to 5 percent patients can have associated traumatic blindness.[25-29] In unconscious patients dilated fixed pupils are considered as 3rd nerve palsy, while it may be really due to optic nerve injury. Hence, in suspected patients, VEP (Visual Evoked Potential) is necessary to establish the diagnosis.[28,29] Mostly, the blindness is due to ischemic necrosis of the nerve in the optic canal. Timely injection of corticosteroid and if necessary, optic canal decompression can improve the chance of visual recovery and prevent the blindness. Hence, early diagnosis, steroid therapy and, if indicated, surgery is likely to reduce the visual problem in head injured patients.

COGNITIVE ABNORMALITIES IN HEAD INJURY

Cognitive abnormalities are the important factors preventing integration of patients in head injury. Large number of cognitive abnormalities are encountered in head injury patients.[9,11,14,15,18,30-32] Surprisingly, cognitive function abnormalities are not limited to severe head injury. A significant number of patients with minor head injury do have short-term or long-term cognitive function derangement.[1,13,16,32,33]

The role of magnetic resonance imaging, specifically magnetic resonance spectroscopy (MRS) and susceptibility-weighted imaging (SWI) has emerged in evaluation of cases with TBI for better predictability. Specifically the number and volume of hemorrhagic diffuse axonal injury (DAI) lesions as well as changes in spectral metabolites such as reduced N-acetylaspartate or elevation in choline related compounds correlate with neurological disability and impairment of global intelligence, memory and attention.[66]

In the recent years considerable interest has been generated in remediation of cognitive deficit following head injury. The mode is by cognitive training and remediation method. However, it is always important to answer whether special education and training skill is enough to correct cognitive deficit. Then the method must be used to improve memory, to perform the work efficiently and to develop skill for better solving of the problems.

The aim of the cognitive rehabilitation is to have a specialized protocol based remedial strategies.[14,17] The specialized strategies must be utilized very early in cognitive rehabilitation. There are evidences that these cognitive defects can improve.[15,16] It is also clear that the recovery of function occurs not by amelioration of damaged function but by adaptation to deficits. Earlier ones adapt to deficit, quicker is the chance of recovery. Hence, it is not absolutely clear whether the attempt to "retrain" memory, attention or problem solving would succeed or not. It is also not clear that a problem is either an additive combination or a component of cognitive process. Many patients with mild but multiple problems may make the entire cognitive deficit more complex and more difficult for correction[15] as compared to severe and single cognitive defect.

Considering above points, it is also important to understand if it is possible to correct the deficit directly. If it is possible, then it is more effective and efficient to remediate a set of deficits independently and then allow the patient to combine them with functional skill or even to educate them in the executive skill.

Rehabilitation is effective in improving functional outcome of after TBI even in persons who have reached stable neurological recovery at 12 or more months following injury. They develop improvement in overall disability, independence, home competency and productivity. In a group of post-acute rehabilitation (>6 months post-injury) independence continuous to occur following discharge.[68]

These strategies are only applicable in particular context to each specific task. Hence, the complex cognitive defects leads to dilemma in rehabilitation strategies. Thus, the boundaries between the intelligence, learning, aptitude, achievement, capacity and skill in learning, etc. delineate the complexities of problems in remediation.

DISORDER OF AROUSAL, SLEEP AND ATTENTION

Arousal and attention defect is a most common cognitive abnormality in head injury. Damage to frontal lobe and reticular activating system play important role in attention. Normal attention requires adequate arousal level throughout the day. The ability to attend particular stimuli in face of potential distractor, provides the ability to maintain prolonged attention. Head injury disrupts the attentional function and reduces the speed of information processing.[34] In head injury there is impaired tonic arousal. Lack of attention is also frequently encountered in patients of minor head injury with post-concussion syndrome. In children, poor attention in classroom is not infrequent. The treatment is basically by behavioral intervention and psychopharmacology. Sometimes, reinforcement of task behavior improves the attentiveness. Rarely, psychostimulants like dextroamphetamine, methylphenidate and pemoline sodium have been used to increase arousal level in lethargic patients.[35,36] However, it is difficult to evaluate the drug response in patients with multiple interacting complex cognitive deficits.

Defects in learning and memory are significant problems in head injury. There is both retrograde and anterograde amnesia. Due to anterograde amnesia, there is considerable difficulty in acquiring new informations. This has tremendous impact in education, professional and vocational point of view.[9,36-38] In head injury, amnesia laterized to both verbal and visuospatial material, and formal testing of memory may be falacious as its validity is limited. Rarely, a certain type of learning is preserved.[36] Chance of improving memory by repetition is remote.[37] Sometimes specific memory enhancing exercise such as (a) drilling patient with a specific piece of information, (b) utilizing memory aid like (diaries, lists and computer and (c) providing limited context such as name of few acquaintances. In school, children need specific attention and extra care for learning.[37]

Anosognosia also prevents quick improvement. Rehabilitation requires patient's effort and will, full participation in exercise, and training process. Many patients lack awareness of their deficits, and do not cooperate in learning exercise. Lack of awareness of deficit leads to lack of motivation. Lack of motivation reduces the learning process and prevents or slower the chance of recovery.[39]

Communication abnormalities are not uncommon. It may either be due to speech problem or due to dysarthria.[40] Cognitive based communication deficit needs speech therapy, using various modalities including videotape and feedback. In communication, education status, language and learning abilities help in recovery of speech.

BEHAVIORAL ABNORMALITIES AND REHABILITATION

Large number of behavioral abnormalities are encountered in head injury patients.[10,12,13,19,31,41-44] The abnormalities can be short-lived or chronic (Table 51.4). These behavioral abnormalities severely limit the reintegration of a head injured patient into his own family, community and working environment. The differences between behavioral and cognitive deficits are artificial as the cognitive problems often contribute to the genesis of behavioral abnormalities.

Aggressive and "agitated" behavior is one of the most frequent abnormality. These aggressive attitudes can lead to homicidal or suicidal tendency and socially and sexually disinhibited behavior. The aggressive

Table 51.4: Behavioral abnormalities in head injury

- Problem in adjustment
  - In family
  - At work place
  - In society
- Aggressive and "agitated behavior"
- Disinhibited behavior
  - Impulsive
  - Hyperexcited
  - Stealing things
  - Making of offensive remarks
- Decreased initiation
- Depression—Lack of interest, depressed mood, lack of motivation.

behavior is a reaction to loss of confidence and depression.

It should be managed by frequent reassurance, and clear information about what is about to happen. If the agitated period is prolonged or severe, treatment with amitriptyline or methylphenidate may help.[45,46] It is believed that the extreme aggressive behavior is due to frontolimbic dysfunction. It may be manifested by epidoside dyscontrol syndrome.[45] Sometimes, carbamazepine is used to increase tolerance to anger. Lithium carbonate and beta blockers such as propranolol have also been used. Usually, conventional neuroleptics are ineffective in controlling aggressive behavior. Proper training, enforcement of certain social behavior may be of benefit.

Sometimes, patients with head injury lack inhibition. They are more impulsive in their work. Frontal lobe plays an important role in disinhibited behavior. Disinhibited sexual behavior is also rarely noticed. Behaviors such as, sexual fondling of strangers, stealing small things like food and making offensive remarks may be observed in patients with head injury. Attempt should be made to decrease the patient's tendency to react by teaching him to "stop and think about the potential consequences".

DECREASED INITIATION AND DEPRESSION

Depression and lack of interest are two very important aspects in head injured patients, which make them sceptic about their activity. Lack of initiation and motivation also hamper in rehabilitation process. These symptoms too, are linked to frontolimbic abnormalities, in which, patient looses link between motivation and action. In some patients there may be only impairment of initiation, but they may have desire to achieve goal and describe the actions required, however, they simply fail to execute them. These patients are benefited from external motivation though structured programs. Motivation programs should be focussed on the successful starting on subsequent steps. Sometimes psychostimulant drugs may also be of some help.

Depression, on the other hand, makes the patient isolated in family and society. In work place, they are unable to mix freely with friends or express freely. Paralysis, fits, other physical disability, and memory disturbances may add to depression. Depression restricts the community involvement and building of new relation, thus, making them maladjusted in environment. Confidence building measures, sympathetic hearing to patient's problem and supportive counseling benefit large number of patients. Role of spouse, children and other family members are important, in bringing the patients out of depression.

REHABILITATION OF CHILDREN

Children pose important problem in rehabilitation. In addition to cognitive and behavioral problems, they also have learning and education problems.[47-49] Greenspan and Mackenzie[48] studied 95 children with head injury. They studied (a) Preinjury status, (b) Postinjury status, (c) Family economic and social status. They reported worse outcome in children with poor socioeconomic status, preinjury ill health and children with lower limb injury. Scott et al[49] studied 43 severely head injured children. Assessment after 13 months showed 42 percent had neurological deficits and 35 percent were identified having a need for special educational support. The score obtained by these children by the parents and teachers showed, significant abnormalities in both health and habits. Middleton[50] studied cognitive and psychological sequelae in children. They found abnormalities at home and in classroom. Children with head injury are neither sick nor mentally handicapped. However, they need rehabilitation that fits their special need. They often acutely aware of their difficulties and loss of freedom, loss of skill and abilities.

There is a sense of fear, anger and frustration. All these parameters must be clearly assessed prior to rehabilitation. In children, parents and teachers play important roles in rehabilitation. Teachers must take extra care and pay a little more attention for these children.

VOCATIONAL REHABILITATION

Gainful re-employment is one of the most difficult aspect in head injury.[16,30,31,51,52] Lack of interest, depression, lack of initiative and motivation hamper their job prospect, in the absence of physical disability. Even, following minor head injury, things are not good. High level of anxiety and stress were noted in 33 percent[16] of the entire head injury group and in 95 percent of the group who returned to work. Kraft et al[51] studied Americans suffered head injury during Vietnam war 15 years later, and only 56 percent gainfully employed and only 64 percent could complete degree courses.

Dikman et al[52] in 1994 studied type and pattern of employment following head injury. They studied 360 patients and analyzed: (a) preinjury employment, (b) injury to rest of the body, (c) severity of head injury and (d) educational status of the patients. In their study 68 percent had returned to work, 93 percent were independent. Vocational rehabilitation depends on several factors including cognitive and neuropsychological recovery. In a study, 17 percent of patients who returned to work had cognitive and personality changes. On the other hand, only 25 percent patients had cognitive defect, in the group who did not go back to work.

Following TBI the type of occupation influences RTW (return to work following TBI) outcome, with best prospect for RTW among people with professional and managerial jobs.[67]

Thus, large number of factors play role in reemployment of patients. Support of family, proper rehabilitation, and adjustment of friends at work place are important for patient's confidence building and reemployment.

POSTCONCUSSION SYNDROME

Minor head injury constitutes around 90 percent of all head injury. Fortunately, mortality, vegetative state and severe physical disability are practically nonexistent with minor head injury. Unfortunately, however, association to cognitive and behavioral problems are considerably high. Over 50 to 60 percent patients do manifest postconcussion problem.[13,14,16] Postconcussion syndrome (PCS) is a condition, characterized by the presence of headache, vertigo, lack of concentration, memory disturbance, loss of appetite and slow reaction. Patient remains depressed and less active with slow reaction. Between 50 to 85 percent patients do have some symptoms and most frequent among them are headache, tiredness and lack of interest to work. In another study 46 percent complained of poor work performance due to depression, poor memory and lack of motivation. Thus, postconcussion syndrome becomes a major public health problem, considering the magnitude of minor head injury and high incidence of postconcussion syndrome. Recently, physiological studies like P300 and cerebral blood flow by transcranial Doppler have shown abnormalities in minor head injury with postconcussion syndrome.[53,54] In their study, Jain and Mahapatra[54] concluded that the abnormality in blood flow velocities by TCD compared well with P300 abnormalities. Both P300 and blood flow abnormalities indicate a diffuse cerebral involvement. There is also a good correlation of P300 wave abnormalities with severity of vertigo. Patients in whom bilateral P300 abnormalities were detected, CT scan also showed cerebral lesions.

Recently, in a series of study from an department has clearly.[54a,54b] Shown low cerebral perfusion in patients with postconcussion syndrome (PCS). Patient with persistent vertigo do have long-term perfusion defect in temporal lobes. SPECT study has shown this perfussion problems, both in adults and children.

Assurance and confidence building measures are the mainstay of treatment. Relaxation training and reduction of stress level are also important. Deep breathing, autogenic training, mediation and control of emotion are likely to increase the working capability and job prospect. Schwatzberg[55] reported use of audiotape and videotape in rehabilitation of head injury patients. He concluded that it is important to accept head injury group as a separate group with specialized training than other problem focussed group. With proper rehabilitation program it is possible to provide better job oriented outcome.

PROBLEMS OF REHABILITATION IN VEGETATIVE PATIENTS

Around 5 to 10 percent of severe head injuries are ultimately vegetative (56-58%).[56,56a] Persistent vegetative state is a social and economic problem. Treatment of vegetative state is an unsolved problem. Moriya et al[56a] reported useful role of median nerve stimulation, in comatose patients. In another study Ueda and Yanagida reported music in awakening respect of comatose patient. Recently, dorsal column stimulation (DCS) has shown improvement in some patients[58] since, 1st report by Kanno, 133 patients in vegetative state have been treated in Japan and USA,[58] clinical improvement was recorded in 57 cases (42-9%). The favorable factors were: (a) young age, (b) head trauma, (c) coma for less than 3 months and CT scan, which show no sign of severe damage. Other significant parametres which indicate chance of recovery are EEG and blood flow improvement following dorsal column stimulation. This leads to unresolved issues regarding the grading of vegetative state. There is no scoring system for chronic unconsciousness. Such a classification should include, cerebral blood flow, EEG and evoked potential. All above will help in selecting patients for spinal cord stimulation.

ENDOCRINAL DYSFUNCTION

All types of endocrinal dysfunction have been reported after severe head injury. In acute head injury with stress, diabetes insipidus and adrenal cortical deficiency may occur. Problem like diabetes insipidus is very obvious and requires judicious management. Chronic endocrinal dysfunctions are by and large of hypothalamic origin.[59-61] Necrosis of pituitary gland and damage to hypothalamus are reported in severe head injury. Amenorrhea or menstrual disorders in females and depressed secretion of testosterone leading the sexual dysfunction are also reported in under hypothyroidism and hypocortisolism require long-term replacement.[59] Hypothalamic disturbances also likely to change sleep cycle[62] (For detail see Chapter 20).

DRIVING AFTER HEAD INJURY

Driving skill is impaired following head injury. Several factors are responsible, which include, physical, visual disability, lack of motivation, poor reaction and loss of confidence.[63-65] Shute and Woodhouse[65] discuss the visual problem and driving ability following head injury. They also considered legal points in relation to visual fitness and driving in patients with head injury. Weakness of limbs, contracture, spasticity and more importantly, post-traumatic epilepsy also create problem following head injury. Galski et al in 1993[64] evaluated driving performance in patients with brain injury. They used combined administration of pre-driver, simulator and behind the wheel evaluation. They analyzed 106 patients and reported that the residual cognitive defects *per se* did not render a person unfit to drive. They also emphasized that the method used was reliable and relatively sensitive to predict the outcome. Overall, the driving becomes a problem in survivors of both severely and mildly head injured patients. Disability, spasticity play important role in severe head injury, as compared to loss of confidence, lack of interest and motivation in patients with minor head injury.

Approximately two-third of screened patients with TBI are able to complete a brief neuropsychologic test battery at 2 to 6 weeks postinjury, regardless of PTA (Post-traumatic amnesia) status. Although, patients out of PTA are less impaired on all test measures. 'Confusion' does not preclude test measures. Early neuropsychological assessment after TBI is feasible for many patients for better rehabilitation.[69]

CONCLUSION

Rehabilitation of head injury has long been neglected. Fortunately, in the recent years things have improved. No doubt rehabilitation is an uphill task in head injury patients due to wide range of involvement, physical, cognitive and behavioral problems. It is a long and tidius process, which needs multidisciplinary approach, and requires dedicated teamwork. Cooperation of patients, sympathetic and supportive role of family and friends help in quicker recovery.

The rehabilitation process must be well designed and a protocol based treatment must be instituted as early as possible. In minor head injuries, confidence building measures, and reassurance play a vital role. Children need a special care, both at home, and at school. In recovery of the children, teachers play important role, in learning and education. In India, things are much worse as the medical and sociocultural systems are different. Overall, the emphasis is on the development and critical evaluation of community based services like, enhancement of social participation, independent living mode in long-term rehabilitation. As the financial burden is immediate and long lasting, the impact on family and community is immense. Hence, it is necessary to develop community based rehabilitation facilities and strategy for active participation in productive, recreational and vocational programs. Thus, knowing the magnitude of the problem, physical, and mental rehabilitation must be considered as an important part in head injury management to improve the overall results.

REFERENCES

1. Jennett B, Teasdale B, Brackman R, et al. Prognosis of patients with severe head injury. Neurosurgery 1979; 4:283-9.
2. Langfitt TW. Gennarelli TA. Can the outcome from head injury be improved? J Neurosurg 1982;56:19-23.
3. Becker DP, Miller JD, Ward JD. The outcome from severe head injury with early diagnosis and intensive management (Class II). J Neurosurg 1977;47:491-502.
4. Jennett B, Teasdale G, Galbraith S, et al. Severe head injury in three countries. J. Neurol Neurosurg Psychiat 1977;40:291-5.
5. Miller JD, Butterworth JF, Gudeman SK, et al. Further experience in the management of severe head injury. J Neurosurg 1981;54:289-99.
6. Jennett B, Bond M. Assessment of outcome after severe brain damage. A practical scale. Lancet 1975;1:480-89.
7. Narayan RK, Greenburg RP, Miller JD, et al. Improved confidence of outcome prediction in severe head injury. A comparative analysis of the clinical examination, multi-modal evoked potential, CT scanning and intracranial pressure. J Neurosurg 1981;54:751-62.
8. Marshall LF. The role of aggressive therapy for head injury: Does it matter? In: Clinical Neurosurgery. William and Wilkin, Baltimore Md 1986; Vol. 34 p. 549.
9. Auerbach SH. Neuroanatomical correlation of attention of behavioural subtype. J Head Trauma Rehabil 1986;1: 1-8.
10. Boll TJ. Behavioural sequelae of head injury. In: Cooper PR (Ed): Head Injury. William and Wilkin, Baltimore 1982; p. 263.

11. Prigatano GP. Psychiatric aspect of head injury. Problem area and suggested guidelines for research. In: Levin HS, Grafman J, Eisenberg HM (Eds). Neurobehavioural Recovery from Head injury. Oxford University Press. New York 1987; p. 215.
12. Levin HS. The neurobehavioural recovery. In: Becker DP, Povlishock JT (Eds): Central Nervous System Trauma Status Report. NIH Bethesda Med 1985; p. 251.
13. Levin HS, Mattis S, Ruff R, et al. Neurobehavioural outcome following minor head injury. A three center study. J Neurosurg 1987;66:234-8.
14. Ben Yishay Y, Diller L. Cognitive defect. In: Rosenthal M, Griffith ER, Bond MR, et al (Ed): Rehabilitation of the head injured adult. FA Davis Company, Philadelphia 1983; p. 163.
15. Hart T, Hyden ME. The ecological validity of Neuropsychological assessment and Mediation. In: Uzzell BP and Gross Y (Eds). Clinical Neuropsychology of Intervention. Martinus Nijhoff Publishing Comp Boston 1986; p. 22.
16. Powel TJ, Collin C, Sulton K. A follow-up study of patients hospitalized after minor head injury. Disability Rehab 1996;18:231-7.
17. Fearnside MR, Cook RJ, McDougall P, et al. The Westrne Head Injury Project. Physical and social outcome following severe head injury. Brit J Neurosurg 1993;7:643-50.
18. Mayer NH, Keating DJ, Rapp D. Skill, routines and activity pattern of daily living. A functional nested approach. In: Uzzell BP, Gross Y (Eds): Clinical Psychology of Intervention, Martinus Nijhoff Publishing, Boston 1986; 205.
19. Mackay LE, Bernstein BA, Chapman PE, et al. Early intervention in severe head injury: Long-term benefits of a formalized progress. Arch Phys Med Rehabil 1992; 73:635-41.
20. Whyte J. Rehabilitation. In NINS, Head Injury Clinical Management and Research. Elizabeth Frost (Ed): AIREN Geneva Switzerland 1990;4:233-48.
21. Moseley AM. The effect of casting combined with stretching of passive ankle dorsiflexion in adults with traumatic head injuries. Physical Therapy 1997;77:240-47.
22. Glenn M, Rosenthal M. Rehabilitation following severe traumatic brain injury. J Head Trauma Rehabil 1986; 1:72.
23. Mital MA, Garber JE, Stinson JJ. Ectopic bone formation in children and adolescents with head injuries, its management. J Ped Ortho 1987;7:83.
24. Spielman G, Gennarelli TA, Rogers CR. Disodium etidronate: Its role in preventory heterotopic ossification in severe head injury. Arch Phys Med Rehabil 1983;64:539.
25. Fukado Y. Microsurgical transethmoidal optic nerve decompression in 700 cases. In: The cranial nerves. Samii M, Jennetta P (Eds): Springer-Verlag, New York 1981; p. 125-28.
26. Gjerris F. Traumatic lesions of visual pathway. In: Vinken PI, Bruyn GW (Eds): Handbook of clinical Neurology, North Holland Publishing Company, Amsterdam 1976; 24:24-57.
27. Walsh FB. Trauma involving anterior visual pathways. Freeman HM (Ed): Ocular Trauma. Apleton-Century-Craft. New York 1979; p. 335-5.
28. Mahapatra AK, Bhatia R. Predictive value of visual evoked potential in unilateral optic nerve injury. Surg Neurol 1989;31:339-42.
29. Mahapatra AK, Tandon DA. A prospective study of 250 patients with optic nerve injury. In: Majid Samii (Ed): Skull base anatomy, radiology and management. S Karger Basel 1994; p. 305-09.
30. Greenwood RJ, McMillan MR, Brooks DN, et al. Effect of case management after severe head injury. BMJ 1994;308:1199-205.
31. Godfrey HP, Bishare SN, Partridze PM, et al. Neuropsychological impairment and return to work following severe closed head injury, implications for clinical management. New Zealand Medical Jour 1993;106:301-93.
32. Gronwall D, Wrightson P. Delayed recovery of intellectual function after minor head injury. Lancet 1974;2:605.
33. Gronwall D. Advances in the assessment of attention and information processing after head injury. In Levin HS, Grafman J, Eisenberg HM (Eds): Neuro-behavioural recovery from head injury. Oxford University Press, New York 1987; p. 335.
34. Van Zomeren AH, Brower WH, Doelman BG. Attention deficit. The riddle of selectivity, special speed and alertness. In Brook SN (Ed): Closed head injury, psychological, social and family consequences. Oxford University Press. Oxford 1984; p. 84.
35. Evans RW, Gualtieri CT. Psycho-stimulant Pharmacology in traumatic brain injury. J Head Trauma Rehabil 1987; 2:29.
36. Nissen MJ. Neuropsychology of attention and memory. J Head Trauma Rehabil 1986;1:13.
37. Gilsky EL, Schacter DL. Remediation of organic memory disorder. Current status and future prospects. J Head Trauma Rehabil 1986;1:54.
38. Hermann DL. Know the memory. The use of questionnaires to assess and study memory. Psychol, Bulletin 1982;92:434.
39. McGlynm SM, Schacter DL. Unawareness of deficit in neuropsychological syndromes. J Clin Exp Neuropsychol 1989;11:143.
40. Sarno M. The nature of verbal impairment after closed head injury. J Nerv Mental Dis 1980;168:685.
41. Lezak MD (Ed): Assessment of the behavioural consequences of head trauma. In: Frontiers of clinical Neurosciences. Alan R Loss Inc, New York 1980; Vol 7.
42. Logue P, Mcearthy SM. Assessment of Neurological disorder. In: Assessment strategies in behavioural Medicine. Keefe KJ, Blumenthal JA (Eds): Grune and Stratton, New York 1982; p. 133.

43. Bond MR. The psychiatry of closed head injury. In Brook N (Ed): Closed Head Injury. Psychological, social and family consequences. Oxford University Press. Oxford 1984; p. 148.
44. Benton AL. Behavioural consequences of closed head injury. In Odom GL (Ed): Central Nervous System Trauma, Research Status Report, National Institute of Health, NIH, Bethesda Med 1979; p. 220.
45. Glenn MB. A pharmacological approach to aggressive and disruptive behaviour after traumatic brain injury (Part 2). J Head Trauma Rehabil 1987;2:80.
46. Jackson RD, Corrigan JD, Arnett JA. Amitriptyline for agitation in head injury. Arch Phys Med Rehabil GG 1985;66:180.
47. Appleton R. Head injury rehabilitation for children. Nursing Times 1994;90:29-31.
48. Greenspan AI, Mac Kenzie EJ. Functional outcome after Pediatric head injury. Pediatrics 1994;94:425-32.
49. Scott JR, Marlow N, Seddon N, et al. Rehabilitation and outcome after severe head injury. Arch Dis Child 1992; 67:222-26.
50. Middleton J. Thinking about head injuries in children. J Chil Psychol Psychiat All Disci 1989;30:663-70.
51. Kraft JF, Schwab KK, Salazar AM, et al. Occupational and educational achievements of head injured Vietnam veterans at 15 years follow-up. Arch Phys Med Rehabi, 1993;74:596-601.
52. Dikman SS, Temkin NR, Machamer JE, et al. Employment following traumatic head injuries. Arch Neurol 1994;51:177-86.
53. Agarwal A, Bama N, Walia BS, Mahapatra AK. P300 wave in patients with post-concussion vertigo: A prospective study of 15 cases. Ind J Otolaryngol Head and Neck Surg 1996;18:121-4.
54. Jain K, Mahapatra AK. P300 and TCD abnormality in minor head injury. A preliminary study. In: Brain protection and neural Trauma, VK Khosla, Kak VK, Sharma BS (Eds): Narosa Publisher, New Delhi 2000;298-305.
54a. Agrawal D, Naveen K, Bal CS, Mahapatra AK. Post-concussion vertigo. Is the cause Central. Correlation with SPECT and CT. Neuroscience Today 2003;7:33-6.
54b. Agrawal D, Naveen K, Bal CS, Mahapatra AV. Post concusion syndrome in Pediatric population. Is medial temporal damage in responsible? Correlation with brain SPECT. A prospective controlled study. Childs Neus Syst 2003;19:628.
55. Schwartzberg SL. Helping factors in a predeveloped support group of persons with head injury. Part I. Participant observer perspective. Ame J Rehabil Occup Therap 1994; 48:297-304.
56. Whyte J. The rehabilitation of the patient in a persistent vegetative state. J Head Trauma Rehabil 1986;1:64.
56a. Moriya T, Noda E, Sakurai J, et al. Neurological evaluation of unconscious patient with median nerve stimulation. 8th Annual Meeting of Society of Coma July, 1999.
57. Michaud LJ, Rivara FP, Grady MS, et al. Predictors of survival and severity of disability after severe head injury in children. Neurosurg 1992;31:254-64.
57a. Ueda K, Yana gida M. Effect of Music on brain in unconscious patient. Paper presented at 8th Annual Meeting of Society for Treatment of Coma-Oita July, 1999.
58. Kanno T, Kamei Y, Yokoyama T. A new treatment for vegetative state after head trauma. Dorsal column stimulation. In Modern trend in the management of neurotrauma. Ramani PS, Sharma A (Eds): Lavanya Printing, Bombay 1994; p. 87-92.
59. Fleischer AS, Rudman DR, Payne NS, et al. Hypothalamic, and hypogonadism in prolonged coma. J Neurosurg 1978;49:550.
60. Hadani M, Findler G, Shaked I, et al. Unusual delayed onset diabetes insipidus following closed head trauma. J Neurosurg 1985;63:456-58.
61. Klingbell GE, Clive P. Anterior hypopituitarysm. A consequence of head injury. Arch Phy Med Rehabil 1985; 66:44.
62. Prigantano GB, Stahl ML, Orrwe, et al. Sleep and dreaming disturbances in closed head injury patients. J Neurol Neurosurg Psychiat 1982;45:78.
63. Van Zomeran AH, Brouner WH, Minderhoud JM. Acquired brain damage and driving. A review. Arch Physic Med Rehabil 1987;68:697.
64. Galski T, Bruno RL, Ehle HT. Prediction of behind the wheel driving performance in patients with cerebral brain damage—a discriminent function analysis. Arne J occup Therapy 1993;47:391-6.
65. Shute RH, Woodhouse JM. Visual fitness to drive after stroke and head injury. Ophthal Physio Optics 1990; 10:327-32.
66. Ashwal S, Babikian T, Gardener-Nichols J, et al. Susceptibility Wt Imaging and proton magnetic resonance spectroscopy in assessment of outcome in pediatric TBI, Arch Phys Med Rehabil 2006;87(12 suppl 2):550-8.
67. Walker WC, Marwitz JH, Kreutzer JS, Hart T, Novack TA. Occupational categories and return to work after traumatic brain injury—a multicenter study. Arch Phys Med Rehabil, 2006;87(12):1576-82.
68. High WM JR, Roebuck-spencer J, Sander AM, et al. Early versus late admissions to post-acute rehabilitation. Impact of functional outcome after TBI, Arch Phys Med Rehabil 2006;87(3):334-42.
69. Kalmar K, Novack TA, Nakase-Richardson R, et al. Feasibility of brief neuropsychological testing during acute patient rehabilitation after traumatic brain injury. Arch Phys Med Rehabil 2008;89(5):942-9.

52 Persistent Vegetative State in Head Injury

AK Mahapatra, Raj Kumar

INTRODUCTION

The persistent vegetative state (PVS) in a neurological condition in which a person is in a state of complete unawareness of self, and environment. This clinical state is also associated with sleep and awake cycle with either partial or complete preservation of hypothalamic and brainstem function.[1-5] Frequently, many patients are in vegetative state and over months, they slowly improve. Hence, this condition may be transient (temporary) or permanent.[1,6,9] Some international studies have reported vegetative state at the end of 6 months.[5,10,11] However, diagnosis of vegetative state after one year of injury, reflects real clinical state as there is failure to recover from acute or chronic head injury. Approximately, 10-14 percent of all severe head injuries develop into PVS.[6] This chapter highlights some aspects of PVS.

Diagnosis of persistent vegetative state is made if patient has no evidence of awareness of self or environment, no evidence of sustained, reproducible, purposeful or voluntary behavioral response to sensory stimulus and critically no evidence of language comprehension. A study by hierarchical functional magnetic resonance imaging (fMRI) auditory processing paradigm was done to determine the extent of retained language processing in PSV cases of an etiologically heterogeneous group. It showed that a subset patient of PSV retain islands of preserved cognitive function, they have evidence of preserved speech processing.[48]

CHARACTERIZATION OF VEGETATIVE STATE

Persistent vegetative state (PVS) is a rare condition. Many synonyms have been used by many authors, such as, vegetative state, persistent vegetative state, apallic syndrome, and coma vigil.[6,7] The clinical characterization is not always enough to establish the vegetative state hence, Grossman and Hegel,[6] suggested additional criteria to distinguish different subjects of vegetative state. They suggested investigative modalities such as CT, magnetic resonance imaging, SPECT and EEG to assess the brain dysfunction. However, all above parameters are only relative indicators of limited predictive value. The clinical criteria for PVS are charted in Table 52.1.[1,2]

Table 52.1: Criteria for diagnosis of vegetative state

- No evidence of awareness of self or environment and no ability to interact with others.
- No evidence of sustained, reproducible, purposeful or voluntary behavior in response to visual, auditory, tactile or noxious stimuli.
- No evidence of language comprehension or expression.
- Intermittent awakefulness manifested sleep-awake cycle.
- Sufficiently preserved hypothalamic, and brainstem autonomic function to survive on nursing care.
- Variably preserved cranial nerves and spinal reflex.
- Finally the bowel and bladder incontinence.

The above clinical criteria, when existing for atleast 12 months following injury, the diagnosis of PVS is tenable.[12-14] Large number of patients those who are diagnosed to be in a vegetative state at 6 to 8 weeks do improve significantly over a period of time.[12,15] Thus, diagnosis of PVS is incorrect at 3 or 6 months following trauma (Table 52.2).

PATHOLOGY IN BRAIN AND PATHOGENESIS OF PVS

Earlier it was presumed that the brainstem injury is the most common cause of PVS. However, neuropathological data do not substantiate the above hypothesis.[16,18] In a MRI study of 42 patients, Kampfl et al[14] reported DAI with lesions in corpus callosum and dorsolateral brainstem to be the key site in post-traumatic PVS. They also proved that the basal ganglia to be the 2nd common site of injury in patients with PVS. In one of classic case Kinney et al,[17] in 1994, suggested the role of thalamus in a patient with post-traumatic coma. Other sites where abnormality can lead to vegetative state are the parahippocampal area and the peduncular lesion of the brainstem. In the MRI study reported by Kampfl et al,[14] all 42 vegetative patients had lesions in the corpus callosum. Similar observations were also made by other authors on MRI.[19,20] However, lesions of

Table 52.2: Incidence of vegetative state

	Year 1979	*No Pt*	*%*
• Jennett et al[10]	International Coma Data Bank	1000	12
• Marshall et al[11]	1991, NIH Traumatic Coma Data Bank	746	42
• Celesia[3]	1996	–	14
• Heindl and Laub[12]	1996	127 Children	5
• Kampfl et all[14]	1998	80 in PYS at 6-8 weeks	42 at 1 yr (50%)

corpus callosum was first identified by Strich in 1956,[21] as a prominent features of DAI. Many of these patients followed by Strich developed severe dementia. In addition to DAI there were deep white matter lesions seen in vegetative patients.[14]

Lesions of the basal ganglia or thalamus were reported in 52 and 40 percent respectively in vegetative patients. In hypoxic-ischemic injury leading to PVS, damage to basal ganglia and thalamus are reported as prominent pathological features on radiological imaging.[5,16,17] Among the corpus callosum lesions, splenium is the most common site. Adam et al,[22] in 1989, in their neuropathological studies demonstrated corona radiata, white matter of the frontal and the temporal lobe involvement in DAI. Another characteristic feature of DAI is the focal lesion of the dorsolateral part of the midbrain, which was also recorded in 74 percent of patients of PVS in MRI, reported by Kamfl et al.[15] In addition to above lesions, they reported tegmental lesion in 17 (8-bilateral), periaqueductal injury in 7 patients and ventral midbrain lesions, in 21 patients (bilateral 14). In 32% patients the midbrain lesions had extended into the pons and in 5 patients medullary lesions were noticed, which were exclusively localized in the olives. Thus, neuropathological and neuroradiological studies suggest DAI, involving basal ganglia, midbrain and splenium of corpus callosum, in vast majority of patients with PVS. Overall, histological picture reveals widespread hypoxic and ischemic damage.[5,16,17]

CT AND MRI FINDING IN PVS

Inspite of PVS being a well known and common entity not much literature is available dealing with CT finding in PVS.[23] However, study by Levin et al[23] reported only supratentorial swelling and midline shift. In their study brainstem injury was uncommon. MRI is far superior to CT scan in detecting DAI, hemorrhagic and nonhemorrhagic contusions in corpus callosum, inferior aspect of frontal and temporal lobes and in the brainstem.[14,15,20,24,25] Moreover, MR imaging shows superior sensitivity in detecting post-traumatic shearing injury in subacute stage of head injury. Due to above reasons, MR considered to be more helpful than CT in localizing and characterizing post-traumatic brain lesions. In PVS, CT and MRI have shown widespread lesions in the brain (Table 52.3). In an MRI study in 42 patients with PSV Kampfl et al[14] reported DAI as the most common pathology, followed by brainstem and corpus callosum injury. Ganglionic lesions were recorded in 22 patients and thalamic lesion in 17 patients with PVS. Supratentorial ventricular enlargement and cortical atrophy were recorded in 28 and 11 patients respectively, while 19 had brainstem atrophy. Thus, the MR imaging at different intervals has helped in finding out the various brain lesions in patients with PVS, which infact is correlated well with the neuropathological findings. Reider-Groswasser et al[26] correlated finding of third ventricle in CT with poor outcome. They reported

Table 52.3: Pathological findings reported in MRI and CT in patients with vegetative state

Site of lesion	*%*
• Rostral brainstem	75
• Basal ganglia	52
• Thalamus	40
• Hippocampus	21
• Parahippocampal gyrus	45
• Cortical contusion	48
• Corpus callocum	70
• Corona radiata	56

poor prognosis in patients having third ventricle width 8 mm and 11 mm distance between septum pellucidum and caudate nucleus (Cerebroventricular index).

TREATMENT OF PERSISTENT VEGETATIVE STATE

The patients with early post-traumatic vegetative state can have recovery when they are followed for longer period. However, accurate prediction of recovery is not possible, and various clinical and laboratory tests fail to predict the recovery. Treatment with multidisciplinary approach has shown better chance of recovery of patients in vegetative state. No doubt vegetative patients need appropriate medical and nursing care.[26,27] There is also a great role of family and their educational status. Family members also need counselling.

After the acute stage, structured protocol based rehabilitation programs helps in faster recovery. Recently, sensory stimulation have been used, based on hypothesis that these stimulations help in fast recovery.[28-33] Those include electric stimulation of dorsal column[30-33] and median nerve stimulation.[31] Both Cooper et al[31,32] and Moriya et al[30] reported improvement in vegetative state following the median nerve stimulation. Recently, deep brain stimulation was also used in patients with PVS.[33,34] Yamamoto et al 1993[34] reported changes in CSF levels of PGD,[2] PGE[2] and monoamines, following deep brain stimulation, in vegetative patients. Cooper et al[31] studied 25 patients and published the efficacy of median nerve stimulation. Some authors have reported value of musical stimulation in recovery of comatose patients.[35,36]

In comatose patients, a pupillary reflex is the strongest prognostic variable, followed by N100 (late auditory evoked potential) and middle latency evoked potentials (MLAEPS). These are reliable models for awakening in comatose patients passing into PSV. Evaluation of primary sensory cortex and higher order process by middle-latency, late and cognitive evoked potentials needs to performed to predict awakening of comatose patients.[47]

PHARMACOTHERAPY IN PERSISTENT COMA

Recently some drugs have been tried in comatose patients. These include aminergic agents, cholinergic agents[37] and Prostaglandin E2.[38] Dopaminergic drugs have also been tried[39-42] they include L Dopa[39,40] and Bromocryptine[40-42] Amphetamine[44] and Amantadine has also been tried. Some authors have tried combination of above drugs in patients in coma. Some reports are available reporting the effect of bromocryptine. These drugs helps in synpatic transmission of dopamine receptors. A combination of Amantadine and Bromocryptine have been shown to increase the release of dopamine. Pharmacotherapy must be started much before cerebral atrophy, as PVS more than 3 months have considerably decreased CBF and $CMRO_2$.

Table 52.4: Points on pharmacotherapy in PSV

- Pharmacotherapy can be started early.
- Onset of effect occurs earlier than other therapies.
- Relatively inexpensive.
- Side effects are only few and mild.
- If ineffective can be discontinued promptly.
- Patients can be selected easily.
- The present pharmacotherapy is quite useful in fascilitating early discharge.

Overall, outcome in patients with cerebral atrophy is poor. Overall, there may a role of pharmacotherapy in treatment of prolonged coma (Table 52.4).

A study was conducted to see the effect of methylphenidate (MPH) on command following and yes/no communication in brain injured patients with severe disorder of consciousness. There were no meaningful effects found either in responsiveness or command following.[46]

Persistent vegetative state is a well known entity in head injury, by and large caused by DAI. Damage to corpus callosum, brainstem and corona radiata is often reported in MRI. Coma and other states of impaired consciousness are signs of extensive dysfunction or injury involving brainstem, diencephalons or cerebral cortex. Management includes prompt stabilization of vital physiological functions to prevent secondary neurological injury, etiological diagnosis and institution of brain directed therapeutics or preventive measures. Prognosis is determined by etiology, clinical signs and physiological tests.[45]

Early physiotherapy, different sensory stimulation, and pharmacological agents can reduce the number of vegetative patients. Recently, spinal cord and deep brain stimulation are under trial and have provided some promising results.

REFERENCES

1. Anonymous. Medical aspects of persistent vegetative state (1). The Multi-society Task Force on PVS. N Eng J Med 1994;330:1499-1508.

2. Anonymous. Medical aspects of the persistent vegetative state (2). The Multi-Society Task Force on PVS Published erratum appears in N Eng J Med 1995;333:130.
3. Celesia GG. Persistent Vegetative state. Neurology 1993; 43:1457-58.
4. Kenard C, Illingworth R. Persistent Vegetative State. J Neurol Neurosurg Psychiat 1995;59:347-55.
5. Doughtery JH, Rawlinson DG, Levy DE, et al. Hypoxic-ischaemic brain injury and vegetative state. Clinical and Neuropathologic correlation. Neurology, 1998;34:991-97.
6. Grossman P, Hagel K. Post-traumatic apallic syndrome following head injury. Part 1. Clinical characteristics. Disbil Rehabil, 1996;18:1-20.
7. Jellinger IC, Seitelberger F. Protracted post-traumatic encephalopathy. Pathology, pathogenesis and clinical implication. J Neurol Sci 1970;10:51-94.
8. Child NC, Mercer WN, Child HW. Accuracy of diagnosis of persistent vegetative state. Neurology, 1993;43:1465-67.
9. Andrews K, Murphy L, Munday R, et al. Misdiagnosis of the vegetative state: Retrospective study in a rehabilitation unit BMJ 1996;313:13-16.
10. Jennett B, Teasdale G, Braakman R, et al. Prognosis of patients with severe head injury. Neurosurgery 1979;4: 283-89.
11. Marshall LF, Gautille T, Klauber MR, et al. The outcome of severe closed head injury. J Neurosurg 1991;75:528-53.
12. Heindl UT, Laub MC. Outcome of persistent vegetative state following hypoxic or traumatic brain injury in children or adolescents. Neuropediatrics 1996;27:94-100.
13. Wade TD. Misdiagnosis of the vegetative state: Persistent vegetative state should not be diagnosed until 12 months from onset of coma BMJ 1996;313:943-4.
14. Kampfl A, Franz G, Aichner F, et al. The persistent vegetative state after closed head injury: Clinical magnetic resonance imaging findings in 42 patients. J Neurosurg 1998;88:809-16.
15. Kampfl A, Schmutzhard E, Franz G, et al. Prediction of recovery from post-traumatic vegetative state with cerebral MRI. Lancet 1998;35:1763-7.
16. Kinney HC, Samuels MA. Neuropathology of persistent vegetative state. A review. J Neuro-pathol Exp Neurol, 1994;53:548-58.
17. Kinney HC, Korein J, Panigraphy A, et al. Neuropathological findings in the brain of Karen Ann Qumlan. The role of the thalamus and the persistent vegetative state. N Eng J Med 1994;330:1469-75.
18. Peters G, Rothemund E. Neuropathology of traumatic apallic syndrome. In Dalle OveG, Gerstenbrand F, Lucking CH (Eds): The Apallic Syndrome. Berlin; Springer-Verlag 1977;PV 78-87.
19. Gentry LR, Thompson B, Godersky JC. Trauma to the corpus callosum: MR features. AJNR 1988;9:1129-38.
20. Mendelsohn BD, Levis HS, Haward H, et al. Corpus callosum lesions after closed head injury in children. MRI, clinical features and outcome. Neuroradiology 1992;34:384-88.
21. Strich SJ. Diffuse degeneration of the cerebral white matter in severe dementia following head injury. J Neurol Neurosurg Psychiat 1956;19:163-85.
22. Adam JH, Doyle D, Ford I, et al. Diffuse axonal injury in head injury: definition, diagnosis and grading. Histopathology 1989;15:49-59.
23. Levin HS, Saydijari C, Eisenberg HM, et al. Vegetative state after closed head injury. A Traumatic Coma Data Bank report. Arch Neuro 1991;l48:580-85.
24. Gentry LR. Imaging of closed head injury. Radiology 1994;191:1-17.
25. Gentry LR, Godersky JC, Thompson BH. Traumatic brainstem injury: MR Imaging. Radiology 1989;171: 177-87.
26. Reider-Groswasser I, CostefF HB, Sazbon L, et al. CT findings in Persistent vegetative state following blunt traumatic brain injury. Brain Injury 1997;11:865-70.
27. Grossman P, Hagel K. Post-traumatic apallic syndrome following head injury, Part 2: Treatment Disability & Rehab 1996;18:57-68.
28. Kanno T. Neurostimulation for a case of unconsciousness of chronic stage. Brain and Nerve 1995;47:643-49.
29. Moriya T, Noda E, Sakurai J, et al. Neurological evaluation of unconscious patients with median nerve stimulation 8th Annual meeting of the Society of Treatment of Coma. July 30,1999.
30. Yokoyama T, Kamei Y, Shoda M, et al. Treatment of vegetative status with Dorsal Column stimulation. Neurol Surg (Tokyo) 1990;18:39-45.
31. Moriya T, Hayashi A, Sakurai A, et al. Median nerve stimulation method for severe brain damage with its clinical improvement. In: Proceedings of the 8th Annual meeting of Society of Treatment of coma. Hori S & Kanno T (Eds) 1999;111-14.
32. Cooper JB, Jane JA, Alves WM, et al. Right median nerve stimulation to hasten awakening from coma. Brain Injury 1999;13:261-67.
33. Matsui T, Fujiwara S, Takahashi H, et al. Indication of electrical deep brain or dorsal column stimulation and new scoring system for prolonged impaired consciousness. J Neurosurg (Tokyo) 1998;7:14-23.
34. Yamamoto J, Fukuya J, Hiramaya T, et al. Deep-brain and spinal stimulation therapy in PVS. Changes in PGD_2, PGE_2 and monoamine in CSF. Proceedings of 6th Annual meeting of Society of Treatment of Coma. Neuron Publishing Co.Ltd. 1993;6:63-70.
35. Ueda K, Yana gida M. Effect of music on brain in the unconscious patients. Paper presented at 8th Annual meeting of Society for Treatment of Coma. Beppu, Oita July 30, 1999.
36. Ijichi K, Tsutsu A, Maeda T, et al. Musical exercise therapy for patients with persistent disturbance of consciousness. Presented at the 8th Annual meeting of the Society for treatment of coma. Beppu, Oita July 30, 1999.
37. Maeda T. Neural mechanism of sleep. Advances in Neurological Sciences (Tokyo) 1995;39:7-15.

38. Matsumura H. Prostaglandins and sleep. Advances in Neurological Science (Tokyo) 1995;39:60-80.
39. Di Rocco C. L dopa treatment of comatose state due to cerebral lesion. J Neurosurg Sci, 1974;7:169-76.
40. Yoshizawa T, Kikuechi H, Karasawa J, et al. Bromocryptine treatment in patients with prolonged disturbances of consciousness and mentality. Shinryo to Shinnyaku. 1984; 21:115-25.
41. Saitosh H, Kurisu A, Shinohara Y. Effect of Bromocryptine on patients' with aphasia due to cerebrovascular disease. Shinkeinaikachiryo 1991;8:543-47.
42. Nishino K. Facilitated effect of L dopa on recovery of prolonged consciousness disturbances and motor aphasia in a patient of cerebral stroke. Prog Med 1998;18:1513-20.
43. Sitsu N. A computer assisted EEG study on Psychiatric properties of antiparkinsonian drugs. Seishin Shinkeigaku Zassi 1992;94:238-62.
44. Chrisostomo AD, Duncan PW, Propst MA. Evidence that amphetamine with physical therapy promotes recovery of motor function in stroke patients. Annl Neurol 1988;23:94-97.
45. Stevens Rd, Bhardwaj A. Approach to comatose patient, Crit Care Med 2006;34(1):31-41.
46. Martin RT, Whyte J. The effect of methylphenidate on command following and yes/no communication in person with severe disorders of consciousness: A meta-analysis of n-of-1 studies, Am, J, Phys Med Rehabil 2007; 86(8):613-20.
47. Fischer C, Luaute J, Adeleine P, Morlet D. Predictive value of sensory and cognitive evoked potentials for awakening from coma, Neurology 2004;2463(4): 169-73.
48. Coleman MR, Rodd JM, Davis MH, Johnsrude IS, et al. Do vegetative patients retain aspect of language comprehension. Evidence from fMRI brain 2007;130(Pt 10):2482-3.

53 Prevention of Head Injuries

P Sarat Chandra, AK Mahapatra

Concern for man himself and his fate must always form the chief interest of all technical endeavors; never forget this in the midst of your diagrams and equations. —***Albert Einstein***

Head injury management places a lot of stress on the managing personnel, on the patients and their attendees. Most of the serious head injuries not only require immediate intensive management, but also long-term physical and cognitive rehabilitation. Even patients with minor head injuries suffer from significant disabling cognitive and somatic symptoms for a considerable period of time. All this causes a lot of drain on personal and national resources, a lot of psychological strain on the immediate family members and cripples the national work force. It thus becomes imperative that more importance should be placed at the root level itself, i.e. prevention.

The most common cause of road traffic accidents is two-wheeler accidents.

Pediatric bicycle related hospitalization are the significant public health problem. The morbidity, mortality among children and economic costs to society are large.[17]

Motor bike accidents are dangerous and a motorcyclist is eight times more likely to be fatally injured than the occupant of the car on the basis of per unit distance travelled. Delhi, which has one of the heaviest traffic in the world, has recorded a phenomenal growth in the number of accidents. The number of accidents recorded in 1995 were 9216 of which 2000 were fatal in nature. The total number of accidents escalated to a total of 13000 in 1997 of which about 2176 were fatal accidents. The trend of increase in number of transport vehicles is serious and the escalation in the number of accidents places a considerable strain on the already existing meager medical facilities. Epidemiology of gymnastics related injury amongst the children in United States showed the number of injuries sustained per 1000 gymnastics participants per year for pediatric population was 4.8. The injuries were greater for ages 12 to 17 years (>4). The place where injuries occurred included school (40%), a place of recreation or sport (39.7) home (14.5%) or on other public property (5.8%). Injuries were strain/sprain/fracture/dislocation, abrasion/contusion, laceration/avulsion, closed head injuries (1.7%), and others. Monitoring of gymnastic injuries can be helpful in prevention.[19]

The following chapter will deal briefly on safety precautions required for head injury prevention.

CRASH INJURIES—BIOMECHANICAL ASPECTS

As early as 1949, Sergeant Elmer Paul of the Indianapolis, United States made his observations with regard to fatal accidents occurring in rural areas and indicated that many of these fatalities resulted in what he judged to be survivable crashes, and that the deaths were needlessly due to poor automotive design. Paul developed a technique of accident reporting which incorporated three basic principles: vehicle report, medical report, and pictures, a unique accomplishment in the annals of comprehensive police reporting.[1]

Moore in 1953 reported certain observations, which hold well even today.

1. In 50 percent of the injury producing accidents one or more doors opened during the impact.
2. Thirty percent of the occupants have been ejected, which more than doubles the risk of moderate to fatal head injury. This generally occurs even if there is 9/16 inch separation between the door and the door frame.[2]
3. Cases are hit in front in approximately 51 percent of the time on the right.
4. Most of the persons are hurt "all over", not simply in one place.
5. 75 percent of the injuries are usually over the face and the neck.
6. Over 56 percent of the causes of the injuries are contributed by ejection, contact against instrument panel, windshield and steering wheel.

Most of the injuries are still hold true in India, as often the safety regulations are still not followed.

Since there are no "isolated systems" but man-machine pathomechanical combinations, it is appropriate to relate such engineering idioms to man. Several classifications of failure have been described.[2,3]

Rupture: A good example is rupture of a bone.

Buckling: This refers to eccentric compressive force applied to the edges of a plate or column, and is analogous to compression fractures of the anterior margins of the vertebral bodies due to loading applied to it in the forward position.

Excessive deformation: This is related to "whip lashing" injuries of the neck and the back. It is more easily visualized in connection with fractures and dislocations exhibiting marked displacement of fragments; and avulsive injuries of the soft parts, including internal organs and their attachments.

Stress raisers: This term refers to "nonuniform surface discontinuities on the member such as screw threads, shoulders, notches, etc". The stress raiser effect is a local affair. It is illustrated by so called pathological fractures in the bone cysts, bone atrophy and the like. Also, because of pathomechanical behavior of a joint due to disease or other acquired condition, greater forces may be transmitted to other functionally related anatomical structure. This is illustrated in the case of "flexion" fracture of the spine incident to a stiff hip.

CRASH HEAD INJURIES—MECHANISMS

Medical reports place the frequency incidence of crash head injuries of all kinds in round figures at between 50 to 80 percent. Among these, high frequency of skull injuries are not surprising in view of experimental studies that linear fractures can be produced by minimal input energy levels of 400 inch pounds.[4-6] Skull fractures may also result from energy input as low as 50 inch pounds, if the head impacts an unyielding sharp edge or projection.

The skull is a spheroid structure containing semi-liquid contents including brain, blood, and cerebrospinal fluid. This closed cavity feature of the head is a major consideration.[4-6] The cranial dura is intimately attached to the inner aspect of the skull. At the craniospinal junction however, the dura and the bone are not intimately apposed. For this reason, large deformations can occur which tend to prevent a pressure build-up in the spinal canal.

However, a sudden increase in intracranial pressure results in pressure gradients through the regions of the brainstem and cerebellum in the direction of the foramen magnum.[5,6]

Linear fractures produced in the drop tests arise from the failure of the bone because of the tensile strain in the outer surface of the skull. The fracture is initiated some distance from the site of the impact and then propagates both toward and away from the impact site. The fracture line propagates toward the site of impact because at the instant of impact the area of inbending is actually under compression. The rebounding of the bone creates tensile strain with its greatest magnitude at the centre of the impact area. From this center point onwards the tensile strain decreases rapidly in all directions.[7,8]

ROLE OF PHYSICIANS IN ACCIDENT PREVENTION

The physician's responsibility becomes very important in evaluating the person's fitness for driving. This medical point of view is significant in view of these three basic propositions.

1. *Human failure overshadows all other factors in the production of highway accidents:* Accident causation is rooted in basic interaction between the driver, highway and the vehicle. Paradoxically enough automation, push button and other inventions designed to offer greater ease of driving do not eliminate the need to exert vigilance and split second timing to maneuver these vehicles in traffic with efficiency and safety. On the contrary, the driver must be in proper physical and mental condition to safely control and maneuver modern responsive high-speed vehicles. There can be no doubt that poor judgment, lack of physical ability, including impairment of sense organs are responsible for accidents.
2. *Human failure may stem from abnormal physiological states, pathological states, pathological conditions, emotional disturbances and the use of drugs and alcohol.* It is not always easy to ascertain the physical, mental, emotional or physiological impairments of an individual. It is therefore, not always easy to arrive at a decision in these cases where possible and probable deterrents to safe driving practices may exist. Few patients realize that small amounts of alcohol is required to impair dangerously, the driving ability and almost 50 percent of fatal motor accidents occur because of alcohol.
3. *The key to ultimate success in motor-vehicle accident prevention lies in the driver.* This means his intelligence, his sense of personal and social responsibility, his reactions to various stimuli in normal conditions and under stress, his ability in good health and in illness. The medical and other implications in regard to driver screening for licensure are obvious, but cannot be overstated, particularly in the domains of his psychosomatic mechanical

capabilities. There is a real need to improve the medical and related standards for driver licensing, including civilian, commercial vehicle and public transportation vehicles.

PREVENTION OF HEAD INJURIES IN TWO-WHEELER OCCUPANTS

Use of crash helmets is useful in reducing head injury in two-wheeler riders.[9-13] The ICMR head injury study, conducted at AIIMS, during 1977-79 showed either lack of use or improper use of helmet leading to head injury. A study from South Australia[12,13] had shown that 38 percent two-wheeler victims did not use helmet, another 54 percent used only poorly designed helmets and only 8 percent victims had used a proper crash helmet. Prospective study at AIIMS during 1981-82, on two-wheeler accidents had revealed improper use or poorly designed helmets.

Prevention of head injury in two-wheeler accidents is centered on the use of the helmet. In 1970, a legislation passed in Queensland, Australia made the use of crash helmet compulsory.

Motorcycle helmet reduce the risk of death and injury in motorcycle riders who crash. Though a well conducted research is required to determine the effect of helmet and different types of helmets on mortality, head, neck a facial injuries.[18]

In Delhi, the use of helmet was introduced in mid seventies, which to some extent reduced the severe head injury in two-wheeler riders. Furthermore, with the widespread use of helmets has eventually led to difference in helmet design and production. Vaughan[13] discussed the use of various types of helmets. Original standard helmet (resembled a building site hat) offered much less protection. A jet helmet (resembling a pilot helmet) does not provide facial and lower jaw protection. The newer full-face helmet is more ideal and reduces the chance of facial injury. The use of jet helmet predisposes to facial injury, which not only disfigures the face but also may cause airway impairment.

Use of helmet for the pillion rider must be enforced, as such rules are not yet imposed in most of the cities in India. A large number of pillion riders are exposed to vehicular injury, as they do not use a helmet. Recently, more concern has been placed in the use of helmets in two-wheelers. In the US, 400,000 people are injured due to cycle accidents every year and about 1000 die[14] among the victims, over 70 percent are children and maximum incidence of bicycle injury has been reported from New York.[15] Although the official figures are not available in India, the figures are expected to be similar, especially in the metropolitan cities.

PREVENTION OF HEAD INJURIES IN CAR OCCUPANTS

With the introduction of small, low budget cars and many middle class families are also opting for four-wheelers, it is thus imperative that accidents involving cars and other four-wheelers will also escalate. The use of following measures will lower the incidence of car accidents:

1. *Use of seat belts for both drivers and passengers:* This considerably reduces both the incidences of serious and fatal injuries. Studies have shown that wearing seat belts prevents serious acceleration-deceleration and dash-board injuries like facial injuries, compressive chest injuries, hip joint dislocation and patellar and tibial fractures.[16]
2. *Car mechanics:* Use of other modern safety constructs and gadgets in the car, for instance the presence of crumple zone, high impact side beams, high tensile steel grinders for the passenger cabin, collapsible steering and autoinflatable balloons significantly reduce the incidence of severe and fatal head injuries.
3. *Other measures:* These include:
   - The use of speed limits near school, institutional and hospital zones.
   - The proper placement of speed breakers, and the proper installation of traffic signals.
   - Good quality roads, use of parallel roads for different vehicular speeds, use of road dividers and on the spot fines for traffic violaters".
   - Enforcement of education at school and college levels for following traffic rules and inducting a sense of moral responsibility in following a safe traffic conduct.

CONCLUSION

Head injuries account for one quarter to one-third of all trauma deaths. But of deaths that occur in patients, who reach hospitals, two-thirds are due to head injuries. Of greater concern is that these head injuries are the most common cause of lifelong disability after trauma. There is an interesting paradox in the amount of knowledge people have about spinal injuries and how little one tends to hear about permanent disability after head injury, in fact 40 times more common. In a study from UK, about 200 patients arriving in a neurosurgical unit in coma from head injury, one-third arrived without any care of the airway at all, and lying flat on their backs. This is a common scene' in our emergency rooms in India.

In terms of disability, we have lost years of work, not only by the patient but also often by the family, a member of which has often given up work or sold land, property, etc. to support the permanently disabled family member. It is the right time that we focus our attention on **injury prevention**.

REFERENCES

1. Kulowski J. Crash injuries: The integrated medical aspects of automobile injuries and deaths. lllinois, Springfield 1960.
2. Plant HF Fractures of the atlas resulting from automobile accidents. Am J Roentgenol 1938;40:867.
3. Platt FN Highway transportation problems, organization and evaluation. Traffic Quarterly, pp 64-82, Jan 1957.
4. Gurdjian ES, Webster JE. Experiences in the surgical management of intracranial crash injuries. Surg Gyanec and Obst 1957;104:205.
5. Gurdjian ES, Webster JE. Trauma of the Central Nervous System, Baltimore, William and Wilkins, 1945.
6. Gurdjian ES. Acute brain injuries. Surgery 1943;13:333.
7. Evan FC. Stress and Strain in Bones, Springfield, Thomas, 1957.
8. Evans JP. Acute Head injuries, Springfield, Thomas, 1950.
9. Harrington T. Helmet, Head injury and Motorcycles. Ariz Med 1984;41:802-4.
10. Krantz KP. Head and neck injury to motorcycle and moped riders with special regards to effect of protective helmets. Injury 1985;16:253-58.
11. Motorcycle injury and crash helmet (Editorial). Brit Med J 1977;1:1491-2.
12. Jamieson KG, Kelly DA. Med J Aust 1973;2:806-88.
13. Vaughan RG. Med J Aust 1977;1:125.
14. Callahan D. Legislating Safety-How far one should go? (Editorial). N Eng J Med 1981;320:1412-3.
15. Bader M. Helmet for child bicyclists. (letter-comments) JAMA 1990;26:1914-15.
16. Fredricks RH. Safety in automotive transportation: Presented to American Association of Motor Vehicle Administrators (AAMVA). Detroit, Mich, June 23rd 1988.
17. Shah S, Sinclair SA, Smith GA, Xiangh H. Pediatric hospitalization bicycle-related injuries, Inj Drev 2007; 13(5):316-21.
18. Liu BC, Ivers R, Norton R, et al. Helmet for preventing injuries in motorcycle riders. Cochrane database syst Rev 2008;23,(1): and (2) Cd 004333.
19. Singh S, Smith GA, Fields SK, et al. Gymnastics related injuries to children treated in emergency department Pediatric 2008;121(4):954-60.

54 Newer Trends in Management of Neurotrauma

AK Mahapatra

INTRODUCTION

As the morbidity and mortality of the patients with severe head injury is very high, there is a continuous search for better management of head injury to reduce the mortality and morbidity. No doubt, prevention of head injury is most important. However, it is an uphill task, as it involves large number of factors from construction and maintenance of road, traffic sense, issue of driving licence, to use of helmet, etc. Over the years, large number of monitoring and investigative facilities have been developed, which to some extent has helped in reducing the mortality. ICU care is one of the new protocol of management.[1-2] Drug treatment like calcium channel blockers and free radical scavengers have raised the hope of having some breakthrough in the management of head injury (Table 54.1).

INVESTIGATIONS

Not long ago, investigations of choice in severe head injury was carotid angiography, which was not only difficult, time consuming, but also invasive and frequently required anesthesia. In last 2 decades, the availability of CT, MRI have changed the outlook of investigation. CT scan is easy, quick and give much more information than what one could have even imagined. Even in minor head injury, when there is doubt of intracranial hematoma, no one hesitates to undertake a CT scan, rather than taking any chances. CT scan has also proved the possibility of developing a new hematoma, which might not be present in the initial CT scan.[4] Hence, repeating the CT scan 2-3 times may be a need rather than a luxury in selected situations. Rarely, MRI scan may show pathology, which even CT scan failed to detect. Thus, neurosurgeons today are more confident regarding the extent of brain damage and predicting the outcome from the beginning.

PATHOGENESIS

In the recent years, more and more evidences have accumulated in our understanding of dynamic brain damage in head injury. The basic problems are hypoxic and ischemic damage. Over the last decade we have realized that large number of chemicals, neurotransmitters, free radicals are involved in the process of membrane damage and altered brain metabolism.[5,8] Damage to the lipid peroxidation, liberation of glutamate, oxygen free radical and nitric oxide synthetase have the damaging effect on cell membrane and receptors, resulting in opening of calcium channel and damage to sodium and potassium pump.

Prevention of above changes by using specific agents like free radical scavengers[11,12] NMDA receptor antagonist[13,14] and superoxide dismutase[5,12] can brighten the overall outcome by preventing cell. damage. Role of calcium channel blocker has not been encouraging. However, further studies are necessary.[15]

ICU MANAGEMENT

Over the last 2 decades the critical ICU care has become an integral part of severe head injury management. Unfortunately, due to lack of facility, this

Table 54.1: Newer modalities

A. **In investigation**
- CT and role of repeat CT
- MRI scan
- SPECT
- PET scanning

B. **In knowledge of pathogenesis**
- Role of free radical
- Calcium channel
- Role of NMDA receptor antagonist

C. **In ICU management**
- ICP monitoring (TCP)
- Jugular venous saturation ($SJVO_2$)
- Barbiturate coma
- Hyperventilation
- Hypothermia

D. **Management of severely disabled**
- Protocol based rehabilitation
- Dorsal column stimulation in vegetative
- Brain pacemaker

is not possible in most of the neurosurgical units in India, except few. ICU management provides intensive monitoring and, if necessary, newer modalities of treatment like barbiturate coma, elective hyperventilation and cerebral microdialysis,[16-20] in selected cases.

ROLE OF BARBITURATE IN HEAD INJURY

There are sufficient data supporting the role of barbiturate reducing cerebral metabolism. It may be considered in hemodynamically stable severe head injury patients with uncontrolled ICP. Around 15 percent severe head injury patients may have intractable raised ICP, with mortality ranging from 85 to 100.[21,22]

Barbiturates exert cerebral protective effect and reduce ICP through many mechanisms: (a) alter cerebral vascular tone, (b) inhibit free radical mediated lipid peroxidation, and (c) reduce cerebral metabolism. Hence, there is reduced cerebral oxygen demand. The use of barbiturate is based on: (1) it can have long-term control of ICP when other modalities have failed, and (2) it is well known that the adequate ICP control improves the outcome.

Among 275 publications on barbiturate, only 27 were relating to ICP control in severe head injury and only 3 among them were Class I studies (prospective, randomized control trials). One of the study by Ward et al in 1985[16] reported no beneficial effect of barbiturate in treated group as compared to controls. Several studies have shown a doubtful role (Table 54.2). Dose prescribed is pentobarbital 10 mg/kg over 30 minutes as a loading dose and 5 mg/ kg every hour 3 doses, then followed by 1 mg/kg hourly.

High dose barbiturate effectively lowers the ICP in severe head injury and reduces the mortality in patients with intractable raised ICP. However, use of barbiturate as prophylaxis to control raise ICP is not recommended. Therefore, routine use of barbiturate is harmful, as improving the quality of outcome has not been proved. There is a need for further randomized control trials.

Table 54.2: Barbiturates vs mortality

Series	*Number of patients*	*Mortality rate*
1. Eisenberg et al 1988	37	83%
2. Lobato et al[18] 1988	47	100%
3. Nordstrom et al[9] 1988	19	63%

ROLE OF HYPOTHERMIA SEVERE HEAD INJURY

Cerebral protective role of hypothermia is well described.[23,24] Deliterious effect of severe hypothermia prevented the use of this modality in head injury. However, recent studies in severe head injury utilizing mild hypothermia has shown beneficial effect.[23] Hypothermia, reduces cerebral metabolism and thereby reduces cerebral consumption of oxygen. Hence, prevents hypoxic and ischemic damage. In a recent randomized trial Marion et al[3] had shown lowering of brain temperature and reduction of CBF with a 40 percent reduction of intracranial pressure. They used cooling blanket and maintained the body temperature between 33 and 34°C. The further study on mild hypothermia is necessary, so that the clinicians can confidently use this non-expensive modality in the management of severe head injury.

ROLE OF CEREBRAL MICRODIALYSIS IN HEAD INJURY

The concept of cerebral microdialysis is relatively new.[11,20,25] Recently, large number of workers have been able to sample and infuse small amount of fluid through microcatheter into brain and try to analyze the extracellular neurochemicals to study the microenvironment of the cells. The fluid is collected by the second lumen of the microcatheter. This process of analyzing and washing out the toxic chemicals from the extracellular space in brain is termed as cerebral microdialysis. This method not only provides a golden opportunity to study the biochemical and neurotransmitter changes but also provides the scope for correcting the microenvironment. Kantha and Shuaib[11] reported a very high concentration of glutamate, glycine and Gamma-aminobutyrate in severe head injury. Excitatory amino acid elevation correlated most closely with potassium elevation and raised ICP. Isolated elevated lactate did not correlate with hypoperfusion or poor outcome.

Langemann et al[25] measured brain glucose, lactate and pH in the effluent retrieved through microcatheter, in 4 head injury patients. The glucose and lactate ratio fairly correlated with clinical course.

Microdialysis appears to be a promising field in monitoring and correcting the neurochemical changes following head injury. At present, it is in an experimental phase and is very expensive. If the cost can be reduced, the use of microdialysis may well become one of the future modalities of monitoring in severe head injuries.

ROLE OF DRUGS IN SEVERE HEAD INJURY

Over last decade, with proper understanding of the role of neurotransmitters and free radicals in mechanism of brain damage, several drugs have been developed to prevent some of these pathogenic mechanisms. Such as liberation of glutamate and damage to cell membrane by lipid peroxidation.[6-8,10,12,26,27]

Elevated acetylcholine level has been reported in head injury. Anticholinergic agents like scopolamine was tried by Saija et al,[26] in head injury. In head injury NMDA receptors have been damaged by excitatory amino acids, like glutamate and aspartate. Hence, NMDA receptor antagonists have been tried in head injury to prevent brain damage.[6-8,13] Commonly tried ones are Phencyclidine, MK-801 and dextromethorphan. Substantial side effect has been noticed in clinical trial by using MK-801 and Phencyclidine, however, dextromethorphan is less toxic and likely to have good future.

Faden and Saltzman in 1992[27] used Polyamines such as spermine and spermidine to block the channel at higher concentration by competitive antagonism, while ketamine blocks NMDA receptor directly.[13] Muizelaar et al in 1993[12] showed promising results, in a Phase II trial, using Polyethylene glycol conjugated superoxide dismutase. Various antioxidants and free radical scavengers can reduce the adverse effects of pathological lipid metabolism and likely to improve the outcome in severe head injury. Anderson et al, 1985[28] had shown the role of vit E, selenium and superoxide dismulate in spinal cord and brain injury. Thus, there is a good prospect of these drugs in improving the outcome of head injury in future, when given timely.

ROLE OF DORSAL COLUMN STIMULATION

Large number of severe head injury patients do survive and ultimately land in a severely disabled or vegetative state.[29] Treatment of persistent vegetative state is an unsolved problem. Recently, role of dorsal column stimulation (DCS) has been shown to have some role in the management of intractable pain or spasticity. Many patients treated for above problems had shown increase in activity and EEG improvemen.[30,31] Subsequently, role of DCS was established to have effect on cerebral blood flow, catecholamine metabolism and EEG activity.

Kanno et al in 1994[32] reported role of DCS in persistent vegetative state. They studied 42 patients among whom, 23 had head injury. They considered 7 criterias: (1) autonomic function, (2) incontinence, (3) emotional state, (4) oral feeding, (5) eye movements, (6) response to simple command and (7) speech. The scoring were recorded prior to and following DCS. Eighteen of 42 patients showed good clinical improvement. However, CBF improved in 22 patients and EEG improved in 23 patients. Improvement was much better in head injury patients as compared to CVA. The factors influencing outcome in vegetative patients are many (Table 54.3). Few among them are of young age and duration of vegetative state. Miyamoto et al in 1982[33] reported a single case in whom cervical epidural stimulation resulted improvement in vegetative state. However, 42.9 percent improvement in vegetative state reported by Kanno et al[32] is an important observation providing hope for vegetative patients in future.

Post-traumatic hypopituitarism is quite frequent and has high incidence which often remained under diagnosed. There remains high frequency of hypothalamic pituitary hormone deficiencies amongst the long-term survivors of TBI with approximately 25 percent having one or more pituitary hormonal deficiencies, marked changes are found in acute phase of TBI with 80 percent cases showing evidence of gonadotropin deficiency, 18 percent growth hormone deficiency and 16 percent corticotrophin, 40 percent demonstrating vasopressin abnormalities resulting into diabetes insipidus or SIADH. Some of these are transient. Most of these cases remain undiagnosed. The data suggests that timely identification and management of hormonal deficiencies can optimize the recovery of patients of TBI it can avoid long-term consequences also.[34]

Table 54.3: Outcome following dorsal column stimulation

	Favorable	*Unfavorable*
1. Age	Less than 20 years	Over 50 years
2. Cause of coma	Head injury	Stroke or hypoxic injury
3. Duration of vegetative state	Less than 3 months	More than 1 year
4. Prestimulation score	Not significant	Not significant
5. In EEG, CBF	Improvement	CBF<20 mlm/min
6. CT scan	No severe damage	Severe damage

Hypopituitarism is a common complication in TBI and aneurysmal subarachnoid hemorrhage, it might contribute to morbidity and poor outcome.[35]

Large doses of propofol are commonly used to control intracranial pressure in ICU, whereas vasopressors are administered to augment cerebral perfusion pressure. A propofol infusion syndrome is a known complication because of overdosing for large time. It is characterized by lactic acidosis, rhabdomyolysis and cardiovascular collapse. The basis of syndrome lies, an imbalance between energy utilization and demand resulting in cell dysfunction, and ultimate necrosis of cardiac and peripheral muscle cells. It is a lethal complication and in patients with risk factor like TBI, an infusion rate of 4 mg/kg per hours should not be exceeded. Early warning signs are unexplained lactic acidosis, lipemia and Brugada like ECG changes.[36]

CONCLUSION

No doubt, the outcome of severe head injury is depressing. Over the years, improved ICU care and availability of some drugs have changed the outcome to some extent. Use of barbiturate, mild hypothermia and hyperventilation have a very limited role in given situations. Initial studies on DCS, have shown promising results in vegetative state, which may become a useful tool in future.

REFERENCES

1. Ghajar J, Harisi RJ, Narayan RK, et al. Survey of critical care management of comatose head injured patients in the United States. Crit Care Med 1995;23:560-7.
2. Muizelaar JP, Schroder ML. Overview of monitoring of cerebral blood flow and metabolism after severe head injury. Can J Neurol Sci 1994;21:56-11.
3. Chan KH, Dearden NM, Miller JD, et al. Multimodality monitoring as a guide to treatment of intracranial hypertension after severe brain injury. Neurosurg 1993; 32:547-53.
4. Labato RD, Rivas JJ, Gomez P. Head injury patients who talked and deteriorated into coma. Analysis of 211 cases studied with CT. J Neurosurg 1991;75:256-61.
5. Kontos HA, Wei EP. Superoxide production in experimental brain injury. J Neurosurg 1986;64:803.
6. Choi OW. Ionic dependence of glutamate neurotoxicity. Neurosciences 1987;7:379-83.
7. Katayama Y, Backer OP, Jamara T, et al. Increase in extracellular glutamate and associated ionic influx following concussion brain injury. J Neurosurg 1940;73:889-900.
8. Faden A, Oemedick P, Panter S, et al. Role of excitatory amino acids and NMDA receptor in traumatic brain injury. Science 1989;244:298-300.
9. Bakshi A, Nagi C, Wadhawa S, Mahapatra AK, Sarkar C. Expression of nitric oxide synthetase in human brain tumour and peritumoral areas. J Neurol Sci 1998;155: 196-203.
10. Bullock R, Zanner A, Myseros JS, et al. Evidence for prolonged release of excitatory amino acids in severe human head trauma. Relationship to clinical events. Ann Ny Acd Sci 1995;705:290-7.
11. Kanthan R, Shuaib A. Clinical evaluation of extracellular amino acid in severe head trauma by intracellular *in vivo* microdialysis. J Neurol Neurosurg Psychiat 1995; 59:326-7.
12. Muizelaar JP, Marmarou A, Yough HE, et al. Improving the outcome of severe head injury with oxygen radical scavenger polyethylene glycol conjugated superoxide desmutase. A Phase II trial. J Neurosurg 1993;78:375-82.
13. Wong EHF, Knight AR, Woodruff GN. 3[H] MK 801 labels at site on NMA receptor channel complex in rat brain membranes. J Neurochem 1988;50:274-81.
14. Wolfe L. Eicosanoids prostaglandins, thromboxans, leukotrienes and other derivatives of carbon 20-unsaturated fatty acids. J Neurochem 1982;38:1-14.
15. Cohadon F. Brain Protection. In: Advances in technical standard in Neurosurgery. L-Symon (Eds) Springer Verlag (Wien), Vol 1994;21.
16. Ward JO, Becker OP, Miller JO, et al. Failure of prophylactic barbiturate coma in the treatment of severe nead injury. J Neurosurg 1985;62:383-8.
17. Villanueva PA. Barbiturate coma and head injuries, present status. In: Modern trends in the management of neurotrauma. PS Ramani and Alok Sharma (Eds) Labanya Print. Bombay 1994;81-3.
18. Labato RO, Sarabia R, Cordobes C, et al. Post-traumatic cerebral hemispheric swelling. Analysis of 55 cases, studied by CT. J Neurosurg 1988;68:417-23.
19. Nordstrom GH, Masseter K, Sundberg B, et al. Cerebral blood flow, vasoreactivity and oxygen consumption during barbiturate therapy in severe traumatic brain lesions. J Neurosurg 1988;68:424-31.
20. Perrson L, Valtysson J, Enblad P, et al. Neurochemical monitoring using intracerebral microdialysis in patients with subarachnoid haemorrhage. J Neurosurg 1996;89: 606-16.
21. Langfitt TW, Genarelli TA. Can the outcome from severe head injury be improved? J Neurosurg 1982;50:19-25.
22. Miller JO, Butterworth JP, Gudeman SK, et al. Further experience for the management of severe head injury. J Neurosurg 1982;54:289-99.
23. Marion OW, Obrist WO, Carliner PM, et al. The use of moderate therapeutic hypothermia for patients with severe head injuries—a preliminary report. J Neurosurg 1993;79:354-62.
24. Shiozaki T, Sugimoto H, Taneda M, et al. Effect of mild hypothermia on uncontrolled intracranial hypertension after severe head injury. J Neurosurg 1993;79:363-8.
25. Langemann H, Mendelowitsch A, Landolt H, et al. Experimental and clinical monitoring of glucose by microdialysis. Clin Neurol Neurosurg 1995;97:149-55.

26. Saija A, Hayes R, Lyeth B, et al. The effect of scopolamine in traumatic brain injury on cholinergic neurons. J Neurotrau 1988;5:161-70.
27. Faden AI, Saltzman S. Pharmacological strategies in CNS trauma. Trends in Pharmacol Sci 1992;13:29-35.
28. Anderson D, Saunders R, Demediwk P, et al. Lipid hydrolysis and perioxidation in injured spinal cord, partial protection with methylprednisolone, or Vito E and Selenium. Centra Nevs Syst Trauma 1985;2:257-67.
29. Janett WB, Plum I. Persistent vegetative state: a syndrome in search of a name. Lancet 1972;1:734-7.
30. Kanno T, Kamei Y, Yokoyama T, et al. Neurostimulation for patients in vegetative status. Pace 1987;10:207-28.
31. Matsui T, Nagata K, Johsita H. Electrical spinal cord simulation. Its possibility of clinical application for restoration of impaired consciousness. Cardiostim Monaco, 1988.
32. Kanno T, Kamei Y, Yokoyama T. A new treatment for vegetative state after head trauma. Dorsal column stimulation. In: Modern trends in the management of Neurotrauma. PS Ramani and Alok Sharma (Eds) Lavanya Printer, Bombay 1994;87-92.
33. Miyamoto E, Komai N, Funahashi K. Cervical epidural stimulation for akinetic mutism: Case report. Appl Neurophysiol (Abstract) 1982;46:310-11.
34. Behan LA, Phillips J, Thompson CJ, Agha A. Neuroendocrine disorders after TBI. J Neurol Neurosurg Psychiat 2008;79(7):753-9.
35. Schneider HJ, Kreistschmann-Andermahr I, et al. Hypothalamopituitary dysfunction following traumatic brain injury and aneurysmal subarachnoid hemorrhage: a systemic review JAMA 2007;26:298(12):1429-38.
36. Otterspoor LC, Kalkman CJ, Cremer OL. Update on propofal infusion syndrome in ICU management of patients with head injury. Curr Opin Anaesthesiol 2008; 21(5):544-51.

55 Genetic Influences in Traumatic Brain Injury

Raj Kumar, Priyanka Kawal, AK Mahapatra

The role of genetic factors in the traumatic brain injury and vulnerability of brain response to trauma is emerging as a new concept in neurotraumatology.[1]

There are reports to show a poor outcome and selective brain vulnerability in cases carrying the APO4E allele. How does such a susceptibility occur is not understood, but the role of genetic expression, patient's own genetic profile and features expressed following injury in outcome of acute brain injury are described.[1] APOE3 and APOE4 gene regulation predicts functional consequences and effects on inflammatory process, cell growth and proliferation to suggest a poor recovery in post-TBI.[7]

In the same way, the roles of cytokines like TNF α and IL-β upregulation following traumatic brain injury (TBI) has been proposed to have a detrimental role in TBI and their antagonism may reduce post-traumatic damage. The work done on genetically engineered mice had added information about the complexity of post-traumatic inflammatory response.[2] When knock-out mice for TNF α gene are subjected to controlled cortical impact brain injury and compared with wild littermates, they exhibited attenuated congnitive deficits and motor dysfunction during the first week after injury. Wild type mice with mild TBI showed marked recovery over time, whereas TNF mice displayed persistent motor deficits up to 4 weeks after injury.

A significantly larger injury cavity was also observed in TNF α (-/-) mice at 2 and 4 weeks after injury, suggesting deleterious effect of cytokines during acute post injury period. It may have a beneficial role in long-term behavioral recovery in tissue repair in more chronic period after brain injury.[3] IL-6 knockout mice showed a reduced recruitment of astrocytes, monocytes or macrophages at the site of injury and a greater cell loss in injured cortex compared with their wild type littermates.

In addition, over the two weeks after injury, IL-6 mice showed less cellular infiltration, neovascularization and more necrosis. In contrast, overexpression of IL-6 was associated with greater cellular infiltration, restoration of normal appearing tissue and neovascularization suggesting IL-6 plays a role in healing of brain.[2]

Regeneration of injured neurons is recognized now, which involves several steps like survival of injured neurons, regeneration assoicated gene expression, expression of permissive or inhibitory matrix molecules for growth activity, axonal regeneration, remyelination of axon and functional synapse formation of surface targeted neurons.[4]

The Nogo gene (NI 35 and NI 250) is present in oligodendrocytes. The Nogo 66 has been shown to bind a specific neuronal receptor and it is hypothesized that this interaction regulates neuronal plasticity and regeneration following injury.

Administration of monoclonal antibodies IN-1 directed against Nogo A has shown to induce the regeneration of transected spinal cord axons after 2 weeks and to enhance functional recovery over 5 weeks period following spinal cord injury.[5] The studies suggest that modulation of Nogo gene activity might be promising therapeutic strategy following CNS injury.

Vascular endothelial growth factor (VEGF) is found to increase *de novo* hippocampal neurogenesis in TBI. Recently, it was found in experimental studies that VGF signaling occurs through FLK1 (VGF receptor 2) and that FLK1 is expressed both by neuroblasts in subgranular layer (SGL) and by maturing granule neurons in adult dentate gyrus (DG) of hippocampus. It is suggested that VEGF is a part of molecular signaling network that mediates *de novo* hippocampal neurogenesis. After TBI, it also mediates survial of *de novo* granule neurons rather than proliferation of neuroblasts in injured brain.[6]

Results of experimental studies on mice have shown the role of FGF-2 on regulation of neurogenesis and cell loss in granule cell layer (GCL) of hippocampal dentate gyrus after experimental TBI. FGF-2 upregulates neurogenesis and protects neurons against degeneration in adult hippocampus after TBI and that FGF-2 supplementation via gene transfer can reduce GCL degeneration after TBI.[8]

Recombinant human erythropoietin (EPO) treatment has been found to promote functional outcome after TBI and stroke, suggesting that endogenous EPO/

or erythropoietin receptor (EPOR) system plays an important role in neuroprotection and neurorestoration in experimental animals.[9] It was observed that less cortical neurogenesis and sensorimotor functions impairment occurred in EPOR null mice after TBI.[9]

Micro RNAs are known to influence many important cellular processes, including proliferation, apoptosis, neurogenesis, angiogenesis and morphogenesis, all processes that are involved in TBI pathophysiology. Experimental work indicated that multiple protein targets and biological processes involved in TBI pathophysiology may be regulated by MRNAs.[10] However, further studies and clinical trials in future may prove the role of different genetic influences in treatment and outcome of TBI.

REFERENCES

1. Teasdale G, Nicoll JAR, Murray G, Fidee M. Association of apolipoprotein E polymorphism with outcome after head injury. Lancet 1997;350:1069-71.
2. Loghi L, Saatman K, Raghupati R, et al. Cellular basis of injury and recovery from trauma in textbook of Neurological Surgery (youmans). H Richard Winn (Ed), with edition (vol. 4). Sounders Publication Philadelphia 1996;323.
3. Scherbel U, Raghupati R, Nakamura M, et al. Differential acute and chronic response of tumor necrosis factor deficient mice to experimental brain injury. Proc Nat Aca Sci USA 1999;96:8721-6.
4. Horner PJ, Gage FH. Regenerating the damaged central nervous system. Nature 2000;963-70.
5. Merkler D, Metz GA, Raineteau O, et al. Locomotor recovery in spinal cord-injury rat treated with antibody neutralizing the myelin associated neural growth inhibitor Nogo-A. J Neurosci 2001;21:3665-73.
6. Lee C, Angoston DV. Vascular endothelial growth factor is involved in mediating increased *de novo* hippocampal neurogenesis in response to TBI. J Neurotrauma 2010; 27:(3/541/53).
7. Crawford F, Wood M, Ferguson S, et al. Apolipoprotein E genotype dependent hippocampal and cortical response to traumatic brain injury. Neuroscience 2009; 159(4):1349-62.
8. Yoshimura S, Termato T, Whalen MJ, et al. FGF2 regulates neurogenesis in differentiation in dentate gyrus after TBI in mice. J Clini Invt 2003;112(8):1202-10.
9. Xiong Y, Mahmood A, Lu D, Qu C, et al. Histological and functional outcomes after TBI in mice null for erythropoietin receptor in CNS. Brain Res 2008;16:1230-247-57.
10. Rendell JB, Liv Y, Dask PK. Traumatic brain injury alters expression of hippocampal micro RNAs, potential regulators of multiple pathophysiological processes. J Neuros Res 2009;87:(61 1435-48).

56 Brain Death: Indian Law on Organ Transplant

A Jindal, AK Mahapatra

INTRODUCTION

The concept of brain death is now well accepted by the medical professionals. The first description of brain death was given in 1950 by Mollaret and Goulon who identified this condition as 'coma depasse.[1] The set of criteria which define brain death vary from country-to-country with one basic aim, that is to demonstrate the absence of all brainstem functions. Therefore, brain death is actually better defined as "brainstem death". During past 2 decades, confirmatory paraclinical tests have been progressively abandoned and the clinical examination has become more and more important to establish brain death. A better understanding of brain death has led to increased number of patients in whom the mechanical ventilation has been electively stopped, avoiding excessive amount of money wasted in intensive care on these cases. The concept of brain death became a legal issue and in India it was defined in 1995 in "The Transplantation of Human Organ Act, 1995". Variety of criteria used differ around the world. The only controversy is now about the use of EEG/ cerebral angiography being used as essential criteria for brain death. As discussed later in the chapter, these tests are useful in difficult situations.

Clinical examination regarding brainstem reflexes is the most important tool for establishing brain death. The other key point is demonstration of significant irreversible damage to brainstem/brain and identifying the cause of death (e.g. severe head injury, etc.).

ESTABLISHING BRAIN DEATH

Brainstem death and brain death are although practically same with regard to concept of organ donation but remain technically different. Brain death mandates irreversible cessation of all functions of entire brainstem and brain, while brainstem death signifies irreversible damage to brainstem. As per the Indian law brainstem death is a legal requirement and not brain death.[15]

Neurological examination is aimed at detecting persisting brainstem function.

Light Reflex

Fixed dilated or intermediate size pupils with absent light reflex is a very important criteria. The light and oculocephalic reflexes can be obtained reliably only after 32 weeks of gestation and hence, caution should be taken in evaluating premature babies.[2]

Absent Corneal Reflex

Tested by touching the periphery of cornea with soft cotton. One should look for absence of blinking and related reflexes (oculopupillary, etc.).

Absent Oculocephalic Reflex

Cervical spine trauma should be ruled out by X-ray cervical spine before testing this reflex. Tested by rapidly turning the head from side-to-side (also called Doll's eye response).

Absent Oculovestibular Reflex (Cold Caloric Test)

External auditory canal needs to be examined for blood, cerumen and perforated drum before performing this test. Ice cold water can be used and if no reaction is obtained with 50 ml water (either a slow deviation of eyes or any nystagmus) a larger volume should be used.

Absent Gag Reflex

Tested by stimulating posterior pharyngeal wall, tonsils, base of tongue. Both sides need to be tested. Suction catheter through endotracheal tube can be used in intubated patients. The response consists of elevation and constriction of pharyngeal muscles with retraction of the tongue.

Apnea Test

Hypoxia must be avoided during apnea test. Different techniques have been used. Continuous oxygenation during the test by placing a cannula into endotracheal tube and giving oxygen[3,4] 6-7 lit/min. The use of a positive end expiratory pressure (PEEP) is an alternative to the cannula technique to prevent hypoxia (but PEEP is not possible in all types of ventilators, e.g. Medisys System used frequently in India). Ideally, first an arterial blood sample is drawn to establish baseline $PaCO_2$ and PaO_2 (150 mm Hg). The oxygen cannula is placed with adequate oxygen flow. ABG samples are repeated every two minutes until $PaCO_2$ reaches 60 mm Hg or and stopped when following conditions appear (arterial oxygen saturation <80%; PaO_2 <50 mm Hg or severe cardiac arrhythmias). Spinal respiratory-like movements can be observed during apnea test[4,5] but they are not effective in ventilation and disappear on repeat examination. Total duration of apnea test when serial ABGs are not available is restricted to 5 min.

No Reaction to Deep Central Painful Stimuli

No movement should be seen during the painful stimulation. Spontaneous movements of spinal reflex origin do occur in brain dead patients often referred as Lazarus' sign,[6] Their origin is supposed to be spinal and they simulate primitive reflexes exhibited by newborns such as Moro reflex. Such movements are more frequent when patient is off the ventilator. The delay in appearance of spinal automatisms usually ranges between 6 to 72 hours. This delay, longer than the usual observation period for brain death, explains why such movements are not seen in every brain dead patient with intact spinal cord. Another explanation is occurrence of spinal shock concurrent with abrupt rise in intracranial pressure which often occurs during brain death.

Absence of Deep Tendon Reflexes

Absence of DTR was initially included in brain death criteria, but, since these reflexes are now thought to be of spinal origin, they are irrelevant in the diagnosis of brain death.

Conditions which can Interfere with Brain Death Diagnosis

1. Hypothermia (range varies 32.2°C in USA to 35°C in UK).
2. Hypoxia can be ruled out by ABG.
3. Drugs, for example, alcohol, muscle relaxants, sedatives, narcotics, barbiturates (ruled out by toxicology screening).
4. Hypotension—(systolic blood pressure <90 mm Hg)
5. Metabolic/endocrine disturbances.

Table 56.1: Proposed investigations
1. Brain imaging by CT/MRI
2. Chest X-ray
3. Cervical spine X-ray
4. ECG
5. Electrolytes, blood glucose, renal function test, LFT
6. Arterial blood gas analysis
7. Urine toxicology screening

In case of any doubt, one should wait and do repeat examinations (never diagnose brain death when in doubt).[9]

Etiology of Brain Death must be Clearly Established

This condition is of crucial importance and must be fulfilled. All relevant investigations (Table 56.1) should be carried out to demonstrate irreversible damage to the brain.

Irreversible brain damage establishment is more important in children where head injury and intracranial hemorrhage are less common causes of brain death.[10]

OBSERVATION PERIOD

The duration of observation is still a matter of controversy. Neurological examination must not be done within 30 minutes of cardiopulmonary resuscitation. It is proposed that if structural brain damage has been established then repeat examination after 6 hours will suffice. Otherwise, the observation period should be prolonged.[11] One should be very careful while evaluating children younger than 5 years. of age. Vecchierini et al in 1992 suggested a simple guideline for observation period.

1. 6 hours for children older than 1 year.
2. 24 hours for infants > 3 months.
3. 48 hours for infants < 3 months. However, such duration is not stated in Indian law and 2 examinations 6 hours apart are suggested for establishing brain death.

PARACLINICAL CONFIRMATORY TESTS

No paraclinical confirmatory test is required if the previous points are fulfilled. EEG, cerebral angiogram, cerebral radionuclide angiogram, cerebral blood flow using stable xenon, transcranial Doppler, ICP monitoring, evoked potentials, digital cerebral angiogram with venous injection all have been used to establish low or absent cerebral circulation but none is required in Indian law to diagnose brain death.

Diabetes insipidus is frequently observed finding in brain dead patients. The condition is diagnosed by the presence of polyuria (urine, output >7 ml/kg/hr or >200 ml/hr), serum hyperosmolality (>310 mos mol/lit) hypernatremia (> 150 mEq/lit) and low urine specific gravity (<1004). Reasons for this conditions are:

i. ADH is no longer produced in dead cells.
ii. Produced ADH is not transported to posterior pituitary.
iii. ADH from posterior pituitary is not released into systemic circulation.

But all patients with brain death do not develop DI. All patients once diagnosed as brain dead go into cardiac asystole within 12 hours to few days time.[12,13] Head injury and intracranial hemorrhage are the two most frequent conditions responsible for brain death. Jennett et al[9] in 1981 found 55 percent of patients with head injury as primary cause of brain death, whereas intracranial bleed was responsible for 28 percent cases of brain death.

The Transplantation of Human Organ Act passed by Indian parliament in 1994 was subsequently ratified by state legislative of Tamil Nadu in May 1995. It accepted brain death as form of death and prohibited commerce of organs of kidney were performed at Sir Ram Chandra Medical College Tamil Nadu, India, thereafter creating a positive public attitude, early brain death identification and certification, prompt consent for organ donation, adequate hospital infrastructure are the prerequisites for successful organ transplantation.[16]

INDIAN LAW AND ORGAN TRANSPLANTATION[14]

The Transplantation of Human Organ Act, 1995 defines the conditions to be fulfilled by the hospitals, medical practitioners and patients before any organ transplantation can be done. Hospitals should be established for at least 2 years, must have obtained a registration under this Act, should possess the essential personnels and equipment as specified in the rules.

Brain death certificate includes:

A. *Patient's details:* Name, age, sex, address, hospital number, name and address of next of kin, consent for transplant.
B. *Preconditions:*

1. *Diagnosis:* Any condition/ illness/accident that led to irreversible brain damage:
   - Date and time of accident/onset of illness.
   - Date and time of non-responsive coma.
2. Findings of board of medical experts:
   a. Following reversible causes of coma have been excluded—intoxication, CNS depressant drugs, muscle relaxants, primary hypothermia, hypovolemic shock, metabolic/endocrine dis-orders.
      - First medical examination—date and time.
      - Second medical examination—date and time.
   b. Tests for absence of brainstem functions:
      - Pupillary size.
      - Pupillary light reflexes.
      - Doll's eye movement.
      - Corneal reflexes.
      - Motor response in any cranial nerve distribution, any response to stimulation of face, limb or trunk.
      - Gag reflex.
      - Cough reflex.
      - Eye movements on caloric testing B/L.
      - Any respiratory movements.
      - Apnea test as specified.
      - Date and time of first and second examination to be mentioned.
3. Doctors entitled to certify brain death
   a. Medical administrator I/C of the hospital.
   b. Authorized specialist.
   c. Neurologist/Neurosurgeon.
   d. Medical officer treating the patient. Minimum time interval between the first and second testing should be six hours.

CONCLUSION

Severe head injury is the most common cause of brain death. All neurosurgeons, neurophysicians must be well aware of rules and regulations and essential criteria required for the diagnosis of this condition. Each brain dead patient is a potential organ donor. Motivation of family members of brain dead patient is important for cadaveric organ transplantation. Patients with cardiac problem, kidney and liver failure will vastly benefit from cadaver transplant program.

REFERENCES

1. Pallis C. From brain death to brainstem death. Br Med J 1982;285:1487-90.
2. Vecchierini-Blinkeau MF, Moussalli SF. Diagnostic de La Mort cerebrale chc$_3$ le nouveaune et l'entant. Neurophysiol Clin 1992;22:179-90.
3. Benzel EC, Gross CD, Hadden TA, Kesterson L, et al. The apnea test for the determination of brain death. J Neurosurg 1989;71:191-4.
4. Marks SJ, Zistein J. Apnoeic oxygenation in apnoea tests for brain death: A control trial. Arch Neurol 1990;47: 1066-8.

5. Ropper AH, Kennedy SK, Russel L. Apnoea testing in the diagnosis of brain death: clinical and physiological observation. J Neurosurg 1981;55:942-6.
6. Mandel S, Arenas A, Scasta D. Spinal automation in cerebral death. N Eng J Med, 1982;307:501.
7. Ropper AH. Unusual spontaneous movements in brain dead patients. Neurology 1984;34:1089-92.
8. Turmel A, Roux A, Bojanwski MW. Spinal man after declaration of brain death. Neurosurgery 1991;28:298-302.
9. Jennett B, Gleve J, Wilson P. Brain death in three neurosurgical units. Br Med J 1981;282:533-9.
10. Freeman JM, Ferry PC. New brain death guidelines in children: Further confusion. Pediatrics 1988;81: 301-3.
11. Black PM, Zervas NT. Declaration of brain death in neurosurgical and neurological practice. Neurosurgery 1984;15:170-4.
12. Black PM. Brain death (Part I of 2). N Eng J Med 1978; 299:338-44.
13. Black PM. Brain death (Part II of 2). N Eng J Med 1978; 299:393-401.
14. Chaubey PC. Medical ethics and health legislation and patient care in India. Chaubey PC (Ed). Saurabh Publishers, New Delhi 1998;258-99.
15. Sethi NK, Sethi PK. Brain stem death, implication in India J Assoc Physicians India 2003;51:910-1.
16. Prabhakar MR, Soundarajan P. Cadeveric renal transplantation: The Chennai experience, Transplant Proc 2008;40(4):110-7.

Index

Page numbers followed by *f* refer to figure and *t* refer to table

O

P

R

S

T